(*continued on back*)

(continued from front)

Statistical Methods
for the Analysis
of Biomedical Data

Statistical Methods for the Analysis of Biomedical Data

ROBERT F. WOOLSON

The University of Iowa
Iowa City, Iowa

JOHN WILEY & SONS

New York • Chichester • Brisbane • Toronto • Singapore

Library of Congress Cataloging in Publication Data:

Woolson, Robert F.
  Statistical methods for the analysis of biomedical data.

  (Wiley series in probability and mathematical
statistics. Applied probability and statistics,
ISSN 0271-6356)
  Includes bibliographies and index.
  1. Medical statistics. 2. Biometry. I. Title.
II. Series.

RA409.W62 1987   610′.21   87-6069
ISBN 0-471-80615-3

Printed in the United States of America

10 9 8 7 6

To my wife, Linda;
my parents, Sallie and the late Willard Hagey;
and my children, Robert and Sandra

Preface

I have written this book with two audiences in mind. First, the book may fill the needs of medical researchers who would like to reference a book that is more substantial than an introductory biostatistics text. Second, the book may be used as a textbook for an introductory sequence in biostatistics, particularly for majors in biostatistics and statistics. With regard to the first audience, I have attempted to cover many topics that are ordinarily interspersed in a variety of specialty statistics textbooks. For instance, this book includes an introduction to methods for the analysis of survivorship data and an introduction to methods for the analysis of epidemiologic data. In addition, topics on categorical data analysis are included as either special chapters or integrated with the other text material. Finally, it may also be noted that the usual procedures for nonparametric data analysis are also covered in this text but are set side by side with the usual parametric test procedures. The book intends to survey a number of statistical topics commonly used in the analysis of biological and medical data. As a textbook for a biostatistics program, the book would be suited to those students who are pursuing a master's degree and who wish to be exposed to a wide variety of topics in the field. The only mathematical prerequisite is algebra.

This book evolved from notes that I have developed from several courses that I have taught at the University of Iowa. Much of the material in the earlier chapters comes from the basic biostatistics course, while much of the material in the later chapters is derived from an applied course in categorical data analysis and a course in methods for epidemiology. The book is not a theoretical text but rather intends to describe statistical procedures by presenting worked examples for each procedure introduced. In this manner the text may be used as a reference text as the user may locate the relevant statistical procedure and follow the illustration that accompanies the discussion of the procedure. It should also be noted that many of the procedures discussed in the text are those I have found particularly useful in my experience as a statistical consultant, both at the University of Iowa and while a graduate student at the University of North Carolina.

Thus, it is hoped that the book will accomplish two objectives: first, to serve as a reference text for those individuals engaged in the analysis of their own biological or medical data and, second, as an introductory text to the field of biostatistics for those individuals who intend to study the field more seriously.

Statistical Methods for the Analysis of Biomedical Data is organized in the following way:

Chapter 1 is an introductory chapter that describes a number of issues that arise in the testing of a very simple hypothesis. The chapter is nontechnical but serves to motivate the use of statistics and, in particular, statistical inference through an example in psychiatric diagnosis.

Chapter 2 deals with the topic of descriptive statistics and introduces many of the important procedures for summarizing numerical data. The chapter includes the discussion of procedures for handling ungrouped and grouped data and also discusses appropriate statistics for summarizing central tendency and variability in the data sets. A brief discussion of graphical procedures is also included in Chapter 2.

Chapter 3 introduces a number of basic probabilistic concepts. After defining probability and illustrating its use with several examples, several useful rules, including the addition rule and multiplication rule for combining probabilities, are discussed.

Chapter 4 is essentially a continuation of Chapter 3, and several important probability distributions are discussed. In addition, the concepts of population, samples, and sampling distributions are introduced.

Chapter 5 is an introduction to the concepts of confidence interval estimation and statistical tests of hypotheses. Examples and illustrations for several common testing and estimation problems are provided.

Chapter 6 describes a series of tests and estimation procedures for the comparison of two groups. Both parametric and nonparametric statistical procedures are discussed.

Chapter 7 is essentially a continuation of the problem of comparison of two groups, except the response variable here is assumed to be a categorized response and the tests compare rates or proportions.

Chapter 8 describes a series of statistical procedures for the assessment of association between two random variables. The usual Pearson correlation coefficient and a number of nonparametric measures are described.

Chapter 9 deals with the topic of linear regression and in particular addresses the question of predicting one variable from another.

Chapter 10 introduces the topic of the analysis of variance for the comparison of more than two groups. Several types of analyses of variance are described, multiple comparison procedures are introduced as well.

Chapter 11 is a continuation of Chapter 10; however, the focus is on nonparametric analysis of variance procedures rather than on procedures that rely on the normal distribution.

Chapter 12 as well may be viewed as a continuation of Chapters 10 and 11, but here the response variable is a categorical variable and the tests are procedures for the comparison of groups based on the chi-square distribution.

Chapter 13 deals with a number of special topics in the analysis of epidemiologic data. After describing some basic study designs, a number of statistical procedures for the analysis of odds ratios are described.

Chapter 14 deals with the problem of estimation and comparisons of survivorship curves and introduces several statistical tests for these comparisons.

It should be emphasized that this book is primarily a text on statistical analysis, and very little is discussed in regard to experimental design. There are some exceptions, however. For example, we discuss the concepts of matching, stratification, and various types of epidemiologic study designs. In addition, a considerable amount of attention is devoted to the question of sample size determination associated with a number of the statistical tests in the text. Finally, the issue of randomization and random assignment of subjects to treatment groups is also described, although somewhat briefly, in one of the earlier chapters.

ROBERT F. WOOLSON

Iowa City, Iowa
June 1987

Acknowledgments

I am grateful to a number of publishers and authors for permission to cite their work or use various tables as appendices for use in conducting the various statistical tests. The specific citations are noted at the foot of tables or in the cited data from publication articles.

I would like to thank the Literary Executor of the late Sir Ronald A. Fisher, F.R.S., Dr. Frank Yates, F.R.S., and the Longman Group Ltd., London for permission to reprint Tables III and IV from their book *Statistical Tables for Biological, Agricultural and Medical Research* (6th Edition 1974).

I am also indebted to Professor Dana Quade for permission to utilize portions of material that he used in a course in nonparametric statistics while I was a student at the University of North Carolina. I especially want to credit him with the ideas in my discussion in Chapter 8 dealing with Kendall's tau A, B, and D.

I also deeply appreciate the invaluable assistance provided by Ms. Karla Schlesselman and Ms. Patricia Francisco, who typed many versions of the manuscript. I am extremely grateful for their patience and diligence in accomplishing this task. Beatrice Shube, senior editor of Wiley-Interscience, has been extremely valuable in providing guidance and assistance along the way in producing this manuscript.

I also wish to thank a number of pharmacology graduate students who have provided examples and problem sets for me over the years. These individuals provided assistance during the first few years I taught a University of Iowa course entitled "Biometrics and Bioassay." This group also provided several illustrations, including many of those that were used to introduce statistical methods in the various chapters of this text, particularly, Chapters 5, 6, 9, and 10.

A very special thanks is to be extended to Mr. Steve Hillis and Mr. Patricio Rojas. Mr. Hillis assisted with a number of editorial aspects in connection with this text and served as a critical reviewer of the text during the last few months of its completion. Mr. Rojas also assisted in many aspects of this text, in particular checking arithmetic computations, formulae, and most importantly he created virtually all of the problem sets included at the end of these chapters. Mr. Rojas also developed the examples in Chapter 14 and wrote computer programs which generated tables 1, 2, 3 and 6 of the appendix. I deeply appreciate the efforts of Mr. Rojas and Mr. Hillis in the development of this text.

I am indebted to the many colleagues and collaborators I have had at the University of Iowa. I owe a special thanks to Dr. Ming Tsuang, Dr. Peter Lachenbruch, Dr. Robert Wallace, and Dr. Peter Isacson. These individuals have supported the completion of this task in many ways and I owe a debt of gratitude to each of them.

Finally, I would like to thank my entire family, but especially my wife, Linda, for invaluable encouragement and support.

Contents

**11. Comparing More Than Two Groups of Observations:
     Rank Analysis of Variance for Group Comparisons   364**

Statistical Methods
for the Analysis
of Biomedical Data

CHAPTER 1

Introduction

1.1 OVERVIEW OF STATISTICS

Statistics often refers to a set of numbers or quantitative facts summarized in the form of charts, tables, and graphs. This conception of statistics is far too narrow, since the subject of statistics is concerned not only with the numbers but also with the *methods* for collecting, organizing, and interpreting data.

Broadly defined, *statistics* is the field of study concerned with the methods of obtaining, summarizing, and drawing inferences from data derived from groups of individuals. *Descriptive statistics* is that branch of statistics dealing with techniques for summarizing and presenting data, while *statistical inference* is that portion of statistics that deals with methods for assessing uncertainties in inductive inferences. A major focus of statistics is the development and application of techniques for making inductive inferences about a large group called a *population* from the study of a subgroup called a *sample*. Much of this text is devoted to statistical inference and its application to common problems in medical and biological research. The theoretical and applied statistical methods that have particular significance for biomedical data are commonly labeled biostatistics; these techniques are emphasized in this text.

Statistical reasoning is commonly employed in the analysis of biological and medical data, and rather than formally describing such reasoning at this point, we consider several hypothetical examples that illustrate the use of such statistical concepts.

Example 1.1.1. A recent issue of a journal reports the results of a therapeutic study of women with breast cancer. It states that women treated with both adjuvant chemotherapeutic agents as well as conventional radio-

1

therapy have significantly longer survival times than those who receive the radiation therapy alone. The report goes on to indicate that the finding is "statistically significant."

Example 1.1.2. Another study in the same journal reports the results of a comparison between two different chemotherapies for the treatment of multiple myeloma. It states that the survival differences between the two groups were not statistically significant at the 5% level. The failure to find a statistically significant difference was explained by the fact that so few patients were available for study in each group.

Example 1.1.3. In a mental health journal, a report authored by two psychiatric researchers describes a study of the major psychoses. The researchers independently diagnosed each patient in a group of 100 patients. The two psychiatrists reportedly agreed on diagnoses 91% of the time, while the expected agreement due to chance alone was 46%. Once again, the report declares the agreement results to be statistically significant and concludes that the two psychiatrists tend to agree on diagnoses.

Example 1.1.4. Elsewhere in the psychiatric journal, the prevalence of psychotic disorders in an urban community is reported to be higher than in a corresponding rural community. Once again, statistically significant differences are reported, and the ratio of prevalence rates is estimated to be 2.4 with a confidence interval of $(1.8, 2.9)$.

Example 1.1.5. A mortality study reports that the risk of death due to accidents and suicides is three times greater for depressive patients than it is for schizophrenic patients. Once again, the finding is annotated as statistically significant.

In each of these examples, it is evident that a scientific question or *hypothesis* is being examined. The first study tested the hypothesis that the combination of chemotherapy and radiation treatment increased patient survival time relative to the time expected for those receiving only the radiation treatment. A similar hypothesis could be set forth for the second example. In the third example, the psychiatrists undoubtedly hypothesized that their diagnostic agreement rate would exceed some "expected" amount of agreement. Analogously, hypotheses are being examined in the remaining two examples.

The usual statistical procedure for testing hypotheses and the meaning of the term *statistical significance* are questions introduced by these examples. In the next section, some statistical terms similar to those in these examples will be introduced by way of a simple hypothesis-testing situation. We consider a statistical testing problem that will serve to illustrate the use of probability and statistics in a simple experiment. It will also emphasize some key questions that must be addressed in designing a study.

1.2 A DESIGNED EXPERIMENT

Consider the following situation. A medical student who has just completed her rotation in psychiatry asserts that she is able to differentiate schizophrenic patients from purely depressed patients using a specified structured interview form which she has designed. This interview schedule consists of a set of questions regarding a person's psychiatric history, and it has been designed to differentiate persons with schizophrenic illness from those with a major depressive illness. Suppose that you, as the student's preceptor, would like to test the validity of her assertion. Statistical methods can be used to design a study to test the validity of her assertion. How do we design a study to test her claim? What data from the study would lead one to conclude that she does have this differential diagnostic ability? And what data would negate the assertion?

A reasonable approach to this problem would be to select several persons, each of whose diagnosis is known to be either schizophrenia or depression. Further, suppose that you and the medical student have agreed to the following ground rules (*protocol*) for the experiment:

(a) Six patients will be selected from the inpatient ward by you: three schizophrenics and three depressives.

(b) The medical student will have the knowledge that three patients are schizophrenic and three are depressive but will not know which diagnosis goes with which person.

(c) The medical student will interview, using her structured interview form, the six patients in an order determined by you. At the end of the interviews, the medical student will construct two lists of three patients each. The patients within a list are those she claims share the same diagnosis.

(d) If the group of six patients have been correctly divided into two subgroups, you would conclude that the medical student's interview schedule has the ability to differentiate the two diagnostic groups.

(e) If the patients have been incorrectly divided, you would conclude that the medical student's interview schedule did not have the claimed discriminatory ability.

We now turn to several issues related to this experiment.

1.2.1 Order of Interviewing (Randomization)

For convenience, denote the three schizophrenic patients by S_1, S_2, and S_3 and the depressive patients by D_1, D_2, and D_3. In what order should the patients be interviewed by the medical student? It is possible to consider various *systematic* arrangements, for example, a schizophrenic patient followed by a depressive. With a systematic arrangement, the possibility exists that the medical student may detect the pattern and correctly make the diagnosis without utilizing the structured interview form.

A way to avoid this difficulty is to construct a scheme whereby each possible ordering of the six patients has an equal chance to be selected. A simple way to achieve such a scheme is through the use of a single die. Let the number 1 correspond to S_1, 2 to S_2, 3 to S_3, 4 to D_1, 5 to D_2, and 6 to D_3. Roll the die once; the first person interviewed is the person whose number appeared on the roll of the die. The die is rolled again to determine the second person to be interviewed. Of course, if the second roll yields the same number that arose on the first roll, the die must be rolled again. One proceeds in this fashion until the order for all six is determined. Once completed, we have produced a *random* ordering of the patients. This is an example of the process of *randomization*. Among other things, it means an ordering has been chosen by a procedure that is completely free from bias or any prejudices that could influence the selection of the ordering. At the start of this process, each of the possible orderings of interviews has the same opportunity to be the one chosen.

1.2.2 Possible Outcomes of the Experiment (Sample Space)

Before actually conducting the experiment, it would be instructive to enumerate beforehand all of the possible groupings of the six patients into two groups of three each. There are 20 such outcomes, and they are listed in Table 1.1.

If the medical student has no ability to differentiate the two diagnostic groups from one another, she chooses at random one of the 20 possible outcomes. Therefore, with 20 outcomes possible, and each one occurring with equal probability, each outcome in Table 1.1 has a 1 in 20 chance of being her selection. Thus, if the student has no discriminatory ability, each outcome or event in Table 1.1 has a $\frac{1}{20}$ probability of occurring in the actual experiment. For simplicity, denote by O_1 the first outcome listed in Table 1.1, by O_2 the second outcome listed in Table 1.1, and so on until, O_{20} designates the twentieth outcome listed in Table 1.1. Hence, if we wish, we can refer to the *probability* of O_1 by the notation $\Pr(O_1)$, the probability of O_2 by the notation $\Pr(O_2)$, and so on, until the probability of O_{20} is given

Table 1.1. Outcomes Possible in Diagnostic Experiment[a]

Outcome	Group 1	Group 2
1	$S_1 S_2 S_3$	$D_1 D_2 D_3$
2	$S_1 S_2 D_1$	$S_3 D_2 D_3$
3	$S_1 S_2 D_2$	$D_1 S_3 D_3$
4	$S_1 S_2 D_3$	$D_1 D_2 S_3$
5	$S_1 D_1 S_3$	$S_2 D_2 D_3$
6	$S_1 D_2 S_3$	$D_1 S_2 D_3$
7	$S_1 D_3 S_3$	$D_1 D_2 S_2$
8	$D_1 S_2 S_3$	$S_1 D_2 D_3$
9	$D_2 S_2 S_3$	$D_1 S_1 D_3$
10	$D_3 S_2 S_3$	$D_1 D_2 S_1$
11	$D_1 D_2 S_1$	$D_3 S_2 S_3$
12	$D_1 S_1 D_3$	$D_2 S_2 S_3$
13	$S_1 D_2 D_3$	$D_1 S_2 S_3$
14	$D_1 D_2 S_2$	$S_1 D_3 S_3$
15	$D_1 S_2 D_3$	$S_1 D_2 S_3$
16	$S_2 D_2 D_3$	$S_1 D_1 S_3$
17	$D_1 D_2 S_3$	$S_1 S_2 D_3$
18	$D_1 S_3 D_3$	$S_1 S_2 D_2$
19	$S_3 D_2 D_3$	$S_1 S_2 D_1$
20	$D_1 D_2 D_3$	$S_1 S_2 S_3$

[a] Group 1 (2) is the set of three patients that the medical student says belong together in the same diagnostic group.

by the notation $Pr(O_{20})$. Two things should be clear:

1. $Pr(O_i) = \frac{1}{20}$ for $i = 1, 2, \ldots, 20$,

and

2. $Pr(O_1) + \cdots + Pr(O_{20}) = 1$.

For any outcome in the set of possible outcomes, its probability of occurring in the actual experiment is 0.05. The second statement indicates that the sum of these probabilities associated with each possible outcome is unity. At this point, we should add that the set of all possible outcomes, as in Table 1.1, is generally termed the *sample space* of the experiment. It is an enumeration of all of the outcomes that could occur.

It is evident from the ground rules of the experiment that if outcomes O_1 or O_{20} are observed, the medical student has correctly separated the patients into two groups. Hence, by the ground rules, we would concede discriminatory ability to the medical student if the experiment results in O_1 or O_{20}. We should examine more carefully now the consequences of such an action.

As previously stated, even if the medical student has no discriminatory ability, the chance of observing each outcome in Table 1.1 is $\frac{1}{20}$. As both O_1 and O_{20} cannot simultaneously occur, the probability that O_1 or O_{20} occurs can be shown to be the sum of the probabilities, that is, $\frac{1}{10}$. Thus, even if the medical student has no ability to differentiate the diagnostic groups, there is 1 chance in 10 that outcomes O_1 or O_{20} would arise when guessing. Put another way, we would reject or discard the "no-ability" hypothesis 10% of the time when, in fact, no ability existed. Clearly, this is an error since we would concede ability when none existed. If we term the no-ability hypothesis the *null* (or working) *hypothesis*, then we are falsely rejecting the null hypothesis 10% of the time. This type of error is called the *type I error*, or an *error of the first kind*, and its probability of occurrence is called the *level of significance*, which is usually denoted by α. Hence, $\alpha =$ Pr[Type I error] = Pr[Rejecting a true null hypothesis]. If we conducted the experiment and either O_1 or O_{20} was observed, we would reject the null hypothesis and state that the result is *statistically significant* at the 10% level. The interpretation of a statistically significant result is clear from this example. We are saying that if the probability of observing a particular event is sufficiently small under the null hypothesis, we will reject this null hypothesis in favor of the alternative hypothesis.

The alternative to the null hypothesis in this experiment specifies discriminatory ability on the part of the medical student. Notationally, it is convenient to use the symbol H_0 for the null hypothesis and H_a for the alternative hypothesis; in this case:

H_0: no ability to separate the diagnostic groups.

H_a: ability to separate the diagnostic groups.

The alternative hypothesis is the hypothesis of interest to both the student and the preceptor, while the null hypothesis is the counterclaim. Note that the previous computations of probabilities of various outcomes in the sample space were done under the assumption that the null hypothesis was true. The alternative hypothesis here is a general nonspecific alternative as it is presently written. For this experiment, we could make H_a more precise.

One alternative hypothesis would propose that the student has the ability not only to differentiate the diagnostic groups but also to correctly *identify* the diagnostic groups. Hence, referring to Table 1.1, if group 1 represents those patients diagnosed by the medical student as schizophrenic while group 2 are those she diagnosed as depressives, only O_1 represents correct identification of diagnoses; O_{20} represents correct separation but incorrect diagnostic labeling or identification. If points (c)–(e) of the ground rules are appropriately modified to require the medical student to correctly identify each patient's diagnosis, only O_1 would lead to the rejection of the no-ability null hypothesis. The level of significance for this particular test would be $\frac{1}{20}$, not $\frac{1}{10}$, as only O_1 leads to rejecting the null hypothesis. As a result, the alternative hypothesis, which supposes the medical student can *identify* the diagnostic groups, is termed a *one-sided alternative hypothesis*: it is "one-sided" or one-half of the general alternative hypothesis of discriminatory ability.

Corresponding to the one-sided alternative hypothesis, the decision rule or test procedure has been modified by definition to exclude those outcomes that are consistent with a general alternative hypothesis but inconsistent with the one-sided alternative hypothesis; such a test procedure is termed a *one-tailed procedure*. For example, the "tail" involving O_{20} does not lead to rejecting the null hypothesis, while the tail involving O_1 does lead to rejecting the null hypothesis.

Returning now to the general two-sided alternative hypothesis of discriminatory ability, we note what effect the sample size may have on the experiment. Suppose the experiment was to involve only four patients: two schizophrenics and two depressives. Using the same arguments as before, we can enumerate the list of six possible outcomes, each with probability $\frac{1}{6}$ under the hypothesis of no real ability. Hence, the outcomes $O_1' = \{ S_1 S_2$ in group 1; $D_1 D_2$ in group 2$\}$ and $O_6' = \{ D_1 D_2$ in group 1; $S_1 S_2$ in group 2$\}$, which represent correct discrimination, have a $\frac{1}{3}$ chance of occurring under the null hypothesis of no ability. To reject the null hypothesis on the basis of this would result in a type I error probability of 0.33, which is surely an unacceptable level. On the other hand, the medical student can do no better than O_1' or O_6'; these outcomes represent perfect discrimination of the two diagnoses. The difficulty here, of course, is that four patients are insufficient to provide a reasonable test of the null hypothesis. Even a well-experienced psychiatrist could not substantiate a claim of diagnostic ability with only four patients and a significance level less than 0.33. This point is extremely crucial to bear in mind with data analysis. Limited sample sizes mean limited ability to detect real alternative hypotheses.

In this section, we have introduced the reader to some basic statistical terminology frequently encountered in the medical literature. The concepts of statistical significance, randomization, and one-tailed and two-tailed tests appear quite regularly in the published medical literature. As the reader progresses through the text, these concepts will be seen again; the diagnostic classification experiment should be kept in mind as a convenient review of these concepts. We shall return to these issues in Chapter 5, where they will be presented formally.

1.3   SCOPE AND ORGANIZATION OF BOOK

This book is intended as an introductory text on the topic of statistical data analysis. It is intended primarily for researchers in the medical and biological sciences, although it may fill the needs of other researchers as well. There are three points that should be remembered in using this book. First, the book is one on data *analysis*; there is very little material in this text on the design of studies. This omission is intentional. It is my own view that the design questions such as sample size determination for complex randomized designs require consideration as a separate topic. The book, *The Planning of Experiments* by D. R. Cox, provides an excellent account of the fundamentals of experimental design. In the present text, various design pointers are briefly discussed; however, our scope is limited on this topic.

The second point is that this text is one of applied statistical techniques and not a theoretical text. The goal in writing this book was to provide an account of many of the useful statistical techniques and to put them into directly useful form for the researcher. Mathematical derivations are kept to a minimum and often omitted entirely. Finally, this book is primarily limited to data analyses regarding a single response variable.

The book is essentially organized into two parts. The first part covers the basic principles required to apply statistical methods. This ends with Chapter 5. Chapter 6 begins the second portion of the text, which deals specifically with data analysis tools.

To the experienced statistician, the topic selection may surprise you. For example, topics discussed include observer agreement, tests for relative risk, and survival data analysis—topics that do not appear in most introductory books. I have selected these topics since, in my own experience, they have arisen regularly, and many of these analyses can be performed by the medical investigator. My goal is that this text will assist these investigators in accomplishing and understanding these analyses.

REFERENCES AND SELECTED READINGS

Armitage, P. (1977). *Statistical Methods in Medical Research*, 4th ed., Blackwell, Oxford.

Bliss, C. I. (1967). *Statistics in Biology*, Vol. 1, McGraw-Hill, New York.

Cochran, W. G., and G. Cox (1957). *Experimental Designs*, 2nd ed., Wiley, New York.

Cox, D. R. (1958). *Planning of Experiments*, Wiley, New York.

Fisher, R. A. (1970). *Statistical Methods for Research Workers*, 14th ed., Oliver and Boyd, Edinburgh.

Mainland, D. (1963). *Elementary Medical Statistics*, Saunders, Philadelphia, PA.

Snedecor, G., and W. Cochran (1967). *Statistical Methods*, 6th ed., Iowa State University Press, Ames.

Steel, R., and J. Torrie (1960). *Principles and Procedures of Statistics*, McGraw-Hill, New York.

CHAPTER 2

Descriptive Statistics

2.1 INTRODUCTION

Although each data point is valuable in an experiment or an epidemiologic study, the investigator generally wants to present the entire data in summary form. In this chapter, we introduce *descriptive statistics*, the branch of statistical methodology that deals with data summarization. We deal with the simplest situation: the case of a single response variable. Most studies, however, involve a multiple set of response variables, making a summary of such data more difficult. On the other hand, the reporting of such multivariate data involves a combination of single-variable summaries along with a set of figures describing the relationship between the variables. Thus, single-variable techniques do have applicability to more complex studies.

What follows is a discussion of some common methods for describing a single response variable.

2.2 CLASSIFICATION OF VARIABLES

The observations in an investigation are the specific values of the variable of interest. Since statistical techniques of description appropriate for one type of variable may be inappropriate for another, it is important to consider common classification schemes for variables.

A straightforward system for classifying a variable is on the basis of the presence or absence of a numerical scale, that is, *quantitative* or *qualitative*, respectively. A variable such as a psychiatric diagnosis is a qualitative variable because it can take a diagnostic value of schizophrenia, mania, neurosis, and so forth, to which there is no corresponding set of numbers. Another qualitative variable is marital status, where the responses include single, widowed, married, divorced, and separated. For both of these variables, no clearly defined numerical values correspond to the various categories of response.

If the observations correspond to responses of a measurable magnitude, then the variable is termed a *quantitative variable*.

Quantitative variables may be continuous or discrete. A quantitative variable is said to be a *continuous variable* if it can take any value in a certain interval. For example, the body weight of a full-term newborn child could assume any value from 1 lb to 15 lb. A *discrete variable* is one that is noncontinuous; it can take on only a countable number of distinct values. In a genetic study of psychiatric disorders, the number of psychiatrically ill relatives of a schizophrenic patient would be a discrete variable. It is evident that the variable can assume the nonnegative integer values $0, 1, 2, \ldots$, but a noninteger value, such as $1\frac{1}{2}$, is impossible.

An alternative classification scheme is the one frequently used in the social sciences and was introduced by Stevens (1946). This scale classifies a variable as nominal, ordinal, interval, or ratio. A *nominal variable* is purely a "name" variable with no ordering of values. Ethnic group, religious preference, marital status, and sex are nominal-scale variables: no order relationship exists between the values of each. For example, there is no order relationship between the religious group categories of Catholic, Jewish, Protestant, and so on.

An *ordinal variable* may be a name variable, but it also has a rank-order relationship among the categories of the variable. Behavior ratings of a person's irritability or their agitation would be examples of ordinal-scale variables. In this case, the rating might take values of absent, mild, moderate, and severe degrees of irritability; an order relationship is clearly understood with this variable, since mild is worse than absent but not as bad as moderate or severe. It is characteristic of the ordinal scale that a rank ordering is achieved but the actual distance between categories is unknown. We know that severe is higher on the irritability scale than moderate, but we cannot state how much higher.

If in addition to a meaningful order relationship the actual distance or difference between successive values is defined in measured units, then the variable is an *interval-scale* variable. For an interval-scale variable, the ratio of different values may not have a clear interpretation. Temperature, when measured on the centigrade scale, is an interval-scale variable since a difference of two temperatures is defined in measured degree units; however, the ratio of two temperatures (e.g., 40° and 20°C) does not imply that 40°C is twice as hot as 20°C. Since 0°C does not correspond to the absence of temperature, the ratio of temperatures lacks a clear meaning.

In contrast to temperature, 0 lb of body weight *implies* no body weight, that is, the absence of the characteristic. Accordingly, the ratio of two body weights, 200 to 100 lb, has the interpretation that the one person is twice as heavy as the other. Such variables are termed *ratio-scale* variables.

For this text, we will consider a variable to be a qualitative variable if it is a nominal or ordinal variable and to be a quantitative variable if it is an interval-scale or ratio-scale variable.

2.3 REPRESENTING DATA WITH NOTATION

To simplify the presentation and development of statistical methods, it is useful to consider notational shorthand for variables and observations. A variable is generally represented by an uppercase letter of the alphabet, most often X, Y, or Z. Values of a variable are usually represented by lowercase letters.

Where a set of data consists of a value of X for one person and another value of X for another person, it is useful to add a subscript to the variable. For five values of the variable X, we denote these observations by

$$x_1, x_2, x_3, x_4, \text{and } x_5. \tag{2.1}$$

We also refer to the collection of observed values as the *sample*, the *data*, or the *observations*. If we place a subscript i on the variable X, then the set of observations (2.1) can be written

$$\{x_i: \text{for } i = 1, 2, 3, 4, 5\}. \tag{2.2}$$

More generally, we would like to permit the sample size to be any positive integer, say n. Thus, we can write a sample of size n as

$$\{x_i: \text{for } i = 1, 2, \ldots, n\}. \tag{2.3}$$

Example 2.3.1. An experiment* was performed to determine the blood alcohol level (mg/mL) required to cause respiratory failure in rats. The experimenter directly assays the alcohol level required, by continuous intravenous feeding, until respiratory failure. At respiratory failure, the blood alcohol level is measured. Seven rats are studied with observed blood alcohol levels (mg/mL) of 9.0, 9.7, 9.4, 9.3, 9.2, 8.9, and 9.0. Here $n = 7$ is the sample size and $x_1 = 9.0$, $x_2 = 9.7$, $x_3 = 9.4$, $x_4 = 9.3$, $x_5 = 9.2$, $x_6 = 8.9$, and $x_7 = 9.0$ are the seven observations.

---

*Goldstein (1971) describes and cites an experiment similar to this. The seven observations here were chosen arbitrarily from his Figure 2.3.

In experiments like Example 2.3.1, it may be helpful to characterize the data with one or two summary numbers.

Definition 2.3.1.   A single number describing some feature of the data is called a *descriptive statistic.*

Two characteristics, central tendency and the variability, are often valuable descriptors of a data set. Other characteristics may be used to describe the data, but we restrict consideration to these two in the following sections.

2.4   CENTRAL TENDENCY OF A SET OF DATA

Central tendency refers to the center or the middle of the data set. There are many measures that describe central tendency, but the most widely used measure of location or central tendency is the sample mean. This quantity is simply the arithmetic sum of the observations divided by the number of observations.

Definition 2.4.1.   The *sample mean* is the arithmetic sum of the observations divided by the number of observations.

In notational terms, the sample mean is defined by

$$\frac{x_1 + x_2 + \cdots + x_n}{n}. \qquad (2.4)$$

Example 2.4.1.   Consider the data described in Example 2.3.1. The sample mean is $(9.0 + 9.7 + 9.4 + 9.3 + 9.2 + 8.9 + 9.0)/7$, or 9.21. Ordinarily, the 9.21 would be rounded* to 9.2 as the original data were recorded to the nearest 0.1 mg/mL.

The sample mean (also called arithmetic mean) is used so frequently that it is convenient to give it the symbol $\bar{x}$, read as "x bar." The numerator of (2.4) is the sum of *n* observations. It is convenient to use summation notation for such expressions. When the summation operator Σ is written to the left of the variable *x* (i.e., Σx), then this notation is shorthand for "add the *x*'s." Since a subscript is associated with each *x*, the expression Σx does not precisely define which particular *x*'s to add. This is resolved by the

---

*Throughout the text, when rounding, we adopt the convention of "rounding down" any figure whose last digit is less than 5 and "rounding up" otherwise. For example, 9.34 becomes 9.3, while 9.35 becomes 9.4.

notation

$$\sum_{i=1}^{n} x_i, \tag{2.5}$$

read as "summation of x sub i from i equals 1 to n." Translated, this means "add the x's starting from x_1 and ending at x_n." The expression $\sum_{i=2}^{4} x_i$ translates "add the x's starting from x_2 and ending at x_4." Clearly, the summation operator is a useful shorthand notation for sums of observations or partial sums of observations.

It follows from the introduction of the symbol Σ that the sample mean $\bar{x}$ is defined most concisely by

$$\bar{x} = \frac{\sum_{i=1}^{n} x_i}{n}. \tag{2.6}$$

Clearly, the sample mean may not be computed for nominal-scale data or for nonnumerical ordinal-scale data.

It is also instructive to examine the effect that extreme observations have on the sample mean. In Example 2.3.1, suppose that the largest observation had been 13.2 mg/mL instead of 9.7 mg/mL. This changes the sample data to 9.0, 13.2, 9.4, 9.3, 9.2, 8.9, and 9.0. The mean for these data is $\bar{x} = (9.0 + 13.2 + 9.4 + 9.3 + 9.2 + 8.9 + 9.0)/7 = 9.7$. Notice that six of the sample observations are less than the sample mean while only one is greater than it. The extreme observation of 13.2 has "pulled" the sample mean away from the bulk of the data values. In general, the sample mean is very sensitive to extreme data points. With extreme data points, one must check the extreme points to see if they are recording or technical errors. If they are not, then measures of central tendency other than the sample mean may be required to describe the location of the data. This is not to be regarded as a condemnation of the sample mean, but merely a cautionary note regarding its use. For Example 2.3.1, the sample mean appears to be a reasonable measure of the center of the data; for the modified Example 2.3.1, the sample mean is a misleading measure of the center of concentration of the data. Therefore, other measures of expressing central tendency are needed.

One such alternative is the sample median.

Definition 2.4.2. The *sample median* is that value in the sample such that no more than one-half of the observations are less and no more than one-half of the observations are greater than it.

The median is the 50th percentage point in the data and is a useful figure since it represents the point at which half the data lie to either side of it. In some cases, more than one number qualifies as the sample median. For example, consider a set of four observations that are the ages of onset of schizophrenia in four persons. The ages recorded are 17, 20, 23, and 29. One notices that 21 satisfies our definition of a sample median. For the same reason, 22 also satisfies our definition of a median. In fact, any value between 20 and 23 meets the definitional criterion. To avoid ambiguity in referring to the sample median in such situations, it is conventional to compute the midpoint of the interval of medians. Hence, for this example, $(23 + 20)/2$, or 21.5, would be termed the sample median.

The general procedure for computing a sample median from a set of observations $x_1, x_2, \ldots, x_n$ is to first arrange the observations from smallest to largest in order. These ordered observations are denoted $x_{(1)}$, $x_{(2)}$, $\ldots, x_{(n)}$, where $x_{(1)} \leq x_{(2)} \leq \cdots \leq x_{(n)}$, that is, $x_{(1)}$ is less than or equal to $x_{(2)}$, which is less than or equal to $x_{(3)}, \ldots$, which is less than or equal to $x_{(n)}$. Therefore, $x_{(1)}$ is the smallest value of x among $x_1, \ldots, x_n$ while $x_{(n)}$ is the largest. The next step is to simply observe if n is odd or even. If n is odd, then the $\frac{1}{2}(n + 1)$th ordered x is the sample median, that is, the sample median is $x_{((n+1)/2)}$. If n is even, then any number between the $(n/2)$th and $(n/2 + 1)$th ordered x is a sample median. The sample median when n is even is taken by our convention to be

$$\frac{x_{(n/2)} + x_{(n/2+1)}}{2}.$$

For the age-of-onset example given earlier, the ordered observations are $x_{(1)} = 17$, $x_{(2)} = 20$, $x_{(3)} = 23$, and $x_{(4)} = 29$. As $n = 4$ and is even, the sample median is one-half the sum of $x_{(4/2)}$ and $x_{(4/2+1)}$, that is, $\frac{1}{2}(x_{(2)} + x_{(3)}) = \frac{1}{2}(20 + 23) = 21.5$.

Example 2.4.2. Continuing Example 2.3.1, the ordered observations are $x_{(1)} = 8.9$, $x_{(2)} = 9.0$, $x_{(3)} = 9.0$, $x_{(4)} = 9.2$, $x_{(5)} = 9.3$, $x_{(6)} = 9.4$, and $x_{(7)} = 9.7$. Since n is odd, the sample median is the $\frac{1}{2}(7 + 1)$th ordered observation, that is, $x_{(4)} = 9.2$. Also notice in this example that the two 9's are indistinguishable, but in any case are the second and third ordered observations.

The sample median for the modified Example 2.3.1 data, in which 13.2 replaced 9.7, is also 9.2. The sample median, unlike the sample mean, is not as strongly affected by the one extreme data point. It is generally true that the sample median is a better measure of location than the sample mean for data sets with a few extreme observations.

Finally, like the sample mean, the sample median can be computed for ratio-scale or interval-scale data. Furthermore, the sample median also may be determined for ordinal-scale data. For example, if 10 psychiatric patients are evaluated on the severity of a depressive symptom and 3 report no symptom, 1 reports mild severity, 2 report moderate severity, and the remaining 4 report extreme severity of the symptom, then the sample median is the moderate-severity category.

Another measure of central tendency is the sample mode.

Definition 2.4.3. The *sample mode* is the most frequently occurring value of the variable in the sample.

In some cases, there may be several values of the variable that satisfy the definition and qualify as modes. In these situations, it is a matter of judgment on the part of the investigator as to whether to report these modes or utilize an alternative measure of location, for example, the sample mean or median. In practice, the reporting of many (three or more) modes is not useful. On the other hand, bimodal (having two modes) situations frequently arise in medical settings and may indicate two different population groups. Here it would be appropriate to report both modes and to present a graphical data display as well.

Example 2.4.3. In an epidemiologic study of psychiatric disease, 200 persons were diagnosed as schizophrenic, 225 as depressive, and 100 as manic. The modal diagnosis in this case is depression.

Example 2.4.4. In Example 2.3.1, 9.0 occurs twice while each other value appears once. Hence the mode is 9.0.

Example 2.4.3 illustrates that the mode may be determined for any type of variable. The variable may be nominal, ordinal, ratio, or interval; it may be qualitative or quantitative. In this sense, the mode is a more general measure of location because it does not require an ordering of values. Accordingly, the mode is most often used for nominal-scale variables but not for ordinal, ratio, or interval scales since the mode does not utilize their quantitative features, just the frequency of occurrence. The sample mode is a simple quantity to compute and is occasionally employed in situations where a quick summary of the data is required.

The *sample midrange*, another measure of central tendency, is one-half the sum of the largest and smallest sample observations: $(x_{(1)} + x_{(n)})/2$. It can also be determined rather quickly from a set of data. It has the drawback of only using two of the sample observations in its computation and is therefore not used frequently. Since it depends entirely on the extreme ends of the data set, it is strongly affected by these two data points.

Numerous other measures can be used for determining the central tendency of a data set. Two that have been used to summarize data involving rates or ratios are the *sample geometric mean* and the *sample harmonic mean*. We shall have little occasion to use them in this book.

Before concluding this section, it would be helpful to introduce formally the concept of a sample *percentile*. It was noted earlier that the median is the 50th percentile. Other percentiles may also be important to consider in a study as well. For instance, the 25th or the 90th percentiles might be wanted to describe the lower and the upper parts of the data. We formulate the following definition.

Definition 2.4.4.   The pth percentile ($0 < p < 100$) for a sample is that value such that no more than p percent of the sample are less than it and no more than $100 - p$ percent of the sample are greater than it. If more than one number satisfies this condition, then the mean of these numbers is defined to be the pth percentile.

Percentiles provide a convenient summary of a data set, and often an investigator may choose to present the deciles (the pth percentiles where p is a multiple of 10), or quartiles (25th, 50th, and 75th percentiles) of the data in addition to or in place of various other summary measures.

2.5   VARIABILITY IN A SET OF DATA

The use of "averages" is so common in newspapers and magazines that most of us feel comfortable with the notion of central tendency. On the other hand, variability or dispersion of a set of observations is a concept that is less familiar to us.

One particular notion of spread or variability easily comprehended is that of the sample range.

Definition 2.5.1.   The *sample range* is $x_{(n)} - x_{(1)}$, the largest sample observation minus the smallest sample observation.

This quantity is definitely easy to compute; however, it utilizes only two of the sample observations, the smallest and the largest.

Example 2.5.1.   In Example 2.3.1, $n = 7$, $x_{(7)} = 9.7$, and $x_{(1)} = 8.9$. Hence the sample range is $9.7 - 8.9 = 0.8$.

Because only two of the sample observations are used, the sample range is not often used except as a rough, easy-to-compute measure of variation.

Let us consider alternatives to the sample range. But first, what characteristics should a measure of variability have? Several seem reasonable. The measure of variability should be small if all of the observations are close to the central tendency of the data, while the measure should increase in magnitude if the observations are more distant from the central value. It is also reasonable to define the measure so that it is in the same units as the original data; for example, if body weight is measured in pounds, then the variability measure should be in pounds. One further requirement is that the measure should remain the same even if the magnitude of the observations changes by adding a constant to each observation. For example, the data set consisting of the observations 8.9, 9.0, 8.7, and 9.4 has the same spread (variability) as the data set consisting of 18.9, 19.0, 18.7, and 19.4. The latter set results from merely adding 10 to each number in the first set. Finally, the measure should be computed from most of the sample and not be restricted to only two observations, as is the range.

Before considering other specific measures, we examine one seemingly plausible measure of variability, namely, the arithmetic sum of the differences of the observations from their sample mean:

$$\sum_{i=1}^{n} (x_i - \bar{x}) = (x_1 - \bar{x}) + \cdots + (x_n - \bar{x}).$$

As an example consider $x_1 = 8.9$, $x_2 = 9.0$, $x_3 = 8.7$, and $x_4 = 9.4$. We see that $\bar{x} = 9.0$; therefore, $(x_1 - \bar{x}) = -0.1$, $(x_2 - \bar{x}) = 0$, $(x_3 - \bar{x}) = -0.3$, and $(x_4 - \bar{x}) = +0.4$. Their sum, zero, would suggest no variability. Nevertheless, these x_i's are different. Therefore, the quantity $\sum_{i=1}^{n}(x_i - \bar{x})$ is not a measure of variability, at least for this example.

Close inspection of $\sum_{i=1}^{n}(x_i - \bar{x})$ reveals, however, that it is zero for all samples. Put another way, the negative deviations from the sample mean are balanced by the positive deviations about the sample mean. Algebraically, by rules of summation, this can be shown by

$$\sum_{i=1}^{n} (x_i - \bar{x}) = \sum_{i=1}^{n} x_i - \sum_{i=1}^{n} \bar{x} = \sum_{i=1}^{n} x_i - n\bar{x}, \qquad (2.7)$$

and from (2.6) it follows that $\sum_{i=1}^{n} x_i = n\bar{x}$; thus, $\sum_{i=1}^{n} x_i - n\bar{x} = 0$.

This calls for consideration of other measures of variability. One approach is to disregard the sign of each difference $(x_i - \bar{x})$, that is, take its absolute value. For the cited example, the respective quantities are 0.1, 0, 0.3, and 0.4, and the sum is 0.8. The mean of these absolute differences is 0.2. This mean is defined as the *mean deviation* or *absolute mean deviation* and is a measure of dispersion. It is defined algebraically by

$$\frac{\sum_{i=1}^{n} |x_i - \bar{x}|}{n}$$

where $|x_i - \bar{x}|$ is the absolute value of the deviation $x_i - \bar{x}$. While this is a measure of dispersion that satisfies the various properties set forth in the preceding discussion, it is not used frequently in data analysis for several reasons. First, it is not possible to determine the mean deviation of the combined group of several groups from the mean deviations of these groups alone. Second, the mean deviation has not been used frequently in statistical inference, that component of statistics that deals with using a sample to draw conclusions about a larger group of which the sample is a subset.

There is another alternative for retaining the size of a $x_i - \bar{x}$ deviation, while avoiding the sign of the deviation. In particular, the sum of squares (SS) of the deviations defined by

$$SS = \sum_{i=1}^{n} (x_i - \bar{x})^2 \tag{2.8}$$

has been proposed as a measure of sample dispersion.

Definition 2.5.2. The *sum of squares* (denoted SS) of a set of observations is defined by $\sum_{i=1}^{n}(x_i - \bar{x})^2$. Since $\bar{x}$ has been subtracted from each x_i, the sum of squares is sometimes called the *corrected sum of squares* to distinguish it from the *uncorrected sum of squares* defined by $\sum_{i=1}^{n}x_i^2$.

The quantity SS utilizes all of the sample observations and increases in magnitude with the expression $(x_i - \bar{x})^2$.

It seems natural to compute a "mean" SS by dividing SS by n; however, the following discussion will explain why this is not done. While computationally there are n components in SS, one of the deviations is completely determined by the other $n - 1$ deviations. This fact follows immediately from (2.7) and is illustrated by the following example. Consider the set of data, $x_1 = 8.9$, $x_2 = 9.0$, $x_3 = 8.7$, and $x_4 = 9.4$; then $\bar{x} = 9.0$, $x_1 - \bar{x} = -0.1$, $x_2 - \bar{x} = 0$, $x_3 - \bar{x} = -0.3$, and $x_4 - \bar{x} = +0.4$. Notice that any selected deviation from the sample mean is equal to the negative of the sum of the remaining three deviations, namely, $-0.1 = -[0 + (-0.3) + 0.4]$, $0 = -[0.1 - 0.3 + 0.4]$, $-0.3 = -[-0.1 + 0 + 0.4]$ and finally $0.4 = -[-0.1 + 0 - 0.3]$. This is no accident, as (2.7) shows

$$(x_1 - \bar{x}) + (x_2 - \bar{x}) + \cdots + (x_{n-1} - \bar{x}) + (x_n - \bar{x}) = 0.$$

Hence, any deviation equals the negative sum of the remaining $n - 1$ deviations; for example,

$$x_n - \bar{x} = -[(x_1 - \bar{x}) + \cdots + (x_{n-1} - \bar{x})].$$

In general, with n observations, one of the sample deviations can be expressed by the other $n - 1$ sample deviations. Therefore, even though a sum of squares is written in a form

$$(x_1 - \bar{x})^2 + \cdots + (x_n - \bar{x})^2 \qquad (2.9)$$

which shows each and every observation making their contribution to the sum, it is understood that one of these deviations can be written in terms of the remaining $n - 1$ deviations.

Therefore, the sum of squares (2.8) is in actuality a sum of $n - 1$ independent squared deviations plus one completely dependent one. Consequently, it is more appropriate to divide SS by $n - 1$ rather than n. (There are other reasons why $n - 1$ rather than n should be the divisor; these have to do with unbiasedness and related technical matters, which will be discussed in Chapter 4.)

Dividing SS $= \sum_{i=1}^{n}(x_i - \bar{x})^2$ by $n - 1$ leads to a quantity that is termed the sample variance and denoted by s^2.

Definition 2.5.3. The *sample variance*, denoted by s^2, is defined by

$$s^2 = \frac{\sum_{i=1}^{n}(x_i - \bar{x})^2}{n - 1}. \qquad (2.10)$$

The denominator of (2.10) is given the label *degrees of freedom*. Hence, the sample variance s^2 is the sample sum of squares SS divided by its degrees of freedom ($n - 1$).

The sample variance (2.10) is in the square of the units of the observations. The positive square root of s^2 is termed the sample standard deviation, denoted s.

Definition 2.5.4. The *sample standard deviation*, denoted by s, is defined by

$$s = \sqrt{\frac{\sum_{i=1}^{n}(x_i - \bar{x})^2}{n - 1}}. \qquad (2.11)$$

This is by far the most often used measure of variability. Consider the following example:

Example 2.5.2. A given data set consists of the integers 5, 6, 8, 10, 12, 14, and 15. We want to determine the sample sum of squares, sample variance, and sample standard deviation.

We easily obtain the sample mean of $\bar{x} = 10$. The following are the computations for the measures of dispersion:

i	x_i	$x_i - \bar{x}$	$(x_i - \bar{x})^2$
1	5	-5	25
2	6	-4	16
3	8	-2	4
4	10	0	0
5	12	$+2$	4
6	14	$+4$	16
7	15	$+5$	25
			$\sum_{i=1}^{7}(x_i - \bar{x})^2 = 90$

The sample sum of squares is 90, the sample variance is 15 ($= 90/6$), and the sample standard deviation is 3.87 ($= \sqrt{15}$).

In Example 2.5.2, if the magnitude of the observations had been changed to 105, 106, 108, 110, 112, 114, and 115 by adding 100 to each of the original observations, then the sample mean would be $\bar{x} = 110$, but the sample sum of squares, sample variance, and sample standard deviation would be identical to those obtained in Example 2.5.2. This suggests that these three measures of dispersion are invariant to adding a constant to each observation. This fact may be shown to be true in general.

The procedure for computing the sum of squares may be simplified by performing some algebraic manipulations on (2.8). In particular, it can be shown that

$$\sum_{i=1}^{n}(x_i - \bar{x})^2 = \sum_{i=1}^{n} x_i^2 - \frac{\left(\sum_{i=1}^{n} x\right)^2}{n}. \tag{2.12}$$

Frequently the left-hand side of (2.12) is regarded as the definitional formula for the sum of squares, while the right-hand side is termed the *computing formula*. The term $(\sum_{i=1}^{n} x_i)^2/n$ is occasionally termed the *correction term for the mean* or *correction factor*. The SS given by the right-hand side of (2.12) is the computation form of the SS; both $\sum_{i=1}^{n} x_i$ and $\sum_{i=1}^{n} x_i^2$ are normally obtainable from calculators in a single step.

Example 2.5.3. Use the data of Example 2.5.2 and determine the sample sum of squares, sample variance, and sample standard deviation using the computing formula. We have $n = 7$:

$$\sum_{i=1}^{n} x_i = 5 + 6 + 8 + 10 + 12 + 14 + 15 = 70;$$

$$\sum_{i=1}^{n} x_i^2 = 25 + 36 + 64 + 100 + 144 + 196 + 225 = 790;$$

$$SS = \sum_{i=1}^{n} x_i^2 - \frac{\left(\sum_{i=1}^{n} x_i\right)^2}{7} = 790 - \frac{(70)^2}{7} = 790 - 700 = 90;$$

$$s^2 = \frac{90}{6} = 15;$$

$$s = \sqrt{15} = 3.87.$$

Computer programs are available that will compute these summary statistics directly; however, the computing form given in (2.12) is often the algorithm used to compute the requisite sum of squares.

We may raise other questions about variability. For example, $\bar{x}$, the sample mean, computed from one sample of size 7 will probably differ from the computed sample mean in another sample of size 7. One could select several samples of size 7, compute the sample mean for each, and then determine the sample variance of these sample means as a measure of the variability of the sample means. This alternative, based on different samples of size 7, requires repetitive experimentation, which is impractical. Fortunately, the variance of the sample mean can be estimated directly from one sample. In fact, it is estimated directly from the sample variance s^2 and the sample size n.

Definition 2.5.5. The *sample variance of the sample mean* is denoted by $s_{\bar{x}}^2$ and is defined by

$$s_{\bar{x}}^2 = s^2/n, \tag{2.13}$$

where s^2 is defined by (2.10).

The variation between the sample means will not be as great as the variation between individual values in a sample. The sample standard deviation of the mean, that is, the square root of (2.13), is called the sample standard error of the mean.

Definition 2.5.6. The *sample standard error of the sample mean* is denoted by $s_{\bar{x}}$ and is defined by

$$s_{\bar{x}} = \sqrt{s^2/n} = s/\sqrt{n}. \tag{2.14}$$

Thus, $s_{\bar{x}}$ is the sample standard deviation of the sample mean $\bar{X}$. It is a measure of the dispersion of $\bar{X}$ while s is a measure of dispersion for X. We shall discuss the interpretation of $s_{\bar{x}}^2$ and $s_{\bar{x}}$ in more detail in a later chapter.

Example 2.5.4. For the data of Example 2.3.1, determine the sample mean, sample variance, sample standard deviation, sample variance of $\bar{x}$, and sample standard error of $\bar{x}$.

The computations yield the following: $n = 7$, $\sum_{i=1}^{7} x_i = 64.5$, and $\sum_{i=1}^{7} x_i^2 = 594.79$, with

$$SS = 594.79 - \frac{(64.5)^2}{7} = 0.4686;$$

$$s^2 = 0.4686/6 = 0.0781;$$

$$s = 0.28 \text{ mg/mL};$$

$$s_{\bar{x}}^2 = 0.0781/7 = 0.0112;$$

$$s_{\bar{x}} = \sqrt{0.0112} = 0.1058 \text{ mg/mL}.$$

All of the variability quantities that have been discussed are absolute measures of variation. Apart from the squaring operations, the measures are expressed in the units of the original data. Some situations require a measure of relative variation which is *unit free*. One such quantity, defined for positive-value data, is the coefficient of variation. Because it is independent of the units of measurement, it can be used to compare the relative variations of several data sets. For example, the variability in serum drug level measures taken at one laboratory can be compared with that of another.

Definition 2.5.7. The *coefficient of variation*, denoted CV, is defined by

$$CV = 100(s/\bar{x})\%. \tag{2.15}$$

Example 2.5.5. Consider the data of Example 2.3.1 and the same data with a magnitude of 100 added to each observation. The sample standard deviation is 0.28 for each data set while the means are 9.21 and 109.21, respectively. Hence, the coefficients of variation are $100(0.28/9.21) = 3.04\%$ for the original data set of Example 2.3.1 and $100(0.28/109.21) = 0.26\%$ for the modified data of Example 2.3.1 with 100 added to each observation.

This tells us that the relative variation of the first data set is approximately 12 times the relative variation of the second data set. This quantity is useful for quality control purposes where data from several laboratories are compared, and it is useful to compare the within-laboratory variation from one laboratory to another.

To conclude, some general comments are in order. First, common sense must prevail in the summary of any data. To apply these summary computations blindly to a set of data will only serve the cause of confusion and will be, at best, uninformative and, at worst, misleading. Second, for some data there are no summary statistics that can entirely represent the experiment fairly. In these situations, the entire data set must be presented either graphically or in tabular form. In some situations, the best that can be done is to obtain a summary of percentiles (100 equal parts) or deciles (10 equal parts) of the raw data. Third and finally, the statistical tools for the summary of data, if used carelessly, may hide more than they reveal about the raw data.

2.6 PICTORIAL DATA REPRESENTATION

A graph or other device for visual display of data can helpfully describe one's data set. Perhaps the foremost advantage of graphical presentation is that complex relationships can be easily demonstrated. It is far easier to notice relationships from a carefully prepared graph than from a detailed tabulation, although in many cases both are required. Large quantities of data can be presented more efficiently with a graph than through most any other means. From the standpoint of visual impact, a more lasting impression is ordinarily made on an audience with a graph. A graph with striking colors and boldface figures can also attract attention to certain points. This may be an advantage, depending on which points are emphasized; however, the reader may have difficulty in objectively assessing the total situation due to the bias introduced by emphasis of selected points.

Other disadvantages of graphs include the tendency to oversimplify a data set by showing only crude variations in the data. In contrast to a table, a certain amount of precision is lost with a graph. The effects of these problems can be minimized if good graphing principles are followed. Finally, graphs are not as flexible as tabulations when many groups are compared. An illustration may clarify this point. Suppose a graph has been prepared in which the incidence rates of schizophrenia have been graphed as a function of age for males, and on the same graph an incidence curve for females has been plotted. Furthermore, suppose that there is a graph for each of six different geographical regions of the United States. Clearly, male–female comparisons within geographical region would be simple to make, while it would be difficult to compare geographical regions with the two sexes combined into a single group. In most cases like this, new graphs or new plots would be required.

In the preparation of graphs, certain general points should be followed. Cox (1978) cites six points to improve graphical clarity. First, all axes should be clearly labeled, including variable names and measurement units. Second, any scale breaks, that is, false origins, must be indicated on the graph. Third, if comparison of related diagrams is to be undertaken, then one should use identical scales on the axes and the figures should be drawn side by side. Fourth, the scales should be arranged so that systematic and approximately linear relationships are plotted at roughly 45° to the horizontal axis. Fifth, any legends or keys should make diagrams as self-explanatory, that is, as independent of the text as is feasible. Finally, interpretation should not be prejudiced by the presentation technique, for example, by superimposing thick, smooth curves on scatter diagrams of faintly reproduced plots of the points.

The axes of reference or frames of reference of a graph are generally of three types: the *rectangular* coordinate system (x and y axes), the *polar* coordinate system, and the *geographical* coordinate system. The rectangular coordinate system consists of an x and a y axis referred to as the abscissa (x) and the ordinate (y), respectively. Generally, the abscissa is used for the independent variable (e.g., age group) while the ordinate is for the dependent variable (e.g., incidence rate of schizophrenia). In medical studies, the x axis is commonly used for the age of individual, the dosage of an agent, or the time of exposure, while the y axis may represent the incidence rate of disease or level of the response variable of interest. For example, to study blood pressure as a function of age, age would be the independent, or x, variable and blood pressure the dependent, or y, variable. In Figure 2.1, we have an example of a rectangular coordinate system. The dependent variable has been incremented so that equal changes in distance in the x direction indicate equal amounts of changes in the y variable. For example, a change in one unit indicates an absolute change of 1000 grams (g). This graph has been plotted on an *arithmetic* scale; that is, the y axis measures the *amount* of change.

Quite often one wishes to compare *rates* of change in a variable, so we use a *logarithmic* scale. Graph paper with a logarithmic scale on the y axis

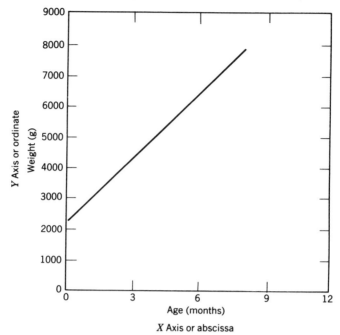

Figure 2.1. Relation of weight (g) on age (months).

and arithmetic scale on the x axis is called semilog paper. This is useful to compare the proportionate rate of change in deaths. In Figure 2.2, we have an example of data plotted on semilog paper. A positive change of one unit on the y axis represents a 10-fold increase in the number of deaths.

With polar coordinates, the frame of reference is the circle. Given an angle of rotation and a radius, one can plot a point in two dimensions. The *pie chart* is a graph that uses this frame of reference. This graph is useful to show how the whole is divided into its component parts; however, it is not useful for comparing groups. Suppose the typical physician in a department of a university spends 35% of his time in clinical work, 30% in teaching, 25% in research, and 10% in miscellaneous activities. The graph in Figure 2.3 is a quick way to present these figures. Since there are 360° in the circle, each percentage point represents 3.6°. Thus, to obtain the angle required, multiply each percentage in the graph by 3.6. It is customary to start with either vertical or horizontal lines and proceed in a clockwise manner to plot the various components in decreasing order.

Geographical coordinates have as a frame of reference a map of a certain geographical area. This is a useful graphical procedure for describing the

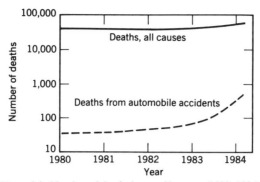

Figure 2.2. Number of deaths by specific cause (1980–1984).

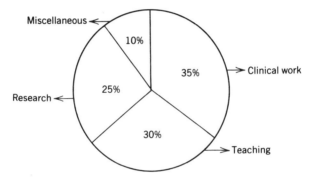

Figure 2.3. Time distribution of university physician.

path of an epidemic or the number of cases by area. This graph is called a *spot map*. This procedure is used often in epidemiologic studies of chronic and infectious diseases.

Caution should be used in the interpretation of spot maps because the points (cases) are affected by population size in the respective areas. For this reason, rates are normally computed, and these figures are classified as low, medium, and high. These are then indicated by different markings on the key. For example, one might use

☐   Low disease rate

▨   Moderate disease rate

▧   High disease rate

to represent disease rates.

One innovative use of such geographical charts has been the color mapping of cardiovascular disease mortality rates of the United States. These maps, provided by the Bureau of the Census, consist of county-by-county plots of rates colored from pink to deep red as low goes to high. The more interested reader may refer to Fienberg (1979) for a number of these illustrations and a more detailed discussion of such graphical statistical techniques.

We have mentioned the pie chart, and the reader may note that it may be used for nominal or ordinal data. Another graph that is ideal for nominal- and ordinal-scale data is the *bar chart*. An example of a bar chart is shown in Figure 2.4. Since there was no time or scale involved on the x axis, the data have been plotted in descending order of magnitude. For proper comparison, the bars should start from a common baseline. A scale break or false origin should never be used in the bar chart; it is the lengths of the vertical bars that are being compared. For example, in Figure 2.4, we note that comparisons may be made between sexes within cause of death and also between causes of death within sexes. Both sets of comparisons can be made because the bars have a common baseline. One type of variation of the bar chart is the *pictorial chart*. In place of vertical columns, each unit (or number of units) is represented by a figure (e.g., a hospital bed, doctor, nurse, man, woman, etc.).

A restriction of the pie chart is the difficulty in comparison of two groups. For example, it is difficult to compare how the physician at University A spends his time in medical activities as compared to the physician at University B. A more useful graph for this type of comparison

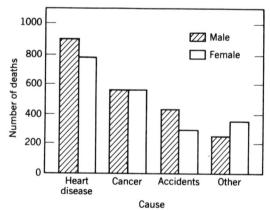

Figure 2.4. Number of deaths by specific cause in a given year.

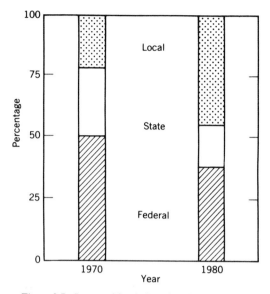

Figure 2.5. Source of funds for a health department.

is the *component band chart*. An example is the chart comparing sources of funds for a local health department presented in Figure 2.5. Again, this graph is suited for both nominal- and ordinal-scale data.

In Section 2.8, we discuss several other means of graphical display that are particularly useful for grouped continuous data. These are the histogram, frequency polygon, and cumulative frequency polygon.

The final graph to mention here is the *scatter diagram*. This is used to point out the relationships between two variables. These relationships are not necessarily causal in nature. Examples of scatter diagrams may be found in the text in the discussion of regression and correlation analysis, and we shall return to these diagrams at that point.

For the reader interested in further details of graphical display, the recent text of Tufte (1983) and the papers of Wainer (1984) and Fienberg (1979) are recommended.

2.7 SAMPLE DESCRIPTION WITH GROUPED DATA

For some data sets it is convenient for the interpretation of the data to have it represented in the simplified form of a *frequency table*. Large quantities

Table 2.1. Ages of Onset of First Illness for 123 Male
Manic-Depressive Patients

Age of Onset in Years	Number of Men
10–20	15
20–30	37
30–40	21
40–50	28
50–60	19
60–70	3

of data often require this kind of table. For example, suppose that in a study of the age of onset of first illness among male manic-depressive patients, it was determined that of the 123 men, 15 had ages of onset between 10 but less than 20 years of age, 37 had ages of onset between 20 but less than 30 years of age, 21 had ages of onset between 30 but less than 40 years of age, 28 had ages of onset between 40 but less than 50 years of age, 19 had ages of onset between 50 but less than 60 years of age, and 3 had ages of onset between 60 but less than 70 years of age. Table 2.1 is a frequency table of the data.

Table 2.1 is also an example of *grouped data* since the ages are grouped in 10-year intervals. For the data of Table 2.1 the grouping was constructed from the individual observations; however, this need not always be the case. In some studies, the data may be gathered according to groups. For example, a questionnaire might ask you to record your annual income as less than $10,000, between $10,000 and $30,000, between $30,000 and $50,000, or greater than $50,000.

In any case, once data like that in Table 2.1 have been gathered, two further questions must be answered: How should the information in the table be presented—either graphically or tabularly—and how does one compute the measures of central tendency and dispersion for the data? We have discussed analogous problems with ungrouped data.

Before addressing these two questions, we first discuss the question of determining the intervals for grouping data. Having decided that grouping is necessary, the first question is to determine the number and the size of the class intervals. Common sense and good judgment are the best tools for making this decision. If too many intervals are used, then the grouping has not really served to simplify the presentation. Conversely, too few intervals represent too gross a categorization of the data. One must bear in mind that the principal reason for grouping the data is to simplify the presentation. Nevertheless, the grouping should not prevent the audience from seeing the data as it was originally collected. Often the intervals are chosen to be equal; however, the nature of the problem under investigation should determine the interval size.

For those who prefer a rule of thumb for determining the number of class intervals, the guideline of Sturges (1926) may be used. In particular, if the sample size n is fairly large (e.g., greater than 50), then the number of class intervals K is the nearest integer to $1 + 3.322 \log_{10} n$, where $\log_{10}$ is the logarithm base 10.

Example 2.7.1. Determine the number of class intervals from the sample size of 123 from Table 2.1 using Sturges's rule. First, calculate $\log_{10} 123 = 2.09$. Substituting this into the formula, we have $1 + 3.322(\log_{10} 123) = 7.94$. The number of classes is 8.

From the computation in Example 2.7.1, we have apparently used too few intervals (assuming we should follow Sturges's rule rigorously).

Once the value of K has been determined, the width of each class interval would be the range divided by K. This would yield K intervals of equal width. In Table 2.1, the minimum and maximum ages of onset that were observed in this study were 12 and 68, respectively. If one applied the result of Sturges's rule and used equal-sized class intervals, then the width of each interval should be $(68 - 12) \div 8$, or 7, years. The intervals would be $12 - 19$ years, $19 - 26$, $26 - 33$, and so on. Ten-year intervals, starting with age 10, are a more workable set of intervals and were chosen for that reason. Once again, this sort of judgment is required by someone who is deciding on the number of class intervals and depends very much on the data. For example, age-of-onset data of psychotic illness frequently has a wide initial class interval starting from zero to, say, 20. Following this, a series of equally spaced smaller intervals is terminated by an interval, which is of the form 60 years and older, that is, open ended on the right.

2.8   TABULATION AND GRAPHING OF GROUPED DATA

We now turn to the question of graphical and tabular display of grouped data and consider hypothetical data that was gathered in an ocular vascular clinic. The data consist of the intraocular pressure in one eye of each of 238 patients. The data are in Table 2.2.

In Table 2.3, we show the same data but grouped into categories of intraocular pressure. The table shows 17 patients had a recorded intraocular pressure of 12 or 13, 20 had a pressure of 14 or 15, and so forth. In actual fact, intraocular pressure is recorded to the nearest integer; for example, 10.1 is recorded as 10 and 22.9 is recorded as 23. The measuring instrument,

Table 2.2. Intraocular pressure (IOP) (mm Hg) for 238 Patients Visiting an Ocular Disease Clinic

Patient ID	IOP	Patient ID	IOP	Patient ID	IOP	Patient ID	IOP	Patient ID	IOP	Patient ID	IOP
1	23	41	17	81	19	121	19	161	22	201	19
2	21	42	19	82	16	122	21	162	23	202	18
3	13	43	20	83	21	123	31	163	18	203	24
4	20	44	18	84	18	124	15	164	22	204	20
5	18	45	20	85	19	125	19	165	19	205	14
6	22	46	21	86	17	126	23	166	12	206	25
7	21	47	20	87	20	127	21	167	17	207	9
8	10	48	20	88	21	128	19	168	27	208	17
9	19	49	20	89	17	129	23	169	18	209	18
10	18	50	13	90	19	130	19	170	12	210	12
11	17	51	17	91	16	131	17	171	14	211	16
12	14	52	17	92	21	132	12	172	23	212	15
13	20	53	15	93	16	133	21	173	17	213	17
14	19	54	23	94	19	134	19	174	14	214	21
15	25	55	19	95	21	135	16	175	18	215	22
16	16	56	20	96	20	136	23	176	19	216	27
17	12	57	19	97	20	137	20	177	18	217	14
18	18	58	18	98	19	138	22	178	20	218	15
19	19	59	22	99	12	139	21	179	21	219	12
20	17	60	18	100	20	140	20	180	19	220	23
21	22	61	16	101	18	141	16	181	17	221	15
22	14	62	21	102	12	142	21	182	22	222	31
23	17	63	21	103	18	143	17	183	20	223	14
24	16	64	24	104	16	144	18	184	18	224	16
25	18	65	15	105	21	145	20	185	17	225	19
26	18	66	20	106	19	146	21	186	19	226	21
27	21	67	23	107	15	147	18	187	16	227	18
28	19	68	25	108	17	148	21	188	17	228	20
29	21	69	14	109	20	149	13	189	19	229	20
30	22	70	25	110	18	150	12	190	16	230	21
31	23	71	25	111	21	151	20	191	17	231	18
32	16	72	15	112	21	152	14	192	20	232	12
33	12	73	17	113	20	153	17	193	16	233	21
34	22	74	16	114	15	154	11	194	21	234	22
35	19	75	18	115	19	155	16	195	20	235	17
36	22	76	18	116	23	156	18	196	19	236	18
37	13	77	20	117	19	157	14	197	21	237	20
38	16	78	19	118	18	158	16	198	20	238	18
39	17	79	17	119	33	159	15	199	12		
40	18	80	18	120	19	160	19	200	13		

Table 2.3. Intraocular Pressure in 238 Patients
with Ocular Vascular Disease

Intraocular Pressure (mm Hg)	Number of Patients
8–9	1
10–11	2
12–13	17
14–15	20
16–17	43
18–19	63
20–21	57
22–23	23
24–25	7
26–27	2
28–29	0
30–31	2
32–33	1
	238

in this case the applanation tonometer, is only capable of providing data to the nearest whole integer. The measurement instrument always places limits on the degree of precision that can be obtained in the measurement process.

This limitation imposed by the measuring instrument has implications for interpreting a recorded value. For example, a recorded value of 8 is a number that could apply to a whole array of true values of the intraocular pressure. A true value of 7.9 or 8.1 would probably be read by the tonometer as an 8.0. In fact, it seems quite sensible to assume that all true intraocular pressures from 7.5 up to, but not including, 8.5 would be recorded as 8. This holds true for all values of the pressure; for example, an 11 is the recorded value corresponding to real pressures of 10.5 up to but less than 11.5, and so forth. Hence, Table 2.3 can be rewritten in the form of Table 2.4.

Table 2.4, therefore, represents the intraocular pressure variable viewed as a *continuous variable*. The fact that only integer values are recorded as a result of the tonometry is a technical limitation of the measuring instrument and is not an indication that the pressure variable is a discrete variable. The true *class limits* in Table 2.4 represent a more realistic interpretation of the data.

The number of patients in each class interval is more generally referred to as the *frequency* in the interval, denoted f_i for the ith class interval.

Table 2.4. Intraocular Pressure in 238 Patients with Ocular Vascular Disease

i	Intraocular Pressure (mm Hg)	Number of Patients (Frequency)	Relative Frequency (%)	Cumulative Relative Frequency (%)
	Class Limits From To			
1	7.5– 9.5	1	0.42	0.42
2	9.5–11.5	2	0.84	1.26
3	11.5–13.5	17	7.14	8.40
4	13.5–15.5	20	8.40	16.80
5	15.5–17.5	43	18.07	34.87
6	17.5–19.5	63	26.47	61.34
7	19.5–21.5	57	23.95	85.29
8	21.5–23.5	23	9.67	94.96
9	23.5–25.5	7	2.94	97.90
10	25.5–27.5	2	0.84	98.74
11	27.5–29.5	0	0.00	98.74
12	29.5–31.5	2	0.84	99.58
13	31.5–33.5	1	0.42	100.00
		$\overline{238}$		

Definition 2.8.1. The frequency f_i divided by the total number of individuals in the sample is called the *relative frequency*. Multiplication of this proportion by 100 places it on a percentage basis.

Thus, the relative frequency is the proportion of the observations falling in a particular interval. In Table 2.4, the relative frequencies of the intervals are given.

Definition 2.8.2. The *cumulative relative frequency* for the ith interval is the sum of the relative frequencies of the intervals that precede the ith interval plus the relative frequency in the ith interval. It is often expressed as a percentage.

Hence, the cumulative relative frequency for the second interval is the relative frequency for the first interval plus that for the second interval. From Table 2.4, this is 0.42 + 0.84, or 1.26%. This number is the percentage of observations less than the upper limit in that class interval. Hence, 1.26% of the observations are less than 11.5 mm Hg, while 61.34% are less than 19.5 mm Hg, and so forth.

One graphical procedure for presenting the data of Table 2.4 is the *histogram*, which was mentioned briefly in Section 2.6. This graph plots the

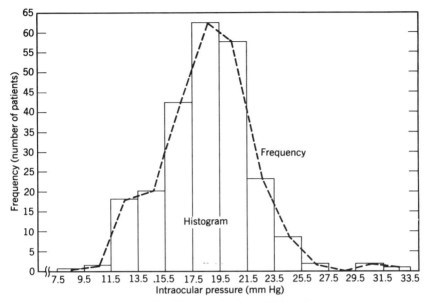

Figure 2.6. Histogram for data of Table 2.4.

frequency (or the relative frequency) divided by the width of the class interval on the y axis. Each class interval is plotted as a rectangle. The width of the rectangle is the width of the ith interval in millimeters of mercury, while its height is the frequency divided by the width of the class interval. Hence, the height of the histogram bar is proportional to frequency/(interval width). However, for *equal-class intervals*, the height is proportional to the frequency, and thus the frequency (or relative frequency) may be plotted against intervals in this case.

In Figure 2.6, a histogram is drawn in which the frequency is plotted against the intraocular pressure. The dotted line in Figure 2.6 is the path determined by connecting the midpoints of the class intervals at the top of the histogram. The resulting polygon (i.e., many-sided figure) is termed a *frequency polygon*; it is an alternative to the histogram as a form for graphical presentation. In Figure 2.6, both the histogram and frequency polygon are shown on the same graph. Most data presentations show one or the other but not both. Also, in Figure 2.6, we used a *scale break* on the x axis because the intraocular pressures do not begin for these data until 7.5 mm Hg.

Figure 2.7 plots the *relative frequency polygon*. This figure is the graph of the relative frequency plotted at the midpoint of the class interval followed

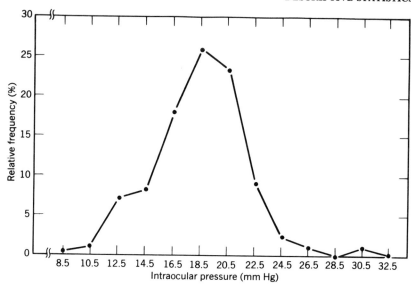

Figure 2.7. Relative frequency polygon for data of Table 2.4.

by the connection of adjacent points. The relative frequency polygon (sometimes called frequency polygon) is a convenient graph to use for comparative purposes. For example, if data from another ocular vascular clinic were available, unless the two sample sizes were equal, it would be difficult to compare results with only a graph like Figure 2.6 from each clinic. Clearly, comparison of relative frequencies is appropriate with the relative frequency polygons because scales for the *y* axis are identical. It should be noted that, in general, for unequal interval widths, the relative frequency would be divided by the width of the interval, and this ratio would be plotted on the *y* axis.

The *cumulative relative frequency* may also be plotted, and this graph is most appropriately prepared by plotting the cumulative relative frequency on the *y* axis and the variable on the *x* axis. For example, Figure 2.8 is a plot of the cumulative relative frequency curve for the data of Table 2.3. The cumulative relative frequency is plotted at the right-hand or upper endpoint of its class interval; the cumulative relative frequency represents the percentage of the observations less than this upper value. This type of graph is very useful for determining the percentiles of the data. The dotted line in Figure 2.8 shows how easily the median (50th percentile) can be derived from the curve. Other percentiles could be determined just as easily.

While the preceding graphs are useful for the presentation of data, they do not begin to exhaust the set of all possible graphical aids. Nevertheless,

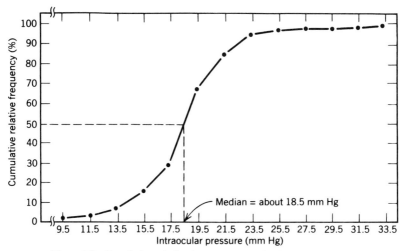

Figure 2.8. Cumulative relative frequency curve for data of Table 2.4.

the preceding three graphs represent a sufficiently broad scope to include many applications.

The computation of summary statistics to determine location and variability characteristics, which we discussed earlier, is an additional aspect of presenting and describing grouped data. We turn to this aspect in the next section.

2.9 SUMMARY STATISTICS FOR GROUPED DATA

For ungrouped data, three measures were described for the central tendency of a sample: the sample mean, sample mode, and sample median. These quantities also may be determined for grouped data.

The sample mode is determined in much the same manner as it is for ungrouped data.

Definition 2.9.1. The *sample mode* for grouped data is defined as the most frequently occurring class interval.

If many intervals satisfy the criterion, it might be wise to state that no modal class exists.

Example 2.9.1. For the data of Table 2.1, the modal class is 20–30 years of age, since 37 men are in this category.

Example 2.9.2. The modal class for the data of Table 2.4 is 17.5–19.5 mm Hg.

Definition 2.9.2. The *sample median* for grouped data is the 50th percentile based on the cumulative relative frequency. The sample median is that value such that no more than one-half the data is less than it and no more than one-half of the data is greater than it.

In the previous section, the median was discussed in connection with Figure 2.8, where a graphical approach was employed to locate the median. A linear interpolation (method of obtaining intermediate terms) could also be used to determine the median from Figure 2.8. Specifically, let us consider the example of Table 2.4 once again in analytical terms. From Table 2.4, 34.87% of the data are less than 17.5 mm Hg, while 61.34% are less than 19.5 mm Hg; hence, the 50th percentile is somewhere between 17.5 and 19.5 mm Hg. A linear interpolation is a procedure whereby one simply draws a straight line between the two points and then finds the desired value from the line. Accordingly, the two points from Figure 2.8 are $(17.5, 34.87)$ and $(19.5, 61.34)$. The slope of the line connecting these two points is $(61.34 - 34.87)/(19.5 - 17.5) = 13.235$. The median is that value of x such that the point $(x, 50)$ is on the line connecting the two points $(17.5, 34.87)$ and $(19.5, 61.34)$. Thus, using the formula for slope, it is clear that $(50 - 34.87)/(x - 17.5)$ is equal to 13.235. Solving for x yields a sample median of 18.64 (i.e., $[(50 - 34.87)/13.235] + 17.5$). It may be noted that other percentiles may be determined in an analogous manner.

The sample mean is also quite straightforward to obtain from grouped data. The procedure is to take the midpoint of an interval and form its product with the frequency in the interval. The sample mean is then computed as the sum of those products across all the class intervals divided by the total sample size (i.e., the sum of the frequencies). We denote the midpoints of the ith class interval by x_i for $i = 1, 2, \ldots, k$ (where k is the number of intervals) and the respective class interval frequencies by f_i for $i = 1, 2, \ldots, k$.

Definition 2.9.3. The *sample mean* for grouped data is defined by

$$\bar{x} = \frac{\sum_{i=1}^{k} f_i x_i}{n}, \tag{2.16}$$

where n is the sample size, that is, $n = \sum_{i=1}^{k} f_i$, and k is the number of intervals.

For the data of Table 2.4, the sample mean is given by $\bar{x} = [1(8.5) + 2(10.5) + 17(12.5) + \cdots + 2(30.5) + 1(32.5)]/238 = 4411/238 = 18.5$ mm

Hg, which is quite close to the sample median. Another way of interpreting the sample mean, when it is computed for grouped data, is to think of its as the ungrouped sample mean in which each observation in an interval is replaced by the midpoint of that interval. This way of thinking is also useful in describing the computations for the grouped data sample variance.

Definition 2.9.4.   The *sample variance* for grouped data is defined by

$$s^2 = \frac{\sum_{i=1}^{k} f_i (x_i - \bar{x})^2}{n - 1}. \tag{2.17}$$

As in the ungrouped situation, the positive square root of (2.17) denoted by s is the sample *standard deviation*, while $s/\sqrt{n}$ is the *sample standard error of the mean* and is denoted by $s_{\bar{x}}$ since it is the sample standard deviation of the sample mean $\bar{x}$. Similarly, $s_{\bar{x}}^2 = s^2/n$ is the *sample variance of the sample mean*. From a computational standpoint, the numerator of (2.17) is computed more easily by using its equivalent computing form of

$$\sum_{i=1}^{k} f_i (x_i - \bar{x})^2 = \sum_{i=1}^{k} f_i x_i^2 - \frac{\left(\sum_{i=1}^{k} f_i x_i\right)^2}{n}. \tag{2.18}$$

Table 2.5. Sample Variance Computations for the Data of Table 2.4

Class Interval (mm Hg)		Midpoint x_i	Frequency f_i	$f_i x_i$	$f_i x_i^2$
7.5	9.5	8.5	1	8.5	72.25
9.5	11.5	10.5	2	21.0	220.50
11.5	13.5	12.5	17	212.5	2,656.25
13.5	15.5	14.5	20	290.0	4,205.00
15.5	17.5	16.5	43	709.5	11,706.75
17.5	19.5	18.5	63	1,165.5	21,561.75
19.5	21.5	20.5	57	1,168.5	23,954.25
21.5	23.5	22.5	23	517.5	11,643.75
23.5	25.5	24.5	7	171.5	4,201.75
25.5	27.5	26.5	2	53.0	1,404.50
27.5	29.5	28.5	0	0	0
29.5	31.5	30.5	2	61.0	1,860.50
31.5	33.5	32.5	1	32.5	1,056.25
			238	4,411.0	84,543.50

$k = 13, \qquad n = 238, \qquad \sum_{i=1}^{k} f_i x_i = 4,411 \qquad \sum_{i=1}^{k} f_i x_i^2 = 84,543.5$

Example 2.9.3. To illustrate the computations, we continue with the data of Table 2.4. Three additional columns are helpful in conducting the calculations: x_i, $f_i x_i$, and $f_i x_i^2$. Therefore, we have listed the summary computations in Table 2.5. Consequently,

$$s^2 = \frac{\left[84{,}543.5 - (4{,}411)^2/238\right]}{237} = 11.7795$$

$$s = \sqrt{11.7795} = 3.4321$$

$$s_{\bar{x}}^2 = 11.7795/238 = 0.0495$$

$$s_{\bar{x}} = \sqrt{0.0495} = 0.2225$$

are the summary figures that describe the sample's variability.

2.10 SUMMARY

In this chapter, we have introduced some basic forms of data description. With the exception of selected topics in the discussion of graphs, the emphasis on the first sections has been exclusively on the problems associated with summarizing ungrouped data, that is, data that consist of individual observations as opposed to data condensed into a table of frequencies.

The last sections describe the procedures for the statistical presentation and summary of grouped data. While a computer obviously can be directed to conduct the various tedious arithmetic steps, the choice of a final presentation format of a data set depends entirely on the analyst's judgment. The methods outlined in this chapter provide some of the alternatives available for grouped data analyses.

For further reading on the topic of graphs, the reader may turn to the recent articles of Fienberg (1979) and Cox (1978). Fienberg provides some interesting graphical examples of geographical maps of disease rates.

PROBLEMS

2.1. Classify each of the variables below using each of the schemes: (i) qualitative or quantitative; (ii) discrete or continuous; and

(iii) nominal, ordinal, ratio, or interval. The variables are
(a) the number of cancer deaths in Iowa during 1985,
(b) the letter grade (A, B, C, D, or F) received in a college course,
(c) the systolic blood pressure of a child,
(d) the sex of a child,
(e) annual family income,
(f) age of a man,
(g) the marital status of a woman, and
(h) the number of times a woman has married in her lifetime.

2.2. Given that

$$x_1 = 11 \qquad x_2 = 12 \qquad x_3 = 13 \qquad x_4 = -10$$

$$y_1 = 9 \qquad y_2 = 7 \qquad y_3 = 5 \qquad y_4 = 3$$

find:

(a) $\sum_{i=1}^{4} x_i$ (b) $\sum_{i=1}^{4} x_i^2$

(c) $(\sum_{i=1}^{4} x_i)^2$ (d) $\sum_{i=1}^{4} x_i y_i$

(e) $(\sum_{i=1}^{4} x_i)(\sum_{j=1}^{4} y_j)$ (f) $(\sum_{i=1}^{3} x_i)(\sum_{j=2}^{4} y_j)$

2.3. A sample of 10 women athletes between ages 23 and 27 reported their current weight, age at menarche, and menstrual status [current amenorrhea (A) or regular menses (R)]:

Woman No.	Menstrual Status	Age at Menarche	Current Weight (kg)
1	R	12	57
2	R	14	65
3	A	10	51
4	R	9	52
5	A	12	48
6	A	12	50
7	A	11	49
8	R	10	59
9	A	10	50
10	R	16	61

(a) Compute the mean and standard deviation for age and weight within each of the menstrual status categories.

(b) Which category has more dispersion in their ages?

(c) Strenuous exercise has been related to menstrual irregularities and weight loss. Do these data support this statement? Why?

2.4. The data in the following table represent selected clinical and laboratory characteristics of chronic lymphocytic leukemia patients.

Patient	Age (yr)	Total Leukocytes ($\times 10^9$/L)	Lymphocytes (%)	Serum Immunoglobulin (IU/mL)	
				IgG	IgM
1	76	69.3	92	30	18
2	50	151.8	95	38	33
3	68	125.0	93	50	13
4	64	17.7	78	58	50
5	83	32.1	57	75	19
6	62	12.8	75	44	44
7	50	88.1	96	33	14
8	67	20.3	85	35	202
9	70	44.5	90	95	50

Source: Lamberson et al. (1984). *Cancer,* **53**, 2481–2486. Copyright © 1984, by the American Cancer Society, Inc. J. B. Lippincott Company.

(a) Compute the sample mean, median, and mode for each variable.

(b) Compute the range, sample variance, and standard deviation for each variable.

(c) Which measures of central tendency and of variability seem more appropriate for each variable?

(d) Compare the variability of the levels of the immunoglobulin using the coefficient of variation.

2.5. In a randomized prospective trial to measure the anxiety-reducing efficacy of a certain oral premedication for pediatric outpatient surgery, 81 children received the premedication and 77 children received a placebo. The following table shows the evaluation of preanesthetic and postanesthetic mental state.

| Location/Observation | Scale | Frequency | |
		Placebo	Premedication
Holding Area			
State of consciousness	Excited/agitated	1	2
	Awake	64	61
	Drowsy	12	16
	Asleep	0	2
Attitude	Resistant	2	0
	Mildly resistant	8	5
	Apprehensive	6	6
	Mildly anxious	61	70
	Cooperative	0	0
Operating Room Arrival			
State of consciousness	Excited/agitated	12	11
	Awake	53	51
	Drowsy	12	18
	Asleep	0	1
Attitude	Resistant	10	5
	Mildly resistant	7	4
	Apprehensive	13	13
	Mildly anxious	5	10
	Cooperative	42	49
Recovery Room			
State of consciousness	Excited/agitated	15	9
	Awake	8	13
	Drowsy	23	17
	Asleep	31	42
Attitude	Resistant	9	8
	Mildly resistant	5	5
	Apprehensive	5	2
	Mildly anxious	4	6
	Cooperative	54	60

Source: Brzustowicz et al. (1984). *Anesthesiology*, **60**, 475–477. Copyright © 1984, by Lippincott/Harper & Row.

Produce a pie chart and a component band chart for each location. Which appears to be more useful for drawing conclusions about the effect of premedication?

2.6. The following data are the ages of 48 tennis players from a community recreation center, who suffer from lateral humeral epicondylitis, also known as "tennis elbow":

37	28	55	47	34	24	53	41
12	39	35	28	55	44	39	33
26	21	46	48	45	53	34	54
55	48	51	31	18	42	49	47
49	37	41	44	49	36	38	39
43	48	46	37	48	41	39	43

(a) Compute the sample mean, sample median, and sample standard deviation for this data set.

(b) Determine the 25th and the 75th percentiles for this sample.

(c) Using categories of 10–15, 16–20, ..., 51–55, construct a frequency distribution. Determine the true class limits and then plot the histogram and cumulative frequency distribution. Compute the sample mean and sample standard deviation from the grouped data in the frequency table.

2.7. To identify poor metabolizers of a certain antihypertensive drug, 25 healthy subjects took the drug and had serial urine samples examined every 2 hr. In the first sample, the observed metabolic ratios, expressed in common logarithms rounded to the nearest one-hundredth, are

Log (metabolic ratio)	Frequency
− 0.70, − 0.29	5
− 0.30, 0.09	8
0.10, 0.49	7
0.50, 0.89	3
0.90, 1.29	0
1.30, 1.69	2

(a) Compute the sample mean.

(b) Compute the sample variance.

(c) Compute the sample standard error of the mean.

(d) Produce a plot of the cumulative relative frequency and a histogram.

2.8. In general, a linear transformation of a variable x to the variable y can be written as $y = ax + b$ for some constants a and b. For example, if x represents temperature in the Celsius scale and y is temperature in the Fahrenheit scale, then the linear transformation relating x and y can be written

$$y = \tfrac{9}{5}x + 32.$$

(a) Given that the temperatures in the Celsius scale of five patients are $x_1 = 38.2$, $x_2 = 41.1$, $x_3 = 37.5$, $x_4 = 40.8$, and $x_5 = 39.2$, obtain the mean and standard deviation of the temperatures in Fahrenheit degrees.

(b) Without transforming the temperatures from Celsius to Fahrenheit degrees, confirm the results obtained in (a) with the formulas

$$\bar{y} = \tfrac{9}{5}\bar{x} + 32 \quad \text{and} \quad s_y = \tfrac{9}{5}s_x.$$

(c) Prove that in general

$$\bar{y} = a\bar{x} + b \quad \text{and} \quad s_y^2 = a^2 s_x^2.$$

2.9. The following data presents the level of astigmatism in 36 patients before and after a special cataract extraction operation.

(a) Compute the mean and the standard deviation for the preoperative and postoperative levels of astigmatism.

(b) Compute the mean and standard deviation of the change in level of astigmatism, that is, postoperative minus preoperative astigmatism.

(c) Group the data in a frequency table using the change variable, and compute the mean, the median, and the standard deviation of this variable using $k = 8$ intervals and $k = 4$ intervals from -2 to $+2$. Which value of k provides a better summary of the data? Why?

(d) Plot the relative frequency polygon when $k = 8$.

	Astigmatism (Diopters)	
Patient No.	Postoperative	Preoperative
1	1.12	1.50
2	0.63	1.37
3	0.67	1.87
4	0.00	0.13
5	1.25	2.13
6	1.25	1.12
7	0.50	1.37
8	0.37	1.13
9	0.50	1.37
10	0.88	0.75
11	1.00	0.50
12	0.25	0.87
13	1.25	1.25
14	0.75	1.50
15	1.13	1.25
16	0.62	0.87
17	1.67	1.12
18	0.25	1.25
19	1.50	1.87
20	0.00	0.38
21	0.62	0.75
22	1.88	3.00
23	1.13	1.75
24	1.75	1.00
25	0.27	0.50
26	0.25	2.13
27	1.88	2.25
28	3.37	4.25
29	0.63	0.87
30	2.88	2.33
31	2.00	2.38
32	1.13	1.00
33	1.25	2.25
34	0.25	0.25
35	1.87	2.00
36	3.12	1.25

Source: Girard et al. (1984). *Am. J. Ophthal.*, **97**, 450–456.

Published with permission from the *American Journal of Opthalmology.* Copyright © by the Ophthalmic Publishing Company.

REFERENCES

Brzustowicz, R. M., D. A. Nelson, E. K. Betts, K. R. Rosenberry, and D. B. Swedlow. (1984). Efficacy of oral premedication for pediatric outpatient surgery, *Anesthesiology*, **60**, 475–477.

Cox, D. R. (1978). Some remarks on the role in statistics of graphical methods, *Appl. Statist.*, **27**, 4–9.

Fienberg, S. E. (1979). Graphical methods in statistics, *Am. Statist.*, **33**, 165–178.

Girard, L. J., J. Rodriguez, and M. L. Mailman. (1984). Reducing surgically induced astigmatism by using a scleral tunnel, *Am. J. Opthalmol.*, **97**, 450–456.

Goldstein, A. (1971). *Biostatistics: An Introductory Text*, The MacMillan Company, New York.

Lamberson, H. V., F. R. Davey, C. M. Schreck, K. Zamkoff, and A. S. Kurec. (1984). Lymphocyte response to pokeweed mitogen in chronic lymphocytic leukemia, *Cancer*, **53**, 2481–2846.

Stevens, S. S. (1946). On the theory of scales of measurement, *Science*, **103**, 677–680.

Sturges, H. A. (1926). The choice of a class interval, *J. Am. Statist. Assoc.*, **21**, 65–66.

Tufte, E. R. (1983). *The Visual Display of Quantitative Information*, Graphics Press, Cheshire, CT.

Wainer, H. (1984). How to display data badly, *Am. Statist.*, **38**, 137–147.

CHAPTER 3

Basic Probability Concepts

3.1 INTRODUCTION

The previous chapter dealt with aspects of data description and ignored entirely the question of testing a hypothesis on the basis of the observed data. Generally, data have been gathered to test a hypothesis or to make a statement regarding the population from which the data were selected. For example, a published report (Woolson et al., 1980) concluded that a group of schizophrenic and manic-depressive persons had shortened survival relative to individuals who were free of these psychiatric disorders. This statement was made on the basis of a sample of 200 schizophrenics, 325 manic-depressives, and 160 nonpsychiatric controls. While this sample outcome is interesting, what is important is whether this is a general finding that will apply to other schizophrenics, manic-depressives, and controls. If it is a result that pertains only to the sample of 685 persons involved in this one study, it may naturally have little value. What can be said about this issue of generalizing the sample result to a larger group?

It is evident that the data analyst must know a great deal about the 685 persons in the sample and must also know how these persons were chosen for inclusion in the sample. Furthermore, it is clear that we require a conceptual framework to study this issue. Probability theory and sampling theory provide such a basis.

To begin to address this issue, we must consider an appropriate population as a frame of reference; the term *population* refers to the group from which the sample is chosen. In the foregoing example, the population might be the collection of all persons who are either schizophrenic, manic-depressive, or free of these disorders. Alternatively, the population might be conceived of as the collection of all such persons in the state of Iowa during a certain period of time. Clearly, several populations could be envisioned.

However, typically, the population is defined by the theoretical question of interest. For example, if one wished to determine if psychotic persons hospitalized at some time during the years 1935–1945 have increased mortality rates relative to a group of psychiatrically symptom-free surgical patients hospitalized during the same time frame, then the population would be all persons satisfying this criterion. The population, then, is generally defined by the substantive question at hand.

In general, a *population* is defined as a collection or totality of a set of objects or persons with one or more characteristics in common. A *sample* is a subset of that population.

In the mortality example, the 525 psychiatric patients represented a sample or subset of the psychotic patient population, while the 160 controls represented a sample from the nonpsychiatric patient population.

The next question is that of sample selection. Specifically, how was the subset of persons chosen for inclusion in the sample? Obviously, if the process by which the sample was chosen cannot be described, then it is generally not possible to make a statement or draw conclusions regarding the population.

By now we see the sequence of events: first, a theoretical question arose in psychiatry; then a population was naturally defined; and finally—since it was impractical to study the entire population—a sample was selected. The problem then becomes one of using the sample information to make a statement about the population that answers our theoretical question. We therefore want to make an *inference*, that is, we want to use the sample data to infer something about the population. Making inferences is, in fact, the central issue in the field of statistics.

It is apparent that what one infers about the population on the basis of the sample may be an incorrect conclusion since the entire population has not been studied. However, to impose the requirement that one is absolutely certain of the conclusion is far too stringent considering the fact that only a portion of the population is studied. Rather than requiring certainty of conclusion, a probabilistic approach can be taken. With this approach, we are able to quantify the degree of uncertainty associated with the inductive inference.

We shall see that when the process of *random sampling* is used to select a sample from the population, then the tools of probability may be used to evaluate the uncertainty of our inferences. In essence, random sampling is a process that generates the sample in a way such that each sample, or subset of the population, has the same opportunity to be the one chosen for study. Intuitively, one can see that the ability to evaluate uncertainties in inference is intimately tied to the process of sampling. In order to discuss sampling from populations, the use of random samples, and the evaluation of uncertainties, we must have some understanding of probability theory. With this overview as background, we proceed to a discussion of basic probability since this forms the conceptual framework for statistical inference.

3.2 PROBABILITY

The terms *probability*, *chance*, and *likelihood* are so commonplace that most of us have some notion of their meaning. If a fair coin is tossed the probability that heads appears is $\frac{1}{2}$. If a balanced six-sided die is rolled the probability that a 3 appears is $\frac{1}{6}$. The probability of a particular outcome is a number that measures the likelihood of the outcome's occurrence. A number close to 0 suggests little chance of occurrence, while a number close to 1 indicates a great chance of occurrence. Thus, the probability of a particular outcome is a number between 0 and 1 that indicates the chance or likelihood of the occurrence of that outcome.

3.2.1 Probability Defined

One way to define and to conceptualize probability is by way of a long-run relative frequency notion. For example, if a fair coin is tossed n times and m of these result in the outcome "heads," then m/n is the relative frequency of occurrence of heads. If n is small, then m/n may not be very close to the true probability of $\frac{1}{2}$; however, in the long run, as n increases without limit, the relative frequency m/n would be expected to approach $\frac{1}{2}$. Figure 3.1 is a graph of the relative frequency of heads plotted against the number of tosses that were observed for this random experiment. Note that the relative frequency approaches $\frac{1}{2}$ as n increases. We formulate the following definition.

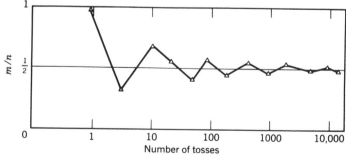

Figure 3.1. Relative frequency of occurrence of heads in n tosses of a fair coin.

Definition 3.2.1.1. If an experiment is performed n times and if m of these result in the outcome E, then the *probability of E occurring* is defined as the limiting ratio, m/n, as n increases without bound, that is, $\lim_{n \to \infty}(m/n)$.

We should note that Definition 3.2.1.1 indicates that the experiment should be conducted an infinite number of times in order to determine a probability. This is impossible; however, one can estimate a probability by choosing a large n. The important point is that Definition 3.2.1.1 provides a basis for a conceptualization of probability rather than directly providing an algorithm for computing probabilities.

Several points may be noted from this definition of probability. First, underlying this discussion is a *random experiment*: a trial to be performed where the outcome depends on chance. The flip of a coin or roll of a die are examples of such random experiments.

Definition 3.2.1.2. An experiment or process where the outcome depends on chance or probability is called a *random experiment*.

Second, there is the collection of all possible outcomes of a random experiment.

Definition 3.2.1.3. The collection of all possible sample outcomes is called the *sample space* and is denoted by the symbol Ω.

Third, there are the events.

Definition 3.2.1.4. An *event* is defined as a subset of the sample space; events are usually denoted by symbols like E, F, or A. We say an event *occurs* if the outcome of the random experiment is included in the event.

Thus, an event is a collection of outcomes. The following example illustrates the concepts of random experiment, event, and sample space.

Example 3.2.1.1. Consider a population of individuals in which 100 are males with schizophrenia, 150 are females with schizophrenia, 200 are male depressives, and 300 are female depressives. Suppose that one person is selected from this population *at random*, that is, each person in the population has an equal and independent chance of being selected. The random experiment or process we are considering is the random selection of a person from the population. The *sample space* Ω consists of all possible outcomes of this *random experiment*. Denoting the 100 male schizophrenics by $MS_1, MS_2, \ldots, MS_{100}$, the 150 female schizophrenics by FS_1, $FS_2, \ldots, FS_{150}$, the 200 male depressives by $MD_1, MD_2, \ldots, MD_{200}$, and the 300 female depressives by $FD_1, FD_2, \ldots, FD_{300}$, then the sample space consists of 750 (i.e., $100 + 150 + 200 + 300$) points or possible outcomes. Each of these outcomes by definition has probability $\frac{1}{750}$ of occurrence. One could consider various events or subsets of this sample space.

The simplest events are those defined as the individual sample outcomes. In this case, we could define 750 events, one corresponding to each possible outcome: $E_1 = \{MS_1$ is selected$\}$, $E_2 = \{MS_2$ is selected$\}$, ..., $E_{750} = \{FD_{300}$ is selected$\}$. It would probably be of greater interest to consider composite events like the following:

$$A_1 = \{\text{a male schizophrenic is selected}\},$$

$$A_2 = \{\text{a female schizophrenic is selected}\},$$

$$A_3 = \{\text{a male depressive is selected}\},$$

$$A_4 = \{\text{a female depressive is selected}\}.$$

Alternatively, it may be of interest to consider only the two events

$$B_1 = \{\text{a schizophrenic is selected}\},$$

$$B_2 = \{\text{a depressive is selected}\},$$

or the two events

$$C_1 = \{\text{a male is selected}\},$$

$$C_2 = \{\text{a female is selected}\}.$$

Clearly, there are many classes of events that can be considered even for this rather simple experiment. One special property of some classes of events is that the events are mutually exclusive—that is, these are events that cannot occur simultaneously.

Definition 3.2.1.5. Two events A and B are *mutually exclusive* if they have no sample outcomes in common; hence, they cannot occur simultaneously.

In Example 3.2.1.1, we see that A_j ($j = 1, 2, 3, 4$) are mutually exclusive events. On the other hand, A_1 and B_1 are not mutually exclusive events; in fact, A_1 is itself a subset of B_1 because if a male schizophrenic is selected, then it is clear that a schizophrenic is selected. Figure 3.2 is a graphical representation of two mutually exclusive events A and B. Note that there is no overlap between these two events.

From Definition 3.2.1.1 and Example 3.2.1.1, it may be noted that probabilities satisfy certain properties. We state two such properties here. First, for any event E the probability of its occurrence, denoted $Pr[E]$, is a number between 0 and 1.

PROPERTY 1.

$$0 \leq Pr[E] \leq 1, \tag{3.1}$$

for any event E.

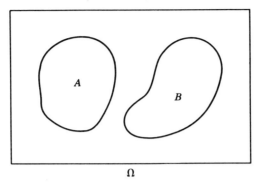

Ω

Figure 3.2. Example of two mutually exclusive events A and B.

The second property concerns the computation of the probability of the occurrence of the event E_1 or the event E_2 or both. If it is known that these events are mutually exclusive, then the joint event, $[E_1$ or $E_2]$, has probability equal to the sum of $\Pr[E_1]$ and $\Pr[E_2]$, and we therefore have

PROPERTY 2.

$$\Pr[E_1 \text{ or } E_2] = \Pr[E_1] + \Pr[E_2] \tag{3.2}$$

or in other notation, $\Pr[E_1 + E_2] = \Pr[E_1] + \Pr[E_2]$ if E_1 and E_2 are mutually exclusive events.

Example 3.2.1.2. Consider a large population of men who have been classified on the basis of smoking habits and chronic respiratory problems. In this population, it is known that 5% of the men have chronic respiratory problems and are nonsmokers, 15% have chronic respiratory problems and are smokers, 50% do not have chronic respiratory problems and are nonsmokers, and 30% do not have chronic respiratory problems and are smokers. Suppose we choose a man at random (i.e., each man has an equal chance of being selected) from this population. For convenience define the events A, B, C, and D as follows:

$A = \{$the man chosen has chronic respiratory problems and is a non-smoker$\}$

$B = \{$the man chosen has chronic respiratory problems and is a smoker$\}$

$C = \{$the man chosen does not have chronic respiratory problems and is a nonsmoker$\}$

$D = \{$the man chosen does not have chronic respiratory problems and is a smoker$\}$

Thus, $\Pr[A] = 0.05$, $\Pr[B] = 0.15$, $\Pr[C] = 0.5$, and $\Pr[D] = 0.3$. Notice that no two of these events can occur simultaneously when one man is chosen and therefore the events are mutually exclusive. For example, since A and B are mutually exclusive, we have $\Pr[A \text{ or } B] = \Pr[A] + \Pr[B] = 0.05 + 0.15 = 0.20$.

For most probability applications, we require computation of probabilities of various combined events. For this reason, it is useful to discuss certain types of events and the ways in which the events might be combined.

It is important to understand two operations that can be applied to sets. These are the union of events and the intersection of events.

Definition 3.2.1.6. The *union* of two events A and B is defined as the set of sample outcomes that belong to A or B or to both A and B.

Definition 3.2.1.7. The *intersection* of two events A and B is defined as the set of sample outcomes belonging to both A and B.

For notational convenience, the union of A and B is denoted by $A \cup B$, while the intersection of A and B is denoted by $A \cap B$ or by AB. The shaded area of Figure 3.3 depicts the union of two events A and B, while the shaded area of Figure 3.4 shows the intersection of A and B. For more than two sets, the union is defined as the set of sample outcomes in at least one of the sets, while the intersection is defined as the set of sample outcomes in all of the sets.

Note that the event $A \cup B$ occurs if either A or B occurs, while the event $A \cap B$ occurs if both A and B occur. Thus, $A \cup B$ is often referred to as "A or B," and AB is often referred to as "A and B."

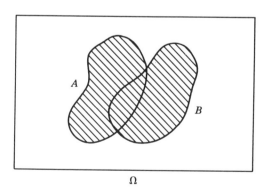

Figure 3.3. Union of two events A and B.

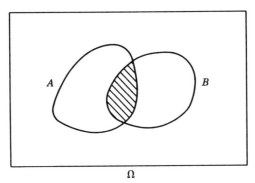

Ω

Figure 3.4. Intersection of two events A and B.

Example 3.2.1.3. In Example 3.2.1.1, the following set relationships exist: $A_1 \cup A_2 = B_1$, that is, the event that a male or a female schizophrenic is chosen is the event that a schizophrenic is chosen, and $A_1 B_1 = A_1$, that is, the event that both a male schizophrenic is chosen and a schizophrenic is chosen is the event that a male schizophrenic is chosen.

If two sets have no sample outcomes in common, then their intersection is the *empty set*, that is, the set with no outcomes in it. The empty set is denoted by the symbol $\varnothing$. Since $\varnothing$ never occurs, we have that $P(\varnothing) = 0$. As may be seen in Figure 3.2, the intersection of two mutually exclusive events is the empty set. Therefore, if A and B are mutually exclusive, then $P(A \cap B) = 0$ since $A \cap B = \varnothing$. In Example 3.2.1.1, since A_1 and A_2 are mutually exclusive events, $P(A_1 A_2) = 0$.

The final special event we describe is the complementary event.

Definition 3.2.1.8. For an event E, the *complement* of E, denoted by $\overline{E}$, is the event that E does not occur.

For example, in Example 3.2.1.1, the complement of B_1 is the event that a schizophrenic is not chosen, which we denote by $\overline{B}_1$.

This background greatly facilitates our use of probability. We have already noted that if E is any event in Ω, then $0 \le \Pr[E] \le 1$, where $\Pr[E]$ means the *probability that the event E occurs*. It is also evident that $\Pr[\Omega] = 1$, since every outcome is included in Ω, and that $P[\varnothing] = 0$ since no outcome is included in $\varnothing$. Furthermore, if $E_1, E_2, \ldots, E_n$ is a collection of mutually exclusive events, then from (3.2) it follows that $\Pr[E_1 + E_2 + \cdots + E_n] = \Pr[E_1] + \cdots + \Pr[E_n]$, since the events do not overlap.

Finally, it may be noted that $\Pr\{\overline{E}\} = 1 - \Pr\{E\}$, where $\overline{E}$ is the complement of E, indicating that E does not occur; that is, the probability that E does not occur is 1 minus its probability of occurrence.

3.2.2 Addition Rule

A useful rule for the computation of the probability of the union of two events is the *addition rule*. In Figure 3.3, the area shaded with lines represents the union of the events A and B. To compute the probability of this union, we may use the following rule.

PROPERTY 3 (ADDITION RULE).　For any two events A and B,

$$\Pr[A \cup B] = \Pr[A] + \Pr[B] - \Pr[AB]. \tag{3.3}$$

That is, the probability of the event A or B is the probability of A plus the probability of B less the probability of their intersection. Inspection of Figure 3.3 justifies the addition rule. In particular, the region common to both A and B has been counted in both $\Pr[A]$ and $\Pr[B]$; hence, it should be subtracted from their sum in order to yield $\Pr[A \cup B]$. Recall that if A and B are mutually exclusive, then $\Pr[AB] = 0$, and hence $\Pr[A \cup B] = P[A] + P[B]$.

Example 3.2.2.1.　In Example 3.2.1.1, let $C_1 = \{$a male is selected$\}$, $C_2 = \{$a female is selected$\}$, with A_1, A_2, A_3, A_4, B_1, and B_2 defined as before. We have $\Pr[C_1 \cup B_1] = \Pr[C_1] + \Pr[B_1] - \Pr[C_1 B_1]$ by the addition rule. Since $\Pr[C_1] = \frac{300}{750}$, $\Pr[B_1] = \frac{250}{750}$, $\Pr[C_1 B_1] = \frac{100}{750}$, then $\Pr[C_1 \cup B_1] = \frac{300}{750} + \frac{250}{750} - \frac{100}{750} = \frac{450}{750}$. This result can also be directly verified since the event $C_1 \cup B_1$ is the event that either a male or a schizophrenic is selected, and we see directly that 450 of the 750 possible sample outcomes satisfy this criterion. Applying the addition rule to the mutually exclusive events A_1 and A_4, we have that $\Pr[A_1 \cup A_4] = \Pr[A_1] + \Pr[A_4] - \Pr[A_1 A_4] = \Pr[A_1] + \Pr[A_4]$, since $\Pr[A_1 A_4] = 0$.

　　Combining (3.1) and (3.3), we note that for any two events A and B, $\Pr[A \cup B] \le \Pr[A] + \Pr[B]$. More generally, for any events $E_1, E_2, \ldots, E_n$, we have that $\Pr[E_1 \cup E_2 \cup \cdots \cup E_n] \le \sum_{i=1}^{n} \Pr[E_i]$. This result is termed *Boole's inequality* (See Feller, 1967), which will be referred to later.

PROPERTY 4 (BOOLE'S INEQUALITY).　For any events $E_1, \ldots, E_n$,

$$\Pr[E_1 \cup E_2 \cup \cdots \cup E_n] \le \sum_{i=1}^{n} \Pr[E_i].$$

3.2.3 Conditional Probability and Multiplication Rule

For some problems, it is meaningful to compute the probability of a particular event given the knowledge that another event has occurred. For

Table 3.1. Probabilities for Example 3.2.1.2

	Nonsmoker $\bar{S}$	Smoker S	
No Respiratory Problems $\bar{R}$	$0.50 = \Pr(\bar{S}\bar{R})$	$0.30 = \Pr(\bar{R}S)$	$0.80 = \Pr(\bar{R})$
Respiratory Problems R	$0.05 = \Pr(\bar{S}R)$	$0.15 = \Pr(SR)$	$0.20 = \Pr(R)$
	$0.55 = \Pr(\bar{S})$	$0.45 = \Pr(S)$	

instance, in Example 3.2.1.2, it may be useful to know the probability that a man with chronic respiratory problems is chosen given the knowledge that the man chosen is a smoker. For convenience, we describe the probabilities from Example 3.2.1.2 in Table 3.1.

In addition, we use the notation S for the event that a smoker is selected, $\bar{S}$ for the event that a nonsmoker is selected, R for the event that a person with respiratory problems is selected, and $\bar{R}$ for the event that a person with no respiratory problems is selected. The probability we seek is the probability that R occurs *given* S occurs, that is, the probability that a person with respiratory problems is selected given that a smoker is selected. This probability is termed a *conditional probability* and denoted by $\Pr[R|S]$, where | is read "given." The probability in question can be computed from the figures in the second column of Table 3.1. In particular, the probability of being a smoker is $0.30 + 0.15 = 0.45$. We note that $0.30/0.45$ of the smokers do not have respiratory problems while $0.15/0.45$ of the smokers do have respiratory problems. Hence, it follows that $\Pr[R|S] = 0.15/0.45 = 1/3$ and $\Pr[\bar{R}|S] = 0.30/0.45 = 2/3$. That is,

$$\Pr[R|S] = \frac{\Pr[RS]}{\Pr[S]} \quad \text{and} \quad \Pr[\bar{R}|S] = \frac{\Pr[\bar{R}S]}{\Pr[S]}.$$

Returning now to the general situation with any two events A and B, we define the conditional probability of A given B to be

$$\Pr[A|B] = \Pr[AB]/\Pr[B] \tag{3.4}$$

provided $\Pr[B] > 0$. From this follows the *multiplication rule* for computing probabilities. This is a handy device for computing the probabilities of joint events like AB.

PROPERTY 5 (MULTIPLICATION RULE). For any two events A and B, the following relationship holds:

$$Pr[AB] = Pr[A|B]Pr[B] = Pr[B|A]Pr[A]. \qquad (3.5)$$

In (3.4) and (3.5), $Pr[A|B]$ is the probability that the event A occurs *given* the knowledge that B occurs.

Example 3.2.3.1. Let A_1, B_1, C_1 be as defined in Example 3.2.1.1; hence, $Pr[A_1] = \frac{100}{750}$ and $Pr[B_1] = \frac{250}{750}$ and $Pr[C_1 B_1] = Pr[A_1] = \frac{100}{750}$ since $C_1 B_1 = A_1$. The *conditional probability* of C_1 given B_1 is the probability that the person selected is a male given that the person is schizophrenic. By (3.4),

$$Pr[C_1|B_1] = \frac{Pr[C_1 B_1]}{Pr[B_1]} = \frac{100/750}{250/750} = \frac{100}{250}.$$

Therefore, from the multiplication rule we have

$$Pr[C_1 B_1] = Pr[C_1|B_1]Pr[B_1] = \frac{100}{250}\frac{250}{750} = \frac{100}{750},$$

which agrees with what was obtained by direct vertification.

In some situations, it may be that $Pr[A|B] = Pr[A]$, that is, the probability of A given the event B is the same as the probability of the event A. This means that knowledge of the occurrence of event B contributes nothing to our knowledge regarding the likelihood of A's occurrence. In such a case, the events A and B are said to be independent events.

If A and B are independent, then $Pr[AB] = Pr[A|B]Pr[B] = Pr[A]Pr[B]$, since $Pr[A|B] = Pr[A]$. Thus, we have the following definition.

Definition 3.2.3.1. Two events A and B are *independent events* if $Pr[AB] = Pr[A]Pr[B]$.

Thus, if $Pr[AB] = Pr[A]Pr[B]$, we say that A and B are independent events, while if $Pr[AB] \neq Pr[A]Pr[B]$, we say that A and B are *dependent events*.

Example 3.2.3.2. If we consider the population given in Example 3.2.1.1, where B_1, B_2 and C_1, C_2 are defined events in the sample space, we note that $Pr[C_1|B_1] = \frac{100}{250}$, but

$$Pr[C_1] = \frac{100 + 200}{750} = \frac{300}{750} = \frac{100}{250}.$$

Hence, C_1 and B_1 are independent, and knowledge of B_1 does not alter the probability of C_1. We also note that

$$\Pr[C_1]\Pr[B_1] = \frac{300}{750}\frac{250}{750} = \frac{100}{750} = \Pr[C_1 B_1],$$

and thus by Definition 3.2.3.1, we have that C_1 and B_1 are independent.

The concept of independence can be extended to more than two events.

Definition 3.2.3.2. The events $A_1, A_2, \ldots, A_n$ are *mutually independent* events if $\Pr[A_1 A_2 \cdots A_n] = \Pr[A_1]\Pr[A_2] \cdots \Pr[A_n]$.

As a final comment, we should clarify the relationship between mutually exclusive events and independent events. Mutually exclusive events A and B satisfy the condition that $\Pr[AB] = 0$; therefore, two mutually exclusive events A and B are not independent unless either $\Pr(A) = 0$ or $\Pr(B) = 0$. Otherwise, they are clearly dependent as $\Pr[A]\Pr[B] > 0$ if both $\Pr[A] > 0$ and $\Pr[B] > 0$, and thus $\Pr(AB) \neq \Pr(A)\Pr(B)$ since $\Pr(AB) = 0$. Thus, mutually exclusive events are dependent events except in the trivial cases when $\Pr[A] = 0$ or $\Pr[B] = 0$.

3.3 BAYES'S THEOREM: A USEFUL RESULT FROM PROBABILITY THEORY

The confirmation of many chronic diseases is a complex and expensive task; accordingly, less complicated diagnostic tests are constantly sought. In addition, for large-scale epidemiologic studies, it is often necessary to propose screening tools that can be rapidly and economically applied to many people.

For instance, open-angle glaucoma is a condition generally confirmed only after extensive ophthalmologic examination including visual field assessment and angiography. Both of these procedures are costly and time-consuming.

This disease, however, is also often accompanied by elevated intraocular pressure; hence, one procedure commonly used to screen for glaucoma is to measure the intraocular pressure with the applanation tonometer. This is a comparatively easy test to perform in the clinic and in community surveys. Since glaucoma is most often accompanied by elevated eye pressure, it is common to classify each screened individual as having elevated or non-elevated pressure. Thus, it is reasonable for large population surveys to use the intraocular pressure as a screening device for glaucoma.

To evaluate the usefulness of the intraocular pressure test as a screening device, a number of questions must be answered:

1. Given an individual has the disease, what is the probability that he will produce a positive (i.e., elevated) screening test outcome?
2. Given an individual does not have the disease, what is the probability that he will produce a negative (i.e., nonelevated) screening test outcome?
3. Given an individual is positive on the screening test, what is the probability that he has the disease?
4. Given an individual is negative on the screening test, what is the probability that he does not have the disease?

The answer to the first question is most often derived by selecting a sample of people known to have the disease and subjecting each person to the test. The second question is answered by choosing a group of people known to be free of the disease and subjecting these people to the test. This is shown by the summary table of frequencies in Table 3.2.

The entries in the table are the numbers of persons: a is the number of positives among the diseased, c is the number of negatives among the diseased, b is the number of positives among the nondiseased, and d is the number of negatives among the nondiseased.

The ratio $a/(a + c)$ estimates the *sensitivity* of the test procedure: it is an estimate of the probability of a positive test result given that the disease exists. The ratio $d/(b + d)$ estimates the *specificity* of the test procedure: it estimates the probability of a negative test result given the disease does not exist. The test's sensitivity and specificity are the answers to questions 1 and 2, respectively. Clearly, we would like a screening tool to be highly sensitive and specific.

For convenience, let D be the event that a person has the disease, $\overline{D}$ be the event that a person does not have the disease, T be the event that the

Table 3.2. Typical Results from a Screening Test Evaluation: Entry is the Number of People

		Diagnosis	
		Diseased $\{D\}$	Not Diseased $\{\overline{D}\}$
Test Procedure	Positive $\{T\}$	a	b
	Negative $\{\overline{T}\}$	c	d
	Total	$a + c$	$b + d$

person is classified positive with the test procedure, and $\overline{T}$ be the event that the person has a negative test result.

Definition 3.3.1 (Sensitivity and Specificity). The *sensitivity* of a screening test is defined by $\Pr[T|D]$. The *specificity* of a screening test is defined by $\Pr[\overline{T}|\overline{D}]$.

Thus, the following formulas characterize the probability of positive and negative test results given the known diagnosis:

$$\text{Test sensitivity} = \Pr[T|D],$$
$$\text{Test specificity} = \Pr[\overline{T}|\overline{D}]. \tag{3.6}$$

As stated earlier, the probabilities (3.6) are usually estimated by choosing two independent samples, one of cases and another of controls, and subjecting them to the test procedure. The data for estimating (3.6) are in the form of Table 3.2. An example illustrates the situation and the computations.

Example 3.3.1. A psychiatric researcher wished to evaluate a diagnostic instrument for possible use as a screening tool for major psychotic illness. This test instrument contained 20 questions regarding individual psychiatric symptoms. A positive test result is one in which a score of 16 or greater is attained, that is, if a person reports having at least 16 of the 20 symptoms. A sample of 388 psychotic patients and an independent sample of 690 nonpsychotic patients were administered the test instrument with the following results:

		Diagnosis	
		Psychosis	Not Psychosis
	Positive	374	10
Test			
	Negative	14	680
	Total	388	690

From these results, the sensitivity of the test is estimated at $0.96 = 374/388$, while the specificity is estimated to be $0.99 = 680/690$. The test appears to be both fairly sensitive and specific, although a qualitative judgment regarding acceptability of a given sensitivity or specificity will depend on the intended application.

It is also frequently of interest to know the probability that a patient has the disease given a positive test result, that is, the answer to question 3. This probability is called the *predictive value of a positive test result* and is given by $\Pr[D|T]$.

Definition 3.3.2 (Predictive Value).   The *predictive value positive* is $\Pr[D|T]$, the probability that a person who has a positive test result has the disease. The *predictive value negative* is $\Pr[\bar{D}|\bar{T}]$, the probability that a person who has a negative test result does not have the disease.

These predictive values can be calculated using a result from probability called Bayes's theorem. This result can be developed in the context of the screening test problem.

To begin, we know from the multiplication rule for probability that

$$\Pr[DT] = \Pr[D|T]\Pr[T]. \tag{3.7}$$

Consequently, we have

$$\Pr[D|T] = \Pr[DT]/\Pr[T] \tag{3.8}$$

by dividing both sides of (3.7) by $\Pr[T]$. The event T occurs when a person is classified positive with the test procedure. Since this person either has or does not have the disease, then either D or $\bar{D}$ must also occur. Thus, if T occurs, then either TD (T and D) or $T\bar{D}$ (T and $\bar{D}$) occur, but not both. Therefore, the event T is equal to the union of DT and $\bar{D}T$, which are mutually exclusive events. Hence, the denominator of the right side of (3.8) is

$$\Pr[T] = \Pr[DT] + \Pr[\bar{D}T], \tag{3.9}$$

and by the multiplication rule applied to each term on the right side of (3.9), we obtain

$$\Pr[T] = \Pr[T|D]\Pr[D] + \Pr[T|\bar{D}]\Pr[\bar{D}]. \tag{3.10}$$

The numerator of the right side of (3.8) is, by the multiplication rule, given by

$$\Pr[DT] = \Pr[T|D]\Pr[D]. \tag{3.11}$$

The desired quantity, $\Pr[D|T]$, is, from (3.8), the ratio of (3.11) to (3.10). Thus, we have the following result.

PROPERTY 6 (BAYES'S THEOREM).   If D indicates an event such as disease and T indicates another event such as a positive test result, then

$$\Pr[D|T] = \frac{\Pr[T|D]\Pr[D]}{\Pr[T|D]\Pr[D] + \Pr[T|\bar{D}]\Pr[\bar{D}]}. \tag{3.12}$$

This equality is the algebraic statement of *Bayes's theorem.*

Again, the principal need for this result in the present context is that estimates of $\Pr[T|D]$ and $\Pr[T|\overline{D}]$ are typically available from studies; however, the predictive value of a positive test result is the term of most interest. An example illustrates the use of (3.12).

Example 3.3.2. In Example 3.3.1, we want to determine the probability that a person who is positive by the test has the disease, that is, determine the predictive value of a positive test. First we compute the probability of a positive test result given the disease and the probability of a positive test given no disease:

$$\Pr[T|D] = \frac{374}{388} = 0.964 \quad \text{and} \quad \Pr[T|\overline{D}] = \frac{10}{690} = 0.014.$$

Utilizing (3.12),

$$\Pr[D|T] = \frac{0.964\,\Pr[D]}{0.964\,\Pr[D] + 0.014\,\Pr[\overline{D}]} \quad \text{or}$$

$$\Pr[D|T] = \frac{0.964\,\Pr[D]}{0.964\,\Pr[D] + 0.014(1 - \Pr[D])} \tag{3.13}$$

as $\Pr[\overline{D}] = 1 - \Pr[D]$.

In general, the predictive value of a positive test result depends on the rate of disease in the population to which the screening test is to be applied.

At first glance, it may be surprising that $\Pr[D]$ remains in (3.13); however, the data of Example 3.3.1 provide no means of estimating the rate of psychotic illness in the general population. Note that the data was taken from two *predetermined* sample sizes of 388 and 690, respectively, and therefore, $388/(388 + 690)$ is *not* an estimate of $\Pr[D]$ in the general population. This point cannot be overemphasized.

Typically, we would evaluate (3.13) for certain assumed values of $\Pr[D]$. This approach is helpful in understanding the behavior of the quantity $\Pr[D|T]$. In Table 3.3, the expression (3.13) is evaluated for different hypothetical values of $\Pr[D]$.

Table 3.3. Values of (3.13) For Selected Disease Rates

$\Pr[D]$	0.00001	0.0001	0.001	0.01	0.1
$\Pr[D|T]^a$	0.0007	0.007	0.0645	0.4102	0.8844

[a] Defined by (3.13).

We see that the predictive value of a positive test result can be quite small if the overall disease rate is small. Clearly, the sensitivity and specificity of the test are not sufficient to evaluate the potential usefulness of a screening instrument in a population; the disease rate is also important.

Before concluding this section, note that we have not yet addressed question 4, the probability that an individual does not have the disease given the test is negative. This was termed the predictive value negative in Definition 3.3.2 and was denoted $Pr[\overline{D}|\overline{T}]$. Replacing D by $\overline{D}$ and T by $\overline{T}$ in (3.12), we have that

$$Pr[\overline{D}|\overline{T}] = \frac{Pr[\overline{T}|\overline{D}]Pr[\overline{D}]}{Pr[\overline{T}|\overline{D}]Pr[\overline{D}] + Pr[\overline{T}|D]Pr[D]}. \qquad (3.14)$$

Not only is Bayes's theorem a very important and commonly used tool for evaluating screening tests and diagnostic instruments but it is also useful in a number of other applications. We shall later find it useful in our discussion of the analysis of epidemiologic data.

3.4 PROBABILITY DISTRIBUTIONS AND RANDOM VARIABLES

Recall that a random experiment is one in which the outcome depends on chance; that is, the outcome may be different when the experiment is repeated under identical conditions. Also recall that the sample space corresponding to a random experiment is the collection of all possible sample outcomes. For example, the random experiment in Example 3.2.1.1 is the selection of a person at random from the set of 750 persons; consequently, the sample space consists of these 750 possible persons, or "outcomes."

In many situations, it is of interest to define a function that contains the information in the sample space in a more usable form. In this example, in which a single person is selected at random from the 750 persons, it is possible to consider a number of functions. Perhaps the investigators only wanted to know if the person selected was a schizophrenic. Therefore, one can define the function X where X takes the value 1 if the person selected is a schizophrenic and 0 if the person is not a schizophrenic. As X is a variable defined for this random experiment, the value of X is not completely predictable, and thus we say that X is a random variable.

Definition 3.4.1 (Random Variable). A *random variable* is a function defined on the sample space that associates each sample outcome with a number.

Each value of X has a probability of occurrence. These probabilities jointly form the *probability distribution* of X.

In our example, X can take two values: 0 or 1. The probability distribution of the random variable X is therefore given by

$$\Pr[X = 1] = \frac{250}{750}, \quad \Pr[X = 0] = \frac{500}{750}. \tag{3.15}$$

To avoid confusing a random variable with the values it may assume, a random variable will be notated by an uppercase letter, and values of the random variable will be notated by lowercase letters. For example, using this notation, the probability distribution of X is given by

$$\Pr[X = x] = \begin{cases} \dfrac{250}{750} & \text{if} \quad x = 1, \\ \dfrac{500}{750} & \text{if} \quad x = 0. \end{cases}$$

The random variable described in (3.15) is an example of a discrete random variable. In general, X is a *discrete random variable* if it can take a countable number of distinct values $x_1, x_2, \ldots$, with respective probabilities $p_1, p_2, \ldots$, where $p_i = \Pr[X = x_i]$, $i = 1, 2, \ldots$. The set of expressions $p_i = \Pr[X = x_i]$, $i = 1, 2, \ldots$, is the probability distribution of X. Clearly, $\sum_i p_i = 1$, that is, the sum of the probabilities is 1. The graph of the probability distribution of a discrete random variable X follows the form given in Figure 3.5. It consists of a series of spikes, one at each value of x_i.

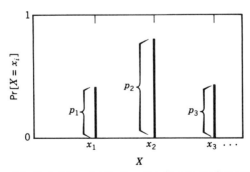

Figure 3.5. Probability distribution of a discrete random variable.

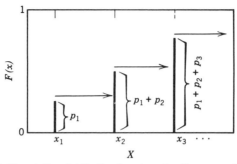

Figure 3.6. Cumulative distribution function of a discrete random variable.

The *cumulative distribution function* of X is $\Pr[X \le x]$, denoted $F(x)$, and is given by

$$F(x) = \Pr[X \le x] = \sum \Pr[X = x_i], \qquad (3.16)$$

where the sum is over all x_i such that $x_i \le x$.

The cumulative distribution function for a discrete random variable results in a graph similar to Figure 3.6.

For a random experiment, it is often possible and of value to define certain random variables that are of direct interest to the investigator. From the underlying probabilities for the original experiment, one may compute the corresponding probabilities induced by a random variable. This results in a probability distribution for the random variable and its cumulative distribution function.

The probability distribution and cumulative distribution function for a discrete random variable are illustrated in the following example.

Example 3.4.1. Thirty percent of the persons first hospitalized with a certain psychiatric disease have at least one subsequent inpatient admission. Suppose two patients are released from the hospital. We shall assume that the probability of one person's readmission is not influenced by the other person's outcome, that is, we assume independence between these two events. Determine the probability distribution and cumulative distribution function for X where X is the number among these two persons who are readmitted.

Clearly, X can take only three values: 0, 1, or 2. Let

$$A_1 = \text{event that patient 1 is readmitted,}$$

$$\overline{A}_1 = \text{event that patient 1 is not readmitted,}$$

$$A_2 = \text{event that patient 2 is readmitted,}$$

$$\overline{A}_2 = \text{event that patient 2 is not readmitted.}$$

Then $\Pr[A_1] = \Pr[A_2] = 0.3$ and $\Pr[\overline{A}_1] = \Pr[\overline{A}_2] = 0.7$. Accordingly, the probability distribution of X is

$$\Pr[X = 0] = \Pr[\overline{A}_1\overline{A}_2] = \Pr[\overline{A}_1]\Pr[\overline{A}_2] = (0.7)(0.7) = 0.49,$$

$$\Pr[X = 1] = \Pr[\overline{A}_1 A_2 \cup A_1\overline{A}_2] = \Pr[\overline{A}_1 A_2] + \Pr[A_1\overline{A}_2]$$

$$= (0.7)(0.3) + (0.3)(0.7) = 0.42,$$

$$\Pr[X = 2] = \Pr[A_1 A_2] = \Pr[A_1]\Pr[A_2] = (0.3)(0.3) = 0.09,$$

and its cumulative distribution function is

$$F(0) = \Pr[X \le 0] = \Pr[X = 0] = 0.49,$$

$$F(1) = \Pr[X \le 1] = \Pr[X = 0] + \Pr[X = 1] = 0.91,$$

$$F(2) = \Pr[X \le 2] = \Pr[X = 0] + \Pr[X = 1] + \Pr[X = 2] = 1.00.$$

The probability distribution and the cumulative distribution function of X are graphed in Figures 3.7 and 3.8, respectively.

In addition to the probability distribution of X, it is generally useful to determine summary numbers that describe the location of the distribution and its dispersion or variability. Two quantities are often of interest, the mean and the variance of the random variable, denoted μ and σ^2, respectively. The mean for a discrete random variable is a weighted average of the

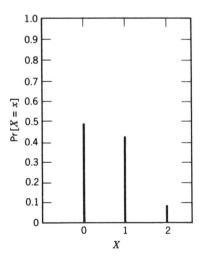

Figure 3.7. Probability distribution for X in Example 3.4.1.

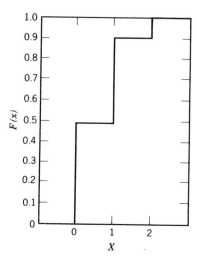

Figure 3.8. Cumulative distribution function for X in Example 3.4.1.

values of X. The weights are the p_i, which represent the probability of occurrence of the X_i.

Definition 3.4.2. The *mean* μ of a discrete random variable X that has probability distribution $\Pr[X = x_i] = p_i$, $i = 1, 2, \ldots$, is given by

$$\mu = \sum_i x_i \Pr[X = x_i] = \sum_i x_i p_i. \tag{3.17}$$

We observe that μ is simply a weighted average of the x_i where the weights are the probabilities p_i.

Definition 3.4.3. The *variance* σ^2 of a discrete random variable is defined by

$$\sigma^2 = \sum_i (x_i - \mu)^2 \Pr[X = x_i] = \sum_i (x_i - \mu)^2 p_i. \tag{3.18}$$

This is a weighted average of squared deviations from the mean. The standard deviation of the discrete random variable X is the positive square root of σ^2 and is denoted by the symbol σ. From (3.18), it is evident that σ^2 and σ are measures of dispersion of the random variable. Similarly, from (3.17), it is clear that μ is a measure of location of the random variable.

Example 3.4.2. The mean and the variance of the random variable defined in Example 3.4.1 are $\mu = 0(0.49) + 1(0.42) + 2(0.09) = 0.60$ and $\sigma^2 = (0 - 0.6)^2(0.49) + (1 - 0.6)^2(0.42) + (2 - 0.6)^2(0.09) = 0.1764 + 0.0672 + 0.1764 = 0.42$. Also, the standard deviation is $\sigma = \sqrt{0.42} = 0.65$.

For some problems, the random variable under study can take any value in a certain interval. In Chapter 2, we referred to such variables as continuous variables. Thus, a random variable that can take any value in a certain interval is called a *continuous random variable*. For example, the systolic blood pressure of a woman aged 30 can take any value within some interval, say, from 100 to 200 mm Hg. Body weight, height, serum cholesterol, and serum triglycerides are examples of other random variables that can assume any value within some interval and thus are continuous random variables.

For continuous random variables, the function that describes its probability of occurrence is a continuous curve. For the continuous random variable X, this function is denoted $f(x)$ and is called the *probability density function*, or *pdf*. The probability density function is not a set of discrete spikes like the probability distribution of a discrete random variable (see Figure 3.5). A typical graph of the probability density function of a continuous random variable X is shown in Figure 3.9. To be a proper *pdf* the area between the curve and the x axis must equal 1.

For continuous random variables, $\Pr[a \leq X \leq b]$ is equal to the area under the curve $f(x)$ from a to b. Consequently, using the curve in Figure 3.9 as an example, the shaded area in Figure 3.10 represents the probability

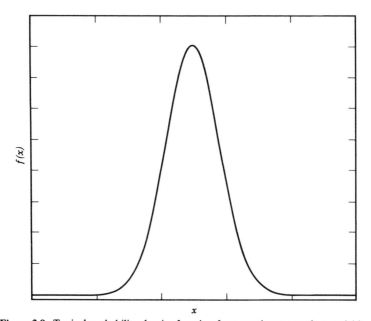

Figure 3.9. Typical probability density function for a continuous random variable.

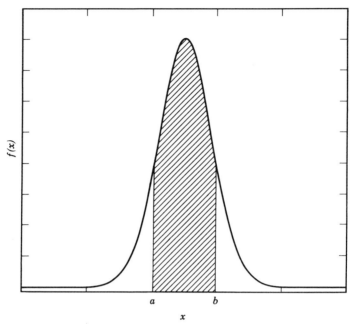

Figure 3.10. Representation of area under the curve as $\Pr[a \leq x \leq b]$. The shaded area is $\Pr[a \leq X \leq b]$.

that X is between a and b. Except for some simple special cases, the computation of $\Pr[a \leq X \leq b]$ would require integral calculus in order to determine areas like that shown in Figure 3.10.

Fortunately, most practical statistical problems require knowledge of only four basic continuous distributions, and in practice, the desired probability can be determined from extensive tables of the distributions. The most commonly used continuous distributions are the *normal, chi-square, t,* and *F* distributions, which are tabulated in the Appendix. These specific distributions will be introduced and discussed in Chapter 4.

A continuous random variable also has a cumulative distribution function $F(x) = \Pr[X \leq x]$; this probability is the area under the curve $f(X)$ to the left of x. The tables in the Appendix can be used to compute these types of probabilities. A typical cumulative distribution function for a continuous random variable is plotted in Figure 3.11 and may be contrasted to that in Figure 3.6.

The mean and variance of a continuous random variable are denoted by μ and σ^2—the weighted averages of x and $(x - \mu)^2$—with the weights now being $f(x)$. Formally, the two quantities are defined in Definition 3.4.4.

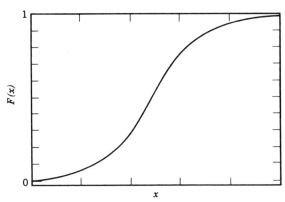

Figure 3.11. Cumulative distribution function of a continuous random variable.

Definition 3.4.4. The *mean* and *variance* of a continuous random variable X, with probability density function $f(X)$, are $\mu = \int xf(x)\,dx$ and $\sigma^2 = \int (x - \mu)^2 f(x)\,dx$, respectively.

In Definition 3.4.4 the symbol $\int$ is the integral or calculus "sum" operator. These two quantities are measures of location and dispersion, respectively. We shall not need to evaluate μ and σ^2 from the definition directly in our applications, but we will need to utilize properties for certain distributions that will be discussed in subsequent chapters.

3.5 SUMMARY

In this chapter, probability is introduced as a tool for inference. Many of the statistical tools used in the analysis of data rely heavily on these basic concepts. A number of new terms have been introduced: the probability of an event, probability distribution, random variable, and conditional probability, among others. Further understanding can be obtained by constructing various examples in the reader's own area of study in which these concepts arise.

In addition, the more mathematically inclined reader is encouraged to refer to a more in-depth treatment of these topics in such texts as Hogg and Craig (1965), Feller (1967), or Freund (1962).

PROBLEMS

3.1. If 0 represents a nonresponse or incomplete response to a mailed health questionnaire and 1 represents a total response, represent the

sample space corresponding to possible outcomes to four questionnaires.

3.2. A certain manufacturing company produces medical supplies. A
worker tests syringes as they are produced and continues testing
until he finds one defective. Describe the sample space of possible
outcomes for the testing process.

3.3. Let $\Omega = \{1, 2, 3, 4, 5\}$, $A = \{1, 2, 3\}$, $B = \{3, 4\}$, and $C = \{2, 3, 4, 5\}$.
Describe the following events:

(a) AB (b) $A \cup C$ (c) $\overline{A} \cup \overline{C}$

(d) $(\overline{A} \cup C)\overline{B}$ (e) $A\overline{C}$

3.4. A special medical center has records of 500 patients. It is known
from the records that

300 patients suffer from rheumatoid arthritis (R),

200 patients have asthma (A),

50 patients have cirrhosis (C),

20 have R and C,

30 have A and C,

20 have R and A,

10 have R, A, and C.

How many patients

(a) have exactly two of these three diseases?

(b) have at least one of the three diseases?

(c) have A if they have R?

(d) have R or A?

3.6. Let $P(A) = 0.5$, $P(B) = 0.8$, and $P(AB) = 0.4$

(a) Are A and B mutually exclusive events? Why?

(b) Are A and B independent events? Why?

(c) Compute $P(A \cup B)$.

(d) Compute $P(A|B)$ and $P(B|A)$ if $P(AB) = 0.2$.

3.6. In a group of 20 physicians, 8 are males and 9 are general practitioners. Of the 8 males, 3 are general practitioners. If a random
selection of 1 physician is made, what is the probability of selecting
a female physician who is not a general practitioner?

3.7. A family has four children, and assume that male and female
children are equally probable and successive births are independent.

Let M stand for male and F for female.

(a) List all elements in the sample space.

(b) Let A be the event that both sexes appear. Find $P(A)$.

(c) Let B be the event that there is at most one girl. Find $P(B)$.

(d) Are the events A and B independent?

3.8. Medical records in a hospital show that 15% of the patients with some disease will die within two years. If four cases are admitted recently at the hospital, find the probability that:

(a) none will die from the disease within this time period;

(b) exactly one will die during the time period.

3.9. The following table shows results of the evaluation of screening tests for some disease. Three-hundred forty patients with this disease and an independent sample of 800 normal subjects were chosen for the evaluation.

| | True Diagnosis | |
| | With Disease | Without Disease |
Screening Test		
Positive	256	48
Negative	84	752
Total	340	800

(a) Determine the sensitivity of the test.

(b) Determine the specificity of the test.

(c) If Pr[Disease] = 0.003, what is the predictive value positive of the test?·

(d) Is 340/1140 a good estimate of Pr[Disease]? Explain your answer.

3.10. The following information pertains to a national symposium held in a medical school with 1100 physicians in attendance.

NUMBER OF PHYSICIANS BY REGION

Physician	North	South	East	Midwest
Family practice	155	50	135	110
Obstetrics	90	65	40	90
Gynecologists	50	50	30	85
Pathologists	35	35	15	65

If a name is selected randomly for an interview, what is the probability that:

(a) it is a southern gynecologist physician?

(b) it is a midwestern physician?

(c) it is a pathologist?

(d) it is an eastern physician if he is known to be a family practice physician?

(e) Are region and type of physician independent?

3.11. A diagnostic test for a particular disease has a sensitivity of 0.96 and a specificity of 0.84. A single test is applied to each subject in a population in which the proportion of persons with the disease is 0.003. Compute the probability that a person positive to this test has the disease.

3.12. In a large population, 35% of the subjects are under 21 years of age, 45% are between 21 and 65 years of age, and the remainder are older than 65 years of age. Suppose that the probability of contracting a certain disease is $\frac{2}{100}$ for those under 21, $\frac{1}{20}$ for those between 21 and 65, and $\frac{1}{7}$ for those older than 65 years of age. If a person is chosen at random from this population:

(a) Compute the probability that the person is 21 years of age or older.

(b) Compute the probability that the person is under 21 years of age and has the disease.

(c) Compute the probability that the person has the disease.

(d) Are the events "age under 21" and "disease" independent or dependent events? Verify your answer numerically.

(e) Are the events "age under 21" and "age over 65" mutually exclusive? Why?

3.13. If a family has two children, let X be the random variable that indicates the number of girls. The probability distribution of X is $\Pr[X = 0] = p_0 = \frac{1}{4}$, $\Pr[X = 1] = p_1 = \frac{1}{2}$, and $\Pr[X = 2] = p_2 = \frac{1}{4}$. Compute (a) the mean of X, (b) the variance of X, and (c) the distribution function of X.

3.14. Let X be the number of trials it takes to properly prepare equipment for a specific laboratory test, and the probability distribution for X is $\Pr[X = x] = (6 - x)/15$, $x = 1, 2, \ldots, 5$.

(a) Show that this is a probability function, that is, show that $\sum_x \Pr[X = x] = 1$ and $\Pr[X = x] \geq 0$ for all x.

(b) What is the probability that it will take exactly three trials to prepare the equipment?

(c) What is the probability that it will take at least two trials but not more than four trials?

(d) Find the cumulative distribution function of X.

(e) What is the probability that it will take at most three trials?

(f) What is the probability that it will take more than two trials?

3.15. Which of the following are valid probability functions?

(a) $\Pr[X = x] = x/2$, for $x = -1, 0, 1, 2$.

(b) $\Pr[X = x] = (6 - 2x)/14$, for $x = 0, 1, 2, 3$.

(c) $\Pr[X = x] = (x^2 - x + 1)/46$, for $x = 0, 1, \ldots, 5$.

REFERENCES

Feller, W. T. (1967). *An Introduction to Probability Theory and its Application*, Vol. I, Wiley, New York.

Freund, J. E. (1962). *Mathematical Statistics*, Prentice-Hall, Englewood Cliffs, NJ.

Hogg, R. V., and A. T. Craig. (1965) *Introduction to Mathematical Statistics*, Macmillan, New York.

Woolson, R. F., M. T. Tsuang, and J. A. Fleming. (1980). Utility of the proportional-hazards model for survival analysis of psychiatric data, *J. Chron. Dis.*, **33**, 183–195.

CHAPTER 4

Further Aspects of Probability for Statistical Inference: Sampling, Probability Distributions, and Sampling Distributions

4.1 INTRODUCTION

In Chapter 3, basic probability and the notions of probability distributions, means, and variances of a random variable were introduced. This chapter is an elaboration of these concepts. In addition, selected probability distributions that are commonly used for statistical data analysis will be presented.

4.2 POPULATIONS, SAMPLES, AND RANDOM SAMPLES

Basic to the field of statistics are the concepts of population and sample. For many biomedical studies, the population we want to study consists of a large number of individuals. For example, the population of interest might be all cardiac patients over 60 years of age or the entire population of the United States. Both of these examples correspond to the everyday view of a population. For some problems, a more conceptual view of a population is required. For instance, if serum ferritin is measured for an individual, then the population of reference might very well be the set of all possible values of serum ferritin that could be obtained for that individual under identical test conditions. This is a purely conceptual population; however, it is useful as a frame of reference and may serve as a probability model for serum ferritin measurements of the individual. Thus, our notion of a population is sufficiently broad to include a group of people or things as well as a group of hypothetical measurements, observations, or numerical values.

We formulate the following definition.

Definition 4.2.1. A *population* is a group of elements that share some common characteristics; most often the population is the reference group we wish to study.

An important part of most statistical analyses is the specification of the population. This requires a statement describing the characteristics that define the population. If a population is defined too broadly, it may include too many heterogeneous subpopulations, and therefore it may be difficult to study. On the other hand, too narrow a definition of a population may limit generalizing the results of the study. It is crucial to carefully define the reference group for a study.

It would be ideal to study each and every element of a population. To do this, however, is generally impractical or impossible for several reasons. The most obvious reason is the size of the population. Often the population is so large that the cost of observing every member would be prohibitive. For a hypothetical population like the serum ferritin measures, it is literally impossible to observe all conceivable values for an individual under identical test conditions. Thus, several factors often preclude the possibility of observing an entire population. Accordingly, the best we can usually do is to study a subset of the population, that is, a selected part of the population. The selection process whereby a subset is chosen is called sampling, and the subset selected is called the sample.

Definition 4.2.2. A *sample* is a subset of a population.

In Figure 4.1, the population is depicted by all of the figures, and the sample consists of the encircled figures. Naturally there are many different samples that could be chosen from this population. This leads us to discuss the methods for sample selection.

The population is the group we wish to study; yet we are usually forced to study it through a sample of that population. For this reason, we want to choose a method for sampling that will permit us to make statements about the population. Our ideal, of course, is to choose a sample that is representative of the entire population. One way to choose a sample of size n that provides a good opportunity for representativeness is to require that each sample of size n have the same opportunity of being chosen—this sampling method is called random sampling.

Definition 4.2.3. A *random sample* of size n from a population of size N is a sample chosen such that all possible samples of size n have the same chance of selection.

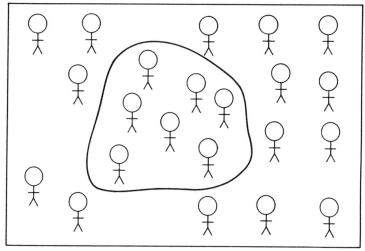

Figure 4.1. Description of a sample as subset of a population.

Random sampling can be done *with* or *without replacement* in the population. In sampling with replacement, a member is chosen, observed, and then replaced in the population for possible reselection in the sample. Sampling with replacement from a finite population is therefore equivalent to sampling from an infinite population since each member of the finite population can appear over and over again in the sample. In sampling without replacement, a member can be chosen for the sample only once. The following example illustrates this distinction.

Example 4.2.1. Consider an urn containing 10 marbles: 3 yellow and 7 black. Suppose a sample of size 2 is to be chosen from this urn. The probability that the first marble chosen is yellow is $\frac{3}{10}$, and if it is replaced, then the probability that the second marble chosen is yellow is also $\frac{3}{10}$. Thus, the probability of selecting two yellow marbles when sampling with replacement is $(\frac{3}{10})(\frac{3}{10})$, or $\frac{9}{100}$. Note that sampling this urn with replacement is equivalent to sampling from an infinite population because sampling with replacement permits us to view the population as an urn of infinitely many marbles, of which 30% are yellow and 70% are black.

In sampling without replacement, the probability of choosing a yellow marble on the first draw is still $\frac{3}{10}$, but now the probability of choosing a yellow marble on the second draw is $\frac{2}{9}$ if the first marble chosen was yellow, or is $\frac{3}{9}$ if the first marble chosen was black. Thus, the probability of selecting a yellow marble on the second draw is dependent on the outcome of the first selection. The probability of two yellow marbles being selected is $\frac{3}{10} \times \frac{2}{9} = \frac{6}{90}$ when sampling without replacement.

Having described the concept of random sampling, we now turn to the mechanics of choosing a random sample. The simplest way to construct a random sample is to use a randomization chart, of which an example is given in the table of random numbers (Table 1 in the Appendix).

This computer-generated table consists of a string of the digits 0–9. The first digit printed in the table was chosen from digits 0–9 in such a way that each of the 10 possible digits had an equal chance of selection, that is, the probability of selection was $\frac{1}{10}$. The second printed digit was chosen in a similar manner, and so on.

To use this chart, begin by first numbering each object in the population serially with 0 up to $N - 1$, where N is the total number of objects in the population. If the last object numbered has, for example, a four-digit number as its number, then the number of the first object should be written as 0000, the number of the second object as 0001, and so forth. To select a random sample, arbitrarily point to a spot in the table of random numbers, and then begin reading digits by proceeding in any direction, either left to right, right to left, or down or up the page. Having read a long string of such digits, then group them by fours to match the number of digits assigned to each object in the population. We then use this string of four-digit numbers to select the random sample in the following way.

Select the object that has the same number as the first four-digit number in the string, select the object that corresponds to the second four-digit number in the string, and so forth, until a sample of the desired size has been selected. If a four-digit number in the string does not correspond to an object (i.e., the number is greater than $N - 1$), then just ignore it and go on to the next number. If sampling without replacement is desired, then once an object has been selected for the sample, it cannot be selected again. Thus, the corresponding four-digit number should be ignored if it is encountered in the string after the object has once been selected. In this way a random sample is selected.

Example 4.2.2.   Consider selecting a random sample of size 10 from the 100 most recent schizophrenic inpatient admissions to a psychiatric unit.

As a first step, we number the 100 inpatient admissions serially from 00 to 99. Thus, for example, the first of the 100 admissions is labeled 00, the second is labeled 01, the one-hundreth is labeled 99. This step only requires a unique number for each patient. Next turn to the table of random numbers (Table 1 of the Appendix). Choose one of the four pages randomly, for example, by flipping a coin twice. If the outcome is a head followed by a head, then choose page 1; if the outcome is a head followed by a tail, then choose page 2; if tail followed by head, then choose page 3; if two tails, then choose page 4. Suppose page 3 of the four pages is chosen. Turn to page 3 of Table 1 in the Appendix; then, with eyes closed, point to any location in the table. Suppose we pointed to the digit 4 in row 15, column 65. We then read across the row to the right; at the end of the row, go up one row and read across to the left, and so on. This gives the following random string of digits:

$$4029544390830432609080201029344926082324 4\ldots$$

Since we required two digits to number our pool of patients, we arrange our chosen string of random numbers into pairs, obtaining 40, 29, 54, 43, 90, 83, 04, 32, 60, 90, 80, 20, 10, ... Our random sample of size 10 consists therefore of patients 40, 29, 54, 43, 90, 83, 04, 32, 60, 80. Notice that the second 90 is discarded since that patient was already chosen as the fifth person in the sample, and sampling without replacement is desired for this example.

It should be evident that random sampling gives all members of the population an equal opportunity to be included in the sample. Accordingly, statistical inference for random-sampling schemes can be quantified by applying probability theory. Thus, random sampling provides a basis for applying the statistical inference techniques in this text.

We will know how to draw an inference when data are gathered through random-sampling methods. However, sometimes it is impractical to obtain a true random sample. For example, a researcher who wants to test the effect of a drug on cancer patients may be restricted to administering the drug only to patients in a certain hospital. Clearly, this group of patients has not been randomly selected from the population of all cancer patients. Yet in order to generalize the results of the study, one may cautiously assume that this group of patients is representative of a population of patients and thus can be considered to be like a random sample. In general, random sampling is assumed for the inference techniques discussed in this and other chapters.

Finally, it should be noted that random sampling is a special case of probability sampling. For probability sampling, the probability of choosing a particular element from the population is known for each element in the population. In random sampling, these probabilities for all elements are equal. In general, as long as these probabilities are known, then statistical inference techniques can be applied, although the probabilities of inclusion in the sample must be incorporated into the analysis.

4.3 PARAMETERS AND STATISTICS

In Chapter 2, we presented quantities computed for samples, including the sample mean and the sample variance. Summary numbers computed from a sample are called *statistics*. For a population, there are also several summary numbers that are useful in describing the probability distribution of a random variable, such as the mean and variance of the random variable. Such summary population numbers are termed *parameters* in order to distinguish them from the sample statistics.

Example 4.3.1. A blood pressure study of women aged 30–35 years is conducted by selecting a random sample of 10 women and measuring their diastolic blood pressures (mm Hg) under similar conditions. The ten values are 88, 84, 85, 80, 82, 87, 84, 86, 83, and 81 mm Hg. The sample mean of these 10 figures is $\bar{x} = 84$. Since $\bar{X}$ is a summary number computed from the sample, it is a statistic. The sample variance s^2 is also a statistic.

The reference population for this problem is the set of diastolic blood pressures for women aged 30–35 years. If every such pressure were taken and recorded, a mean could be calculated that would be a summary number for the entire reference population and therefore a parameter. The sample mean $\bar{x} = 84$ might be viewed as an estimator of this unknown population parameter.

The example describes a common use of statistics, namely, the estimation of parameters. Since the population in this example cannot be studied in its entirety, the sample provides summary numbers for us, and these in turn are used to infer something about the corresponding population numbers.

In the previous chapter, we discussed random variables and certain quantities computed from them: the mean (μ) and variance (σ^2). For a given population, there is usually a random variable of interest to us. In Example 4.3.1, the random variable X is the diastolic blood pressure of women aged 30–35, and for this population of women, there is a probability distribution corresponding to X. It might look something like the probability density function in Figure 4.2. In Figure 4.2, μ is the population mean of X and is a population parameter.

Both μ and σ^2 are examples of population parameters. Their counterparts in the sample are the sample mean $\bar{x}$ and the sample variance s^2, which are examples of sample statistics.

In Sections 4.5 and 4.6, we shall present some population probability models commonly used as the basis for biostatistical analysis. Before discussing these topics, it is beneficial to develop some results that are

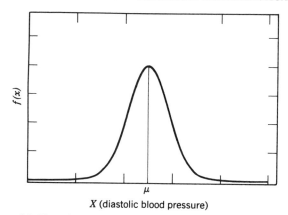

Figure 4.2. Hypothetical probability density function for Example 4.3.1.

useful for computing certain probabilities. To those familiar with the concepts of permutations and combinations, the next section may be omitted.

4.4 PERMUTATIONS AND COMBINATIONS: FACTORIAL NOTATION

The discussion of several distributions requires knowledge of permutations, combinations, and factorial notation. Suppose we have n objects, all distinguishable, and we would like to compute the number of different ways that we can arrange these in a row. If we think of n positions to be filled, then there are n ways to fill the first position, $n - 1$ to fill the second position (since one was already chosen to fill the first), $n - 2$ ways to fill the third, and one way to fill the last. That is, there are $n(n - 1)(n - 2) \cdots 1$ ways to arrange these objects.

Definition 4.4.1. The symbol $n!$ is read "n factorial" and denotes the product of all the integers from 1 up to and including n; that is, $n! = n(n - 1)(n - 2) \cdots 1$. We define $0! = 1$.

Definition 4.4.2. The number of ways to order n distinguishable objects is called the *number of permutations* of n *things taken n at a time* and is given by $n!$.

Example 4.4.1. Suppose four techniques are to be used in a study to evaluate visual acuity. Each study participant is to be tested with each of the four methods. In how many different orders can the techniques be administered to a patient? Each person can be tested with any of the four methods first, then any of the remaining three methods second, then any of the remaining two methods third, and the final one last. There are 4! = 4 × 3 × 2 × 1, or 24, permutations of these four techniques.

Now consider the case when there are r slots ($r < n$) and we can fill each slot with one of the n objects. Each different arrangement is called a permutation of n things taken r at a time. Reasoning as before, we see that the number of such permutations is given by $n(n - 1) \cdots (n - r + 1)$. For convenience, we may multiply and divide by $(n - r)!$ which leads to $n!/(n - r)!$.

Definition 4.4.3. The number of ways to order n distinguishable objects taken r at a time is called the *number of permutations of n things taken r at a time* and is given by $n!/(n - r)!$.

Example 4.4.2. Suppose only two of the four techniques in Example 4.4.1 will be used for each study participant. In how many ways can we order these four techniques taken two at a time? Using the preceding, it follows that there are $4!/2!$, or 12, ways to order these four techniques taken two at a time.

Frequently, applications arise in which it is important to know the number of ways that a subgroup of size r can be selected from n distinct objects without regard to order. For example, suppose a litter of four animals, A_1, A_2, A_3, and A_4, are available for an experiment and we wish to choose two from this litter. In how many ways can this be done? In Table 4.1, the 12 ($= 4!/2!$) permutations of these four animals taken two at a time are individually enumerated.

We note that permutations 1 and 2 result in the same outcome: animals A_1 and A_2 are chosen. The two permutations differ only in the order in which the animals were chosen. The same holds for permutations 3 and 4 together, 5 and 6 together, and so forth. Thus, if the order in which the animals are chosen is not considered, then the number of ways to choose two animals from among the four is 6, that is, one-half of the 12 permutations shown in Table 4.1.

More generally, the number of ways to choose r objects from n objects is given by the number of permutation of n things taken r at a time $[= n!/(n - r)!]$ divided by the number of ways that the r chosen objects can be ordered ($= r!$).

Definition 4.4.4. The number of ways of choosing r objects from n without regard to order is given by $n!/(n - r)!r!$ and is called the *number of combinations of n things taken r at a time.*

Table 4.1. Permutations of Four Animals Taken Two at a Time

Permutation	Animal Chosen First	Animal Chosen Second
1	A_1	A_2
2	A_2	A_1
3	A_1	A_3
4	A_3	A_1
5	A_1	A_4
6	A_4	A_1
7	A_2	A_3
8	A_3	A_2
9	A_2	A_4
10	A_4	A_2
11	A_3	A_4
12	A_4	A_3

The number of combinations of n things taken r at a time is sometimes denoted $\binom{n}{r}$, that is,

$$\binom{n}{r} = \frac{n!}{(n-r)!r!}.$$

Finally, this expression is also useful in a slightly different context. In particular, suppose we wish to consider the number of distinguishable permutations of n objects in the situation where r of the objects are indistinguishable from one another and the other $n - r$ objects are distinguishable from the r objects but not from one another. For example, suppose a person is going to plant 10 rose bushes in a row, and 3 bushes are white and 7 bushes are red. Furthermore, the person wants to know how many distinguishable permutations are possible. In this case, $n = 10$ and $r = 3$. Then each permutation will correspond to a combination of the numbers 1–10 taken three at a time. That is, a permutation is defined by where the white bushes are planted: $(1, 4, 5)$ means that white bushes are planted in the first, fourth, and fifth spots, and so forth. Thus, the number of distinguishable permutations is $\binom{10}{3}$, or, more generally, $\binom{n}{r}$.

Definition 4.4.5. The number of distinguishable permutations of n objects in the situation where r are indistinguishable from one another and $n - r$ are distinguishable from the r but not from one another is

$$\binom{n}{r} = \frac{n!}{(n-r)!r!}.$$

Example 4.4.3. Consider five tosses of a coin in which two are heads and three are tails. From Definition 4.4.5 there are $\binom{5}{2} = 5!/3!2!$ ways (i.e., 10 ways) in which this could happen. These are:

heads on toss 1 and toss 2,
heads on toss 1 and toss 3,
heads on toss 1 and toss 4,
heads on toss 1 and toss 5,
heads on toss 2 and toss 3,
heads on toss 2 and toss 4,
heads on toss 2 and toss 5,
heads on toss 3 and toss 4,
heads on toss 3 and toss 5, or
heads on toss 4 and toss 5.

Thus, there are 10 distinguishable permutations of 2 heads and 3 tails.

4.5 SOME DISCRETE PROBABILITY DISTRIBUTIONS

At this point, we continue the topic of discrete random variables first introduced in Chapter 3. The focus in this section is to discuss selected discrete probability distributions. For the most part, we deal in this section with the number of events of a certain type, for example, cures or cases. Emphasis is on those distributions used later in the text. For a fuller account of discrete distributions, refer to Johnson and Kotz (1969).

4.5.1 Binomial Distribution

The binomial distribution is one of the most widely used distributions in statistics. An easy way to explain this distribution is with a coin-tossing example.

Consider the experiment where a coin will be tossed $n = 3$ times. Define the random variable X to be the number of heads that appear during the experiment. Suppose $p = 0.4$ is the probability of observing a head on any one toss; since it is the same coin being tossed each time, clearly p will be the same for each toss. Each toss of the coin will be called a *trial*.

The event of a head on the first toss will be denoted H_1, the event of a head on the second toss will be denoted H_2, and the event of a head on the third toss will be denoted H_3. Now if $X = 2$, that is, if two heads appear during the three trials, then either $H_1 H_2 \overline{H}_3$ or $H_1 \overline{H}_2 H_3$ or $\overline{H}_1 H_2 H_3$ will occur; that is, either the two heads appear on trials 1 and 2, or on trials 1 and 3, or on trials 2 and 3. Thus, $\Pr(X = 2) = \Pr(H_1 H_2 \overline{H}_3 \cup H_1 \overline{H}_2 H_3 \cup \overline{H}_1 H_2 H_3) = \Pr(H_1 H_2 \overline{H}_3) + \Pr(H_1 \overline{H}_2 H_3) + \Pr(\overline{H}_1 H_2 H_3)$, since these three events are mutually exclusive.

Clearly, knowledge of the outcome of one trial does not contribute to knowledge of the likelihood of the outcome of another trial; hence, events associated with different trials are mutually independent, and the trials are said to be *independent trials*. For example, H_1, H_2, and H_3 are mutually independent events since each event corresponds to a different trial. Thus, $\Pr(H_1 H_2 \overline{H}_3) = \Pr(H_1)\Pr(H_2)\Pr(\overline{H}_3) = (0.4)(0.4)(0.6) = (0.4)^2(0.6)$. Similarly, $\Pr(H_1 \overline{H}_2 H_3) = \Pr(H_1)\Pr(\overline{H}_2)\Pr(H_3) = (0.4)(0.6)(0.4) = (0.4)^2(0.6)$, and $\Pr(\overline{H}_1 H_2 H_3) = (0.6)(0.4)(0.4) = (0.4)^2(0.6)$. Thus, $\Pr(X = 2) = 3(0.4)^2(0.6)$. Note that $\Pr(X = 2)$ is equal to the number of distinguishable permutations of two heads in three trials, $\binom{3}{2} = 3$, times the probability of each distinguishable permutation of two heads in three trials, $(0.4)^2(0.6)$. We can write $\Pr(X = 2) = \binom{3}{2}(0.4)^2(0.6) = \binom{n}{2}p^2(1 - p)^{n-2}$, where $n = 3$ is the number of trials. A similar argument shows that $\Pr(X = x) = \binom{n}{x}p^x(1 - p)^{n-x}$ for $x = 0, 1, \ldots, n$, since $\binom{n}{x}$ is the number of distinguishable permutations of x heads in n trials and $p^x(1 - p)^{n-x}$ is the probability of each distinguishable permutation of x heads in n trials. In this example, X is a binomial random variable.

In general, the binomial random variable originates when the following conditions prevail:

(i) there are n independent trials;

(ii) the outcome of each trial must result in only one of two mutually exclusive events, which will be referred to as "success" and "failure" (e.g., head or tail, diseased or nondiseased);

(iii) the probability of success is constant from trial to trial and is given by p $(0 < p < 1)$.

The binomial random variable X is the number of successes in these n independent trials, and its probability distribution is given by

$$\Pr(X = x) = \binom{n}{x}p^x(1 - p)^{n-x} \quad \text{for } x = 0, 1, \ldots, n, \qquad (4.1)$$

where n is the sample size. This distribution depends on two parameters, n and p. Recall that $\binom{n}{x} = n!/x!(n - x)!$, where $\binom{n}{x}$ is the number of combinations of n things taken x at a time. In Figure 4.3, several binomial random variables are plotted for selected values of p.

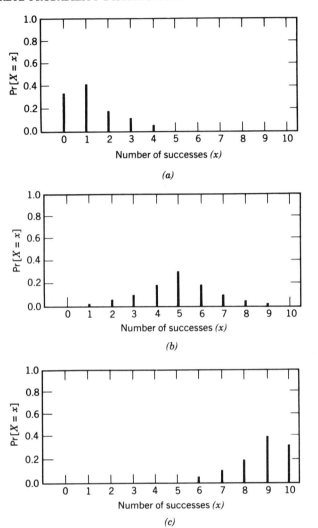

Figure 4.3. Probability distribution for three binomial random variables: (a) $p = 0.1$, $n = 10$; (b) $p = 0.5$, $n = 10$; (c) $p = 0.9$, $n = 10$.

The cumulative distribution function of X is given by

$$\Pr[X \le x] = \sum_{i:\, i \le x} \binom{n}{i} p^i (1-p)^{n-i} \quad \text{for all nonnegative } x, \quad (4.2)$$

where the summation is over all integers i such that i is less than or equal to x. The expression $\Pr[X \le x]$ has been tabulated in Table 2 of the Appendix for selected values of n and p.

The mean and the variance of the binomial random variable may be computed from expression (4.1) with the following results:

$$\mu = np \tag{4.3}$$

and

$$\sigma^2 = np(1 - p), \tag{4.4}$$

respectively.

Since the probability of success on one trial is p, it is not surprising that the mean number of successes in n trials is $\mu = np$, the number of trials times the probability of success for each trial.

The binomial random variable is useful in the study of disease rates. For example, a very large population of people may be known to contain a proportion p who are afflicted with a certain disease. Suppose we select n persons at random from this population and define X to be the number of persons in our sample of size n who have the disease. We can consider the process of selecting the sample to be composed of n independent trials, where one person is selected on a trial. Clearly, the probability that on any given trial the person selected will have the disease is equal to p if we sample with replacement and is also equal to p when sampling without replacement if this population is so large that p is not altered by the selection of a finite sample. Thus, X is a binomial random variable, and the probability distribution for the random variable X—the number of persons with the disease in this sample—is given by expression (4.1) since X has a binomial distribution.

Example 4.5.1.1. Suppose the probability that a child selected at random is left-handed is 0.20. For a random sample of five children, what is the probability that two are left-handed? If we let X be the number of left-handed children in our sample, then X will have a binomial distribution with $n = 5$, $p = 0.2$. Then from (4.1) we have that

$$\Pr[X = 2] = \binom{5}{2}(0.2)^2(0.8)^3 = \frac{5!}{2!3!}(0.04)(0.512)$$

$$= 10(0.04)(0.512) = 0.2048.$$

What is the probability that two or less are left-handed? This probability is

$$\Pr[X \le 2] = \Pr[X = 0] + \Pr[X = 1] + \Pr[X = 2]$$

$$= \frac{5!}{0!5!}(0.2)^0(0.8)^5 + \frac{5!}{1!4!}(0.2)^1(0.8)^4 + \frac{5!}{2!3!}(0.2)^2(0.8)^3$$

$$= (0.8)^5 + 5(0.2)(0.8)^4 + 10(0.2)^2(0.8)^3$$

$$= 0.94208;$$

that is, in a random sample of five children, there is a 0.94208 chance that two or fewer of the five will be left-handed.

This figure could also be obtained directly from Table 2 of the Appendix. In addition, $\Pr[X = 2]$ could be obtained from Table 2 by observing that

$$\Pr[X = 2] = \Pr[X \le 2] - \Pr[X \le 1]$$

$$= 0.94208 - 0.73728$$

$$= 0.2048,$$

as we obtained before. For large n, the use of the table or more extensive tables is recommended.

Finally, for this example, the mean number of left-handed children is $np = 5(0.2) = 1$ while the variance is $np(1 - p) = 5(0.2)(0.8) = 0.8$.

The binomial distribution is used in situations where each individual in a population can be classified by the presence or absence of a certain attribute. That is, a fraction p $(0 < p < 1)$ of that population possesses some characteristic and the remaining fraction $(1 - p)$ does not have the characteristic. This population is shown in Figure 4.4. For example, in studies of a chronic disease such as lung cancer, each person in a defined population can be classified as having or not having lung cancer. Other examples include populations classified on the basis of sex (male or female), age (< 45 or ≥ 45), marital status (married or not married), and so on. Simpler examples arise in games of chance such as coin tossing, in which the outcome of each toss is either heads or tails.

The binomial probability model can be used when a random sample is selected by replacement from a population of any size, like the one shown in Figure 4.4, or when a random sample is selected without replacement from an infinite population. In particular, if we define X as the number of

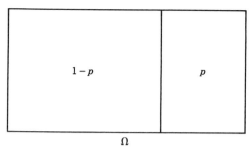

Figure 4.4. Population dichotomized with proportion (p) having a characteristic.

individuals in our sample with the characteristic, then X will have a binomial distribution provided conditions i–iii hold.

4.5.2 Poisson Distribution

Another probability distribution of interest is the Poisson distribution.

Definition 4.5.2.1. The random variable X has a *Poisson distribution* if

$$\Pr[X = x] = \frac{e^{-\lambda}\lambda^x}{x!}, \qquad x = 0, 1, 2, \ldots . \tag{4.5}$$

The mean and the variance of the Poisson random variable are given by $\mu = \lambda$ and $\sigma^2 = \lambda$, respectively. It is assumed that $\lambda > 0$.

Note that the mean and the variance of the Poisson random variable are equal. The cumulative distribution function of (4.5) is

$$\Pr[X \le x] = \sum_{i:\, i \le x} \frac{e^{-\lambda}\lambda^i}{i!} \quad \text{for all nonnegative } x, \tag{4.6}$$

where the summation index i is over all integers i such that i is less than or equal to x.

The quantity e in equations (4.5) and (4.6) is $2.718\ldots$, the base of the natural, or *Naperian*, logarithm. Tables for the cumulative distribution function of the Poisson random variable are given in Table 3 of the Appendix. If in the binomial situation n is very large while p is very small, then the distribution for the number of cases is approximated by a Poisson distribution with $\lambda = np$. This fact simplifies calculations.

The Poisson distribution may be viewed as an approximation to the binomial as described above; however, it also arises more directly. Suppose there is an interval of time, say a year, and during this time the number of occurrences of a certain event is to be observed. Suppose also that the following assumptions hold:

(i) The probability of one event in a very small interval of time, for example, a minute of the year, is proportional to the size of the small interval, (i.e., Pr[one event in the interval $(t, t + h)$] $\doteq \alpha h$, where h is the interval size and α is the rate parameter);

(ii) the probability of two or more events in a very small interval is negligible; and

(iii) the occurrences in one interval are independent of those in any other interval;

then letting X be the number of events over the entire time period $(0, T)$, the distribution of X is given by

$$\Pr[X = x] = \frac{(\alpha T)^x e^{-\alpha T}}{x!}, \qquad x = 0, 1, 2, \ldots,$$

which is the Poisson distribution with $\lambda = \alpha T$. This distribution is quite appropriate for use when studying rare diseases.

Example 4.5.2.1.   Suppose there are typically five cases of bladder cancer per year among Iowa men 35–40 years of age. Let X be the number of cases observed during a year. Then the above three assumptions are reasonable, and thus X will have a Poisson distribution with $\lambda = 5(1) = 5$. For a given year, compute the probability of zero, one, and two cases. From (4.5), we compute

$$\Pr[X = 0] = \frac{e^{-5}(5)^0}{0!} = e^{-5} = 0.00674,$$

$$\Pr[X = 1] = \frac{e^{-5}(5)^1}{1!} = 5e^{-5} = 0.03369,$$

$$\Pr[X = 2] = \frac{e^{-5}(5)^2}{2!} = 12.5e^{-5} = 0.08422.$$

From Table 3 of the Appendix, the probability of two or fewer cases is 0.12465, the sum of the three computed probabilities.

The final example demonstrates how the expected number of cases must be computed to reflect the population size and time period in question.

Example 4.5.2.2. Suppose that the annual incidence rate of leukemia in the state of Iowa is 11.2 cases/100,000 population. If 100,000 people are followed for one year, what is the probability of no new cases of leukemia? If 1000 people are followed for one year what is the probability of no new cases?

In order to answer these two problems, we must first compute the rate of new cases in one year for each of these two hypothesized populations. For 100,000 people the rate of new cases is 11.2, and hence, for X defined as the number of new cases in a year among 100,000 people,

$$\Pr[X = 0] = \frac{(11.2)^0 e^{-11.2}}{0!} = 0.0000137.$$

On the other hand, for 1000 people, the rate of new cases is 0.112 [i.e., $(11.2/100,000)1000$]; hence, for X defined as the number of new cases in a year among 1000 people,

$$\Pr[X = 0] = \frac{(0.112)^0 e^{-0.112}}{0!} = 0.89.$$

Thus, the rate of new cases must be adjusted to account for the size of the population. In a similar manner, if the population were to be followed for two years rather than one year, the respective rates of new cases would be 22.4 and 0.224, which are double the rates for one year.

In general, the incidence rate is reported in new cases per population size per time period, and this rate is adjusted to account for the population size and time period relevant to the intended application.

4.5.3 Hypergeometric Distribution

The hypergeometric distribution is closely related to the binomial distribution. It differs primarily as a result of the assumed population. For the binomial situation, if sampling without replacement was done, then it was assumed that the population sampled was much larger than the sample. Consequently, the value of p did not vary from trial to trial.

On the other hand, suppose the population is not large, with N being the size of the population. Furthermore, assume that each of these items in the population either has or lacks a certain characteristic (e.g., disease). Let D be the number in the population who have the characteristic. If we choose a random sample of size n from the entire population ($n \leq N$) by sampling without replacement, then the random variable X, defined as the number of items in the sample that have the characteristic, is a *hypergeometric random variable*. The hypergeometric probability distribution is given by

$$\Pr[X = x] = \binom{D}{x}\binom{N-D}{n-x}\bigg/\binom{N}{n} \quad \text{for } x = 0, 1, \ldots, \text{minimum}(D, n).$$
(4.7)

This expression arises since we only need to compute the number of ways of choosing samples of size n from N and then divide this number into the number of these samples that satisfy the condition that x have the characteristic and $n - x$ do not. The number of ways to choose a sample of size n from among N is $\binom{N}{n}$ while the number of these that satisfy the condition that x of the n have the characteristic $\binom{D}{x}\binom{N-D}{n-x}$ and expression (4.7) follows.

Example 4.5.3.1. A sample of 5 is to be chosen from a group of 10 people, 4 men and 6 women. What is the probability that 2 women will be in the chosen sample? Using expression (4.7), we have $N = 10$, $D = 6$, and $n = 5$; therefore,

$$\Pr[X = 2] = \binom{6}{2}\binom{4}{3}\bigg/\binom{10}{5}$$

$$= \frac{6!4!5!5!}{2!4!3!1!10!} = 0.238$$

Notice that the binomial is not an appropriate model for this problem since the probability that a woman is selected is not constant from trial to trial but changes depending on the outcome of previous trials.

Finally, the mean and the variance of X are

$$\mu = n\frac{D}{N} \quad \text{and} \quad \sigma^2 = n\frac{D}{N}\frac{N-D}{N}\frac{N-n}{N-1}, \tag{4.8}$$

respectively.

4.5.4 Multinomial Distribution

There are many other discrete distributions that are useful in medical applications. The reader may refer to texts of Feller (1967) or Johnson and Kotz (1969) for a detailed list. The final discrete distribution considered here is an example of a multivariate distribution (i.e., one with multiple response categories). This distribution is the *multinomial distribution*; it is the natural generalization of the binomial distribution. In the situation where this distribution arises, there are k ($k \geq 2$) mutually exclusive and exhaustive categories. For example, a psychiatric diagnosis may be a psychotic disorder, a nonpsychotic disorder, or no disorder; each person falls into exactly one of these three ($k = 3$) categories. The k random variables are defined as

$$X_1 = \text{number of trials resulting in type 1 outcomes,}$$

$$X_2 = \text{number of trials resulting in type 2 outcomes,}$$

$$X_k = \text{number of trials resulting in type } k \text{ outcomes.}$$

The event $[X_1 = x_1, X_2 = x_2, \ldots, X_k = x_k]$ is the event that x_1 of outcomes are of type 1, x_2 are of type 2, $\ldots$, x_k are of type k.
The *multinomial distribution* is appropriate in the following situation:

(i) there are n independent trials;
(ii) each trial must result in one of k mutually exclusive outcomes called type 1, type 2, $\ldots$, type k; and
(iii) the probability of a type i outcome is p_i and is constant from trial to trial, and $\sum_{i=1}^{k} p_i = 1$.

The multinomial distribution is the distribution of the set of k random variables, $X_1, \ldots, X_k$, which are the number of type $1, 2, \ldots, k$ outcomes respectively in the n trials. Specifically, the distribution of $(X_1, \ldots, X_k)$ is given by

$$\Pr[X_1 = x_1, \ldots, X_k = x_k] = \frac{n!}{x_1! x_2! \cdots ! x_k!} p_1^{x_1} p_2^{x_2} \cdots p_k^{x_k}, \quad (4.9)$$

where $\sum_{i=1}^{k} p_i = 1$ and $x_1, \ldots, x_k$ are nonnegative integers satisfying $\sum_{i=1}^{k} x_i$

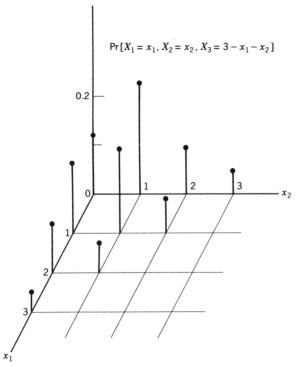

Figure 4.5. Multinomial distribution for $n = 3$, $p_1 = 0.2$, $p_2 = 0.3$: $\Pr[X_1 = x_1, X_2 = x_2] = [3!/x_1!x_2!(3 - x_1 - x_2)!](0.2)^{x_1}(0.3)^{x_2}(0.5)^{3-x_1-x_2}$.

$= n$. The mean of each X_i is given by

$$\mu_i = np_i \tag{4.10}$$

and its variance is given by

$$\sigma_i^2 = np_i(1 - p_i). \tag{4.11}$$

Figure 4.5 is a graph of a trinomial distribution in which $n = 3$, $p_1 = 0.2$, $p_2 = 0.3$, and therefore $p_3 = 0.5$. Note that it is only necessary to plot x_1 and x_2 since $x_3 = n - x_1 - x_2$; thus, given any two of the x_i, the third is determined.

Having described a group of widely applied discrete distributions, we now turn to an example of a continuous distribution.

4.6 NORMAL PROBABILITY DISTRIBUTION

The most widely known and used continuous distribution for data analysis is the *normal distribution*. It is the most important distribution in applied statistics. It is easier to describe this distribution with a picture of the probability density function than to describe it mathematically. The graph shown in Figure 4.6 illustrates a normal probability density function.

In general, the probability density function for any continuous random variable must satisfy two properties: (1) $f(x) \geq 0$ for all values of x and (2) the area between $f(x)$ and the x axis is 1. The normal pdf $f(x)$ not only satisfies these but also other properties: it is symmetric about the point $X = \mu$, that is, it is centered at μ; it approaches zero as x goes to $+\infty$ or $-\infty$; and it is a bell-shaped curve. The *normal probability density function* depends on two parameters, μ and σ^2, the mean and the variance. The mathematical expression for the normal pdf is

$$f(x) = \frac{1}{\sigma\sqrt{2\pi}} \exp\left(-\frac{(x-\mu)^2}{2\sigma^2}\right), \qquad -\infty < x < \infty, \qquad (4.12)$$

where exp is e raised to the power in parentheses, and μ and σ^2 are respectively the mean and the variance of X.

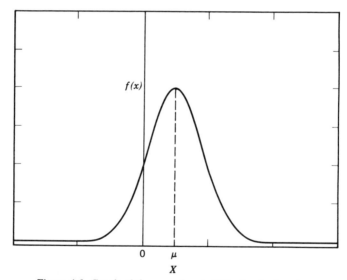

Figure 4.6. Graph of the normal probability density function.

The normal distribution was derived independently by Carl Friedrich Gauss and others; however, it is frequently called the *Gaussian distribution* in his honor. The historical study of this distribution stemmed from interest in studying probability models for random errors. It is easy to imagine a situation in which we desire to determine some true value μ using a measuring instrument for which positive and negative errors are equally likely and for which values closer to μ would occur more frequently than values farther from μ. If the measurement is taken infinitely many times, the relative frequency of occurrence of different values of X, the observed value, might look something like the curve in Figure 4.6. This model accounts for the random errors found in this measuring process and is a model in which the normal probability distribution is frequently used today.

The normal distribution is useful in other contexts. Some biological variables follow a normal probability distribution, while simple functions, such as the logarithm of other biological variables, follow a normal distribution. As an example, several large-scale epidemiologic studies suggest that the serum cholesterol measurements of large populations tend to follow a normal distribution, whereas the logarithm of the serum triglyceride levels tends to be normally distributed. Thus, there are situations in which a biological characteristic is normally distributed. This is not, however, the principal reason for the widespread use of the normal distribution.

The main reason for the widespread use of the normal distribution in the area of statistical inference is the *central limit theorem*. In particular, if a population has been sampled and if the sample size n is large, then the distribution of the sample mean $\overline{X}$ will approximate a normal distribution. This result is called the central limit theorem, and we will discuss this result further in the next section.

From (4.12) we note that the normal distribution is a two-parameter distribution, depending on both μ and σ^2. From (4.12) it is possible to compute the following probabilities for the normal curve:

$$\Pr[\mu - \sigma < X < \mu + \sigma] \doteq 0.68,$$

$$\Pr[\mu - 2\sigma < X < \mu + 2\sigma] \doteq 0.95, \qquad (4.13)$$

$$\Pr[\mu - 3\sigma < X < \mu + 3\sigma] \doteq 0.99.$$

The expressions in (4.13) state that approximately two-thirds of the observations are between plus and minus one standard deviation from the mean, approximately 95% are between plus and minus two standard deviation units from the mean, while nearly all of the observations (99%) lie

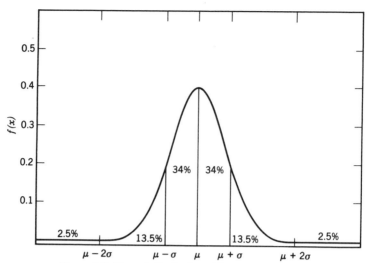

Figure 4.7. Normal distribution with approximate areas.

between $\mu - 3\sigma$ and $\mu + 3\sigma$. The first two of these probabilities in (4.13) are illustrated in Figure 4.7.

If σ decreases for a fixed μ, then we see in Figure 4.8 that the probability density function becomes more peaked at the point μ and has far less probability in the tails. This fact is also seen by a careful inspection of equations (4.13). Hence, σ is a *scale* or dispersion quantity for the normal distribution. The quantity μ is a *location* or shift parameter that moves the whole of the distribution in the direction of μ. Finally, the cumulative distribution function for a normal random variable with a mean of μ and a variance of σ^2 is illustrated by Figure 4.9. It is a sigmoid, or S-shaped, curve.

The notation $N(\mu, \sigma^2)$ is used to denote a random variable that has a normal distribution with mean μ and variance σ^2. That is, a random variable that is $N(\mu, \sigma^2)$ has the probability density function defined in (4.12). It would be impossible to generate probability tables for all values of μ and σ^2. Fortunately, any $N(\mu, \sigma^2)$ random variable X may be transformed to a $N(0, 1)$ random variable, that is, to a normal random variable with mean 0 and variance 1. We shall denote the $N(0, 1)$ variable by Z. The equation that transforms X to Z is given by

$$Z = \frac{X - \mu}{\sigma}. \tag{4.14}$$

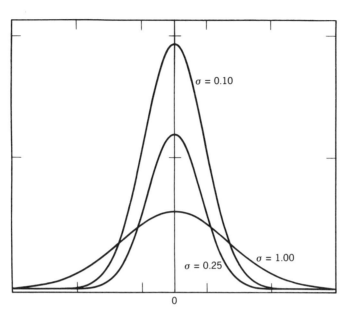

Figure 4.8. Frequency functions for normal distributions with $\mu = 0$ and $\sigma = 0.1$ and $\sigma = 0.25$ and $\sigma = 1.0$.

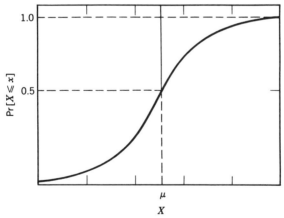

Figure 4.9. Cumulative probability distribution $P[X \leq x]$ for a normal distribution with mean μ and variance σ^2.

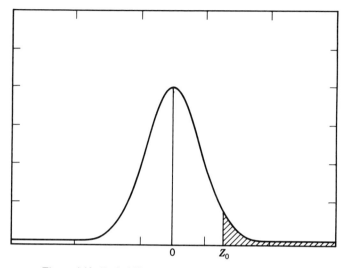

Figure 4.10. Probability listed in Table 4 of the Appendix.

This random variable Z is commonly termed the *standard normal*, or *unit normal*, *variable*. Probabilities that Z exceeds certain values are tabulated in Table 4 of the Appendix. Notice that the values in Table 4 correspond to the shaded area in Figure 4.10. In Table 4, Z_0 is read from the row and the column headings while the probability is found in the body of the table. Notice that the table only lists values for positive Z_0. By the symmetry of the standard normal curve,

$$\Pr[Z < -Z_0] = \Pr[Z > Z_0], \tag{4.15}$$

and therefore the areas corresponding to negative values of Z_0 can be determined.

The cumulative distribution function of Z is denoted by $\Phi(z)$, that is, $\Phi(z) = \Pr[Z < z]$. By the symmetry of the normal curve, we have $\Phi(-z) = 1 - \Phi(z)$, and this facilitates the use of Table 4 in the Appendix.

Example 4.6.1. Consider the standard normal random variable Z and determine the following probabilities: $\Pr[Z > 1]$, $\Pr[Z < -1]$, $\Pr[Z > -2]$, and $\Pr[-1 < Z < 2]$. From Table 4 of the Appendix we can read $\Pr[Z > 1] = 0.1587$ directly. On the other hand, by symmetry of the standard normal curve, we note that $\Pr[Z < -1] = 1 - \Pr[Z < 1]$; therefore, $\Pr[Z < -1] = \Pr[Z > 1]$ and $\Pr[Z < -1] = 0.1587$. In a similar manner, symmetry ensures that $\Pr[Z > -2] = 1 - \Pr[Z > 2]$, and thus $\Pr[Z > -2] =$

$1 - 0.0228 = 0.9772$. Finally,

$$\Pr[-1 < Z < 2] = \Pr[Z < 2] - \Pr[Z < -1]$$
$$= 1 - \Pr[Z > 2] - \Pr[Z > 1]$$
$$= 0.9772 - 0.1587$$
$$= 0.8185$$

The previous example illustrates the use of the table and the symmetry property for the standard normal variable. The following example illustrates the use of (4.14) for any normal variable.

Example 4.6.2. Suppose it is known that the mean blood glucose (mg/mL) in a group of diabetic rats treated with a drug is 1.8 mg/mL with $\sigma = 0.2$ mg/mL. Assuming that the blood glucose follows a normal distribution in this population, compute $\Pr[X > 2]$, $\Pr[X < 1.6]$, and $\Pr[1.65 < X < 1.95]$, where X is the blood glucose level. To solve these problems, we use (4.14) with $\mu = 1.8$ and $\sigma = 0.2$, that is, $Z = (X - 1.8)/0.2$ is a standard normal random variable. From this relationship it is clear that

$$\Pr[X > 2] = \Pr\left[\frac{X - 1.8}{0.2} > \frac{2 - 1.8}{0.2}\right] = \Pr[Z > 1],$$

which is 0.1587 from Table 4 of the Appendix. Similarly, $\Pr[X < 1.6] = \Pr[Z < -1]$, which by symmetry is $\Pr[Z > 1]$, or 0.1587 from Table 4. Also,

$$\Pr[1.65 < X < 1.95] = \Pr\left[\frac{1.65 - 1.8}{0.2} < Z < \frac{1.95 - 1.8}{0.2}\right]$$
$$= \Pr[-0.75 < Z < 0.75] = 1 - 2\Pr[Z > 0.75]$$
$$= 1 - 2(0.2266) = 0.5468.$$

Likewise, the cumulative probability distribution for the $N(0, 1)$ random variable can be computed using Table 4 of the Appendix. Thus, cumulative probabilities for an arbitrary normal variable with mean μ and variance σ^2 are easily determined by applying the relation in Equation (4.14) and using the table. In particular, if X is $N(\mu, \sigma^2)$, then

$$\Pr[X \leq a] = \Pr\left[Z \leq \frac{a - \mu}{\sigma}\right] = \Phi\left(\frac{a - \mu}{\sigma}\right),$$

and this last probability can be determined from Table 4 (Appendix).

Percentiles of a normal random variable X are easily derived by relationship (4.14) and the corresponding percentiles for the standard normal random variable Z. The pth percentile for Z is that value of Z, denoted by z_p, such that $p = \Pr(Z \leq z_p)$. For example, the 50th percentile of Z is denoted z_{50} and is equal to 0 since $\Pr(Z \leq 0) = 0.5$. Other percentiles for Z can be computed from Table 4 of the Appendix. For instance, the 95th percentile of Z is 1.645 since $\Pr(Z \leq 1.645) = 0.95$. In order to determine the corresponding percentile for a normal random variable X, which has a mean of μ and a variance of σ^2, we can use (4.14) to show that the pth percentile of X, denoted by x_p, is equal to $x_p = \mu + z_p\sigma$, where z_p is the pth percentile of Z.

Example 4.6.3.   Compute the 5th, 50th, and 95th percentiles for the blood glucose variable X in Example 4.6.2. From Table 4 of the Appendix, $z_1 = -1.645$, $z_{50} = 0$, and $z_{95} = 1.645$. Since $\mu = 1.8$ and $\sigma = 0.2$, for X it follows that $x_5 = 1.8 - 1.645(0.2) = 1.471$ is the 5th percentile, $x_{50} = 1.8 + 0(0.2) = 1.8$ is the 50th percentile, and $x_{95} = 1.8 + 1.645(0.2) = 2.129$ is the 95th percentile.

Before concluding our discussion of the normal distribution, we should point out that there are many situations in which the actual data may conform quite closely to the normal distribution. It is interesting to refer to the empirical frequency data on intraocular pressure in Chapter 2. Figure 2.7 is the empirical frequency polygon, and it appears to roughly approximate the normal probability density function in Figure 4.6. The empirical cumulative relative frequency in Figure 2.8 also seems to approximate Figure 4.9.

There are three other continuous probability distributions that are quite valuable in applied statistics. These are the *t distribution*, the *chi-square* (χ^2) *distribution*, and the *F distribution*. These distributions are useful when considering the probability distribution of certain statistics from random samples taken from a normal population. Accordingly, these probability distributions are discussed in the context of studying random samples from a normal population. Therefore, we shall introduce the concept of a probability distribution generated by random sampling before discussing these distributions.

4.7 SAMPLING DISTRIBUTIONS: PROBABILITY DISTRIBUTIONS GENERATED BY RANDOM SAMPLING

We have defined a statistic as a number or a quantity that is calculated from a sample of data. Examples of statistics are the sample mean $\overline{X}$ and the sample variance s^2. We shall see in this section that the quantities $\overline{X}$ and s^2 are random variables with probability distributions determined by

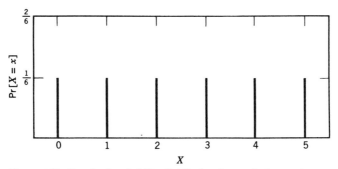

Figure 4.11. Graph of probability distribution for psychotic symptoms.

their values in repeated random sampling. That is, the value of $\overline{X}$ will generally vary from one sample of size n to another sample of size n.

This section covers the probability distributions of $\overline{X}$ and of s^2 when repeated *random* samples are selected from a population. We shall see that the probability distributions of $\overline{X}$ and s^2 are easily studied under the assumption of random sampling. The probability distribution of a statistic generated by repeated random sampling is called the *sampling distribution* of the statistic.

Consider a hypothetical population of people in which each person is classified on the basis of the number of five possible positive psychotic symptoms. Clearly, if X is the number of symptoms positive for a person selected at random, then X can take values of 0, 1, 2, 3, 4, or 5.

Let us suppose that the probability of X taking a given value is $\frac{1}{6}$ for each of the six values. The probability distribution of X is graphed in Figure 4.11.

We can compute the mean and the variance of the random variable X. In particular, employing the general formulas from Chapter 3, the mean of X, denoted by μ_X, is

$$\mu_X = \sum x_i \Pr[X = x_i]$$

$$= \tfrac{1}{6}(0) + \tfrac{1}{6}(1) + \tfrac{1}{6}(2) + \tfrac{1}{6}(3) + \tfrac{1}{6}(4) + \tfrac{1}{6}(5) = 2\tfrac{1}{2} \quad (4.16)$$

while the variance of X, denoted σ_x^2, is

$$\sigma_X^2 = \sum_i (x_i - \mu)^2 \Pr[X = x_i]$$

$$= \tfrac{1}{6}(0 - 2.5)^2 + \tfrac{1}{6}(1 - 2.5)^2 + \tfrac{1}{6}(2 - 2.5)^2 + \tfrac{1}{6}(3 - 2.5)^2$$

$$+ \tfrac{1}{6}(4 - 2.5)^2 + \tfrac{1}{6}(5 - 2.5)^2 = \tfrac{35}{12}. \quad (4.17)$$

It is important to remember that this is a hypothetical problem, at least in the sense that we would not ordinarily know the probability distribution of a random variable. If we did know the distribution of the random variable, then one would not need to draw a sample. This example, however, allows us to study the behavior of certain statistics when drawing samples at random from a population when we know the underlying distribution.

Consider the selection of random samples of size 2 from the population, sampling with replacement. Denote the two sample values of X by X_1 and X_2; that is, X_1 is the number of symptoms positive for the first person in the sample, and X_2 is the number of symptoms positive for the second person in the sample. There are (6)(6), or 36, different samples of size 2 possible. For each sample of size 2, we can compute the sample mean $\bar{x}$ and the sample variance s^2. Clearly, each of the 36 random samples has probability $\frac{1}{36}$ of being the one selected. The 36 samples, sample means, $\bar{x}$, and sample variances, s^2, are summarized in Table 4.2.

For example, the sample (2, 5) is a sample in which the first person chosen had two psychotic symptoms and the second person chosen had five psychotic symptoms. The sample mean $\bar{x}$ is $(2 + 5)/2 = 3.5$ while the sample variance s^2 is $[(2 - 3.5)^2 + (5 - 3.5)^2]/(2 - 1) = 4.5$.

Table 4.2. Thirty-Six Random Samples Possible from the Population of Figure 4.11, $\bar{X}$, and s^2

(x_1, x_2)	$\bar{x}$	s^2	(x_1, x_2)	$\bar{x}$	s^2
(0, 0)	0	0	(3, 0)	1.5	4.5
(0, 1)	0.5	0.5	(3, 1)	2.0	2.0
(0, 2)	1.0	2.0	(3, 2)	2.5	0.5
(0, 3)	1.5	4.5	(3, 3)	3.0	0
(0, 4)	2.0	8.0	(3, 4)	3.5	0.5
(0, 5)	2.5	12.5	(3, 5)	4.0	2.0
(1, 0)	0.5	0.5	(4, 0)	2.0	8.0
(1, 1)	1.0	0.0	(4, 1)	2.5	4.5
(1, 2)	1.5	0.5	(4, 2)	3.0	2.0
(1, 3)	2.0	2.0	(4, 3)	3.5	0.5
(1, 4)	2.5	4.5	(4, 4)	4.0	0
(1, 5)	3.0	8.0	(4, 5)	4.5	0.5
(2, 0)	1.0	2.0	(5, 0)	2.5	12.5
(2, 1)	1.5	0.5	(5, 1)	3.0	8.0
(2, 2)	2.0	0	(5, 2)	3.5	4.5
(2, 3)	2.5	0.5	(5, 3)	4.0	2.0
(2, 4)	3.0	2.0	(5, 4)	4.5	0.5
(2, 5)	3.5	4.5	(5, 5)	5.0	0

Table 4.3. Sampling Distributions of $\overline{X}$ and S^2 from Table 4.2

$\bar{x}$	$\Pr[\overline{X} = \bar{x}]$	s^2	$\Pr[S^2 = s^2]$
0	$\frac{1}{36}$	0	$\frac{6}{36}$
0.5	$\frac{2}{36}$	0.5	$\frac{10}{36}$
1.0	$\frac{3}{36}$	2.0	$\frac{8}{36}$
1.5	$\frac{4}{36}$	4.5	$\frac{6}{36}$
2.0	$\frac{5}{36}$	8.0	$\frac{4}{36}$
2.5	$\frac{6}{36}$	12.5	$\frac{2}{36}$
3.0	$\frac{5}{36}$		
3.5	$\frac{4}{36}$		
4.0	$\frac{3}{36}$		
4.5	$\frac{2}{36}$		
5.0	$\frac{1}{36}$.		

In practice, we would get only one of these 36 samples as our sample of size 2, but because sampling is random, each of the samples in Table 4.2 has probability of $\frac{1}{36}$ of being the one chosen. To determine the sampling distribution of $\overline{X}$ and s^2, we determine for each distinct value of $\overline{X}$ (and of s^2) its probability of occurrence under random sampling. Accordingly, we aggregate the figures in Table 4.2 to obtain the distribution summarized in Table 4.3. These are the *sampling distributions* or the probability distributions of $\overline{X}$ and s^2 in repeated random samples of size 2.

We can now determine the mean and the variance of $\overline{X}$ in repeated random sampling by using the distribution of $\overline{X}$ given in Table 4.3. Denoting the mean of $\overline{X}$ by $\mu_{\overline{X}}$ and its variance by $\sigma_{\overline{X}}^2$, we have

$$\mu_{\overline{X}} = \tfrac{1}{36}(0) + \tfrac{2}{36}(0.5) + \cdots + \tfrac{2}{36}(4.5) + \tfrac{1}{36}(5.0) = 2\tfrac{1}{2}, \qquad (4.18)$$

and

$$\sigma_{\overline{X}}^2 = \tfrac{1}{36}(0 - 2.5)^2 + \tfrac{2}{36}(0.5 - 2.5)^2 + \cdots$$

$$+ \tfrac{2}{36}(4.5 - 2.5)^2 + \tfrac{1}{36}(5.0 - 2.5)^2 = \tfrac{35}{24}. \qquad (4.19)$$

Referring back to μ_X and σ_X^2, the respective mean and variance of X, we note from (4.16), (4.17), (4.18), and (4.19) that $\mu_{\overline{X}} = \mu_X$ and $\sigma_{\overline{X}}^2 = \sigma_X^2/2$. That is, the mean of $\overline{X}$ is the original population mean, while the variance of $\overline{X}$ is the original population variance divided by n, the sample size.

These results are true in general and may be stated formally as the following theorem.

Theorem 4.7.1. *If random samples of size n are drawn with replacement from a population with a mean of μ_X and a variance of σ_X^2, then the mean and variance of $\overline{X}$ are related to the original mean and variance by*

$$\mu_{\overline{X}} = \mu_X \tag{4.20}$$

and

$$\sigma_{\overline{X}}^2 = \sigma_X^2/n. \tag{4.21}$$

If sampling without replacement is done, then these relationships are valid if the population is much larger than the sample.

Put another way, the mean of $\overline{X}$ is the sampled population's mean, while the variance of $\overline{X}$ is the sampled population's variance divided by n, the sample size. This explains why in Chapter 2 we divided the sample variance by n and referred to it as the *sample variance of the sample mean*.

Another important result that has already been indicated in the preceding section is that the actual sampling distribution of $\overline{X}$ closely approximates a normal distribution. This result is illustrated in Figure 4.12, in which the sampling distribution of $\overline{X}$ for the samples of Table 4.2 is graphed. Formally, this result is known as the central limit theorem.

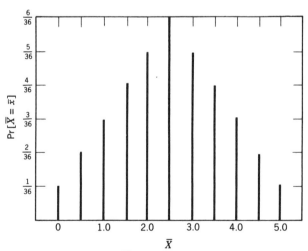

Figure 4.12. Sampling distribution of $\overline{X}$ for random samples of size 2 from population in Figure 4.11.

Theorem 4.7.2 (Central Limit Theorem). *If random samples of size n are drawn with replacement from a population with a mean of μ_X and a variance of σ_X^2 (with $0 < \sigma_X^2 < \infty$), or without replacement from a population that is large compared to the sample, then the sampling distribution of $\sqrt{n}\,(\overline{X} - \mu_X)/\sigma_X$ is closely approximated by the standard normal distribution (with zero mean and variance of 1) if n is large.*

The formal derivation of this can be found in most mathematical statistics texts [e.g., Hogg and Craig (1967)]; however, we get an empirical appreciation for this result by looking at Figure 4.12 and seeing what resulted from Figure 4.11 with a sample size of only $n = 2$.

Theorem 4.7.1 and 4.7.2 regarding $\overline{X}$ from *random sampling* form the theoretical basis for much of statistical data analysis. As stated in Section 4.6, the central limit theorem is the principal reason for the widespread use of the normal distribution in statistics. As a rule of thumb, n should be at least 20 before using the normal approximation; however, the closeness of the approximation in general depends on the distribution sampled.

Frequently, $\overline{X}$ is regarded as a *point estimator* of μ_X. That is, the sample mean is used as an estimator of the population mean. From expression (4.20), we know that the mean of $\overline{X}$ is μ_X. As an estimator of μ_X, $\overline{X}$ is said to be *unbiased* since its mean value in repeated random sampling is μ_X. In statistical estimation problems, this is an attractive property for a given estimator.

Can the same be said for the sample variance s^2? We must determine the value of the sample variance as an estimator of the overall population variance σ_x^2. From Table 4.3, the mean of s^2, μ_{s^2} can be easily computed. We obtain

$$\mu_{s^2} = \tfrac{6}{36}(0) + \tfrac{10}{36}(0.5) + \tfrac{8}{36}(2.0) + \tfrac{6}{36}(4.5) + \tfrac{4}{36}(8) + \tfrac{2}{36}(12.5) = \tfrac{35}{12}$$

$$(4.22)$$

which is σ_X^2. This is a general result. In particular, the statistic s^2 is an *unbiased* estimator of σ_X^2. The average or expected value of s^2 in repeated random sampling is the population variance σ_X^2. This result further explains why we choose to use $n - 1$ rather than n as the denominator in the variance computation in Chapter 2. If we had used n rather than $n - 1$, then the resulting statistic would not be an *unbiased* estimator of σ_X^2.

As a consequence of the findings in this section, various sample quantities would appear to be reasonable *point estimators* for various population quantities when random sampling is used. These are summarized in Table 4.4.

Table 4.4. Population Parameters and Sample Statistics for Random Sampling

Population Parameter		Sample Statistic	
Name	Symbol	Estimator Symbol	Estimator Name
Population mean	μ	$\overline{X}$	Sample mean
Population variance	σ^2	s^2	Sample variance
Population standard deviation	σ	s	Sample standard deviation
Population variance of $\overline{X}$	$\sigma_{\overline{X}}^2 = \sigma^2/n$	$s_{\overline{X}}^2 = s^2/n$	Sample variance of $\overline{X}$
Population standard error (or population standard deviation of $\overline{X}$)	$\sigma_{\overline{X}} = \sigma/\sqrt{n}$	$s_{\overline{X}} = s/\sqrt{n}$	Sample standard error (or sample standard deviation of $\overline{X}$)

Furthermore, if random sampling has been used, it is reasonable to expect the estimators to be good estimators of the population parameters. The main results of this section are worth summarizing. For random samples of size n from a population with mean μ and variance σ^2, the following hold:

1. The mean and variance of $\overline{X}$ are μ and σ^2/n, respectively.
2. The mean of s^2 is σ^2.
3. $\overline{X}$ and s^2 are unbiased estimators of μ and σ^2, respectively.
4. The probability distribution of $\sqrt{n}(\overline{X} - \mu)/\sigma$ may be approximated by the standard normal probability distribution if n is large.

These results hold for virtually all populations; the key requirement is that of random sampling.

We now return to the discussion of other continuous distributions and examine three that derive from randomly sampling a normal population.

4.8 THE t, χ^2, AND F PROBABILITY DISTRIBUTIONS

As mentioned in the previous section, the t, χ^2, and F distributions are appropriate when random samples are selected from a normal population. We stated that $\sqrt{n}(\overline{X} - \mu)/\sigma$ is distributed like a standard normal variable if n is large even if the population is not normal. Furthermore, if samples are drawn randomly from a normal population with mean μ and variance

σ^2, then regardless of the sample size, $\overline{X}$ is a normally distributed variable with the mean of $\overline{X}$ being μ and its variance being σ^2/n. Hence, for random samples of size n from a normal distribution, the exact result

$$\sqrt{n}\,(\overline{X} - \mu)/\sigma = Z \qquad (4.23)$$

is true for any sample size. By the central limit theorem, the result (4.23) is only an approximate relationship for nonnormal populations when the sample size is large.

Example 4.8.1. From Example 4.6.2, suppose a random sample of size 4 is to be selected from the population. We wish to find $\Pr[\overline{X} > 2]$ and $\Pr[\overline{X} < 1.6]$. To determine these probabilities, one notes that since $\mu = 1.8$ and $\sigma = 0.2$ and the population is normal, then $\overline{X}$ is $N(1.8, 0.04/4)$; hence,

$$\Pr[\overline{X} > 2] = \Pr\left[\frac{\overline{X} - 1.8}{\sqrt{0.01}} > \frac{2 - 1.8}{\sqrt{0.01}}\right] = \Pr[Z > 2.0] = 0.0228.$$

Similarly,

$$\Pr[\overline{X} < 1.6] = \Pr\left[\frac{\overline{X} - 1.8}{\sqrt{0.01}} < \frac{1.6 - 1.8}{\sqrt{0.01}}\right] = \Pr[Z < -2.0]$$

$$= \Pr[Z > 2.0] = 0.0228.$$

The t distribution arises quite naturally when samples are randomly drawn from a normal distribution. Perhaps most common is the situation in which a random sample of size n is drawn from a $N(\mu, \sigma^2)$ population. If σ^2 is not known, then we must estimate it, and one possibility is to use s^2. If we consider a ratio like the left side of Equation (4.23) with s replacing the unknown σ, that is, $\sqrt{n}\,(\overline{X} - \mu)/s$, the question arises of what is its probability distribution.

The distribution of $\sqrt{n}\,(\overline{X} - \mu)/s$ is called the t distribution.

Definition 4.8.1. If a random sample of size n is chosen from a normal population with mean μ and variance σ^2, then $\sqrt{n}\,(\overline{X} - \mu)/s$ is said to have a t *distribution with* $n - 1$ *degrees of freedom*, denoted as

$$t(n - 1) = \sqrt{n}\,(\overline{X} - \mu)/s. \qquad (4.24)$$

In (4.24), $\overline{X}$ and s^2 are the sample mean and sample variance, respectively; this ratio is essentially the Z-type ratio (4.23) in which σ is estimated from the sample. See Table 5 in the Appendix for percentage points of the t distribution.

Use of the table is illustrated with the following example.

Example 4.8.2. Compute the probability that a t random variable with eight degrees of freedom is larger than 1.108. From Table 5 of the Appendix, we find that $\Pr[t(8) > 1.108] = 0.15$ by reading the probabilities listed at the bottom of the table. Note that values of t are in the body of the table, while the corresponding probabilities are listed as the bottom row of the table. The top row of the table is simply 2 times the bottom row and is the probability that the t is greater than the tabled t or less than the negative of the tabled t. For example, $\Pr[t(8) > 1.108] + \Pr[t(8) < -1.108] = 0.30$, from the top of the table.

It is also possible to determine values of t that correspond to certain probabilities—for example, the value of $t(12)$ such that $\Pr[t(12) > t_0] = 0.05$ is 1.782. This is located by finding 0.05 at the bottom of the table and then locating the 12-degrees-of-freedom row in the left column. This row and column intersect at the value 1.782. The reader may use linear interpolation if intermediate values are required or check more extensive tables.

The t family of distributions is a one-parameter family, with the parameter being the number of degrees of freedom. Like the standard normal (Z) probability density function, the t probability density function is symmetric about zero and approaches zero as t goes to either $+\infty$ or $-\infty$. It is flatter in shape than the pdf of Z but becomes more like that of Z as the degrees of freedom approach infinity (see Figure 4.13). The t distribution can be used to make an inference on μ when σ^2 is unknown. This is a very useful distribution in statistical applications since the population variance is rarely known. It is useful for inference regarding the means of normal populations and is used extensively in later chapters.

Another one-parameter distribution that arises in random sampling from the normal distribution is the χ^2 distribution. This is a useful distribution for statistical inference regarding the variance of a normal population.

Definition 4.8.2. If a random sample of size n is chosen from a normal population with mean μ and variance σ^2, then $(n-1)s^2/\sigma^2$ follows a χ^2 distribution with $n - 1$ degrees of freedom, and we write

$$\chi^2(n-1) = (n-1)s^2/\sigma^2. \qquad (4.25)$$

A table for the χ^2 distribution is given in the Appendix (Table 6).

Example 4.8.3. Determine the probability that a χ^2 random variable with 14 degrees of freedom is less than 6.57. From Table 6 of the Appendix, we choose the row with 14 degrees of freedom and read across to the value of 6.57. The probability 0.05 at the top of the table is the one sought.

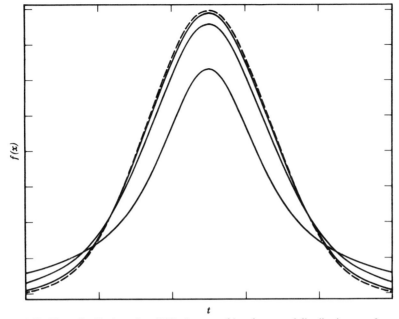

Figure 4.13. The t distributions (in solid line) approaching the normal distribution $\mu = 0$, $\sigma = 1$ (dotted curve) as the degrees of freedom increase.

The most widespread use of the χ^2 distribution is in the area of categorical data analysis, and we shall use this distribution in later chapters. A graph of three χ^2 variates (with 1, 5, and 10 degrees of freedom) is illustrated in Figure 4.14. We note that the χ^2 random variable is a nonnegative valued random variable.

Definition 4.8.3. The F *distribution*, or the variance ratio distribution, follows from the comparison of the sample variances, s_1^2 and s_2^2, of two independent random samples. For independent random samples of sizes n_1 and n_2 from the normal populations $N(\mu_1, \sigma_1^2)$ and $N(\mu_2, \sigma_2^2)$, the quantity

$$F(n_1 - 1, n_2 - 1) = \frac{s_1^2/\sigma_1^2}{s_2^2/\sigma_2^2} \qquad (4.26)$$

is said to follow an F distribution with degrees of freedom $n_1 - 1$ in the numerator and degrees of freedom $n_2 - 1$ in the denominator.

It is a nonnegative valued random variable and is appropriate for comparing variances of normal populations. Table 7 of the Appendix has a selected list of probability values for the F distribution, while Figure 4.15 is a plot of a typical F distribution with two and nine degrees of freedom.

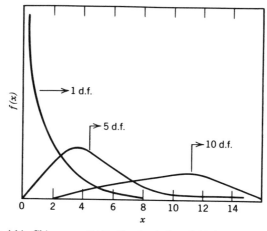

Figure 4.14. Chi-square distribution for 1, 5, and 10 degrees of freedom.

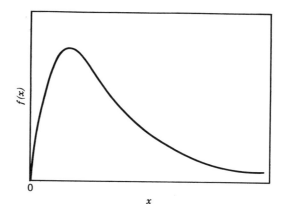

Figure 4.15. The F distribution for $n_1 - 1 = 2$ and $n_2 - 1 = 9$ degrees of freedom.

Example 4.8.4. Determine the probability that an F random variable with five and seven degrees of freedom is greater than 2.88. From Table 7 of the Appendix, this probability is located by finding 2.88 in the table under the column labeled 5 and the row labeled 7. The probability is 0.10.

4.9 SUMMARY

This chapter includes a number of important results for statistical inference. It provides the basis for the application of probability to various problems of data analysis. A major theme in this chapter is that random sampling provides the basis for the application of very powerful statistical inference techniques. In subsequent chapters, we will apply many of these techniques for testing hypotheses and estimating parameters.

PROBLEMS

4.1. From a group of 60 patients, a random sample without replacement of size 12 is desired. Several procedures to obtain the sample are proposed. Determine if the procedures below would yield random samples. Justify your conclusion.

(a) Patients are labeled 00–59. From the table of random numbers (Table 1 in the Appendix), two digit numbers are read. If the number chosen is 00–59, then the corresponding patient is chosen; if the number if bigger than 59, subtract 59 from the number and choose that patient. In either case, if a patient was chosen earlier in the sample, choose another random number.

(b) Same as (a) but discard the number if it is bigger than 59.

4.2. Identify the following as parameters or statistics.

(a) $\bar{X} \pm 2.011s$,

(b) $\sigma / \sqrt{\mu}$,

(c) $2\mu + \bar{X}$,

(d) $\sigma^2 + \sigma - 10$,

(e) $s^2(\sigma^2 + 1)$.

4.3. Verify that

(a) $\binom{n}{0} = \binom{n}{n} = 1$ (b) $\binom{n}{x} = \binom{n}{n-x}$

(c) $\binom{n}{1} = \binom{n}{n-1} = n$

(d) $\binom{n}{x} = \dfrac{n(n-1)\cdots(n-x+1)}{x(x-1)\cdots 3 \cdot 2 \cdot 1}$

4.4. A certain drug reduces pain in 75% of the cases treated. If 9 patients receive this drug, compute the following where X is the number of patients successfully treated.

(a) $\Pr[X \geq 7]$,

(b) $\Pr[X \geq 8]$,

(c) $\Pr[X = 7]$,

(d) $\Pr[X < 4]$,

(e) $\Pr[3 \leq X < 8]$,

(f) $\Pr[2 < X \leq 7]$.

4.5. If $n = 7$ and $p = 0.3$ for a binomial random variable X, calculate the mean μ and the variance σ^2 of X.

4.6. For the random variable X of problem 4.5 compute:
   (a) $1 - \Pr[X < 3]$,
   (b) $\Pr[(X \geq 4)$ and $(X \geq 5)]$,
   (c) $\Pr[X \geq 4]$ and $\Pr[X \geq 5]$.

4.7. Suppose the number of cases of a disease in a certain region is a Poisson random variable with a mean of eight per week and let X be the number of cases in any week. Determine:
   (a) $\Pr[X \leq 2]$,
   (b) $\Pr[X = 3]$,
   (c) $\Pr[X > 5]$,
   (d) $\Pr[4 \leq X < 15]$.

4.8. Twenty identical bottles of a cold medicine are presented to a customer in a drug store to determine the ability of the person to detect if the seal of protection was broken. The customer is informed that 10 of the bottles have been opened (tampered with) and then closed. If X is the random variable that measures the number of successful classifications of "bad" bottles, and an individual has no special ability to distinguish between tampered and untampered bottles, compute:
   (a) the probability of no errors, that is, $\Pr[X = 0]$,
   (b) the probability of one error, that is, $\Pr[X = 1]$.

4.9. If X has a normal distribution with mean $\mu = 100$ and variance $\sigma^2 = 25$, evaluate:
   (a) $\Pr[X > 110.0]$,
   (b) $\Pr[X < 106.8]$,
   (c) $\Pr[X < 88.4]$,
   (d) $\Pr[X > 90.8]$,
   (e) $\Pr[101.7 < X < 112.3]$,
   (f) $\Pr[93.85 \leq X \leq 106.15]$,
   (g) $\Pr[90.15 \leq X \leq 94.65]$.
   (h) If $\Pr[X < X_0] = 0.9115$, find the corresponding X_0 value.

4.10. Draw 10 random samples of size 5 from Table 1 of the Appendix by selecting five two-digit random numbers (00–99). Let X represent a random number. What are μ and σ^2 for the population of two-digit numbers? For each of the 10 samples, compute $\overline{X}$ and s^2. See if the mean of the ten $\overline{X}$ values is close to μ, and if the mean of the ten s^2 values is close to σ^2.

4.11. A random sample of size 25 is selected from a population with mean $\mu = 85$ and standard deviation $\sigma = 4$. Approximate the following probabilities using the central limit theorem:

(a) $\Pr[\bar{X} > 86.645]$,

(b) $\Pr[\bar{X} < 84.340]$,

(c) $\Pr[83.04 < \bar{X} < 86.96]$.

4.12. The sample mean $\bar{X}$ obtained from a population with $\mu = 40$ and $\sigma^2 = 9$ is observed to be 42. Determine the sample size n used if $\Pr[\bar{X} < 41] = 0.75$.

4.13. With a random sample of size $n = 25$ from a population with $\mu = 450$, a sample mean $\bar{X}$ and a sample variance s^2 are obtained as $\bar{X} = 454$ and $s^2 = 121$. Using the sample variance as an estimator for σ^2, compute the probability of obtaining the observed sample mean or a greater value.

4.14. If, in problem 4.13, the population variance is $\sigma^2 = 90$, compute the probability of obtaining the observed sample variance or a greater value.

4.15. Use the tables in the Appendix to determine the following:

(a) $\Pr[t(10) > 2.228]$,

(b) $\Pr[t(10) < -2.228]$,

(c) $\Pr[0.876 < t(11) < 3.106]$,

(d) $\Pr[-1.055 < t(30) < 1.055]$,

(e) value of t_0 such that $\Pr[t(18) > t_0] = 0.025$.

4.16. Use the tables in the Appendix to determine the following:

(a) $\Pr[\chi^2(13) > 4.107]$,

(b) $\Pr[\chi^2(11) < 3.82]$,

(c) value of χ_0^2 such that $\Pr[\chi^2(21) > \chi_0^2] = 0.500$,

(d) $\Pr[12.88 < \chi^2(27) < 18.11]$.

REFERENCES

Cochran, W. G. (1963). *Sampling Techniques*, 2nd ed., Wiley, New York.

Feller, W. (1967). *An Introduction to Probability Theory and its Applications*, 3rd ed., Wiley, New York.

Hogg, R. V., and A. T. Craig. (1967). *Introduction to Mathematical Statistics*, Macmillan, New York.

Johnson, N. L., and S. Kotz. (1969). *Discrete Distributions*, Houghton-Mifflin, Boston.

Confidence Intervals and Hypothesis Testing: General Considerations and Applications

5.1 INTRODUCTION

Nearly always when a study is performed, the major goal is to examine a particular scientific hypothesis. We recognize that although a study is only one experiment, we normally want to generalize the findings. Computations performed on the sample data and summary numbers (i.e., statistics) that are used to describe the sample are to be used to draw a conclusion about the population. Since the sample is only a part of the population, our reasoning is inductive rather than deductive. A conclusion we draw about the population may be incorrect, as it is based on only a sample. *Statistical inference* is that branch of statistics that deals with the evaluation of the uncertainty in inductive inference and the procedures and tools for making these inferences.

There are two major aspects of statistical inference: *estimation of parameters* and *testing of hypotheses*. Often these procedures are both applied in a given problem since they complement one another. In estimation of parameters, a numerical value or a set of values is computed from the sample and is used as our best estimate of the corresponding population parameter. For example, a random sample of 20 girls aged 11–13 years from a given school might yield a mean body weight of 110 lb; thus, we might conclude that the mean in this population of 11–13-year-old girls is 110 lb. We realize that another random sample of 20 girls would probably give a mean different from 110 lb, but we may not know how different. In hypotheses testing, the major focus is on arriving at a yes–no decision regarding certain population characteristics; for example, "Is the mean body weight of girls age 11–13 greater than 105 lb?" As noted, the two concepts of testing and estimation complement each other since a yes–no decision on a hypothesis is more helpful if it is accompanied by an estimate of the magnitude of the effects. For example, if we conclude that the mean body weight of girls age 11–13 is greater than 105 lb, then how much greater than 105 lb do we estimate the true mean to be?

In this chapter, we describe certain features of both of these aspects of statistical inference. For each of these, we apply the techniques to the problem of drawing an inference from a single population. In particular, we consider inference regarding a single continuous population mean and variance. We also study the problem of making an inference about the binomial parameter p.

5.2 ESTIMATION OF POPULATION CHARACTERISTICS: POINT AND INTERVAL ESTIMATION

In estimation, we are interested in making a statement about the value of a parameter, a certain quantity in the population. For example, in the case of the population mean μ, we may wish to make a statement about our best "guess" for the value of μ, and we often use the sample mean as an estimator of the quantity μ. Estimation in which a single sample value is used as the estimator of the parameter is referred to as *point estimation*. This contrasts with another form of estimation termed *interval estimation*, in which an interval is determined from the sample and is used to make a statement about our confidence that the interval includes the parameter. Such intervals are called *confidence intervals*. For instance, we may compute a 95% confidence interval for a population parameter. The correct interpretation of a 95% confidence interval is that in repeated random sampling 95% of the intervals computed in this same way would include the population parameter. This implies that 5% of these intervals would not. In a given study, the data analyst will only have the one interval that has been computed and will not know if this interval actually includes the parameter or not. However, since 95% of the intervals computed by random sampling would include the population parameter, the data analyst would be "95% confident" of the statement concerning the inclusion of a parameter in the interval. There is nothing special about the use of 95% as the confidence coefficient, and values of 99%, 90%, or others may be used depending on the nature of the question.

Definition 5.2.1. A $(1 - \alpha)100\%$ *confidence interval* $(0 < \alpha < 1)$ for a parameter λ is an interval of values determined from the sample whereby the method for determining the interval of values would provide an interval including λ $(1 - \alpha)100\%$ of the time in repeated random sampling. The quantity $(1 - \alpha)100\%$ is termed the *confidence coefficient*, and the interval of values is the *confidence interval*.

Although the general concept of a confidence interval is straightforward, the procedures for computing confidence intervals depend on the type of problem under study and the parameter to be estimated. To illustrate the general principles involved in the determination of a confidence interval, we present in this section the procedures for determining confidence intervals for the mean and variance for a continuous random variable. In addition, we consider the problem of placing a confidence interval on the binomial proportion p.

5.2.1 Confidence Interval for a Population Mean μ with Variance σ^2 Known

We consider the situation in which the random variable in the population follows a normal distribution. Later we note that the assumption is not crucial for placing confidence intervals on the mean, provided the sample size is large, and thus will remove the normality assumption when the sample size is large.

5.2.1.1 *Normal Population*
Consider a random sample $X_1, \ldots, X_n$ from a normal distribution with an unknown mean μ and a known variance σ^2. We assume the sample was drawn with replacement or else that the population is large compared to the sample. Denoting the random variable as X, then X is $N(\mu, \sigma^2)$, and $\overline{X}$, the sample mean, is $N(\mu, \sigma^2/n)$. From expression (4.23), we have

$$\sqrt{n}\,(\overline{X} - \mu)/\sigma = Z, \qquad (5.1)$$

where Z is the standard normal variate. Generally, we want a confidence interval that has a high probability of including the true mean μ (e.g., a 95 or 99% confidence interval). That is, we want a $(1 - \alpha)100\%$ confidence interval, where α is a small number like 0.05 or 0.01. From Table 4 in the Appendix we can find $Z_{1-\alpha/2}$, which is the value of Z such that $\alpha/2$ of the probability is less than $-Z_{1-\alpha/2}$ and $\alpha/2$ of the probability is greater than $Z_{1-\alpha/2}$. We denote such a Z by $Z_{1-\alpha/2}$; that is, $Z_{1-\alpha/2}$ is the value of Z

such that $\Pr[Z \le Z_{1-\alpha/2}] = 1 - \alpha/2$. Hence it follows that

$$\Pr\left[-Z_{1-\alpha/2} < Z < Z_{1-\alpha/2}\right] = 1 - \alpha, \tag{5.2}$$

and setting (5.1) into the middle term in (5.2), one obtains

$$\Pr\left[-Z_{1-\alpha/2} < \sqrt{n}\left(\overline{X} - \mu\right)/(\sigma) < Z_{1-\alpha/2}\right] = 1 - \alpha. \tag{5.3}$$

Further algebraic manipulation of (5.3) shows that

$$\Pr\left[\overline{X} - Z_{1-\alpha/2}(\sigma/\sqrt{n}) < \mu < \overline{X} + Z_{1-\alpha/2}(\sigma/\sqrt{n})\right] = 1 - \alpha. \tag{5.4}$$

That is, $(1 - \alpha)100\%$ of the intervals determined by $(\overline{X} - Z_{1-\alpha/2}\sigma/\sqrt{n}, \overline{X} + Z_{1-\alpha/2}\sigma/\sqrt{n})$ will include μ. As a consequence, we have the following result.

Theorem 5.2.1.1. *If* $X_1, \ldots, X_n$ *is a random sample from a normal population with unknown mean* μ *and known variance* σ^2, *then*

$$\overline{X} \pm Z_{1-\alpha/2}(\sigma/\sqrt{n}) \tag{5.5}$$

is a $(1 - \alpha)100\%$ *confidence interval for* μ. *It is assumed that the random sample is drawn with replacement or that the population is large compared to the sample.*

Example 5.2.1.1.1. To illustrate the use of (5.5), consider the data of Example 2.3.1, which consist of the seven blood alcohol measurements at respiratory failure. We assume that blood alcohol levels are normally distributed in this population, and the population variance is known to be 0.09, that is, $\sigma^2 = 0.09$ (mg/mL)^2. For illustration, we determine 90, 95, and 99% confidence intervals for μ. For a 90% confidence interval, $\alpha/2 = 0.05$, for a 95% interval $\alpha/2 = 0.025$, and for a 99% interval $\alpha/2 = 0.005$ in result (5.5). Hence, recalling that $\overline{X} = 9.21$ in Example 2.3.1, the following confidence intervals are computed.

90% confidence interval: $\quad 9.21 \pm 1.645(0.3/\sqrt{7}) = (9.02, 9.40),$

95% confidence interval: $\quad 9.21 \pm 1.96(0.3/\sqrt{7}) = (8.99, 9.43), \quad (5.6)$

99% confidence interval: $\quad 9.21 \pm 2.58(0.3/\sqrt{7}) = (8.92, 9.50).$

The values of 1.645, 1.96, and 2.58 in (5.6) are determined from Table 4 of the Appendix.

From expression (5.6), we note that the width of the confidence interval increases with an increase in the confidence coefficient. This result is as expected since the confidence coefficient is a reflection of the likelihood that the interval includes the mean μ.

The width of a confidence interval for μ from (5.5) is given by

$$w = \frac{2\sigma Z_{1-\alpha/2}}{\sqrt{n}}. \tag{5.7}$$

Expression (5.7) shows that the width of the confidence interval increases with an increase in σ, the standard deviation, and increases with an increase in the confidence coefficient $(1 - \alpha)$. In addition, Equation (5.7) demonstrates that the width of the confidence interval for μ decreases with an increase in n, the sample size. This means that one can determine the sample size requirements for a given problem by specifying the maximum confidence interval width to be tolerated for a given confidence coefficient.

For example, suppose it is known that $\sigma = 10$, and we want the width of the 95% confidence interval for μ to be less than 5 units. Solving (5.7) for n, we find that

$$n \geq \frac{4\sigma^2 Z_{1-\alpha/2}^2}{w^2} \tag{5.8}$$

is the sample size requirement. Substituting the values of $w = 5$, $\sigma = 10$, and $Z_{1-\alpha/2} = 1.96$ into equation (5.8), we determine that $n \geq 61.47$; therefore, 62 observations would be required.

5.2.1.2 Nonnormal Population

In Chapter 4, the central limit theorem stated that the sample mean $\overline{X}$ of a random sample of size n drawn with replacement from a population with mean μ and variance σ^2 may be approximated by a normal distribution with mean μ and variance σ^2/n. That is, under the central limit theorem, $\sqrt{n}(\overline{X} - \mu)/\sigma$ is approximately a standard normal random variable. Recall that this result is also true if sampling is done without replacement if the population is large compared to the sample. (*Note:* Unless stated otherwise, it will be assumed for the remainder of the text that if sampling without replacement is used, then the population is large compared to the sample.) Hence, provided that n is sufficiently large ($n \geq 20$ is a rule of thumb), then the $(1 - \alpha)100\%$ confidence interval for μ is approximated by (5.5).

The central limit theorem then provides the theoretical basis for using (5.5) as a $(1 - \alpha)100\%$ confidence interval for the mean μ of a random variable with variance σ^2 known even when the population distribution is unknown.

5.2.2   Confidence Interval for a Population Mean μ with Variance σ^2 Unknown

Once again, consider a random sample $X_1, \ldots, X_n$ from a normal population with mean μ but unknown population variance σ^2. From equation (4.24), we know that the t distribution is defined by

$$t(n-1) = (\overline{X} - \mu)/(s/\sqrt{n}), \tag{5.9}$$

where $\overline{X}$ and s^2 are the sample mean and sample variance, respectively. We can determine for a given value of α that value of $t(n-1)$, denoted by $t_{1-\alpha/2}(n-1)$, such that $\Pr[t(n-1) \le t_{1-\alpha/2}(n-1)] = 1 - \alpha/2$, from which it follows that

$$\Pr\left[-t_{1-\alpha/2}(n-1) < t(n-1) < t_{1-\alpha/2}(n-1)\right] = 1 - \alpha. \tag{5.10}$$

Note that (5.10) is analogous to (5.2). Inserting Equation (5.9) for the middle term in Equation (5.10) and performing some algebra, we obtain a $(1-\alpha)100\%$ confidence interval for μ given by

$$\overline{X} \pm t_{1-\alpha/2}(n-1)(s/\sqrt{n}), \tag{5.11}$$

where $t_{1-\alpha/2}(n-1)$ is obtained from Table 5 of the Appendix, with $n-1$ degrees of freedom.

Theorem 5.2.2.1.   *If $X_1, \ldots, X_n$ is a random sample from a normal population with mean μ and unknown variance σ^2, then $\overline{X} \pm t_{1-\alpha/2}(n-1)s/\sqrt{n}$ is a $(1-\alpha)100\%$ confidence interval for μ. If the population is not normal but n is large, then this interval is an approximate $(1-\alpha)100\%$ confidence interval for μ.*

Example 5.2.2.1.   To illustrate, let us consider the following data from a clinical trial of propranolol as a treatment for anxiety neurosis. Each of nine persons with the disorder had their systolic blood pressure recorded while under treatment with propranolol and at another time while being given a placebo treatment. The nine control-treatment differences are (in mm Hg) $+1$, -1, $+20$, -10, $+19$, $+8$, $+6$, -1, and $+3$. Assuming these differences are from a normal distribution, we can calculate a 99% confidence interval for the mean difference in the population. From these data, we compute $n = 9$, $\overline{X} = +5$, and $s^2 = 93.5$. From Table 5 of the Appendix, with eight degrees of freedom, we obtain $t_{0.995}(8) = 3.355$. Hence, following expression (5.11), the 99% confidence interval for the population mean of the differences is: $5 \pm 3.355(\sqrt{93.5/9}) = (-5.8, 15.8)$. This interval has precisely the same interpretation as the interval given by result (5.5), that is, 99% of the intervals generated by this procedure will include the population mean of the differences. Therefore, unless a very unusual sample has arisen, this interval includes the true population mean difference.

From expression (5.11), the width of the $(1 - \alpha)100\%$ confidence interval for μ is

$$w = \frac{2(s)t_{1-\alpha/2}(n-1)}{\sqrt{n}}. \qquad (5.12)$$

Determining the sample size necessary in order to keep the width of a confidence interval less than a certain value involves several complications. From (5.12) we observe that s is unknown prior to the study and $t_{1-\alpha/2}(n-1)$ itself depends on n. One approach is to consider

$$\Pr\left[2t_{1-\alpha/2}(n-1)s/\sqrt{n} \le w\right] = \Pr\left[\frac{(n-1)s^2}{\sigma^2} \le \frac{(n-1)nw^2}{4t_{1-\alpha/2}^2(n-1)\sigma^2}\right]. \qquad (5.13)$$

Recalling from Equation (4.25) that $(n-1)s^2/\sigma^2$ has a $\chi^2(n-1)$ distribution, the right side of Equation (5.13) is equivalent to

$$\Pr\left[\chi^2(n-1) \le \frac{n(n-1)}{t_{1-\alpha/2}^2(n-1)} \frac{w^2}{4\sigma^2}\right]. \qquad (5.14)$$

The solution of this sample size problem then proceeds by trial and error on (5.14) or by direct computation, which is illustrated by the following example.

Example 5.2.2.2. Suppose one would like the 95% confidence interval for μ to have width less than or equal to σ. What is the chance that this would be achieved with 25 observations? Substituting $w = \sigma$ and $t_{1-\alpha/2}(24) = 2.064$ into Equation (5.14), we obtain $\Pr[\chi^2(24) \le 35.21]$, which is approximately 0.93 from the figures in Table 6 of the Appendix.

Trial-and-error solution of Equation (5.14) comes about if one specifies a value of w as a multiple of σ (e.g., $w = \sigma$ or $w = 2.5\sigma$) and then solves Equation (5.14) for n for a certain level of probability. There are criteria for sample size determination other than the ones used in this section; however, if estimation of a population mean is the objective of the study, then the procedures we described here are the proper ones to use.

5.2.3   Confidence Interval for the Variance σ^2 of a Normal Population

Consider a random sample $X_1, X_2, \ldots, X_n$ selected from a $N(\mu, \sigma^2)$ population with μ and σ^2 both unknown. From Equation (4.25), $(n-1)s^2/\sigma^2$ follows a chi-square distribution with $n-1$ degrees of freedom. Accordingly, from Table 6 of the Appendix, we find the values $\chi^2_{\alpha/2}(n-1)$ and $\chi^2_{1-\alpha/2}(n-1)$, which satisfy

$$\Pr\left[\chi^2_{\alpha/2}(n-1) < \chi^2(n-1) < \chi^2_{1-\alpha/2}(n-1)\right] = 1 - \alpha. \quad (5.15)$$

Substitution of $s^2(n-1)/\sigma^2$ for the middle term of Equation (5.15) and conducting some algebraic manipulations, we find

$$\left(\frac{(n-1)s^2}{\chi^2_{1-\alpha/2}(n-1)}, \frac{(n-1)s^2}{\chi^2_{\alpha/2}(n-1)}\right) \quad (5.16)$$

is a $(1-\alpha)100\%$ confidence interval for σ^2, the population variance.

Theorem 5.2.3.1.   *If $X_1, \ldots, X_n$ is a random sample from a normal population with mean μ and variance σ^2, then (5.16) is a $(1-\alpha)100\%$ confidence interval for σ^2.*

Example 5.2.3.1.   Suppose a random sample of size 22 has been selected from a normal distribution, and the sample variance s^2 is 1450. Using (5.16), we can determine a 95% confidence interval for σ^2. From Table 6 of the Appendix, we find $\chi^2_{0.975}(21) = 35.5$ and $\chi^2_{0.025}(21) = 10.3$. Hence, a 95% confidence interval is given by $(21(1450)/35.5, 21(1450)/10.3)$, or $(857.7, 2956.3)$.

The preceding situations exhaust the confidence interval cases for one normal population. Other problems involve the comparison of two or more normal populations or deal with the association of several variables; they will be discussed as they arise in subsequent chapters. We next turn to the problem of placing a confidence interval on a single binomial parameter p.

5.2.4   Confidence Interval for a Binomial Proportion p

Recall that a binomial population is one in which each individual is classified on the basis of having or not having a certain characteristic. It is assumed that p $(0 < p < 1)$ is the proportion of the population with the characteristic.

If p is unknown, a random sample of size n is selected from this population, and the fraction of the sample with the characteristic is a logical point estimator of p. Formally we denote the random sample by $X_1, \ldots, X_n$, where each X_i will be equal to 1 if the ith randomly selected individual has the characteristic and equal to 0 if the individual does not have the characteristic.

The sample mean $\overline{X}$ is defined by $\overline{X} = \sum_{i=1}^{n} X_i/n$ and is simply the proportion of the sample that has the characteristic. The sample sum $\sum_{i=1}^{n} X_i$ is the number of the n sample individuals with the characteristic and follows a binomial distribution with parameters p and n. Furthermore, each X_i can be viewed as a binomial random variable with parameters p and $n = 1$; therefore, the mean μ and variance σ^2 of each X_i are p and $p(1 - p)$, respectively. Thus, if n is large enough, the central limit theorem may be applied to $\overline{X} = \sum_{i=1}^{n} X_i/n$. This is stated in the following result.

Theorem 5.2.4.1. *If $X_1, \ldots, X_n$ is a random sample from a binomial population with parameters p and 1 and if $np(1 - p) \geq 5$, then the sample proportion $\overline{X} = \sum_{i=1}^{n} X_i/n$ has an approximate normal distribution with mean p and variance $p(1 - p)/n$.*

This approximation is fairly accurate if $np(1 - p) \geq 5$. For other situations, the approximation may be seriously in error, and the exact binomial distribution should be used for inference. For convenience, denote the sample proportion $\overline{X}$ by $\hat{p}$; by Theorem 5.2.4.1, $\hat{p}$ is approximately normal with mean p and variance $p(1 - p)/n$. Since p is unknown, then $p(1 - p)/n$ is unknown, but it may be estimated by replacing p by $\hat{p}$; therefore, $\hat{p}$ is approximately normal with mean p and variance $\hat{p}(1 - \hat{p})/n$. Accordingly, $\hat{p}$ may be converted to a standard normal by

$$Z = \frac{\hat{p} - p}{\sqrt{\hat{p}(1 - \hat{p})/n}},$$

and thus a confidence interval for p can be determined, similar to the way (5.5) was derived.

Theorem 5.2.4.2. *If $X_1, \ldots, X_n$ is a random sample from a binomial population with parameters p and 1 and if $np(1 - p) \geq 5$, then $\hat{p} \pm Z_{1 - \alpha/2}\sqrt{\hat{p}(1 - \hat{p})/n}$ is an approximate $(1 - \alpha)100\%$ confidence interval for p.*

Three additional points should be noted in this development. First, the variance of $\hat{p}$ is $p(1 - p)/n$ (i.e., $\sigma/\sqrt{n}$) and is estimated by $\hat{p}(1 - \hat{p})/n$; these are often denoted by $\sigma_{\hat{p}}$ and $s_{\hat{p}}$, respectively. The second point is that the results in Theorems 5.2.4.1 and 5.2.4.2 may be modified to be applied to $n\hat{p}$, the observed total number of successes. In particular, by another version of the central limit theorem, $n\hat{p}$ is approximately $N(np, np(1 - p))$, and an approximate $(1 - \alpha)100\%$ confidence interval for np is $n\hat{p} \pm Z_{1-\alpha/2}\sqrt{n\hat{p}(1 - \hat{p})}$. Finally, there is the question of how large n must be to justify the application of the central limit theorem. If $n\hat{p}(1 - \hat{p}) \geq 5$, then the approximations are generally quite accurate.

If $n\hat{p}(1 - \hat{p}) < 5$, then alternative confidence limit methods are required, and the following theorem provides an exact method.

Theorem 5.2.4.3. *Using the exact binomial distribution, a* $(1 - \alpha)100\%$ *confidence interval for* p *is* (p_L, p_U), *where* p_L *and* p_U *satisfy*

$$\sum_{i=y}^{n} \binom{n}{i} p_L^i (1 - p_L)^{n-i} = \alpha/2,$$

$$\sum_{i=0}^{y} \binom{n}{i} p_U^i (1 - p_U)^{n-i} = \alpha/2,$$

and

$$y = \sum_{i=1}^{n} x_i,$$

the observed number of successes.

Theorem 5.2.4.3 requires computation of the combinatorial terms $\binom{n}{i}$, but fortunately graphs have been developed that simplify the procedure. These graphs are reproduced in Table 8 of the Appendix.

Example 5.2.4.1. A cardiac medication is given to 10 patients in a study and 1 of the 10 patients experiences side effects. We would like to place a 95% confidence interval on the population proportion with side effects.

We first compute $\hat{p} = \frac{1}{10} = 0.1$ and $n\hat{p}(1 - \hat{p}) = 10(0.1)(0.9) = 0.9 < 5$. Thus, the normal approximation is not appropriate and the exact limits of Theorem 5.2.4.3 should be used. Using Table 8 of the Appendix, we obtain $(0.01, 0.45)$ as the 95% confidence interval for p.

Example 5.2.4.2. In a study of 100 patients with an ocular vascular disorder, 50 were found to show improved visual function after a one-month course of systemic steroid therapy. Place a 95% confidence interval on the population improvement rate. Here $n = 100$, $\hat{p} = 0.5$, and $n\hat{p}(1 - \hat{p}) = 25 > 5$ so the normal approximation is valid. The 95% confidence interval is

$$\hat{p} \pm 1.96\sqrt{\hat{p}(1 - \hat{p})/n}$$

or

$$0.5 \pm 1.96\sqrt{0.5(0.5)/100} = (0.4020, 0.5980).$$

We also note that $s_{\hat{p}}^2 = 0.5(0.5)/100 = 0.0025$, and the estimated standard error of $\hat{p}$ is $\sqrt{0.0025} = 0.05$.

For further details on the computation of exact binomial confidence limits, the reader may refer to Conover (1971).

We now leave the topic of estimation and turn to the question of testing statistical hypotheses.

5.3   TESTING STATISTICAL HYPOTHESES

The concept of testing hypotheses is fundamental to statistical inference. As indicated earlier in the chapter, hypothesis testing refers to the body of statistical techniques that can be used to arrive at a yes or no decision regarding a particular hypothesis.

An example best illustrates the nature of statistical tests of hypotheses. The concepts discussed in the following section are general, however, and are central to all statistical tests of hypotheses.

5.3.1   Hypotheses Testing for a Population Mean μ: σ^2 Known

Suppose past experience indicates that a strain of rats treated with 80 mg/kg hexobarbital have a mean sleeping time of 26 min. Furthermore, assume that sleeping time as a random variable is normally distributed with a population standard deviation of 3 min. Accordingly, the graph in Figure 5.1 describes the probability distribution for this random variable.

Suppose an experiment is to be conducted to determine if iproniazid (100 mg/kg) increases the hexobarbital-induced sleeping time in rats. Let us assume further, for purposes of exposition, that the sleeping time distribution is still normal and $\sigma = 3$ for those animals treated with iproniazid and hexobarbital; hence, Figure 5.1 shows the assumed distribution, except that μ might be greater than 26. Thus, we are interested in determining if the distribution of sleeping times is shifted to the right so that μ exceeds 26. The strategy adopted in a statistical approach to test this hypothesis is to assume that iproniazid does *not* increase the mean sleeping time; this hypothesis is discarded only if the sample outcome has a small probability of occurring under this hypothesis of no increase. In this way, the burden of "proof" for discarding this hypothesis of no increase rests

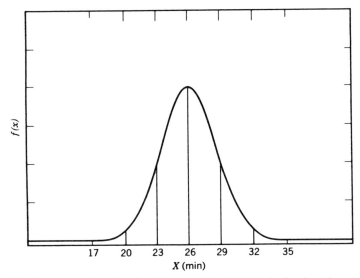

Figure 5.1. Frequency function for the normally distributed sleeping time variable: $\mu = 26$ min; $\sigma = 3$ min.

with the sample data. Consequently, one sets as the "alternative hypothesis" the hypothesis of increased sleeping time. Notationally, we have

$$H_0: \quad \mu = 26 \text{ as the null hypothesis, and}$$

$$\tag{5.17}$$

$$H_a: \quad \mu > 26 \text{ as the alternative hypothesis.}$$

Let us suppose that nine animals have been chosen for study and their observed iproniazid–hexobarbital sleeping times are 25, 31, 24, 28, 29, 30, 31, 33, and 35 min. Assuming these data are a random sample from the population, the statistic $\overline{X}$ has a normal distribution. Furthermore, if H_0 is true, then $\overline{X}$ has a mean of 26 min. On the other hand, if H_a is true, then the mean of $\overline{X}$ is greater than 26 min. In either case, the assumed variance of $\overline{X}$ is $\sigma^2/n = (3)^2/9 = 1$. Thus, the statistic $\overline{X}$ is normally distributed with a variance of 1 and a mean of 26 or greater than 26, depending on which hypothesis is true.* Graphically, the distribution of $\overline{X}$ under the null hypothesis is shown in Figure 5.2.

*Recall that for large n, $\overline{X}$ is approximately normal no matter what the underlying distribution, so the discussion in this section applies to the general situation in which the population distribution is not known but σ^2 is known.

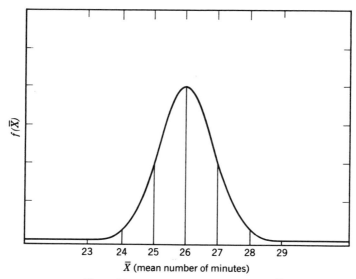

$\overline{X}$ (mean number of minutes)

Figure 5.2. Null hypothesis distribution of $\overline{X}$.

Under the alternative hypothesis, the mean of $\overline{X}$ is greater than 26. What values of $\overline{X}$ should lead us to retain H_0 and what values of $\overline{X}$ should lead us to reject H_0? One procedure to follow is to specify a small probability, say 0.05 or 0.01, and determine from Figure 5.2 the values of $\overline{X}$ that are in the extreme 0.05 or 0.01 of the distribution. For this problem, we would be interested in those values of $\overline{X}$ that are large since these would strongly favor the alternative hypothesis. In Figure 5.3, the set of values of $\overline{X}$ in the upper 0.05 of the null hypothesis distribution in Figure 5.2 is sketched.

Figure 5.3 suggests the following rule for deciding on H_0:

$$\text{Reject } H_0 \text{ in favor of } H_a \quad \text{if } \overline{X} > \overline{X}_{0.95},$$
$$\text{Do not reject } H_0 \qquad\qquad \text{if } \overline{X} \le \overline{X}_{0.95}, \tag{5.18}$$

where $\overline{X}_{0.95}$ is such that $\Pr[\overline{X} < \overline{X}_{0.95}|\mu = 26] = 0.95$. In this case, $\overline{X}_{0.95} = 27.65$. Clearly, if rule (5.18) is followed, then 5% of the time when the null hypothesis is true, it would be rejected. This is an error and is termed the type I error of the test. The probability of this type I error is called the level of significance of the test and is denoted by the symbol α. Hence, in probability notation, the probability of a type I error is

$$\alpha = \Pr[\text{Reject } H_0|H_0 \text{ true}]. \tag{5.19}$$

That is, α is the probability of rejecting H_0 given that H_0 is true.

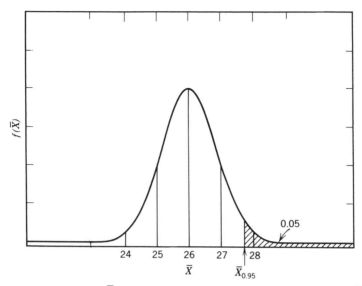

Figure 5.3. Values of $\overline{X}$ in the upper 5% of the null hypothesis distribution of $\overline{X}$.

Definition 5.3.1.1. For testing a null hypothesis H_0 against an alternative hypothesis, the *type I error of the test* is the rejection of the null hypothesis when it is true. The probability of a type I error is called the *significance level of the test* and is usually denoted by α.

If it turns out that the null hypothesis is rejected, it is frequently stated as a "statistically significant result at the $(\alpha)100\%$ level." It is imperative to recall the structure of statistical tests when reading the results of a study that are declared significant. This term has a very precise interpretation in the context of testing a hypothesis. Conversely, a result that is not significant does not "prove" the null hypothesis, since the null hypothesis is assumed to hold unless the data indicate strong evidence to the contrary. Therefore, nonsignificant results should be stated in weaker terms than significant findings. One way to state nonsignificant results is to indicate that the null hypothesis is not rejected, or that there is insufficient evidence for rejection, rather than stating that the null hypothesis is accepted.

How do we determine the region of rejection shown in Figure 5.3? That is, how do we determine $\overline{X}_{0.95}$? In the sleeping time problem we can determine $\overline{X}_{0.95}$ of Figure 5.3 using Equation (4.23): $\sqrt{n}\,(\overline{X}-\mu)/\sigma = Z$. In particular, since $\overline{X}$ is normal, we know that $\sqrt{9}\,(\overline{X}-\mu)/3 = Z$, where Z is the standard normal variate. Then, $0.95 = \Pr(\overline{X} \le \overline{X}_{0.95}|\mu = 26) = \Pr[\sqrt{9}\,(\overline{X}-26)/3 \le \sqrt{9}\,(\overline{X}_{0.95}-26)/3] = \Pr[Z \le \sqrt{9}\,(\overline{X}_{0.95}-26)/3]$, which implies that $Z_{0.95} = \sqrt{9}\,(\overline{X}_{0.95}-26)/3$. From Table 4, of the Appendix,

$Z_{0.95} = 1.645$. Hence, if $\mu = 26$, it follows that $\sqrt{9}(\overline{X}_{0.95} - 26)/3 = 1.645$. Thus, $\overline{X}_{0.95} = 27.65$. Therefore, from decision rule (5.18), the set of values of $\overline{X}$ that lead to rejecting H_0 is the set $\overline{X} > 27.65$; this region is called the critical region. More precisely, it would be termed an α-*level critical region*, since it corresponds to the significance level of α.

Definition 5.3.1.2.   The *critical region* is the set of values of the test statistic that lead to rejection of the null hypothesis.

More generally, if $\mu = \mu_0$, then

$$\sqrt{n}\left(\overline{X} - \mu_0\right)/\sigma = Z \quad \text{and} \quad \sqrt{n}\left(\overline{X}_{1-\alpha} - \mu_0\right)/\sigma = Z_{1-\alpha};$$

thus,

$$\overline{X}_{1-\alpha} = \mu_0 + Z_{1-\alpha}\sigma/\sqrt{n}. \tag{5.20}$$

Hence, for the problem of testing H_0: $\mu = \mu_0$ versus H_a: $\mu > \mu_0$, the α-level critical region is $\overline{X} > \mu_0 + Z_{1-\alpha}\sigma/\sqrt{n}$. Using a similar argument, for the alternative H_a: $\mu < \mu_0$, the α-level critical region is $\overline{X} < \mu_0 - Z_{1-\alpha}\sigma/\sqrt{n}$.

From the sample of nine observations, $\overline{X}$ is computed as 29.56 min; hence, from expression (5.18), the null hypothesis would be rejected, since $29.56 > 27.65$. The conclusion then is that the mean sleeping time of this strain of rats treated with iproniazid and hexobarbital is greater than 26 min ($\alpha = 0.05$).

While one can incur the error of rejecting a true null hypothesis, a similar probability exists of rejecting a false null hypothesis. To illustrate this, let us assume that iproniazid does indeed increase sleeping time to 28 min. What chance do we have of rejecting H_0 if $\mu = 28$? In effect, we must determine the probability that $\overline{X} > 27.65$ if $\mu = 28$. The desired probability is shaded in Figure 5.4. The probability of the shaded region is $\Pr[\overline{X} > 27.65|\mu = 28]$ which, using Equation (4.23), is

$$\Pr[\text{Reject } H_0|\mu = 28] = \Pr[Z > -0.35], \tag{5.21}$$

since $\Pr[\text{Reject } H_0|\mu = 28] = \Pr[\overline{X} > 27.65|\mu = 28] = \Pr[\sqrt{9}(\overline{X} - 28)/3 > \sqrt{9}(27.65 - 28)/3] = \Pr[Z > -0.35]$. This probability is termed the *power of the test* (5.18) when $\mu = 28$. It is our ability to detect a true alternative hypothesis.

The probability of a type II error is the probability of accepting H_0 when H_a is true; hence, the type II error probability of the test (5.18) when

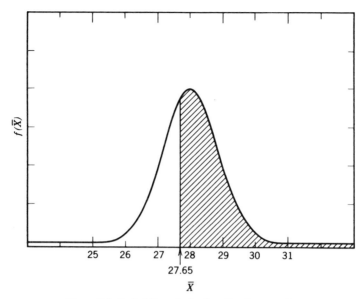

Figure 5.4. Probability of rejecting H_0 when $\mu = 28$.

$\mu = 28$ is given, from Equation (5.21), by

$$\Pr[\text{Accept } H_0 | \mu = 28] = 1 - \Pr[\text{Reject } H_0 | \mu = 28]$$

$$= 1 - \Pr[Z > -0.35] = \Pr[Z < -0.35]. \quad (5.22)$$

The type II error probability is denoted by β and the power is therefore $1 - \beta$.

Definition 5.3.1.3. The *type II error of a test* is the acceptance of the null hypothesis when the alternative hypothesis is true. The probability of a type II error is denoted by β. The *power of the test* is the probability of rejecting the null hypothesis when the alternative hypothesis is true and is equal to $1 - \beta$ since it is 1 minus the probability of a type II error.

From Figure 5.4, it is evident that the power of the test increases as μ increases; hence, the test has a higher probability of detecting the alternative that $\mu = 30$ than it does to detect the alternative $\mu = 28$.

One further term that is useful in hypothesis testing problems is that of a P value. We computed an $\bar{X}$ of 29.56 min while the rejection region consists of those values greater than 27.65. Clearly, the null hypothesis is rejected at $\alpha = 0.05$; however, the observed value of $\bar{X}$ is *so* extreme that it may be of value to quantify its extremeness by computing the probability that an $\overline{X}$ as extreme as 29.56 or more extreme would be observed under H_0. That is, it may be of interest to compute $\Pr[\overline{X} > 29.56 | \mu = 26]$. This quantity would be termed the P value and is simply the probability, under the null hypothesis, of observing a result as extreme or more extreme as the one observed.

Definition 5.3.1.4. The P *value* of a statistical test is the probability of observing a sample outcome as extreme or more extreme as the one observed. This probability is computed under the assumption that the null hypothesis is true.

Hence, the P value for this example is $\Pr[\overline{X} > 29.56 | \mu = 26] = \Pr[\sqrt{9}(\overline{X} - 26)/3 > \sqrt{9}(29.56 - 26)/3] = \Pr[Z > 3.56] \doteq 0.0002$ from Table 4 of the Appendix. The results of this experiment may then be reported as statistically significant with a P value of 0.0002. This is a rather common way of reporting the results of a statistical test.

It should be evident that there are several factors in the hypothesis testing problem: α, β, the null and alternative hypotheses, and the sample size. They are interrelated.

Consider the example we have been considering, and suppose it was desired to set α at 0.01 rather than 0.05. If we do this, then from (5.20) we have $\overline{X}_{0.99} = 26 + 2.33(3)/\sqrt{9} = 28.33$ since $Z_{0.99} = 2.33$, and the decision rule is

$$\text{Reject } H_0: \mu = 26 \qquad \text{if } \overline{X} > 28.33,$$
$$\text{Do not reject } H_0: \mu = 26 \quad \text{if } \overline{X} \le 28.33. \tag{5.23}$$

What effect does rule (5.23) have on the type II error probability? At $\mu = 28$, $\Pr[\overline{X} \le 28.33 | \mu = 28] = \Pr[Z \le (28.33 - 28)/1] = \Pr[Z < 0.33]$. Comparing this to criteria (5.22), the type II error probability has notably increased with the decrease in α, since $\Pr[Z < -0.35] < \Pr[Z < 0.33]$. Thus, the decrease in α has resulted in the power of the test decreasing. This is a general result: for a fixed alternative hypothesis and a fixed sample size, a decrease in α results in an increase in β.

Finally, let us examine the role of sample size in this test. Consider the case in which $\alpha = 0.05$. Suppose n is increased from 9 to 16. In this case, $\sigma/\sqrt{n} = 3/\sqrt{16} = 0.75$, and the critical region becomes $\overline{X} > 27.23$ as $Z_{0.95} = 1.645$ and $\overline{X}_{0.95} = 26 + 1.645(0.75) = 27.23$ by (5.20). The type II error probability of this test at $\mu = 28$ is $\Pr[\overline{X} \le 27.23 | \mu = 28]$. From (4.23) we obtain

$$\Pr[\overline{X} \le 27.23 | \mu = 28] = \Pr[Z \le (27.23 - 28)/(0.75)]$$
$$= \Pr[Z \le -1.03]. \tag{5.24}$$

Comparing equation (5.24) to equation (5.22), it is clear that result (5.24) is smaller since $\Pr[Z < -1.03] < \Pr[Z < -0.35]$. That is, for a fixed alternative hypothesis and α, the increase in sample size has decreased β, which means that the power $1 - \beta$ has increased. This is precisely why sample size is such an important consideration in the planning of a study. The power of the test, or the ability to detect an alternative, increases with n. In general, we specify an alternative hypothesis of interest, and then determine n so that there is a high power to detect this alternative.

Thus, for the general problem of testing a null hypothesis versus an alternative hypothesis, certain relationships exist between α, β, n, and the alternative hypothesis. Two main points are:

1. For a fixed α and alternative hypothesis, an increase in n yields increased power, that is, $1 - \beta$ increases.
2. For a fixed n and alternative hypothesis, an increase in α yields a decrease in β.

The preceding problem is an example of a *one-sided alternative hypothesis* since the alternative specified that μ was greater than 26 min. The test (5.18) is a *one-tailed test* because only large values of $\overline{X}$ lead to rejection of H_0. A *two-sided alternative hypothesis* would be appropriate if one wanted to test if iproniazid *altered* the mean sleeping time without any particular direction stated. In this case, the testing problem would be stated as that of testing

$$H_0: \mu = 26 \quad \text{versus} \quad H_a: \mu \neq 26. \tag{5.25}$$

Note that the alternative includes both $\mu < 26$ and $\mu > 26$ as possible alternative hypotheses. In this situation, both large and small values of $\overline{X}$ should lead to rejecting H_0 in favor of H_a. To construct a 0.05-level two-tailed test of (5.25), we would place 0.025 in each tail of the null hypothesis distribution given in Figure 5.5. Consequently, the critical region would be defined by those values of $\overline{X}$ less than $\overline{X}_{0.025}$ and those values of $\overline{X}$ greater than $\overline{X}_{0.975}$, where $\overline{X}_{0.025}$ and $\overline{X}_{0.975}$ are defined by

$$\Pr[\overline{X} < \overline{X}_{0.025}|\mu = 26] = 0.025,$$
$$\tag{5.26}$$
$$\Pr[\overline{X} > \overline{X}_{0.975}|\mu = 26] = 0.025,$$

and are shown in Figure 5.5. Using (5.20) and Table 4 of the Appendix, we obtain $Z_{0.025} = -1.96$, $Z_{0.975} = +1.96$, and therefore $\overline{X}_{0.025} = 26 - 1.96(1) = 24.04$ and $\overline{X}_{0.975} = 26 + 1.96(1) = 27.96$, since $\sigma/\sqrt{n} = 3/\sqrt{9} = 1$. The

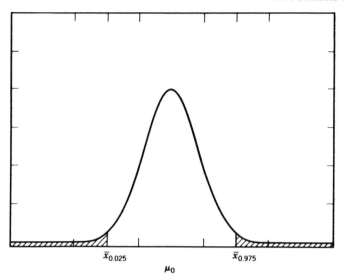

$$\bar{x}_{0.025} \qquad\qquad \bar{x}_{0.975}$$
$$\mu_0$$

Figure 5.5. Two-sided 0.05 critical region for testing (5.25).

decision rule is then

$$\text{Reject } H_0 \qquad \text{if } \bar{X} < 24.04 \text{ or } \bar{X} > 27.96,$$

$$\text{(5.27)}$$

$$\text{Do not reject } H_0 \quad \text{if } 24.04 \le \bar{X} \le 27.96.$$

Moreover, power and type II error could be determined for a particular alternative hypothesis, as we did for the one-sided alternative hypothesis.

Thus far, the decision rules have been in terms of $\bar{X}$; these are summarized in Table 5.1. However, the decision rules can also be expressed in terms of the statistic $Z = \sqrt{n}(\bar{X} - \mu_0)/\sigma$. For example, rejecting H_0 if $\bar{X} > \bar{X}_{1-\alpha} = \mu_0 + Z_{1-\alpha}\sigma/\sqrt{n}$ is equivalent to rejecting H_0 if $Z = \sqrt{n}(\bar{X} - \mu_0)/\sigma > Z_{1-\alpha}$. In Table 5.2, the decision rules given in Table 5.1 are expressed in terms of $Z = \sqrt{n}(\bar{X} - \mu_0)/\sigma$.

Since the standard deviation of $\bar{X}$ is $\sigma/\sqrt{n}$, then $Z = \sqrt{n}(\bar{X} - \mu_0)/\sigma$ is the number of standard deviations that $\bar{X}$ is from μ_0. Thus, rejecting H_0 if $\bar{X}$ is much greater than μ_0 is equivalent to rejecting H_0 if Z is much greater than zero, and rejecting H_0 if $\bar{X}$ is much less than μ_0 is equivalent to rejecting H_0 if Z is much less than zero. Recalling that Z will have a standard normal distribution under the null hypothesis if the population is normal, or an approximate standard normal distribution if the population

Table 5.1. Hypotheses Tests for μ: σ^2 Known (Decision Rules in Terms of $\overline{X}$)

A. Data: Random sample $X_1, X_2, \ldots, X_n$ from a population with mean μ and variance σ^2.
B. Assumption: σ^2 is known.
C. Sample size requirements: If the population is normal, n can be any size; if the population is not normal, n must be large.
D. Computation: $\overline{X} = \sum_{i=1}^{n} X_i/n$.
E. Hypotheses tests:

Hypotheses	Decision rule
H_0: $\mu = \mu_0$ H_a: $\mu > \mu_0$	Reject H_0 if $\overline{X} > \mu_0 + Z_{1-\alpha}\sigma/\sqrt{n}$
H_0: $\mu = \mu_0$ H_a: $\mu < \mu_0$	Reject H_0 if $\overline{X} < \mu_0 - Z_{1-\alpha}\sigma/\sqrt{n}$
H_0: $\mu = \mu_0$ H_a: $\mu \neq \mu_0$	Reject H_0 if $\overline{X} > \mu_0 + Z_{1-\alpha/2}\sigma/\sqrt{n}$ or if $\overline{X} < \mu_0 - Z_{1-\alpha/2}\sigma/\sqrt{n}$

Table 5.2. Hypotheses Tests for μ: σ^2 Known (Decision Rules in Terms of Z)

A. Data: Random sample $X_1, X_2, \ldots, X_n$ from a population with mean μ and variance σ^2.
B. Assumption: σ^2 is known.
C. Sample size requirements: If the population is normal, n can be any size; if the population is not normal, n must be large.
D. Computation: $Z = \sqrt{n}(\overline{X} - \mu_0)/\sigma$.
E. Hypotheses tests:

Hypotheses	Decision rule
H_0: $\mu = \mu_0$ H_a: $\mu > \mu_0$	Reject H_0 if $Z > Z_{1-\alpha}$
H_0: $\mu = \mu_0$ H_a: $\mu < \mu_0$	Reject H_0 if $Z < -Z_{1-\alpha}$
H_0: $\mu = \mu_0$ H_a: $\mu \neq \mu_0$	Reject H_0 if $Z > Z_{1-\alpha/2}$ or if $Z < -Z_{1-\alpha/2}$

is not normal but the sample size is large, then Table 5.2 should be easy to understand.

In the example, we had $\bar{X} = 29.56$, $n = 9$, and $\sigma = 3$. For testing H_0: $\mu = 26$ against H_a: $\mu > 26$ at the 0.05 significance level using the Z statistic, the decision rule then is to reject H_0 if $Z > Z_{0.95} = 1.645$. Since $Z = \sqrt{9}\,(29.56 - 26)/3 = 3.56 > 1.645$, then H_0 is rejected in favor of H_a at the 0.05 significance level.

We now turn to some further examples of one-population testing problems.

5.3.2 Hypothesis Testing for a Population Mean μ: σ^2 Unknown

It is very unusual in practice to *know* the population variance σ^2; when σ^2 is not known, it is generally estimated by the sample variance s^2. Therefore, in place of Z, we use t to formulate our decision rules for the mean, analogous to those developed in the previous section. Specifically, if

$$t = \sqrt{n}\,\frac{\bar{X} - \mu_0}{s}, \tag{5.28}$$

then t has a $t(n - 1)$ distribution under the null hypothesis if the population is normal; if the population is not normal but the sample size is large, then t has an approximate $t(n - 1)$ distribution. Thus, a critical region of size α for testing

$$H_0: \mu = \mu_0 \quad \text{versus} \quad H_a: \mu > \mu_0 \tag{5.29}$$

may be determined by finding $t_{1-\alpha}(n - 1)$ from Table 5 of the Appendix and then solving $t_{1-\alpha}(n - 1) = \sqrt{n}\,(\bar{X} - \mu_0)/s$ for $\bar{X}$. The decision rule for testing H_0 versus H_a in (5.29) would be

$$\begin{aligned} &\text{Reject } H_0 && \text{if } \bar{X} > \mu_0 + t_{1-\alpha}(n - 1)s/\sqrt{n}\,, \\ &\text{Do not reject } H_0 && \text{if } \bar{X} \le \mu_0 + t_{1-\alpha}(n - 1)s/\sqrt{n}\,. \end{aligned} \tag{5.30}$$

Note that (5.30) is similar to the rules given in the prior section, except t replaces Z and s replaces σ. Alternatively, the decision rule can be defined in terms of t statistics. Defining $t = \sqrt{n}\,(\bar{X} - \mu_0)/s$, then the rule equivalent to (5.30) is

$$\begin{aligned} &\text{Reject } H_0 && \text{if } t > t_{1-\alpha}(n - 1), \\ &\text{Do not reject } H_0 && \text{if } t \le t_{1-\alpha}(n - 1). \end{aligned} \tag{5.31}$$

Example 5.3.2.1. Consider the sleeping time data of the previous section in which the nine observations are 25, 31, 24, 28, 29, 30, 31, 33, and 35 min. From these we wish to test at $\alpha = 0.05$,

$$H_0: \mu = 26 \quad \text{versus} \quad H_a: \mu > 26.$$

Suppose that the population variance is unknown and must be estimated from the sample. We assume the nine observations are from a normal population. From these data, we compute

$$\overline{X} = 29.56, \qquad s^2 = 12.53, \qquad s = 3.539.$$

From Table 5 of the Appendix, $t_{.95}(8) = 1.860$, and we reject H_0 if the computed t exceeds 1.860. The computed t is

$$t = \frac{\sqrt{9}\,(29.56 - 26)}{3.539} = 3.02$$

which exceeds 1.860; thus, we reject H_0 in favor of H_a at the 0.05 significance level.

It is evident from the development that a test of the other one-sided alternative hypothesis, that is, $H_a: \mu < \mu_0$, would be based on small values of t, that is, $t < -t_{1-\alpha}(n-1)$. The decision for testing $H_0: \mu = \mu_0$ versus $H_a: \mu < \mu_0$ would be

$$\begin{aligned}
\text{Reject } H_0 \qquad & \text{if } t < -t_{1-\alpha}(n-1), \\
\text{Do not reject } H_0 \quad & \text{if } t \geq -t_{1-\alpha}(n-1).
\end{aligned} \qquad (5.32)$$

In addition, for a two-sided alternative hypothesis $H_a: \mu \neq \mu_0$, the decision rule would be the two-tailed test; that is,

$$\text{Reject } H_0 \qquad \text{if } \begin{cases} t < -t_{1-\alpha/2}(n-1) \\ \text{or} \\ t > t_{1-\alpha/2}(n-1), \end{cases}$$

$$\text{Do not reject } H_0 \quad \text{if } -t_{1-\alpha/2}(n-1) \leq t \leq t_{1-\alpha/2}(n-1).$$

Thus, one- and two-sided alternative hypotheses lead to the same type of decision rules as in the last section, with tests here based on the t rather than the Z distribution. These tests are summarized in Table 5.3.

Table 5.3. Hypotheses Tests for μ: σ^2 Unknown (Decision Rules in Terms of t)

A. Data: Random sample $X_1, X_2, \ldots, X_n$ from a population with mean μ and variance σ^2.
B. Sample size requirements: If the population is normal, n can be any size; if the population is not normal, n must be large.
C. Computation: $t = \sqrt{n}\,(\overline{X} - \mu_0)/s$.
D. Hypotheses tests:

Hypotheses	Decision rule
$H_0: \ \mu = \mu_0$ $H_a: \ \mu > \mu_0$	Reject H_0 if $t > t_{1-\alpha}(n-1)$
$H_0: \ \mu = \mu_0$ $H_a: \ \mu < \mu_0$	Reject H_0 if $t < -t_{1-\alpha}(n-1)$
$H_0: \ \mu = \mu_0$ $H_a: \ \mu \neq \mu_0$	Reject H_0 if $t > t_{1-\alpha/2}(n-1)$ or if $t < -t_{1-\alpha/2}(n-1)$

5.3.3 Hypothesis Testing for a Normal Population Variance σ^2

When discussing confidence intervals for a normal population variance σ^2, we used the chi-square distribution; specifically, we used the property that $(n-1)s^2/\sigma^2 = \chi^2(n-1)$. For testing

$$H_0: \sigma^2 = \sigma_0^2 \quad \text{versus} \quad H_a: \sigma^2 \neq \sigma_0^2 \tag{5.33}$$

we can use $(n-1)s^2/\sigma_0^2$ as the criterion statistic, since under H_0 it follows a chi-square distribution with $n-1$ degrees of freedom. The rejection rule for testing H_0 versus the two-sided alternative in (5.33) would be

$$\text{Reject } H_0 \quad \text{if} \begin{cases} \dfrac{(n-1)s^2}{\sigma_0^2} > \chi^2_{1-\alpha/2}(n-1) \\ \text{or} \\ \dfrac{(n-1)s^2}{\sigma_0^2} < \chi^2_{\alpha/2}(n-1) \end{cases} \tag{5.34}$$

$$\text{Do not reject } H_0 \quad \text{if } \chi^2_{\alpha/2}(n-1) \leq \frac{(n-1)s^2}{\sigma_0^2} \leq \chi^2_{1-\sigma/2}(n-1)$$

where $\chi^2_{\alpha/2}(n-1)$ and $\chi^2_{1-\alpha/2}(n-1)$ may be obtained from Table 6 of the Appendix.

Example 5.3.3.1. Continuing with the sleeping time data, suppose there is interest in testing H_0: $\sigma^2 = 9$ versus H_a: $\sigma^2 \neq 9$ at $\alpha = 0.05$. We have previously computed $s^2 = 12.53$. From Table 6 of the Appendix, $\chi^2_{0.025}(8) = 2.18$ and $\chi^2_{0.975}(8) = 17.53$. We compute $(n - 1)s^2/\sigma_0^2 = 8(12.53)/9 = 11.14$. This number neither exceeds 17.5 nor is less than 2.18; therefore, we have insufficient evidence to reject H_0.

For the one-sided alternative hypothesis H_a: $\sigma^2 < \sigma_0^2$ (H_a: $\sigma^2 > \sigma_0^2$), rejection of H_0 would be decided if $(n - 1)s^2/\sigma_0^2 < \chi^2_\alpha(n - 1)$ ($(n - 1)s^2/\sigma_0^2 > \chi^2_{1-\alpha}(n - 1)$).

5.3.4 Hypothesis Testing for Binomial Parameter p

For a binomial population, it may be of interest to test the hypothesis that the parameter p takes a certain value p_0. Similar to the confidence interval discussion, two procedures are presented. The first is the test based on the exact binomial distribution, while the second test is based on the central limit theorem and uses the normal distribution.

We assume a random sample of size n from a binomial population, and for convenience, we denote the total number of successes by y and the sample proportion by $\hat{p}$, where $\hat{p} = y/n$. Our interest is in testing

$$H_0: p = p_0 \quad \text{versus} \quad H_a: p \neq p_0. \tag{5.35}$$

Similar to problems involving the normal distribution, we determine the critical region by specifying a significance level and then examine the distribution of the test statistic under H_0. Under H_0 the distribution of Y would appear as in Figure 5.6; therefore, we must find that value of Y, call it $y_{\alpha/2}$, so that

$$\Pr\left[Y \leq y_{\alpha/2}\right] = \sum_{i=0}^{y_{\alpha/2}} \binom{n}{i} p_0^i (1 - p_0)^{n-i} = \alpha/2 \tag{5.36}$$

and that value of Y, call it $y_{1-\alpha/2}$, so that

$$\Pr\left[Y \geq y_{1-\alpha/2}\right] = \sum_{i=y_{1-\alpha/2}}^{n} \binom{n}{i} p_0^i (1 - p_0)^{n-i} = \alpha/2. \tag{5.37}$$

Once these values are determined, the critical region is $y \leq y_{\alpha/2}$ and $y \geq y_{1-\alpha/2}$.

Since the probability distribution of Y is discrete, it may not be possible to determine $y_{\alpha/2}$ and $y_{1-\alpha/2}$ to satisfy the equalities in (5.36) and (5.37).

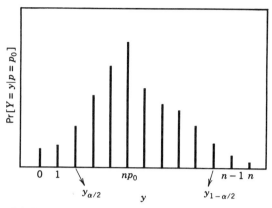

Figure 5.6. Determination of critical region for two-tailed binomial test.

Accordingly, in order to ensure that the size of the critical region is no bigger than α (i.e., $\leq \alpha$), we choose $y_{\alpha/2}$ and $y_{1-\alpha/2}$ to satisfy the following:

$$\sum_{i=0}^{y_{\alpha/2}} \binom{n}{i} p_0^i (1 - p_0)^{n-i} \leq \alpha/2,$$

$$\sum_{i=0}^{y_{\alpha/2}+1} \binom{n}{i} p_0^i (1 - p_0)^{n-i} > \alpha/2,$$

(5.38)

and

$$\sum_{i=y_{1-\alpha/2}}^{n} \binom{n}{i} p_0^i (1 - p_0)^{n-i} \leq \alpha/2,$$

$$\sum_{i=y_{1-\alpha/2}-1}^{n} \binom{n}{i} p_0^i (1 - p_0)^{n-i} > \alpha/2.$$

(5.39)

Table 2 of the Appendix can be used to determine a critical region for certain n and p; more extensive tables can be found in the Documenta Geigy Scientific Tables (1962).

Example 5.3.4.1. Suppose 40% of leukemia patients treated with the conventional therapy improve. In a clinical trial of 25 patients, 14 of the patients showed improvement on a test therapy. Is this sufficient evidence to reject the hypothesis that the improvement rate is 0.40? We shall use H_0: $p = 0.4$, H_a: $p \neq 0.4$, and $\alpha = 0.05$.

From Table 2 of the Appendix, we refer to $n = 25$ and $p = 0.40$ since H_0: $p = 0.40$. From this table, we find $\Pr[Y \leq 4] = 0.00947$ and $\Pr[Y \leq 5] = 0.02936$; therefore, $y_{0.025} = 4$. In addition, $\Pr[Y \geq 16] = 1 - \Pr[Y \leq 15] = 1 - 0.98683 = 0.01317$ and $\Pr[Y \geq 15] = 1 - \Pr[Y \leq 14] = 1 - 0.96561 = 0.03439$ so $y_{0.975} = 16$. Hence, our critical region is $y \leq 4$ or $y \geq 16$, and the actual significance level is $0.00947 + 0.01317 = 0.02264$, which is ≤ 0.05. Since the observed value of Y is 14, we do not have sufficient evidence to reject the null hypothesis.

A test like the one just performed in which the actual significance level (0.02264) is less than the nominal size of 0.05 is called a *conservative* test. In order to ensure the significance level, or validity, of the test, we shall retain H_0 more often than we would like. Naturally, conservative tests are less powerful than their nonconservative counterparts. For discrete probability distributions, the exact desired significance level usually cannot be attained, particularly when n is small, and it is generally recommended to err on the side of keeping the actual significance level less than rather than greater than the desired significance level.

Exact binomial tests for one-sided alternatives may also be performed with the obvious modifications of (5.35), (5.38), and (5.39). For H_a: $p > p_0$, (5.39) is modified by replacing $\alpha/2$ everywhere by α; and for H_a: $p < p_0$, (5.38) is modified by replacing $\alpha/2$ everywhere by α.

If n is sufficiently large so that $np_0(1 - p_0) \geq 5$, then the normal distribution approximation to the binomial may be used to test H_0 since the central limit theorem applies. In particular, the statistic $Z = (\hat{p} - p_0)/\sqrt{p_0(1 - p_0)/n}$ may be compared to the standard normal values of $Z_{1-\alpha/2}$ and $-Z_{1-\alpha/2}$ to test H_0 versus H_a in (5.35). The test criterion is

$$\text{Reject } H_0 \quad \text{if} \begin{cases} \dfrac{(\hat{p} - p_0)}{\sqrt{p_0(1 - p_0)/n}} > Z_{1-\alpha/2} \\ \text{or} \\ \dfrac{(\hat{p} - p_0)}{\sqrt{p_0(1 - p_0)/n}} < -Z_{1-\alpha/2}, \end{cases} \qquad (5.40)$$

$$\text{Do not reject } H_0 \quad \text{if} \quad -Z_{1-\alpha/2} \leq \dfrac{(p - p_0)}{\sqrt{p_0(1 - p_0)/n}} \leq Z_{1-\alpha/2}.$$

Example 5.3.4.2. Continuing the last example, we note that $np_0(1 - p_0) = 25(0.4)(0.6) = 6$, so the normal approximation test criterion (5.40) can be

Table 5.4. Hypotheses Tests for Binomial Parameter p
(Decision Rules in Terms of Z)

A. Data: Random sample $X_1, X_2, \ldots, X_n$ from a binomial population.
B. Sample size requirements: n must be sufficiently large so that $np_0(1 - p_0) \geq 5$; otherwise, the exact test described in the text should be used.
C. Computation: $Z = (\hat{p} - p_0)/\sqrt{p_0(1 - p_0)/n}$
D. Hypotheses tests:

Hypotheses	Decision rule
$H_0: \quad p = p_0$ $H_a: \quad p > p_0$	Reject H_0 if $Z > Z_{1-\alpha}$
$H_0: \quad p = p_0$ $H_a: \quad p < p_0$	Reject H_0 if $Z < -Z_{1-\alpha}$
$H_0: \quad p = p_0$ $H_a: \quad p \neq p_0$	Reject H_0 if $Z > Z_{1-\alpha/2}$ or if $Z < -Z_{1-\alpha/2}$

used. At $\alpha = 0.05$, $-Z_{0.975} = -1.96$ and $Z_{0.975} = 1.96$ from Table 4 of the Appendix. Since $\hat{p} = \frac{14}{25} = 0.56$, we have

$$\frac{0.56 - 0.40}{\sqrt{0.4(0.6)/25}} = \frac{0.16}{0.0979} = 1.63$$

and $-1.96 \leq 1.63 \leq 1.96$, so $H_0: p = 0.4$ is not rejected.

The one-sided alternative hypothesis $H_a: p < p_0$ ($H_a: p > p_0$) is accompanied by the corresponding one-tailed critical region

$$\frac{\hat{p} - p_0}{\sqrt{p_0(1 - p_0)/n}} < -Z_{1-\alpha} \left(\frac{\hat{p} - p_0}{\sqrt{p_0(1 - p_0)/n}} > Z_{1-\alpha} \right)$$

and may be used for situations in which a one-sided alternative is appropriate.

These decision rules for large n are summarized in Table 5.4.

5.4 SUMMARY

In this chapter, we have outlined the general points involved in the testing of hypotheses and in confidence interval estimation. In subsequent chapters, these concepts are used as a basis for many of the analyses. By way of summary, a number of steps are involved, explicitly or implicitly, in testing hypotheses:

1. The null hypothesis H_0 and the alternative hypothesis H_a are specified.
2. The significance level α is chosen.
3. A statistic whose null hypothesis distribution is known is selected for the statistical test.
4. A sample size n is chosen that will yield the power, $1 - \beta$, needed to detect an alternative hypothesis of interest.
5. A critical region is determined.
6. The statistic is computed and compared to the critical region.
7. If the statistic is in the critical region, reject the null hypothesis; otherwise, do not reject it.

Finally, our action is to reject or not reject the null hypothesis; accordingly, if H_0 is true, then its rejection is an error (type I). If H_0 is false, failure to reject it is also an error (type II).

Much of the remainder of this text is devoted to statistical tests and estimators for commonly occurring practical problems. We shall see that testing and estimation go hand in hand for most problems, and where tests are performed, corresponding estimators are also computed. We shall see through applications that hypothesis testing and confidence interval estimation are equivalent concepts in the sense that a $(1 - \alpha)100\%$ confidence interval for a parameter includes all values of that parameter that, if assumed as H_0, would be accepted by the corresponding two-tailed α-level test of H_0. Hence, the concepts of testing and interval estimation are closely related.

PROBLEMS

5.1. A random sample of 49 persons have a total cholesterol mean of $\overline{X} = 240$ mg/dL. Assuming $\sigma = 30$ mg/dL, compute a 95% confidence interval for the population mean.

5.2. In Problem 5.1, determine the sample size necessary to reduce the width of the 95% confidence interval in half.

5.3. Sixteen patients in a medical trial report a mean level of 60 g/week of alcohol consumption and a sample variance of 36. Find a 95% confidence interval for μ. State any assumptions used in solving this problem.

5.4. The white blood cell count in a group of 28 persons has a mean of 6300 with variance equal to 10,000. Obtain a 90% confidence interval for the population variance.

5.5. In an industrial plant, a researcher found lower respiratory tract symptoms in 30 of 40 workers. With this information, obtain a 95% confidence interval for the proportion of symptoms in the population.

5.6. A program to stop smoking expects to obtain a 75% success rate. The observed number of definitive cessations in a group of 100 adults attending the program is 80. Is this sufficient evidence to conclude that the success rate has increased?

5.7. Suppose the average remaining lifetime of a 40-year-old man is 32 years. Thirty men aged 40 are found to live a mean of 35 additional years with standard deviation of 9 years. If the remaining lifetime of a 40-year-old is approximately normally distributed, then test if the expected lifetime of this group is greater than would be expected.

5.8. In Problem 5.7 suppose the population variance is known to be 64, then test the same hypothesis at $\alpha = 0.05$.

5.9. From population mortality data, suppose that 4% of males age 65 die within one year. If it is found that 60 of such males in a group of 1000 die within a year, is this evidence of an increase in mortality in this sample?

5.10. The height of adults living in a suburban area of a large city has a mean equal to 67 in. with a standard deviation of 2.18 in. In a sample of 178 adults living in the inner city area, the mean height is found to be 65 in. Assuming the same standard deviation for the two groups, are the mean heights significantly different?

5.11. If the mean height in the inner city group is known to be 66.5 in, find the power of the test in Problem 5.12.

REFERENCES

Conover, W. J. (1971). *Practical Nonparametric Statistics*, Wiley, New York.

Documenta Geigy Scientific Tables, 6th ed. (1962). Geigy Pharmaceuticals, Division of Geigy Chemical Corporation, Ardsley, NY.

CHAPTER 6

Comparison of Two Groups: *t*-Tests and Rank Tests

6.1 INTRODUCTION

A frequent problem in medical research is the comparison of two groups of individuals. These two groups may be formed in either *observational* or *experimental* investigations—two basic types of medical research studies. They differ in the degree of control the researcher may exercise. A straightforward approach in an experimental study is to use randomization to create the two comparison groups. It is generally impossible, however, to employ randomization in an epidemiologic or observational investigation. In most observational studies, the groups have been created by factors that are not directly under the control of the investigator. Typically, individuals have assigned themselves to various groups, or at least they generally have not been assigned to groups by the investigator. Thus, if there is a significant difference between two diagnostic groups in an observational study, the association may be causal or related to other factors. For example, in a study comparing the academic performance of hyperactive boys to those who are not hyperactive, the differences in academic performance between these two diagnostic groups may be due to hyperactivity or may be due to other factors related to hyperactivity.

On the other hand, in an experimental study the factor under investigation can be controlled. To conduct a therapeutic study of anxiety neurosis, for example, it may be possible for the investigator to control the assignment of the two treatment regimens to the individual patients. In this case, the investigator could employ randomization, in which each person has an equal and independent chance of receiving a given treatment.

For both types of study, differences in outcome between the two study groups may be due to (1) real differences between the effects of the two treatments, (2) differences in the way the groups were handled during the study period, (3) differences between the patients with respect to some initial characteristics, or (4) random chance variations. In an experimental study, it is possible to deal directly with any of these possible explanations for a treatment group difference. In an observational study, it is generally more difficult to completely handle these possible explanations. Explanations 2 and 3 are potentially serious shortcomings of any study. If group differences in the outcome variables are due to differences in the way the groups were handled or due to initial group differences, then these may generally be expected to distort or bias the sample data. Clearly, every attempt should be made in a study to account for and deal with these possible explanations.

Differences due to the manner in which the two groups were managed during the course of a study may be minimized and sometimes entirely discounted by the use of double-blind techniques. These techniques are commonly used in clinical trials, which are experiments involving humans. These trials are often conducted to compare the therapeutic value of a new treatment in contrast to the conventional or standard therapy. A clinical trial is said to be *double blind* if neither the patient nor the person collecting the data knows the treatment the patient is receiving; it is *single blind* if the patient does not know the treatment he is receiving. In some trials, this is not possible; however, for studies involving subjective response data, the technique is invaluable and is almost mandatory. In most studies, a true double-blind study requires more personnel for data collection. If, for example, there simply is no way that the treating physician can avoid knowing the patient's treatment due to ethical considerations, then the study may require an additional person to collect the important response data. In other cases, side effects and other factors may preclude the possibility of this type of study entirely.

In observational studies, it is generally more difficult to deal with this issue of differences in the way groups were handled. In one field follow-up study of psychiatric patients by Tsuang, Woolson, and Simpson (1980), an attempt was made to blind the interviewers from an interviewee's actual diagnosis. In this study, four distinct diagnostic groups of patients were interviewed 40 years after an initial admission for a psychotic illness. The principal device used to blind the field interviewers was to divide the interviewers into two teams, one to arrange the time and place of the interview and the other team to actually conduct the interview.

In general, each study design calls for a careful consideration of the biases that may affect it. It is necessary to consider carefully the possibility of using double- or single-blind techniques, the refinement of data collection instruments, and the possibility of including control or baseline measurements at various points in the study.

The issue of initial differences between the groups can be properly viewed as both a design and analysis question. There are numerous procedures that are used to minimize the effect of this particular problem. One useful device is that of dividing the patients into subgroups of patients so that patients within a subgroup are homogeneous, while those in different subgroups are not. Each subgroup is called a stratum, and hence this procedure is called *stratification* or *frequency matching*. This technique may be applied to both experimental and observational studies. For example, in an observational study where it was of interest to contrast the 40-yr course of illness between paranoid and nonparanoid schizophrenics, it was prudent to first stratify by sex and socioeconomic status. In this manner, the two diagnostic subtypes of schizophrenia can be compared within each sex–socioeconomic status category. Accordingly, from a design standpoint, the planner of such a study would want to be certain that sufficient numbers of patients will be available for study in each sex–socioeconomic status subgroup.

An extreme case of stratification is the *pair-matched* design in which only two persons in each subgroup may be used; if this design had been used in the previously discussed study, each subgroup would have consisted of a paranoid schizophrenic patient and a non–paranoid schizophrenic patient. In a pair-matched design, it is presumed that all of the relevant *confounding variables*—variables that affect the treatment and outcome variables—have been accounted for through the matching. Matching can be a useful technique for an observational study, and it should be noted that there are a number of variations on the matching theme, for example, the use of multiple rather than single controls per case.

In an experimental study, such as a clinical trial, randomization can also be used to create the comparison groups within each subcategory of the stratification variables. In the pair-matched experimental study, for example, the table of random numbers or a coin may be used to decide which person in the pair will be assigned to the first treatment and which to the second. This kind of randomization can ordinarily not be performed in an epidemiologic or other observational study, and differences between outcome variables in the two groups may be due to nonmatched factors that affect both the outcome variables and the criteria of group classification. Dealing with such issues in epidemiologic investigations can be a difficult problem. In experimental studies, the differential effects of such factors are expected to be balanced between the comparison groups through the randomization process. Randomization tends to balance the two groups with respect to unmatched confounding factors. Another feature of randomization is that the assignment of treatments to individual patients is made in an unbiased manner, and patients have an equal opportunity to be assigned to each of the treatment groups. If randomization is not done, it is difficult to rule out the biasing effect of confounding variables as the possible explanation of an observed difference in the response variates.

To summarize, we note that observational and experimental studies differ qualitatively. In an experimental study, it is possible to employ randomization; consequently, the investigator can control or manipulate the factors under study. In this way, antecedent–consequent relationships are more readily studied. Conversely, in an *observational* study, randomization is generally not possible; thus, the control of factors is more difficult. Stratification and other devices are helpful for such studies.

In spite of the differences, statistical estimation and hypotheses testing may be applied to either type of study, although the interpretation of the results can be different. For either type of study, after having done the best that is practicable to remove the effects of explanations 2 and 3, the data analysts are then in a position to deal with the probability or statistical question of assessing the magnitude of the group difference. As one might expect, this assessment depends on both the design of the study and the probability distribution of the outcome variable. For the two-group comparison problem, we shall consider both the matched-pair design and the two-independent-samples design. With regard to the probability distribution of the observations, we shall divide the discussion and presentation into two sections: tests based on the normal distribution (t-tests) and tests using the ranks of the data that do not require the assumption of a normal distribution (rank tests).

6.2   USE OF t-TESTS FOR GROUP COMPARISONS

This class of statistical tests is one of the most widely used in the statistical analysis of medical data. There are two main varieties of the test: the *paired t-test* and the *two-sample t-test*. As one might expect, the paired t-test is applicable to paired data, that is, the matched-pairs design, and the two-sample t-test is for the two-independent-groups design. A common error in using these tests is to apply the two-sample t-test to pair-matched data. This is incorrect since the two-sample t-test requires that the two samples be selected independently of one another. This assumption is not met for the pair-matched design, since one sample is selected to match the other sample on a set of characteristics, and the two samples are therefore dependent. This incorrect application of the two-sample t-test often occurs when the pair-matched data are incomplete, for example, members of some pairs are missing or otherwise fail to provide a response. In this unfortunate situation, it is not appropriate to apply the two-sample t-test to matched-pair data.

Table 6.1. Data Layout for Matched-Pair Studies

Pair	Group 1	Group 2	Differences
1	y_{11}	y_{21}	$y_{11} - y_{21} = d_1$
2	y_{12}	y_{22}	$y_{12} - y_{22} = d_2$
⋮	⋮	⋮	⋮
n	y_{1n}	y_{2n}	$y_{1n} - y_{2n} = d_n$

Both classes of *t*-test, the paired *t*-test and the two-sample *t*-test, require an assumption of an underlying normal distribution. In the case of the paired *t*-test, it is assumed that the pairwise differences are normally distributed; in the case of the two-sample *t*-test, it is assumed that the individual samples are random samples from a normal distribution. We begin with the paired *t*-test.

6.2.1 Paired *t*-Test for Comparing Means: A Test for Matched Pairs

The data for matched-pair studies are generally in the form of Table 6.1, where y_{ij} is the response of the *i*th member of pair *j*.

In order to apply the paired *t*-test procedure properly, we first compute the pairwise differences $d_1, d_2, \ldots, d_n$ which are assumed to be a random sample from a normal distribution. That is, we are assuming that variable *d* has the frequency function given by the expression

$$f(d) = \frac{1}{\sigma_d \sqrt{2\pi}} \exp\left(-\frac{(d - \mu_d)^2}{2\sigma_d^2}\right), \qquad -\infty < d < \infty, \qquad (6.1)$$

where μ_d is the mean and σ_d^2 is the variance of *d*. The inference problem is one of testing the hypothesis that the population mean difference is equal to zero versus either one- or two-sided alternative hypotheses; in addition, we shall consider the problem of estimating μ_d. From the assumption that $d_1, \ldots, d_n$ is a random sample from a normal distribution and recalling that the sample mean from a normal distribution has the same mean as the population sampled and has a variance given by the original population's variance divided by *n*, it follows that the sample mean $\bar{d}$, where $\bar{d} = \sum_{i=1}^{n} d_i/n$, is normal with mean μ_d and variance σ_d^2/n. Thus, $Z = \sqrt{n}(\bar{d} - \mu_d)/\sigma_d$ is a standard normal random variable, and $t = \sqrt{n}(\bar{d} - \mu_d)/s_d$ is a *t* variable with $n - 1$ degrees of freedom, where $s_d^2 = \sum_{i=1}^{n}(d_i - \bar{d})^2/(n - 1)$. Thus, under H_0: $\mu_d = 0$, the statistic $t = \sqrt{n}(\bar{d} - 0)/s_d = \sqrt{n}(\bar{d}/s_d)$ has a $t(n - 1)$ distribution, and a test of H_0: $\mu_d = 0$ can be conducted using

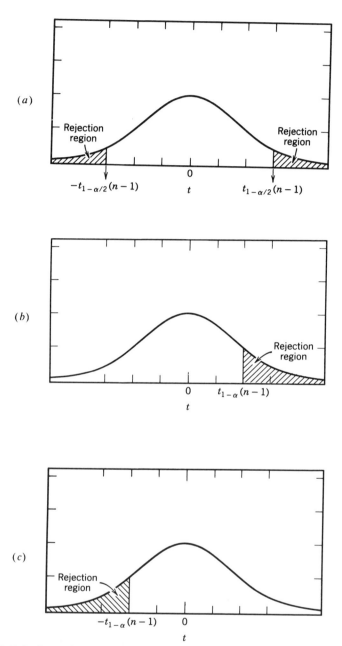

Figure 6.1. Rejection regions for paired t-test: (a) two-tailed α-level test (H_a: $\mu_d \neq 0$; (b) one-tailed α-level test (H_a: $\mu_d > 0$); (c) one-tailed α-level test (H_a: $\mu_d < 0$).

150

Table 6.2. Outline of Paired *t*-Test Procedure for Testing Mean Difference $\mu_d = 0$

A. Data: $d_1, \ldots, d_n$ from Table 6.1.
B. Assumptions: $d_1, \ldots, d_n$ is a random sample from a normal distribution with μ_d and σ_d^2 unknown.
C. Computations:

$$\bar{d} = \sum_{i=1}^{n} \frac{d_i}{n}, \quad \text{the sample mean difference;}$$

$$s_{\bar{d}} = \sqrt{\frac{\sum_{i=1}^{n}(d_i - \bar{d})^2}{n(n-1)}}, \quad \begin{array}{l} \text{the sample standard error of the} \\ \text{mean difference;} \end{array}$$

$$t = \frac{\bar{d}}{s_{\bar{d}}}, \quad \text{the paired } t\text{-statistic.}$$

D. Two-tailed statistical test:
   1. Null hypothesis: $H_0: \mu_d = 0$
   2. Alternative hypothesis: $H_a: \mu_d \neq 0$
   3. Decision rule for an α-level test: Reject H_0 in favor of H_a if t computed in step C is less than $-t_{1-\alpha/2}(n-1)$ or if t is greater than $t_{1-\alpha/2}(n-1)$.
   One-tailed statistical test:
   1. Null hypothesis: $H_0: \mu_d = 0$
   2. Alternative hypothesis: $H_a: \mu_d > 0$ ($H_a: \mu_d < 0$)
   3. Decision rule for an α-level test: Reject H_0 in favor of H_a if t computed in step C is greater than $t_{1-\alpha}(n-1)$ [reject H_0 in favor of H_a if t computed in C is less than $-t_{1-\alpha}(n-1)$].

the t distribution since this testing problem is identical to that presented in Section 5.3.2. For the two-sided alternative hypothesis $H_a: \mu_d \neq 0$, the two-tailed rejection region is depicted in Figure 6.1a. For the one-sided alternative hypotheses $H_a: \mu_d > 0$ and $H_a: \mu_d < 0$, the rejection regions are shown in Figures 6.1b and 6.1c. Note that $t = \sqrt{n}\,\bar{d}/s_d = \bar{d}/s_{\bar{d}}$, where $s_{\bar{d}} = s_d/\sqrt{n}$ is the sample standard error of the mean difference. The statistical test procedure is summarized in Table 6.2.

In Table 6.2, the values $t_{1-\alpha/2}(n-1)$ and $t_{1-\alpha}(n-1)$ are obtained from Table 5 of the Appendix; these values are used to form the statistical test since the ratio $\bar{d}/s_{\bar{d}}$ has a $t(n-1)$ sampling distribution when the null hypothesis that $\mu_d = 0$ is true. Thus, we see that for the matched-pair design the statistical test is based on the t distribution with $n-1$ degrees of freedom.

In addition to the statistical test of the hypothesis that $\mu_d = 0$, it is also possible to construct a confidence interval for μ_d. First, we note that $\bar{d}$ is a point estimator of μ_d, and since

$$t = \frac{\sqrt{n}\left(\bar{d} - \mu_d\right)}{s_d} = \frac{\bar{d} - \mu_d}{s_{\bar{d}}} \tag{6.2}$$

has a $t(n - 1)$ distribution, it follows that a $(1 - \alpha)100\%$ confidence interval for μ_d is given by

$$\bar{d} \pm t_{1-\alpha/2}(n - 1)s_{\bar{d}}, \tag{6.3}$$

where $t_{1-\alpha/2}(n - 1)$ is from Table 5 of the Appendix. Noting that $\Pr[-t_{1-\alpha/2}(n - 1) < t < t_{1-\alpha/2}(n - 1)] = 1 - \alpha$ and substituting (6.2) in for t leads to $\Pr[\bar{d} - t_{1-\alpha/2}s_{\bar{d}} < \mu_d < \bar{d} + t_{1-\alpha/2}s_{\bar{d}}]$ and (6.3) results.

We may note that the confidence interval (6.3) is equivalent to the two-tailed statistical test. Specifically, if 0 is in the interval (6.3), then the two-tailed α-level test of H_0: $\mu_d = 0$ would lead to accepting H_0 since it follows that the computed t satisfies $-t_{1-\alpha/2} < t < t_{1-\alpha/2}$. Conversely, if 0 is not in the interval (6.3), then the two-tailed α-level test of H_0: $\mu_d = 0$ leads to rejecting H_0 since the computed t is either greater than $t_{1-\alpha/2}$ or less than $-t_{1-\alpha/2}$.

Example 6.2.1.1. The effect of propranolol on the drinking behavior of ethanol-habituated rats was examined by studying a sample of seven rats. The rats were allowed to drink from a 20% ethanol solution ad libitum for 10 days. The amounts consumed by each animal during the last 10 hr before propranolol administration (10 mg/kg i.p.) and after administration are recorded in the accompanying tabulation. Is there evidence at the 5% significance level that propranolol decreases the amount of ethanol consumption? In this problem, it is evident that a one-tailed test is in order since a decrease in consumption is hypothesized after propranolol administration. Hence, we are testing H_0: $\mu_d = 0$ versus H_a: $\mu_d > 0$. Table 6.3 presents the worked solution to this problem.

| | Ethanol (mL/hr) | | |
Rat	Before propranolol	After propranolol	d_i
1	0.86	0.25	0.61
2	0.75	0.11	0.64
3	1.26	0.50	0.76
4	1.05	0.60	0.45
5	0.64	0.35	0.29
6	0.34	0.45	−0.11
7	0.79	0.67	0.12

Table 6.3. Worked Solution to Example 6.2.1.1 Using Paired t-Test

A. Data: The differences are $0.61, 0.64, 0.76, 0.45, 0.29, -0.11, 0.12$.
B. Assumptions: The differences in A are a random sample from a normal population.
C. Computations: $n = 7$, $\bar{d} = 0.39$, $s_{\bar{d}} = 0.12$. These figures arise from the following computations:

i	d_i	d_i^2
1	0.61	0.3721
2	0.64	0.4096
3	0.76	0.5776
4	0.45	0.2025
5	0.29	0.0841
6	-0.11	0.0121
7	0.12	0.0144
	2.76	1.6724

$$\sum_{i=1}^{7} (d_i - \bar{d})^2 = \left[\sum_{i=1}^{7} d_i^2 - \frac{1}{7} \left(\sum_{i=1}^{7} d_i \right)^2 \right]$$

$$= 1.6724 - \frac{(2.76)^2}{7} = 0.5842,$$

$$s_{\bar{d}} = \sqrt{\frac{0.5842}{7(6)}} = 0.12 \quad (\text{this is the estimated standard error of } \bar{d}),$$

$$\bar{d} = \frac{2.76}{7} = 0.39 \quad (\text{this is the estimator of } \mu_d),$$

$$t = \frac{0.39}{0.12} = 3.25.$$

D. One-tailed test:
  1. Null hypothesis: H_0: $\mu_d = 0$
  2. Alternative hypothesis: H_a: $\mu_d > 0$
  3. Decision rule for 0.05 level test: Reject if $t > t_{0.95}(6)$.
E. Action taken: From Table 5 of the Appendix, $t_{0.95}(6) = 1.943$; hence, as $t = 3.25 > 1.943$, the null hypothesis is rejected at the 5% level of significance. The P value for 3.25 is determined from Table 5 of the Appendix to be less than 0.01 since $3.25 > 3.143$.

Example 6.2.1.1 is an example of a one-sided alternative hypothesis and a one-tailed statistical test. In many situations, it is the one-sided alternative that is of interest to the investigator. This is frequently, but not always, true of therapeutic trials, in which the test treatment is expected to be at least as good as the conventional mode of therapy. In other situations, the two-sided alternative is of interest.

In Example 6.2.1.1, if a two-sided alternative was of interest rather than the one-sided, then the critical value at $\alpha = 0.05$ of the *t*-test statistic would be $t_{0.975}(6) = 2.447$ rather than $t_{0.95}(6) = 1.943$. In this case, H_0 would be rejected if the computed t was less than -2.447 or greater than 2.447. A two-sided confidence interval in the form of (6.3) is $0.39 \pm (2.447)(0.12)$; hence, a 95% confidence interval for μ_d is $(0.10, 0.68)$. Notice that zero is not in this interval, and hence the two-sided null hypothesis would be rejected at the 0.05 level. This agrees with the conclusion reached when testing against the two-sided alternatives since 3.25 (the computed t in Table 6.3) exceeds 2.447.

We now turn to the question of sample size requirements for a matched-pair study. If a one-sided alternative hypothesis is of interest—say that $\mu_d > 0$—then provided we assume the variance (σ_d^2) is known, it is straightforward to determine the required number of pairs n such that an α-level one-tailed test has power $1 - \beta$. The sample size is determined by noting that $Z = (\bar{d} - \mu_d)/(\sigma_d/\sqrt{n})$ has a standard normal distribution, and

$$\Pr\left[\frac{\bar{d}}{\sigma_d/\sqrt{n}} > Z_{1-\alpha}|\mu_d = 0\right] = \alpha,$$

where α is the required significance level and $Z_{1-\alpha}$ is from Table 4 of the Appendix. The power requirement for the alternative $\mu_d = \mu_d^*$ is

$$\Pr\left[\frac{\bar{d}}{\sigma_d/\sqrt{n}} > Z_{1-\alpha}|\mu_d = \mu_d^*\right] = 1 - \beta.$$

With some algebra these two preceding conditions require that the number of pairs n for power $1 - \beta$ for the alternative that $\mu_d = \mu_d^*$ for a one-tailed α-level test is

$$n = \frac{\sigma_d^2\left(Z_{1-\alpha} + Z_{1-\beta}\right)^2}{\left(\mu_d^*\right)^2},$$

where both $Z_{1-\alpha}$ and $Z_{1-\beta}$ are from Table 4 of the Appendix.

For a two-tailed test, $Z_{1-\alpha}$ is replaced by $Z_{1-\alpha/2}$; otherwise, there are no changes in the formula given. It is important to note that an estimate of the underlying variance σ_d^2 of the differences is required to determine sample size requirements.

In practice, one has data from previous pilot studies that are used to estimate σ_d^2. This is then used as an approximation to σ_d^2 in the foregoing sample size formula. Once again, this is an approximation to the sample size since we have assumed the variance is known; however, for large n this approximation is adequate ($n \geq 20$). If the estimate of σ_d^2 has been based on a small sample, the procedures described in Section 5.2.2 (see Example 5.2.2.2) would be preferred to the above.

Example 6.2.1.2. Suppose a study is to be conducted in which a medication for hypertension is to be given to a sample of middle-aged men. Each man will have his systolic blood pressure (SBP) recorded; then medication will commence for a 14-day period, after which the SBP reading will be taken again. In previous studies of a related medication the before–after difference in SBP has a variance of 400 (mm Hg)^2. Suppose the new medication is of interest if it reduces the mean SBP by 10 mm Hg or more. How many men should be studied in order to have the significance level be 0.05 and also to have a 90% chance of detecting a 10 mm Hg change in mean SBP?

For this problem, a one-sided alternative is of interest, that is, H_a: $\mu_d > 0$, where d is before–after SBP. From Table 4 of the Appendix, we find $Z_{1-\alpha} = Z_{0.95} = 1.645$ and $Z_{1-\beta} = Z_{0.90} = 1.28$ for the level and power requirements, respectively. Therefore, with $\sigma_d^2 = 400$, $\mu_d = 10$, we have

$$n = \frac{400(1.645 + 1.28)^2}{(10)^2} = 34.2.$$

Hence, 35 men should be chosen for the study. If a mean difference of $\mu_d = 5$ is of interest, we would find that

$$n = \frac{400(1.645 + 1.28)^2}{(5)^2} \doteq 137,$$

so the sample size is considerably higher for this alternative hypothesis which is closer to 0. In general, it is important to be able to specify the size of difference that is clinically important, in this case a difference of 10 mm Hg. Once this clinical difference is specified, then sample size can be determined so that an adequate chance to detect this alternative will be achieved.

We may note (as in Chapter 5) that to increase power for a given alternative, n would need to be increased. In particular, for $1 - \beta = 0.95$, $\mu_d = 10$, $\alpha = 0.05$, and $\sigma_d^2 = 400$, the required n is

$$n = \frac{400(1.645 + 1.645)^2}{(10)^2} \doteq 44,$$

in contrast to the 35 required for a power of 0.90.

In summary, we note that the paired *t*-test is a test for the mean of a normal distribution. The test is appropriate if we assume the set of differences are a random sample from the normal distribution. If the differences do not arise from a normal population but from another continuous distribution, then this test may still be fairly accurate if the number of pairs is sufficiently large. Many statisticians would probably regard a sample of 20 pairs as sufficiently large to proceed with the test in spite of nonnormality. As we shall see in later sections, there are other tests that may be applied to these nonnormal cases. Before proceeding to other matched-pair tests, we consider the two-sample version of the *t*-test.

6.2.2 Two-Sample *t*-Test for Comparing Means: A Test for Two Independent Groups

Data for two independent random samples may be represented in the notational form seen in Table 6.4. There are n_1 observations for the first group and n_2 observations for the second group. For the *two-sample t-test*, the following assumptions are required for these two independent random samples:

1. $y_{11}, \ldots, y_{1n_1}$ is a random sample from a normal distribution with mean μ_1 and variance σ_1^2;
2. $y_{21}, \ldots, y_{2n_2}$ is an independent random sample from a normal distribution with mean μ_2 and variance σ_2^2; and
3. $\sigma_1^2 = \sigma_2^2 = \sigma^2$, that is, the variances are equal to some unknown but common variance.

Note, in particular, the third assumption of variance homogeneity. To properly apply the two-sample *t*-test for testing the hypothesis that $\mu_1 = \mu_2$, this assumption is required. Later we discuss a procedure that does not require this assumption.

Table 6.4. Data Layout for Two Independent
(Unmatched) Samples

Group 1	Group 2
y_{11}	y_{21}
y_{12}	y_{22}
$\vdots$	$\vdots$
y_{1n_1}	y_{2n_2}

If the population variances are equal, then the question of estimating this common variance arises. While many estimators can be considered, the preferred estimator on statistical grounds is the pooled variance estimate of σ^2, which is a weighted average of the within-group variances, where the weights are the degrees of freedom. In particular, the estimator is

$$s_p^2 = \frac{(n_1 - 1)s_1^2 + (n_2 - 1)s_2^2}{(n_1 - 1) + (n_2 - 1)}, \tag{6.4}$$

where s_1^2 and s_2^2 are the two respective sample variances; that is, $s_i^2 = \sum_{j=1}^{n_i}(y_{ij} - \bar{y}_i)^2/(n_i - 1)$ (for $i = 1, 2$) and $\bar{y}_i$ is the sample mean for group i.

The *pooled variance* (6.4) is thus a weighted average of the two sample variances where the weights are the sample degrees of freedom. Viewed as an estimator of σ^2, s_p^2 is based on $n_1 + n_2 - 2$ degrees of freedom, $n_1 - 1$ from sample 1 and $n_2 - 1$ from sample 2.

By the assumptions for the two independent random samples, the sample means $\bar{y}_1$ and $\bar{y}_2$ each have normal distributions with means μ_1 and μ_2 and variances σ_1^2/n_1 and σ_2^2/n_2, respectively. It can be shown that $\bar{y}_1 - \bar{y}_2$, the difference of these two independent means, is also normal with mean $\mu_1 - \mu_2$ and variance $\sigma_1^2/n_1 + \sigma_2^2/n_2$. Consequently,

$$Z = \frac{(\bar{y}_1 - \bar{y}_2) - (\mu_1 - \mu_2)}{\sqrt{\sigma_1^2/n_1 + \sigma_2^2/n_2}}$$

is a standard normal variate. If, in addition, $\sigma_1^2 = \sigma_2^2 = \sigma^2$, then we have

$$Z = \frac{(\bar{y}_1 - \bar{y}_2) - (\mu_1 - \mu_2)}{\sqrt{\sigma^2(1/n_1 + 1/n_2)}} \quad \text{or} \quad Z = \frac{(\bar{y}_1 - \bar{y}_2) - (\mu_1 - \mu_2)}{\sigma\sqrt{(1/n_1 + 1/n_2)}}.$$

If σ^2 is estimated by s_p^2, the pooled variance with $n_1 + n_2 - 2$ degrees of freedom, then when $\mu_1 - \mu_2 = 0$ it can be shown that

$$t = \frac{\bar{y}_1 - \bar{y}_2}{s_p\sqrt{1/n_1 + 1/n_2}}$$

has a $t(n_1 + n_2 - 2)$ distribution and a test of the equal-means hypothesis

Table 6.5. Outline of Two-Sample *t*-Test Procedure

A. Data: y_{ij}, $i = 1, 2$; $j = 1, 2, \ldots, n_i$ from Table 6.4.
B. Assumptions: The three assumptions stated at the beginning of this section.
C. Computations: For $i = 1, 2$, compute

$$\bar{y}_i = \sum_{j=1}^{n_i} \frac{y_{ij}}{n_i}, \quad \text{the sample mean,}$$

$$s_i^2 = \sum_{j=1}^{n_i} \frac{(y_{ij} - \bar{y}_i)^2}{(n_i - 1)}, \quad \text{the sample variance.}$$

Then, compute

$$s_p^2 = \frac{(n_1 - 1)s_1^2 + (n_2 - 1)s_2^2}{(n_1 - 1) + (n_2 - 1)}, \quad \text{the pooled variance;}$$

$$s_{(\bar{y}_1 - \bar{y}_2)} = s_p\sqrt{(1/n_1 + 1/n_2)}, \quad \begin{array}{l}\text{the sample standard error of the} \\ \text{mean difference,}\end{array}$$

$$t = \frac{\bar{y}_1 - \bar{y}_2}{s_{(\bar{y}_1 - \bar{y}_2)}}, \quad \text{the two-sample } t\text{-statistic.}$$

D. Two-tailed statistical test:
   1. Null hypothesis: $H_0: \mu_1 = \mu_2$
   2. Alternative hypothesis: $H_a: \mu_1 \neq \mu_2$
   3. Decision rule for an α-level test: Reject H_0 in favor of H_a if t computed in step C is less than $-t_{1-\alpha/2}(n_1 + n_2 - 2)$ or greater than $t_{1-\alpha/2}(n_1 + n_2 - 2)$.

   One-tailed statistical test:
   1. Null hypothesis: $H_0: \mu_1 = \mu_2$
   2. Alternative hypothesis: $H_a: \mu_1 > \mu_2 (H_a: \mu_1 < \mu_2)$
   3. Decision rule for an α-level test: Reject H_0 in favor of H_a if t computed in step C is greater than $t_{1-\alpha}(n_1 + n_2 - 2)$ [reject H_0 in favor of H_a if t computed in C is less than $-t_{1-\alpha}(n_1 + n_2 - 2)$].

can be based on this statistic. The resulting *t*-test statistic is termed the two-sample *t*-test statistic, and the formal test procedure is summarized in Table 6.5.

In Table 6.5, the values $t_{1-\alpha/2}(n_1 + n_2 - 2)$ and $t_{1-\alpha}(n_1 + n_2 - 2)$ may be obtained from Table 5 of the Appendix. The rejection regions are similar to those in Figure 6.1, except here we have a *t* with $n_1 + n_2 - 2$ degrees of freedom.

Since the quantity $[(\bar{y}_1 - \bar{y}_2) - (\mu_1 - \mu_2)]/s_{(\bar{y}_1 - \bar{y}_2)}$ has a *t* distribution with $n_1 + n_2 - 2$ degrees of freedom, it follows that a $(1 - \alpha)100\%$ confidence interval for $\mu_1 - \mu_2$ is given by

$$(\bar{y}_1 - \bar{y}_2) \pm t_{1-\alpha/2}(n_1 + n_2 - 2)s_{(\bar{y}_1 - \bar{y}_2)}. \tag{6.5}$$

The derivation for this interval follows the same line of reasoning as that for the paired *t* interval presented in (6.3). As we noted for the paired *t*-test, this confidence interval may be used to construct the two-tailed statistical test of the hypothesis that $\mu_1 - \mu_2 = 0$. Specifically, if zero is in the interval (6.5), then the two-tailed α-level test of H_0: $\mu_1 = \mu_2$ would lead to acceptance of H_0. Conversely, the alternative hypothesis (H_a: $\mu_1 \neq \mu_2$) would be accepted if zero is not in the confidence interval. In fact, the $(1 - \alpha)100\%$ confidence interval for $\mu_1 - \mu_2$ consists of those values of $\mu_1 - \mu_2$ that, if assumed as H_0, would lead to accepting H_0. Those values are described by (6.5).

Example 6.2.2.1. In a follow-up study of a group of paranoid schizophrenics, the age of onset of each person's illness was determined. For the following data, test the hypothesis that the mean age of onset is the same for each sex. The data are:

Age of Onset in Years

Males	Females
24	22
33	34
23	26
20	31
26	26
32	35
35	25
21	38
25	36
	22
	23
	37

Table 6.6. Worked Solution to Example 6.2.2.1 Using the Two-Sample *t*-Test

___

A. Data: Group 1 observations: 24, 33, 23, 20, 26, 32, 35, 21, 25
    Group 2 observations: 22, 34, 26, 31, 26, 35, 25, 38, 36, 22, 23, 37
B. Assumptions: The age-of-onset distribution for each sex is normally distributed with the same variance. The two samples are two independent random samples from their respective populations.
C. Computations:

	Males	Females
	$n_1 = 9$	$n_2 = 12$
	$\bar{y}_1 = 26.56$	$\bar{y}_2 = 29.58$
	$s_1^2 = 29.78$	$s_2^2 = 38.45$

Thus, $s_p^2 = [8(29.78) + 11(38.45)]/19 = 34.80$ is the pooled estimator of σ^2, and

$$s_{(\bar{y}_1 - \bar{y}_2)} = 5.90\sqrt{\left(\tfrac{1}{9} + \tfrac{1}{12}\right)} = 2.60$$

is the estimated standard error of $\bar{y}_1 - \bar{y}_2$. Since $\bar{y}_1 - \bar{y}_2 = 26.56 - 29.58 = -3.02$, then $t = -3.02/2.60 = -1.16$.
D. Two-tailed statistical test:
    1. Null hypothesis: $H_0: \mu_1 = \mu_2$
    2. Alternative hypothesis: $H_a: \mu_1 \neq \mu_2$
    3. Decision rule for 0.05 α-level test: Reject H_0 if $t < -t_{0.975}(19)$ or $t > t_{0.975}(19)$.
E. Action taken: From Table 5 of the Appendix, $t_{0.975}(19) = 2.093$, and from step C, $t = -1.16$; therefore, at the 5% level of significance, there is not sufficient evidence to reject H_0.

___

We assume that these two samples are independent of one another; this assumption implies that there was no matching. Let us test $H_0: \mu_1 = \mu_2$ versus $H_a: \mu_1 \neq \mu_2$ at $\alpha = 0.05$. The solution is outlined in Table 6.6.

From Table 5 of the Appendix, one also notes that $\Pr[t(19) > 1.16]$ is less than 0.15 but greater than 0.10. Hence, it follows that $\Pr[t(19) < -1.16]$ would also be between 0.10 and 0.15. The P value for a two-tailed test must include both tails of the distribution, hence, $P = \Pr[t(19) > 1.16] + \Pr[t(19) < -1.16]$. The P value for Example 6.2.2.1 could be reported as $0.2 < P < 0.3$, that is, $2(0.10)$ to $2(0.15)$. If interest had been on the one-sided $(\mu_1 < \mu_2)$ rather than the two-sided alternative hypothesis, the P value would be reported as $0.10 < P < 0.15$ since only one tail would be used to perform the test.

A 95% confidence interval for $\mu_1 - \mu_2$ can be computed using (6.5) and by using the summary figures in Table 6.6. In particular, a 95% confidence interval is $-3.02 \pm (2.093)(2.6)$, or $(-8.46, 2.42)$. Notice that zero is in the interval, in agreement with the two-tailed 5% test that led to acceptance of H_0.

Turning to sample size requirements, we proceed as in the paired *t* situation. In particular, we consider the sample size required for an α-level test for the one-sided alternative that $\mu_1 - \mu_2 > 0$ to have power $1 - \beta$. We also assume that the variance σ^2 ($= \sigma_1^2 = \sigma_2^2$) is a fixed and known value and that the sample sizes are equal. Following the argument of the previous section, the number of observations required in each group, n, is given by

$$n = \frac{2\sigma^2 (Z_{1-\alpha} + Z_{1-\beta})^2}{(\mu_1 - \mu_2)^2},$$

where σ^2 is the variance, $Z_{1-\alpha}$ and $Z_{1-\beta}$ are from Table 4 of the Appendix, and $\mu_1 - \mu_2$ is the value of the population mean difference for which the power requirements are desired. For the two-sided alternative hypothesis, $Z_{1-\alpha}$ is replaced by $Z_{1-\alpha/2}$. Furthermore, if n_1 and n_2 are not to be equal but $n_2 = cn_1$, a multiple of n_1 (e.g., $n_2 = 2n_1$ or $n_2 = \frac{1}{2}n_1$), then

$$n_1 = \frac{\sigma^2 (1 + 1/c)(Z_{1-\alpha} + Z_{1-\beta})^2}{(\mu_1 - \mu_2)^2}$$

is the sample size for group 1 for the one-sided alternative hypothesis. The second group sample size is $n_2 = cn_1$.

Example 6.2.2.2. Suppose we wish to plan a study like that described in Example 6.2.2.1. We shall use $\sigma^2 = 36$, and we would like to know what sample size we require in each group in order to be able to detect a difference of 5 years in the mean ages of onset between the sexes with 90% power. We use $\alpha = 0.05$ and a two-tailed test; hence, with equal group size of n per group, we have

$$n = \frac{2(36)(1.96 + 1.28)^2}{(5)^2} = 30.2,$$

and 31 is the number required in each group.

Strictly speaking, the sample size computation for the *t*-test above required knowledge of σ^2. In the practical situation when σ^2 is unknown, the sample size determination can be based on the mean difference in σ units. In Chapter 10, such a graph is presented for the two-sample problem (Figure 10.1).

In Example 6.2.2.1, the two sample variances are fairly close to one another, so the equal population variance assumption seems tenable. On the other hand, we might ask, how far apart can the sample variances be before concluding that the population variances are not equal? The following example illustrates a situation in which the equal-variance assumption is questionable.

Example 6.2.2.3. Twenty-nine male alcoholics suffering from secondary hypertension participated in a study to determine the efficacy of a new antihypertensive agent. The men were assigned at random to either the control group or the treatment group. Those assigned to the control group received placebo tablets, and those assigned to the treatment group received tablets containing the active agent. Blood pressure was determined daily for each person upon awakening. At the end of 30 days a final measurement was made. Data are expressed as mean arterial pressure (i.e., (2 diastolic pressure + systolic pressure)/3, in mm Hg). The hypothesis that the two groups have equal means versus the alternative hypothesis that the test treatment group has a lower mean arterial pressure is to be tested. The data are the following:

Mean Arterial Pressure at 30 Days Posttreated

Placebo Treated		Test Treated	
105	109	92	98
107	119	96	109
110	143	104	106
117	162	119	91
124	91	106	88
153	146	100	94
137	109	93	
174		90	

To test $H_0: \mu_1 = \mu_2$ versus $H_a: \mu_1 > \mu_2$ the sample mean and variance for each sample are required. We find that:

Placebo Treated	Test Treated
$n_1 = 15$	$n_2 = 14$
$\bar{y}_1 = 127.1$	$\bar{y}_2 = 99$
$s_1^2 = 579.8$	$s_2^2 = 77.7$

Before performing a two-sample *t*-test, the magnitude of difference in the sample variances leads us to question the equal-variance assumption. It appears that this assumption is not met in the present case. Two questions arise. First, is there a modification of the two-sample *t*-test that does not require the equal-variance assumption? Second, can we test, in the usual statistical manner, the hypothesis that the population variances are equal? In the following two sections we discuss these two questions in turn.

6.2.3   Cochran–Cox *t*-Test for Equality of Means: A Modified *t*-Test for Two Independent Groups

Statisticians have studied a variety of test procedures for the problem of comparing two means of normally distributed data when the population variances are not assumed to be equal. This section presents one such test procedure that is an approximate *t*-test. Approximation is required since an exact *t*-test procedure is unknown. The test procedure presented is based on a sample statistic whose exact probability distribution can be approximated by the *t* distribution in Table 5 of the Appendix. Cochran and Cox (1957) describe this procedure, and it offers a simple and reasonably powerful test of the equal-means hypothesis; however, there is no single best procedure for this problem.* This method uses the *t* distribution, and it is outlined in Table 6.7. In Table 6.8, Example 6.2.2.3 is analyzed using this modified *t*-test.

This test procedure tends to be *conservative*. In the context of the preceding example, this means that the true level of significance of the test is less than or equal to 0.05. As one might guess, the true level of significance may be less than 0.05 if, in fact, the population variances are equal. This is evident when $n_1 = n_2 = n$ by comparing this approximate *t*-test to the two-sample *t*-test. The two-sample *t*-test would require comparison of the computed *t* to a tabular (Table 5, Appendix) value with $n_1 + n_2 - 2 [= 2(n - 1)]$ degrees of freedom. The Cochran–Cox *t*-test uses a weighted average of the tabular values of *t* with degrees of freedom given by $n_1 - 1$ and $n_2 - 1$. Hence, the degrees of freedom used in this approximate *t*-test $(n - 1)$ is half that used for the two-sample *t*-test $[2(n - 1)]$. A glance at Table 5 of the Appendix indicates that for a given significance level, the magnitude of a tabular *t* required for rejection of a null hypothesis *decreases* with an *increase* in degrees of freedom. Generally, it is easier

---

*Satterthwaite (1946) proposes a different procedure which is produced by many computer packages.

Table 6.7. Outline for Cochran–Cox Two-Sample t-Test Procedure for Comparing Two Normal Means with Unequal Variance

A. Data: $y_{ij} = 1, 2; \ j = 1, 2, \ldots, n_j$ from Table 6.4.
B. Assumptions:
   1. $y_{11}, \ldots, y_{1n_1}$ is a random sample from a normal distribution with mean μ_1 and variance σ_1^2.
   2. $y_{21}, \ldots, y_{2n_2}$ is an independent random sample from a normal distribution with mean μ_2 and variance σ_2^2.
C. Computations: For $i = 1, 2$, compute $\bar{y}_i = \sum_{j=1}^{n_i} y_{ij}/n_i$, the sample mean, and s_i^2, the sample variance. Then compute

$$s_{\bar{y}_1 - \bar{y}_2} = \sqrt{\left(s_1^2/n_1 + s_2^2/n_2\right)}, \quad \begin{array}{l}\text{sample standard error of the mean}\\\text{difference,}\end{array}$$

$$t' = \frac{\bar{y}_1 - \bar{y}_2}{s_{(\bar{y}_1 - \bar{y}_2)}}, \quad \text{the approximate } t\text{-statistic.}$$

For the two-tailed test compute

$$f_{1-\alpha/2} = \frac{\left(s_1^2/n_1\right)t_{1-\alpha/2}(n_1 - 1) + \left(s_2^2/n_2\right)t_{1-\alpha/2}(n_2 - 1)}{s_1^2/n_1 + s_2^2/n_2}$$

for the one-tailed test compute

$$f_{1-\alpha} = \frac{\left(s_1^2/n_1\right)t_{1-\alpha}(n_1 - 1) + \left(s_2^2/n_2\right)t_{1-\alpha}(n_2 - 1)}{s_1^2/n_1 + s_2^2/n_2}.$$

D. Two-tailed statistical test:
   1. Null hypothesis: $H_0: \mu_1 = \mu_2$
   2. Alternative hypothesis: $H_a: \mu_1 \neq \mu_2$
   3. Decision rule for an α-level (conservative) test: Reject H_0 in favor of H_a if t' in step C is less than $-f_{1-\alpha/2}$ or t' in C is greater than $f_{1-\alpha/2}$.
   One-tailed statistical test:
   1. Null hypothesis: $H_0: \mu_1 = \mu_2$
   2. Alternative hypothesis: $H_a: \mu_1 > \mu_2 \ (H_a: \mu_1 < \mu_2)$
   3. Decision rule for an α-level (conservative) test: Reject H_0 in favor of H_a if t' computed in step C is greater than $f_{1-\alpha}$ (reject H_0 if favor of H_a if t' computed in C is less than $-f_{1-\alpha}$).

Table 6.8. Worked Solution to Example 6.2.2.3 Using the Cochran–Cox Two-Sample t-Test

A. Data:
   Placebo: 105, 107, 110, 117, 124, 153, 137, 174, 109, 119, 143, 162, 91, 146, 109
   Test: 92, 96, 104, 119, 106, 100, 93, 90, 98, 109, 106, 91, 88, 94.
B. Assumptions: The mean arterial blood pressure is a normally distributed random variable for both the placebo and test-treated persons. The two samples are independent random samples. (No assumption is made regarding the variances.)
C. Computations:

	Placebo	Test
	$n_1 = 15$	$n_2 = 14$
	$\bar{y}_1 = 127.1$	$\bar{y}_2 = 99$
	$s_1^2 = 579.8$	$s_2^2 = 77.7$

$$s_{\bar{y}_1 - \bar{y}_2} = \sqrt{579.8/15 + 77.8/14} = 6.65 \text{ mm Hg}$$

$$\bar{y}_1 - \bar{y}_2 = 127.1 - 99 = 28.1 \text{ mm Hg}$$

$$t' = \frac{28.1 \text{ mm Hg}}{6.65 \text{ mm Hg}} = 4.23.$$

Since a one-sided alternative is of interest, and from Table 5 of the Appendix $t_{0.95}(13) = 1.771$ and $t_{0.95}(14) = 1.761$, then

$$f_{0.95} = \frac{(579.8/15)(1.761) + (77.8/14)(1.771)}{579.8/15 + 77.8/14} = 1.762$$

D. One-tailed statistical test:
   1. Null hypothesis: $H_0: \mu_1 = \mu_2$
   2. Alternative hypothesis: $H_a: \mu_1 > \mu_2$
   3. Decision rule for 0.05 α-level test: Reject H_0 in favor of H_a if $t' > f_{0.95} = 1.762$.
E. Action taken: Since $t' = 4.23 > 1.762 = t_{0.95}$, the null hypothesis is rejected in favor of H_a. One concludes that at the 5% level of significance the active agent significantly decreases the mean arterial pressure.

to reject a null hypothesis with an increase in degrees of freedom. All of this suggests that this approximate *t* procedure may, in some cases, be a very conservative test procedure. Power or ability to detect an alternative hypothesis may be lost by using this procedure; however, the significance level is guaranteed. On the other hand, if the two-sample *t*-test is used and the assumption of equal variances is not true, then the stated significance level of the two-sample *t*-test may be incorrect. To help decide which test to use, a procedure for testing the hypothesis of equal variances is needed.

6.2.4 The *F*-Test for Equality of Variances: A Test for Two Independent Groups

The *F* distribution was first introduced in Chapter 4. Referring to expression (4.26), recall that it is a distribution formed by the ratio of two quantities. The numerator in this expression is the sample variance divided by the population variance of a normal random sample, while the denominator is the corresponding ratio from an independent random sample. Clearly, if population variances were equal, then the ratio of the two-sample variances follows an *F* distribution. This follows since *F* is $(s_1^2/\sigma_1^2)/(s_2^2/\sigma_2^2)$, which is s_1^2/s_2^2 if $\sigma_1^2 = \sigma_2^2$. This leads directly to a formal statistical test. Table 6.9 outlines the *variance ratio* or *F-test* procedure.

The quantities $F_{1-\alpha}(n_1 - 1, n_2 - 1)$ and $F_{1-\alpha/2}(f_{larger}, f_{smaller})$ are obtained from Table 7 of the Appendix. The two-sided alternative hypothesis is of interest if we want to determine whether the two-sample *t*-test is appropriate for the equal-means hypothesis. In Table 6.10, this two-sided variance ratio test is applied to the data of Example 6.2.2.3.

The main conclusion from Table 6.10 is that the population variances may not be assumed to be equal. If a test of the population means is of interest to the investigators, then the Cochran–Cox *t*-test would be preferred to the two-sample *t*-test. Hence the analysis outlined in Table 6.8 would appear to be the appropriate test procedure for comparing the two means.

Perhaps the reader may find it confusing that the rejection rule for an α-level test procedure using the *F*-test is to reject H_0 in favor of two-sided alternatives if $F > F_{1-\alpha/2}(f_{larger}, f_{smaller})$. The potentially confusing point is that a one-tailed rejection region appears for a two-sided alternative hypothesis. To clarify this issue, we first note that the larger sample variance is the numerator of our test statistic. This is in contrast to using the sample 1 variance divided by the sample 2 variance as the test criterion. For example, we could use the statistic s_1^2/s_2^2 as the ratio and reject H_0: $\sigma_1^2 = \sigma_2^2$ in favor of H_a: $\sigma_1^2 \neq \sigma_2^2$ if s_1^2/s_2^2 is too small or too large. This test would be to

Table 6.9. Outline of *F*-Test Procedure for Equality of Two Variances from Two Independent Samples

A. Data: y_{ij}, $i = 1, 2$, $j = 1, 2, \ldots, n_i$, from Table 6.4.

B. Assumptions:

    1. $y_{11}, \ldots, y_{1n_1}$ is a random sample from a normal distribution with mean μ_1 and variance σ_1^2.

    2. $y_{21}, \ldots, y_{2n_2}$ is an independent random sample from a normal distribution with mean μ_2 and variance σ_2^2.

C. Computations: For $i = 1, 2$ compute

$$\bar{y}_i = \sum_{j=1}^{n_i} \frac{y_{ij}}{n_i}, \quad \text{the sample mean,}$$

$$s_i^2 = \sum_{j=1}^{n_i} \frac{(y_{ij} - \bar{y}_i)^2}{n_i - 1}, \quad \text{the sample variance.}$$

Then determine

$$s_{\text{larger}}^2 = \text{larger of } s_1^2 \text{ and } s_2^2,$$

$$s_{\text{smaller}}^2 = \text{smaller of } s_1^2 \text{ and } s_2^2,$$

$$f_{\text{larger}} = \text{degrees of freedom of } s_{\text{larger}}^2,$$

$$f_{\text{smaller}} = \text{degrees of freedom of } s_{\text{smaller}}^2,$$

and finally compute

$$F = \frac{s_{\text{larger}}^2}{s_{\text{smaller}}^2}.$$

D. Two-tailed statistical test:

    1. Null hypothesis: H_0: $\sigma_1^2 = \sigma_2^2$

    2. Alternative hypothesis: H_a: $\sigma_1^2 \neq \sigma_2^2$

    3. Decision rule for an α-level test: Reject H_0 in favor of H_a if F computed in step C is greater than $F_{1-\alpha/2}(f_{\text{larger}}, f_{\text{smaller}})$.

One-tailed statistical test:

    1. Null hypothesis: H_0: $\sigma_1^2 = \sigma_2^2$

    2. Alternative hypothesis: H_a: $\sigma_1^2 > \sigma_2^2$ (H_a: $\sigma_1^2 < \sigma_2^2$)

    3. Decision rule for an α-level test: Reject H_0 in favor of H_a if s_1^2/s_2^2 computed in step C is greater than $F_{1-\alpha}(n_1 - 1, n_2 - 1)$ [reject H_0 in favor of H_a if s_2^2/s_1^2 is greater than $F_{1-\alpha}(n_2 - 1, n_1 - 1)$].

Table 6.10. Worked Solution to Example 6.2.2.3 to Test for Equality of Variance Using F-Test

---

A. Data:
   Placebo: 105, 107, 110, 117, 124, 153, 137, 174, 109, 119, 143, 162, 91, 146, 109
   Test: 92, 96, 104, 119, 106, 100, 93, 90, 98, 109, 106, 91, 88, 94.
B. Assumptions: The mean arterial blood pressure is a normally distributed random variable for both the placebo and test-treated persons. The two samples are independent random samples. (No assumption is made regarding the variances.)
C. Computations:

$$\begin{array}{cc} \text{Placebo} & \text{Test} \\ n_1 = 15 & n_2 = 14 \\ \\ s_1^2 = 579.8 & s_2^2 = 77.7 \end{array}$$

Hence, it follows that:

$$s_{\text{larger}}^2 = 579.8, \quad s_{\text{smaller}}^2 = 77.7,$$

$$f_{\text{larger}} = 14, \quad f_{\text{smaller}} = 13,$$

and

$$F = 579.8/77.7 = 7.5.$$

D. Two-tailed statistical test:
   1. Null hypothesis: $H_0: \sigma_1^2 = \sigma_2^2$
   2. Alternative hypothesis: $H_a: \sigma_1^2 \neq \sigma_2^2$
   3. Decision rule for a 10% level test: Reject H_0 in favor of H_a if $F > F_{0.95}(14, 13)$.
E. Action Taken: From Table 7 of the Appendix, $F_{0.95}(15, 13) = 2.53$ and $F_{0.95}(12, 13) = 2.60$; therefore $F_{0.95} \doteq 2.55$, while F computed in step C is 7.5; since $F = 7.5 > 2.55 \doteq F_{0.95}(14, 13)$, H_0 is rejected in favor of H_a at the 10% level of significance. The P value for the test is much less than 0.01 as may be seen by inspection of Table 7 of the Appendix.

---

reject H_0 if

$$\frac{s_1^2}{s_2^2} < F_{\alpha/2}(n_1 - 1, n_2 - 1) \quad \text{or if} \quad \frac{s_1^2}{s_2^2} > F_{1-\alpha/2}(n_1 - 1, n_2 - 1). \quad (6.6)$$

Clearly, (6.6) is a two-tailed test procedure. An equivalent two-tailed test procedure could be performed by considering the ratio s_2^2/s_1^2. In this case, the two-tailed test procedure is to reject H_0 if

$$\frac{s_2^2}{s_1^2} < F_{\alpha/2}(n_2 - 1, n_1 - 1) \quad \text{or if} \quad \frac{s_2^2}{s_1^2} > F_{1-\alpha/2}(n_2 - 1, n_1 - 1). \quad (6.7)$$

To show that (6.6) is equivalent to the procedure outlined for the two-sided alternative hypotheses in Table 6.9, we note that the inequality $s_1^2/s_2^2 < F_{\alpha/2}(n_1 - 1, n_2 - 1)$ is the same as $s_2^2/s_1^2 > 1/F_{\alpha/2}(n_1 - 1, n_2 - 1)$, but it is a mathematical fact that $1/F_{\alpha/2}(n_1 - 1, n_2 - 1) = F_{1-\alpha/2}(n_2 - 1, n_1 - 1)$. Hence, (6.6) is equivalent to rejecting H_0 if

$$\frac{s_2^2}{s_1^2} > F_{1-\alpha/2}(n_2 - 1, n_1 - 1) \quad \text{or if} \quad \frac{s_1^2}{s_2^2} > F_{1-\alpha/2}(n_1 - 1, n_2 - 1).$$

$$(6.8)$$

That is, reject H_0 if the larger sample variance divided by the smaller sample variance exceeds the $1 - \alpha/2$ percentile of an appropriate F distribution. Clearly, (6.8) is identical to the rule stated in Table 6.9. A simple repetition of these steps with (6.7) would show that it is equivalent to expression (6.8) as well. Thus, we see the reason for the one-tailed test procedure for a two-sided alternative hypothesis.

Another point that arises from this discussion of testing for variance equality in order to select an equal-means test is that of the significance level to be used to test for equal variances. Although it is difficult to give rigid guidelines, it is preferable to select larger significance levels to avoid the error of using the two-sample *t*-test when variances are unequal. A level of 10% to 15% for the variance ratio test is a value that seems reasonable.

Finally, it should be stated that if the sample variances are not greatly different, then most applied statisticians would probably not perform the *F*-test and would perform the usual two-sample *t*-test. While this author generally agrees with this, we must at least "eyeball" the variances to check for marked differences; we must remember that if variances are greatly different, then the α level stated for the two-sample *t*-test may be incorrect. On the other hand, if the relative sizes of the sample variances are not enormously different, then it probably is not worth worrying about any discrepancy since the two-sample *t*-test is fairly robust to mild inequality of variances.

Another point requiring elaboration is the fact that this variance ratio statistic can be used to place a confidence interval on σ_1^2/σ_2^2. In fact, a $(1 - \alpha)100\%$ confidence interval for σ_1^2/σ_2^2 may be derived directly from (4.26). It is

$$\left[\frac{s_1^2}{s_2^2} \left(\frac{1}{F_{1-\alpha/2}(n_1 - 1, n_2 - 1)} \right), \frac{s_1^2}{s_2^2} F_{1-\alpha/2}(n_2 - 1, n_1 - 1) \right]. \quad (6.9)$$

For Example 6.2.2.3, a 90% confidence interval may be obtained from (6.9). In particular, using Table 7 of the Appendix, $F_{0.95}(14, 13) \doteq 2.55$ and $F_{0.95}(13, 14) \doteq 2.51$, while from Table 6.10 we have $s_1^2/s_2^2 = 7.5$. Hence, $(7.5/2.55, 7.5(2.51)) = (2.94, 18.83)$ is a 90% confidence interval for σ_1^2/σ_2^2. Notice that 1 is not in the interval—the test of equal variances agrees with the confidence interval, as it should.

Besides the Cochran–Cox *t*-test procedure, it is often possible to transform the observations in order to meet the assumption of homogeneous variance. If such a transformation can be found, then the two-sample *t*-test may be applied to the transformed data. We discuss various transformations in the following section.

6.2.5 Transformation of Data To Equalize Variance

In general, the two-sample *t*-test is more robust to departures from the normality assumption than to the homogeneity of variance assumption. That is, if data are not precisely normally distributed, the two-sample *t*-test provides a valid* test of the hypothesis if the data do not depart a great deal from a normal distribution, particularly if n_1 and n_2 are large (each ≥ 20) and the variances are equal. It is the central limit theorem that provides this protection against departures from normality. On the other hand, if the variances are unequal, the two-sample *t*-test may produce an invalid test of the equal-means hypothesis. Accordingly, one may transform the data in order to meet the variance homogeneity assumption. While many transformations are possible, three are most often considered.

The *logarithmic transformation* is frequently applied to data when the investigator suspects that the variability increases with the size of the response variable. For example, this transformation is particularly useful for blood count data such as white blood cell count, lymphocytes, leukocytes, and so on. It is also useful for time response data where the observations are the time to death, time in remission, and so on. Some general points regarding the *logarithmic* transformation include the

---

*By a valid test, we mean that the significance level (α) or P value reported are correct, or if not precisely accurate, then the stated values are no bigger than the true values. A test that lacks such control of α is termed an invalid test since the reported P values may be considerable underestimates of the true ones.

following:

1. Any base of the logarithm may be used, but most analysts prefer to work with base 10.
2. The logarithm may be applied only to positive observations.
3. If an occasional zero arises, it is suggested that $\log(Y + 1)$ be used.
4. The transformation $\log(Y + 1)$ is also preferred to $\log Y$ if values of Y can be in the range from 0 to 10.

The *square root* transformation is appropriate for Poisson count data. In microbiology, bacterial counts per plate are determined, and the square root transformation Y is often considered, where Y is the number of counts per plate. This transformation is also appropriate for the analysis of certain types of mortality data. For example, if the number of suicides or accidental deaths are to be compared between two communities of approximately equal population sizes, then the Poisson distribution is a likely distribution for the number of such deaths. In general, the square root transformation is considered appropriate for data consisting of small integer counts in which the mean and variance are roughly equal.

The *angular* transformation is most appropriate for binomial count data. In practice, the transformation is applied to a proportion p. The precise transformation is defined by $\arcsin(\sqrt{Y})$; it is the radian measure of the angle whose sine is $\sqrt{Y}$. For a fuller discussion of this transformation and others the reader may refer to Box and Cox (1964, 1982).

One final word of caution regarding the use of transformations. The standard deviation of transformed observations may not merely be inverted to determine the standard deviation of the untransformed data. For example, if the standard deviation of the square root transformed data is 4, it does not follow that the standard deviation of the untransformed data is $4^2 = 16$. For example, consider a sample of size 3 consisting of 4, 8, and 12 for which the standard deviation is $\sqrt{\frac{1}{2}\left[(4 - 8)^2 + (8 - 8)^2 + (12 - 8)^2\right]} = 4$. The standard deviation of 16, 64, and 144 is not equal to 16. In fact, it is equal to 64.7. This is an obvious point when you think about it; however, it is easily overlooked when analyzing transformed data.

Although a common reason for transforming is to obtain equal variances, there are others, including an attempt to achieve a simple linear additive model for the data or normality of distribution. These and other reasons are discussed by Box and Cox (1964, 1982) and Bickel and Doksum (1981).

6.3   USE OF RANK TESTS FOR GROUP COMPARISONS

The t-tests for equal means and the F-test for equal variances assume an underlying normal distribution for the data. There are alternative test procedures that do not require such an assumption and that are still valid if the data are normal. Testing and estimation procedures that do not require, or are free, from, the normality assumption are called distribution-free procedures. Strictly speaking, a statistical test procedure is distribution-free if the significance level of the test is valid for any underlying, continuous distribution. That the distribution be continuous is a requirement since it is difficult to derive tests that are distribution free in the class of all distributions, but it is possible to derive distribution-free tests in the subcategory of continuous distributions. In addition to being called distribution-free tests, these tests are also called *nonparametric* tests. A test based on an assumption that the data are normally distributed, such as the t-test, is called a *parametric* test, since the test is focused on a specified parameter like the mean μ. The terms distribution-free and nonparametric appear interchangeably in this text.

Rank tests are distribution-free test procedures that utilize the rank order of the observations in place of the observations; thus, the ranks constitute a transformation of the data. Since only the ordering of the observations is required, rank tests may be applied to ordinal-scale data as well as to interval- and ratio-scale data. Since these nonparametric rank tests provide valid tests for the entire class of continuous distributions, they are valid, in particular, for normally distributed data. Thus, the rank tests compete with the t-tests; furthermore, they would be valid tests even when normality does not hold if continuity holds. In addition, the rank tests also compete with the t-tests because rank statistics are often easier to compute. Historically, the study of the normal distribution and t-tests preceded the study of rank tests. Today, parametric and nonparametric test procedures are each commonly applied to problems of data analysis. If normality assumptions are obviously not met, for example, when the data are ordinal, nonparametric tests are typically applied in preference to the parametric tests.

We begin with a rank test procedure for the matched-pairs design.

6.3.1   Wilcoxon Signed-Rank Test: A Nonparametric Rank Test for Matched-Pair Studies

Wilcoxon (1945) developed several test procedures based on ranks; the signed-rank test is the test he proposed for the matched-pair design. Consider data of the form described in Table 6.1. The hypothesis of

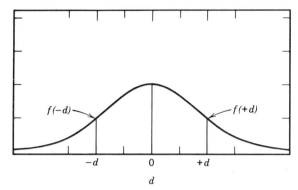

Figure 6.2. Symmetric frequency function of differences.

principal interest is that the first group and second group have identical probability distributions, that is, the set of pairwise differences have a probability distribution that is centered at zero. Furthermore, we assume that the distribution of the differences is symmetric about zero, a reasonable assumption since the first and second group have identical distributions under this null hypothesis. Hence, if the differences arise from a continuous distribution, it follows that the probability density function $f(d)$ for the set of differences is symmetric about zero and is centered at zero when the null hypothesis is true. Graphically, we have the situation described by Figure 6.2 under the null hypothesis. From Figure 6.2, it is evident that a difference of given absolute value has an equal chance of being a positive or a negative difference, that is, $f(-d) = f(+d)$ for all values of d. This statement, of course, holds true for a difference of any size. Given a difference of a given absolute value or ranked absolute value, the probability that the difference is a positive difference is $\frac{1}{2}$. The probability that the difference is a negative difference is also $\frac{1}{2}$. All of these facts hold under the null hypothesis of identical distributions for groups 1 and 2. Thus, under the null hypothesis, one would expect the ranks of the absolute values of the differences to be evenly distributed between negative and positive differences. This suggests using the sum of the ranks associated with the positive differences (or the sum of the ranks associated with the negative differences) as a test statistic. If the curve of Figure 6.2 was shifted to the left, then we would expect the sum of the ranks of the negative differences (positive differences) to be large (small). A shift to the left indicates that the second group has a distribution center greater than that of the first group (see Table 6.1 for direction of differences). Conversely, if the curve was shifted to the right, then we would expect the sum of the ranks of the negative differences (positive differences) to be small (large). A shift to the right suggests that the second group has a center less than that of the first group.

Under the null hypothesis that the differences $d_1, \ldots, d_n$ come from a symmetric distribution centered at 0, the chance that a d_i of a given absolute magnitude is positive is the same chance that it is positive, that is, $\frac{1}{2}$. Hence the probability that a given difference is positive is $\frac{1}{2}$ regardless of the absolute magnitude of the difference. Given the observed values of the absolute differences $|d_1|, \ldots, |d_n|$, there are 2^n possible assignments of signs to the absolute differences. Each of these 2^n assignments is equally likely under the null hypothesis and has probability $\left(\frac{1}{2}\right)^n$. If the differences with positive signs tend to be larger (in absolute value) than those with the negative signs, then this would suggest that the differences are centered at $\mu_d > 0$. In the following example, we illustrate how a test could be performed using this concept of conditioning on the observed magnitude of the differences.

Example 6.3.1.1. A study was conducted in which four pairs of obese children, matched on initial body weight, age, and sex, were placed on weight reduction programs. Two dietary programs were compared, A and B, and one child in each pair was assigned at random to one of the programs. Program B is a dietary plan while A is a dietary plan plus exercise. The amounts of body weight reduction after six months on the two diets are shown in the accompanying table.

| | Program | | |
Pair	A	B	Difference $(A - B)$
1	22	26	-4
2	14	12	$+2$
3	18	11	$+7$
4	11	5	$+6$

It is of interest to test the hypothesis of equal effectiveness in reducing weight against the alternative that A is superior. We may note that the four differences take values 4, 2, 7, and 6 in absolute value. There are 2^4 possible assignments of the sign ($+$ or $-$) to these four differences. One way to construct a statistical test of the equal-effectiveness hypothesis is to enumerate the entire $2^4 = 16$ possible assignment of signs to 4, 2, 7, and 6 and compute the sum of the positive differences for each of these. These are summarized in the following table.

Possible Signs for Differences				Sum of Positive Differences
2	4	6	7	(S_+)
+	+	+	+	19
−	+	+	+	17
+	−	+	+	15
+	+	−	+	13
+	+	+	−	12
−	−	+	+	13
−	+	−	+	11
−	+	+	−	10
+	−	−	+	9
+	−	+	−	8
+	+	−	−	6
−	−	−	+	7
−	−	+	−	6
−	+	−	−	4
+	−	−	−	2
−	−	−	−	0

Thus, for these differences, the sum of the positive differences S_+ can take values from 0 to 19. Since each of the lines in the preceding table has probability $\frac{1}{16}$ under the null hypothesis, we can list the probability distribution of S_+. In particular,

$$\Pr[S_+ = 0] = \tfrac{1}{16} \qquad \Pr[S_+ = 10] = \tfrac{1}{16},$$

$$\Pr[S_+ = 2] = \tfrac{1}{16} \qquad \Pr[S_+ = 11] = \tfrac{1}{16}$$

$$\Pr[S_+ = 4] = \tfrac{1}{16} \qquad \Pr[S_+ = 12] = \tfrac{1}{16}$$

$$\Pr[S_+ = 6] = \tfrac{2}{16} \qquad \Pr[S_+ = 13] = \tfrac{2}{16}$$

$$\Pr[S_+ = 7] = \tfrac{1}{16} \qquad \Pr[S_+ = 15] = \tfrac{1}{16}$$

$$\Pr[S_+ = 8] = \tfrac{1}{16} \qquad \Pr[S_+ = 17] = \tfrac{1}{16}$$

$$\Pr[S_+ = 9] = \tfrac{1}{16} \qquad \Pr[S_+ = 19] = \tfrac{1}{16}$$

For the observed sample, the differences are $+2$, -4, $+6$, and $+7$; hence $S_+ = 15$. It may be noted that this seems favorable to the hypothesis that the differences are centered at $\mu_d > 0$; however, we note that the $\Pr[S_+ \geq$

$15] = \frac{3}{16}$ since $\Pr[S_+ \geq 15] = \Pr[S_+ = 15] + \Pr[S_+ = 17] + \Pr[S_+ = 19]$. The observed outcome is probably not extreme enough to warrant rejection of the null hypothesis since the P value for the observed S_+ is $\frac{3}{16}$.

While the analysis in the example is valid, the computations can be burdensome, particularly if there is a large number of pairs. For larger n and a new set of differences, an entirely new table of differences would have to be generated.

One simplification is to consider the ranks of the absolute differences from 1 to n and consider the possible assignment of signs to these ranks. There are 2^n assignments of signs, each equally likely under the null hypothesis. For a given n, it is possible to generate all possible sign assignments to the ranks of $1, 2, \ldots, n$, and tabulation of the probabilities for each value of the sum of the positive differences is easily done. It follows that the sampling distribution of the sum of the positive ranks (negative ranks) depends only on n and the 2^n permutations of plus and minus signs to the ranks. That is, replacing the absolute values of differences with their ranks yields a statistic whose distribution does not depend on the underlying distribution of the differences. The resulting test procedure is clearly distribution free. The Wilcoxon (1945) signed-rank test procedure is described in outline form in Table 6.11. In this description, μ_d is the location parameter for the distribution of the differences.

In Table 6.11, $Z_{1-\alpha}$ and $Z_{1-\alpha/2}$ are determined in the usual way from Table 4 of the Appendix. On the other hand, $T_{1-\alpha/2}(n)$ and $T_{1-\alpha}(n)$ are determined from Table 9 of the Appendix. For a given sample size n, the cumulative distribution of T_+ (or T_-) is tabulated in Table 9 of the Appendix. The quantity $T_{1-\alpha}(n)$ is defined as that value of T_+ such that, under the null hypothesis,

$$\Pr[T_+ > T_{1-\alpha}(n)] \leq \alpha \quad \text{and} \quad \Pr[T_+ > T_{1-\alpha}(n) - 1] \geq \alpha. \quad (6.10)$$

When using Table 9 of the Appendix, it may be necessary to use the fact that $\Pr[T_+ > i] = \Pr[T_+ < n(n+1)/2 - i]$ and $\Pr[T_- > i] = \Pr[T_- < n(n+1)/2 - i]$ for $i = 1, 2, \ldots, n(n+1)/2$.

The complicated inequalities in expression (6.10) arise because the distribution of T_+ is itself a discrete rather than continuous; hence, it may not be possible to find a value of T_+ such that the exact level of α is obtained. This problem was also noted when we discussed the one-sample binomial test in Chapter 5. For example, for $\alpha = 0.05$, $n = 5$, we find from Table 9 of the Appendix that $\Pr[T_+ > 13] = 0.0625 \geq 0.05$ and $\Pr[T_+ > 14] = 0.0313 \leq 0.05$. Clearly, a one-tailed test in which we require α to be no bigger than 0.05 would require rejection of H_0 if T_+ exceeded 14. The actual level of such a one-tailed test would be 0.0313. Thus, a conservative test would result, since $0.0313 < 0.05$.

Table 6.11. Outline of Wilcoxon Signed-Rank Test Procedure

A. Data: $d_1, \ldots, d_n$ from Table 6.1.

B. Assumptions: $d_1, \ldots, d_n$ is a random sample from a continuous, symmetric distribution centered at μ_d. Assume all d_i are nonzero, i.e., discard zeros.

C. Computations:

1. Compute $|d_1|, \ldots, |d_n|$.

2. Assuming each $|d_i|$ is nonzero, then order them from smallest to largest.

3. Assign a rank of 1 to the smallest quantity, a rank of 2 to the next largest, 3 to the next largest..., n to the largest absolute difference. In the case of absolute differences being "tied" for the same ranks. The mean rank is assigned to each (midranks). If there are many ties, then the procedures in Table 6.13 should be followed.

4. Let T_+ denote the sum of the ranks assigned to the positive differences, T_- denote the sum of the ranks assigned to the negative differences. In actual computations, $T_- = \dfrac{n(n+1)}{2} - T_+$, so once T_+ or T_- is computed, the other is known immediately.

D. Two-tailed statistical test:

1. Null hypothesis H_0: $\mu_d = 0$

2. Alternative hypothesis H_a: $\mu_d \neq 0$

3. Decision rule for an α-level test:

(a) Exact test: Reject H_0 in favor of H_a if $T_+ > T_{1-\alpha/2}(n)$ or if $T_- > T_{1-\alpha/2}(n)$.

(b) Large-sample test: Reject H_0 in favor of H_a if

$$Z_+ = \left[\frac{T_+ - n(n+1)/4}{\sqrt{n(n+1)(2n+1)/24}} \right] > Z_{1-\alpha/2},$$

or if

$$Z_- = \left[\frac{T_- - n(n+1)/4}{\sqrt{n(n+1)(2n+1)/24}} \right] > Z_{1-\alpha/2}.$$

One-tailed statistical test:

1. Null hypothesis: H_0: $\mu_d = 0$

2. Alternative hypothesis: H_a: $\mu_d > 0$ (H_a: $\mu_d < 0$)

3. Decision rule for an α-level test:

(a) Exact test: Reject H_0 in favor of H_a if $T_+ > T_{1-\alpha}(n)$ [reject H_0 in favor of H_a if $T_- > T_{1-\alpha}(n)$].

(b) Large-sample test: Reject H_0 in favor of H_a if

$$Z_+ = \frac{T_+ - n(n+1)/4}{\sqrt{n(n+1)(2n+1)/24}} > Z_{1-\alpha}$$

[reject H_0 in favor of H_a if

$$Z_- = \frac{T_- - n(n+1)/4}{\sqrt{n(n+1)(2n+1)/24}} > Z_{1-\alpha}\,].$$

Table 6.12. Worked Solution to Example 6.2.1.1 Using the Signed-Rank Test

---

A. Data: The differences are 0.61, 0.64, 0.76, 0.45, 0.29, -0.11, and 0.12.
B. Assumptions: The differences are a random sample from a symmetric, continuous distribution.
C. Computations:

Pair	d_i	$|d_i|$	Rank of $|d_i|$
1	0.61	.61	5
2	0.64	.64	6
3	0.76	.76	7
4	0.45	.45	4
5	0.29	.29	3
6	-0.11	.11	1
7	0.12	.12	2

Hence, $T_- = 1$ and $T_+ = 27$.
D. One-tailed statistical test:
  1. Null hypothesis: $H_0: \mu_d = 0$
  2. Alternative hypothesis: $H_a: \mu_d > 0$
  3. Decision rule for .05 level test: Reject H_0 in favor of H_a if $T_+ > T_{0.95}(7)$.
E. Action taken: From Table 9 of the Appendix, $\Pr[T_+ > 23] = \Pr[T_+ \leq 4] = 0.0547$ and $\Pr[T_+ > 24] = \Pr[T_+ \leq 3] = 0.0391$; hence, one should reject if $T_+ > 24$. Clearly, since $T_+ = 27$, we reject H_0; the significance level of this test is equal to 0.0391. The P value is $\Pr[T_+ > 26] = \Pr[T_+ < 28 - 26] = \Pr[T_+ \leq 1] = 0.0156$ from Table 9 of the Appendix. This is also easily computed directly since there is only one arrangement of signs that yields $T_+ = 28$ and one that yields $T_+ = 27$. Of the 128 (2^7) equally likely assignments of signs, the P value is therefore $\frac{2}{128}$, or 0.0156.

Example 6.3.1.2. It may be helpful to reanalyze Example 6.2.1.1 using the signed-rank test procedure. The worked solution appears in Table 6.12.

We note that the large-sample tests in Table 6.11 are based on the normal distribution. These tests follow from a central limit theorem for nonparametric statistics. This central limit theorem arises by considering the 2^n assignment of signs to the ranks and considering the distribution of T_+. This result has broader application for other nonparametric tests as well. For sample sizes in which the number of nonzero differences is at least 20, we may use this large-sample test procedure. This result makes this rank test particularly attractive since the exact distribution involving the 2^n permutations need not be generated for all sample sizes. This is a tremendous savings of work for large n.

Table 6.13. Outline of a Wilcoxon Signed-Rank Test Procedure with Correction for Ties (Large-Sample Test)

A. Data: $d_1, \ldots, d_n$ from Table 6.1.
B. Assumptions: $d_1, \ldots, d_n$ are a random sample from a continuous symmetric distribution with mean μ_d. Assume all d_i are nonzero (discard zero differences).
C. Computations:
   1. Compute $|d_1|, \ldots, |d_n|$.
   2. Rank (excluding the zero differences) the differences from smallest to largest, using midranks for tied differences.
   3. Let

$$t_1 = \text{the number of differences tied at one value of } d,$$

$$t_2 = \text{the number of differences tied at another value of } d,$$

$$\vdots$$

$$t_r = \text{the number of differences in the last tied group.}$$

   4. Let T_+ (T_-) denote the sum of the ranks of the positive (negative) differences.
   5. Let

$$M = \tfrac{1}{4}[n(n+1)],$$

$$s^2 = \frac{2n(n+1)(2n+1) - \sum_{j=1}^{r} t_j(t_j - 1)(t_j + 1)}{48}.$$

   6. $Z_+ = \dfrac{T_+ - M}{s}$, and $Z_- = \dfrac{T_- - M}{s}$.

D. Two-tailed statistical test:
   1. Null hypothesis: $H_0: \mu_d = 0$
   2. Alternative hypothesis: $H_a: \mu_d \neq 0$
   3. Decision rule for an α-level test: Reject H_0 in favor of H_a if Z_+ or $Z_- > Z_{1-\alpha/2}$.
   One-tailed statistical test:
   1. Null hypothesis: $H_0: \mu_d = 0$
   2. Alternative hypothesis: $H_a: \mu_d > (H_a: \mu_d < 0)$
   3. Decision rule for an α-level test: Reject H_0 in favor of H_a if $Z_+ > Z_{1-\alpha}$ (reject H_0 if favor of H_a if $Z_- > Z_{1-\alpha}$).

If there are tied differences, then the large-sample procedure in Table 6.11 can be modified to accommodate this. For small samples, the exact distribution like Example 6.3.1.1 must be generated for the tied ranks, and is not presented here. For large samples, the modified test procedure is straightforward; it is outlined in Table 6.13. As before, $Z_{1-\alpha/2}$ and $Z_{1-\alpha}$ are obtained from Table 4 of the Appendix.

Let us consider another example in which the signed-rank test may be applied.

Example 6.3.1.3. An experiment was conducted to determine the effects of chlormethiazole on the serum prolactin levels of male alcoholics. All men abstained from alcohol during the study. Serum prolactin concentrations were measured via radioimmunoassay at the time of admission and on the seventh day after treatment with chlormethiazole. The data is presented in the accompanying table.

Patient	Serum Prolactin (mV/L) Before	After	d_i	$\lvert d_i \rvert$	Rank $\lvert d_i \rvert^a$
1	330	310	+20	20	2
2	250	190	+60	60	7
3	280	140	+140	140	17
4	180	130	+50	50	5
5	180	180	0	0	—
6	330	250	+80	80	9
7	330	130	+200	200	18
8	250	120	+130	130	15
9	390	180	+210	210	19
10	280	280	0	0	—
11	110	140	−30	30	3
12	280	150	+130	130	15
13	220	170	+50	50	5
14	270	150	+120	120	13
15	210	260	−50	50	5
16	440	90	+350	350	20
17	360	230	+130	130	15
18	210	100	+110	110	12
19	310	210	+100	100	11
20	240	170	+70	70	8
21	330	240	+90	90	10
22	220	230	−10	10	1

[a] Rank of $\lvert d_i \rvert$ after discarding the two zero differences and reducing n from 22 to 20. Patients 4, 13 and 15 are tied at $\lvert d \rvert = 50$; their ranks would have been 4, 5 and 6, so mid-rank $= (4 + 5 + 6)/3 = 5$.

Table 6.14. Worked Solution of Example 6.3.1.3 Using Wilcoxon Signed-Rank Test with Correction for Ties

A. Data: The differences are   20, 60, 140, 50, 0, 80, 200, 130, 210, 0, -30, 130, 50, 120, -50, 350, 130, 110, 100, 70, 90, -10.
B. Assumptions: The differences are a random sample from a symmetric, continuous distribution.
C. Computations: We have $n = 20$.

d_i	$|d_i|$	Rank $|d_i|$	d_i	$|d_i|$	Rank $|d_i|$
20	20	2	130	130	15
60	60	7	50	50	5
140	140	17	120	120	13
50	50	5	-50	50	5
0	0	—	350	350	20
80	80	9	130	130	15
200	200	18	110	110	12
130	130	15	100	100	11
210	210	19	70	70	8
0	0	—	90	90	10
-30	30	3	-10	10	1

$$T_- = 1 + 3 + 5 = 9 \qquad T_+ = 201 \qquad M = 20(21)/4 = 105$$

Since there are three values assigned the midrank 5 and three values assigned the midrank 15, then $t_1 = 3$ and $t_2 = 3$ and thus

$$s^2 = \tfrac{1}{48}[2(20)(21)(41) - (24 + 24)]$$

$$s = 26.77$$

$$Z_+ = \frac{201 - 105}{26.77} = 3.59$$

D. One-tailed statistical test:
  1. Null hypothesis: H_0: $\mu_d = 0$
  2. Alternative hypothesis: H_a: $\mu_d > 0$
  3. Decision rule for a 0.01 level test: Reject H_0 in favor of H_a if Z_+ computed in step C is greater than $Z_{0.99}$.
E. Action taken: From Table 4 of the Appendix, $Z_{0.99} = 2.33$ while our computed value of Z_+ is 3.59; hence, the null hypothesis is rejected. The P value is once again a small quantity, in fact, $P < 0.00001$.

The question of interest is whether the prolactin levels decrease after chlormethiazole.

We consider testing the one-sided alternative hypothesis at the 0.01 level of significance using the test described in Table 6.11. Ignoring the zeros, we would have an n of 20 rather than 22. From the above data, we compute $T_- = 1 + 3 + 5 = 9$ and $T_+ = 2 + 4 + 6 + 7 + \cdots + 20 = 201$. From Table 9 of the Appendix, with $n = 20$, we see that $\Pr[T_+ \geq 201] = \Pr[T_+ \leq (20)(21)/2 - 201] = \Pr[T_+ \leq 9] \doteq 0.00001$. Hence, the P value for the exact test is infinitesimal, and the null hypothesis should be rejected. The large-sample test from Table 6.11 leads to the following computations: $n(n + 1)/4 = 105$ and $n(n + 1)(2n + 1)/24 = 717.5$; thus, it follows that $Z_+ = (201 - 105)/\sqrt{717.5} = 3.58$. From Table 4 of the Appendix, $Z_{0.99} = 2.33$; the large-sample test also leads to rejection of the null hypothesis.

By applying the procedure outlined in Table 6.13, we can correct for the ties in the data. We summarize this alternative, preferred analysis in Table 6.14.

An alternative way to perform the Wilcoxon signed test when the sample size is large is to use the paired t-test procedure, described in Table 6.2, based on the signed ranks. That is, replace the data by the corresponding signed ranks and then follow the procedure outlined in Table 6.2. This method also works when there are ties and is particularly easy when a program for the paired t-test is available. See Iman (1974) for more details.

The preceding analyses describe the use of the Wilcoxon signed-rank test, an alternative to the paired t-test, for testing hypotheses concerning the shift or location parameter μ_d when the data are not normally distributed. A remaining issue is the *estimation* of μ_d when the differences are not normally distributed. In the normal distribution situation, the sample mean $\bar{d}$ is regarded as the best point estimator of μ_d, while expression (6.3), $\bar{d} \pm t_{1-\alpha/2}(n - 1)s_{\bar{d}}$, provides a confidence interval estimator for μ_d. Thus, our discussion of the t-distribution included both tests of hypotheses and estimation procedures. Similarly, for the Wilcoxon signed-rank test, there is a corresponding procedure for estimation of parameters, so that summary statistics along with results of the test procedure can be presented in data analysis.

The procedure for estimating the location of the distribution of the differences is based on the following principle: choose as the point estimator the quantity $\tilde{d}$, where $\tilde{d}$ is an amount subtracted from each and every difference in order to make T_+ equal to T_-. In effect, we determine how much we should subtract from each pairwise difference in order to make the resulting quantities T_+ and T_- conform to the null hypothesis of no difference as closely as possible. Whatever is subtracted would seem to be a reasonable estimator of location, since it is that value that in a sense centers the data. This is, in fact, one way to rationalize our choice of $\bar{d}$ as the estimator of μ_d in the paired t-test. Clearly, if $\bar{d}$ was subtracted from each difference, the resulting adjusted differences $d_i - \bar{d}$ would have a mean of zero, leading to a t value of zero. A t value of zero is as conformable with the null hypothesis as is possible. We shall apply the same principle to the signed-rank test procedure.

To find the estimator $\tilde{d}$, it is convenient to write T_+ in an alternative form. We assume that we have a set of differences $d_1, \ldots, d_n$ in which there are no zeros and no ties among the absolute values of the differences. In this case, it can be shown that T_+ can be rewritten as

$$T_+ = \text{number of } \tfrac{1}{2}(d_i + d_j) \quad \text{that are greater than zero for } i \leq j. \quad (6.11)$$

As a result of (6.11), the statistic T_+ takes the most central value if one-half of $\tfrac{1}{2}(d_i + d_j)$ for $i \leq j$ are greater than zero, while the remaining half is less than zero. Thus, $\tilde{d}$ should be such that one-half of $\tfrac{1}{2}[(d_i - \tilde{d}) + (d_j - \tilde{d})] = [\tfrac{1}{2}(d_i - d_j) - \tilde{d}]$ are greater than zero. The quantity $\tilde{d}$ that achieves this is the median of these averages. Hence, the estimator of location for the signed ranks procedure is $\tilde{d}$, where

$$\tilde{d} = \underset{i \leq j}{\text{median}} \frac{d_i + d_j}{2}. \quad (6.12)$$

There are $\tfrac{1}{2}[n(n+1)]$ averages of the form $\tfrac{1}{2}(d_i + d_j)$ for $i \leq j$.

A simple way to get the estimator is to construct a two-way table for d_i by d_j and enter the sum $d_i + d_j$ in the table. Let us use this method to determine the signed-rank estimator of location using the set of differences of -0.11, 0.12, 0.29, 0.45, 0.76, 0.61, and 0.64 from Example 6.2.1.1. The two-way table is given in Table 6.15. Note that the differences are ordered before they are entered as rows and columns. Since $n = 7$, it follows that the median of the averages $\tfrac{1}{2}(d_i + d_j)$ for $i \leq j$ is the mean of the 14th and 15th ordered averages. From Table 6.15, the signed-rank estimator is the mean of 0.38 $(= .76/2)$ and 0.44 $(= .88/2)$, the mean of the 14th and 15th ordered $\tfrac{1}{2}(d_i + d_j)$. The median is 0.41. This is to be compared to the value of 0.39 found for $\bar{d}$.

The procedure above may also be applied if a few ties are in the data. For data with a few zero differences, it is recommended that the zero differences be discarded and the estimator derived on the basis of the reduced set of differences.

In general, the estimator of location (6.12) should accompany the Wilcoxon signed-rank test in the data presentation. Unfortunately, non-

Table 6.15. Computations for Signed-Rank Estimator of Location for Example 6.2.1.1: Entry is Sum of d_i and d_j

d_i	d_j						
	-0.11	0.12	0.29	0.45	0.61	0.64	0.76
-0.11	-0.22	0.01	0.18	0.34	0.50	0.53	0.65
0.12		0.24	0.41	0.57	0.73	0.76	0.88
0.29			0.58	0.74	0.90	0.93	1.05
0.45				0.90	1.06	1.09	1.21
0.61					1.22	1.25	1.37
0.64						1.28	1.40
0.76							1.52

parametric tests are often reported without the estimators. Very seldom are we only interested in a statistical test. The corresponding estimator is also quite important for proper communication of the study results to others.

A confidence interval may also be determined for μ_d, the center of symmetry of the distribution of differences. By denoting $\frac{1}{2}(d_i + d_j)$ as b and the ordered set of b's as $b_{(1)} < b_{(2)} < \cdots < b_{(n(n+1)/2)}$, then it can be shown that

$$\Pr\left[b_{(i)} < \mu_d \le b_{(i+1)}\right] = \Pr[T_+ = i] \quad \text{for } i = 0, 1, \ldots, \tfrac{1}{2}[n(n+1)],$$

$$(6.13)$$

where $b_{(0)}$ is defined as $-\infty$, and $b_{(n(n+1)/2+1)} = +\infty$, and where the probability on the right side of (6.13) is computed under the hypothesis that $\mu_d = 0$ (thus Table 9 of the Appendix may be used to assist our confidence interval computations). It follows from (6.13) that

$$\Pr\left[\mu_d \le b_{(i)}\right] = \Pr[T_+ \le (i-1)]. \qquad (6.14)$$

This quantity may be used directly to obtain confidence intervals for μ_d. In particular, from Table 9 of the Appendix, we can find, for a given α_1, α_2, and n, the values i and j such that

$$\alpha_1 = \Pr[T_+ \le i-1] = \Pr\left[\mu_d \le b_{(i)}\right] = \Pr\left[\mu_d < b_{(i+1)}\right] \quad (6.15)$$

and

$$1 - \alpha_2 = \Pr[T_+ \le j-1] = \Pr\left[\mu_d \le b_{(j)}\right].$$

Hence,

$$\Pr\left[b_{(i)} < \mu_d \le b_{(j)}\right] = \Pr\left[b_{(i+1)} \le \mu_d \le b_{(j)}\right] = 1 - \alpha_1 - \alpha_2, \quad (6.16)$$

and $[b_{(i+1)}, b_{(j)}]$ is a $(1 - \alpha_1 - \alpha_2)100\%$ confidence interval for μ_d. For larger n ($n \geq 20$), the quantity (6.14) may be approximated by the normal distribution. In particular, the approximate probability (Lehmann, 1975) is

$$\Pr[\mu_d \leq b_{(i)}] = \Pr[T_+ \leq i - 1] \doteq \Pr[Z \leq Z^*], \qquad (6.17)$$

where $Z^* = [2(i - 1) - \frac{1}{2}n(n + 1)]/\sqrt{n(n + 1)(2n + 1)/6}$ and Z is the standard normal variate. Hence, to compute a $(1 - \alpha)100\%$ confidence interval using the large-sample procedure, the interval would be $b_{(i+1)}$ to $b_{(j)}$, where i is found by solving

$$-Z_{1-\alpha/2} = \frac{2(i - 1) - (1/2)[n(n + 1)]}{\sqrt{n(n + 1)(2n + 1)/6}} \qquad (6.18)$$

for i, and j is found by solving

$$Z_{1-\alpha/2} = \frac{2(j - 1) - (1/2)[n(n + 1)]}{\sqrt{n(n + 1)(2n + 1)/6}} \qquad (6.19)$$

for j.

If i is not an integer, then $i + 1$ is taken as the integer immediately above the computed i in (6.18). If j is not an integer, it too is taken as the next integer above the computed value in (6.19). As an example, if $n = 22$ and we desire a $(1 - \alpha)100\%$ confidence for μ_d, then (6.18) is $-1.96 = [2(i - 1) - 22(23)/2]/\sqrt{22(23)(45)/6}$ and $i = 67.1$. Hence, we take $i + 1$ to be 68. Similarly, from (6.19) we have $1.96 = [2(j - 1) - 22(23)/2]/\sqrt{22(23)(45)/6}$ and $j = 187.9$, and we take j to be 188. Hence, the 95% confidence interval would be the interval between the 68th ordered average and the 188th ordered average difference.

Let us now determine confidence intervals for the data of Table 6.15. For Table 6.15, the ordered averages may be obtained; these ordered averages and various probabilities are summarized in Table 6.16. The second column of Table 6.16 is taken directly from Table 6.15, while the last column of Table 6.16 is determined from Table 9 of the Appendix for $n = 7$. From Table 6.16, we note that $\Pr[\mu_d \leq b_{(3)}] = 0.0234$ and $\Pr[\mu_d \leq b_{(26)}] = 0.9766$. Hence, the interval $[b_{(4)}, b_{(26)}]$ is a $0.9766 - 0.0234 = 0.9532$, or 95.32%, confidence interval for the location parameter μ_d. From Table 6.16, $b_{(4)} = 0.12$ and $b_{(26)} = 0.685$; hence, an approximate 95% confidence interval for the center of the distribution is $[0.12, 0.69]$. The paired t in Section 6.2.1 yielded a 95% confidence interval of $[0.10, 0.68]$.

In general, it may not be possible to obtain a confidence interval with an exact coefficient of 95 or 99% due to the discrete nature of the distribution

Table 6.16. Ordered Averages of Differences and Probabilities
for Data of Table 6.15

i	$d_j + d_k$	$b_{(i)} = \frac{1}{2}(d_j + d_k)$	$\Pr[\mu_d \le b_{(i)}] = \Pr[T_+ \le i - 1]$
1	-0.22	-0.11	0.0078
2	0.01	0.005	0.0156
3	0.18	0.09	0.0234
4	0.24	0.12	0.0391
5	0.34	0.17	0.0547
6	0.41	0.205	0.0781
7	0.50	0.250	0.1094
8	0.53	0.265	0.1484
9	0.57	0.285	0.1875
10	0.58	0.290	0.2344
11	0.65	0.325	0.2891
12	0.73	0.365	0.3438
13	0.74	0.370	0.4063
14	0.76	0.380	0.4688
15	0.88	0.440	0.5312
16	0.90	0.450	0.5937
17	0.90	0.450	0.6562
18	0.93	0.465	0.7109
19	1.05	0.525	0.7656
20	1.06	0.530	0.8125
21	1.09	0.545	0.8516
22	1.21	0.605	0.8906
23	1.22	0.610	0.9219
24	1.25	0.625	0.9453
25	1.28	0.640	0.9609
26	1.37	0.685	0.9766
27	1.40	0.700	0.9844
28	1.52	0.760	0.9922

of T_+. In practice, if a 95% interval is desired, one gets as close to 0.95 as possible but generally stays above rather than beneath it.

In many cases, a one-sided rather than two-sided confidence interval is sought. This is readily obtained from Table 6.16. In particular, since $\Pr[\mu_d \le b_{(4)}] = 0.0391$, it follows that $[b_{(5)}, \infty]$ is a 96.09% confidence interval for μ_d. Therefore, we would have the following examples as possible confidence intervals for μ_d:

$[0.17, \infty)$ with confidence coefficient 96.09%;

$[0.205, \infty)$ with confidence coefficient 94.53%.

Thus, the full range of inference—hypotheses testing, point estimation, and confidence interval estimation—are available with the signed-rank procedure. These procedures may be preferable to the paired t procedures since fewer assumptions are required with these signed-rank methods.

Turning to the question of sample size requirements for the signed-rank test, we consider only the large-sample situation. Furthermore, it is assumed that the sample size is to be determined for the one-sided alternative hypothesis that $\mu_d = \mu_d^* > 0$. Even with these restrictions, the required sample size depends on the underlying distribution of the differences. If one assumes that the differences are normally distributed, then the required number of differences n for an α-level test to have power $1 - \beta$ against the alternative hypothesis that $\mu_d = \mu_d^*$ is

$$
n = \frac{\pi \sigma_d^2 \left(Z_{1-\alpha} + Z_{1-\beta} \right)^2}{3 \left(\mu_d^* \right)^2},
$$

where $Z_{1-\alpha}$ and $Z_{1-\beta}$ are from Table 4 of the Appendix, σ_d^2 is the variance of the differences, and π is the number of radians in the half-circle. For the two-sided alternatives, $Z_{1-\alpha}$ is replaced by $Z_{1-\alpha/2}$. We may note that the sample size is $\pi/3$ times the value obtained for the paired t-test in Section 6.2.1. This illustrates that the signed-rank test has efficiency (i.e., ratio of sample sizes to have equal power) $3/\pi = 0.955$ relative to the t-test when the data are normal. Very little additional sample size is required for the signed-rank test to have the same power as the t-test even when the data are normal. For other assumed distributions, the reader may refer to Lehmann (1975).

Let us now turn to a rank test and estimation procedure appropriate for the comparison of two independent samples.

6.3.2 Wilcoxon–Mann–Whitney Rank Sum Test: A Nonparametric Test for Two Independent Groups

The previous section illustrated the usefulness of rank test procedures for matched-pair data. An analogous class of rank test procedures may be applied to data from two independent samples.

Like the matched-pair situation, the procedure for ranking data and for constructing a formal statistical test is straightforward. We assume that we have n_1 observations in the first sample (group 1) and n_2 observations in the second sample (group 2), where the two samples represent independent random samples from their respective populations. To test the hypothesis that the two groups have identical distributions, rank the entire set of $n_1 + n_2$ observations from smallest to largest. Under the hypothesis of equal distribution in the groups, the assignment of ranks to the $n_1 + n_2$ observations is equivalent to a random assignment of the integers $1, 2, \ldots, n_1 + n_2$ into two groups with n_1 in one group and n_2 in the other group. There are

$$\binom{n_1 + n_2}{n_1} = \frac{(n_1 + n_2)!}{n_1! n_2!}$$

ways to divide the set of ranks into two groups of sizes n_1 and n_2 (recall that $n! = n(n-1)(n-2) \cdots 3 \cdot 2 \cdot 1$. Each of these ways is equally likely under the null hypothesis of no group difference; hence, the probability of each grouping of ranks is $n_1! n_2! / (n_1 + n_2)!$

It is quite natural to choose the sum of the ranks in one of the samples as a criterion for detecting differences between the centers of the two populations. For the moment, let us work with the sum of the ranks for the group that has the smaller sample size. If this statistic, call it S, is too small, this indicates that this group may be centered at a point less than the other group's center. Conversely, a large value of S is consistent with an upward shift in this group's center relative to the other group's. To determine the probability distribution of S under the null hypothesis, compute S for each of $(n_1 + n_2)! / n_1! n_2!$ equally likely assignments of ranks. The following example is one in which the rank sum would appear to be a valuable procedure.

Example 6.3.2.1. Chlorpromazine is thought to have antagonistic effects on some of the actions of amphetamine. This study was conducted on pigeons who were trained to peck a lever. Behavioral effects were measured by the number of pecks per hour. Nine pigeons were studied—five assigned at random to the amphetamine group and four assigned at random to the group receiving amphetamine and chlorpromazine. On the basis of the following data, is there sufficient evidence to conclude at the 5% level of significance that chlorpromazine has an antagonistic effect on the action of amphetamine? The data include:

NUMBER OF PECKS PER MINUTE

Amphetamine	Amphetamine + Chlorpromazine
14.5	6.5
11.4	9.1
16.4	8.4
11.9	3.7
10.3	

In this example, it is clear that we have two independent samples. The independence was achieved by the random assignment of the pigeons to groups. It is equally clear that an assumption of a normal distribution is not realistic, since the data are in the form of discrete rates; if sample sizes were larger, this latter point would not be as crucial. We would like a method of testing the hypothesis that does not require the assumption of normality of distribution for its validity. One general test procedure is the *rank sum* test proposed by both Wilcoxon (1945) and Mann and Whitney (1947). The procedure is outlined in Table 6.17. The quantities $T_{\alpha/2}(n_1, n_2)$, $T_{1-\alpha/2}(n_1, n_2)$ and $T_{1-\alpha}(n_1, n_2)$ are obtained from Table 10 of the Appendix, and $Z_{1-\alpha/2}$, $Z_{1-\alpha}$ are from Table 4 of the Appendix.

In Table 6.18, Example 6.3.2.1 is analyzed via the rank sum test procedure.

For large n_1, n_2 the large-sample test procedure described in Table 6.17 may be performed. At a minimum, the smaller of n_1 and n_2 should be at least 10 before using this version of the test. In this case, the nonparametric statistic version of the central limit theorem justifies the use of the approximation

$$Z = \frac{T_1 - (1/2)n_1(n_1 + n_2 + 1)}{\sqrt{(1/12)n_1 n_2(n_1 + n_2 + 1)}}, \qquad (6.20)$$

where Z is the standard normal variate. Hence, the rejection or decision rule for the two-sided alternative in Table 6.17 for large samples is given by: reject H_0 if favor of H_a if Z in (6.20) is greater than $Z_{1-\alpha/2}$ or less than $-Z_{1-\alpha/2}$, where $Z_{1-\alpha/2}$ is from Table 4 of the Appendix.

If there are observations tied for a set of ranks, the large sample procedure in Table 6.17 is modified by using

$$Z = \left[T_1 - \tfrac{1}{2}n_1(n_1 + n_2 + 1) \right]$$
$$\Big/ \sqrt{\left[\tfrac{1}{12}n_1 n_2(n_1 + n_2 + 1) - \frac{n_1 n_2 \sum_{i=1}^{s}\left(t_i^3 - t_i\right)}{12(n_1 + n_2)(n_1 + n_2 - 1)} \right]}, \qquad (6.21)$$

where t_1 = number of observations tied for one set of ranks,

t_2 = number of observations tied for another set of ranks,

$$\vdots$$

t_s = number of observations tied for another set of ranks.

Table 6.17. Outline of Wilcoxon (Mann–Whitney) Rank Sum Test Procedure

A. Data: The data are y_{ij}, $i = 1, 2$, $j = 1, 2, \ldots n_i$, similar to Table 6.4.

B. Assumptions: $y_{11}, \ldots, y_{1n_1}$ is a random sample from a continuous distribution; $y_{21}, \ldots, y_{2n_2}$ is an independent random sample from a continuous distribution. The two continuous distributions are assumed to differ only (or at most) in their locations μ_1 and μ_2, respectively.

C. Computations: For convenience, label the samples so that $n_1 \leq n_2$, i.e., let group 1 refer to the sample with smaller sample size.
1. Order the observations in the two groups combined and assign a rank of 1 to the smallest observation in the two groups, assign a rank of 2 to the next largest observation in the two groups, and so forth. In the case of tied observations, assign the midrank to each.
2. Let T_1 denote the sum of the ranks in group 1 (the group with the smaller sample size), T_2 the sum of the ranks in group 2.

D. Two-tailed statistical test:
1. Null hypothesis: $H_0: \mu_1 = \mu_2$
2. Alternative hypothesis: $H_a: \mu_1 \neq \mu_2$
3. Decision rule for an α-level test:
   (a) Exact test: Reject H_0 in favor of H_a if $T_1 - \frac{1}{2}n_1(n_1 + 1) < T_{\alpha/2}(n_1, n_2)$ or if $T_1 - \frac{1}{2}n_1(n_1 + 1) > T_{1-\alpha/2}(n_1, n_2)$.
   (b) Large-sample test: Reject H_0 in favor of H_a if

$$\frac{T_1 - \frac{1}{2}n_1(n_1 + n_2 + 1)}{\sqrt{\frac{1}{12}n_1 n_2(n_1 + n_2 + 1)}} > Z_{1-\alpha/2}$$

or if

$$\frac{T_1 - \frac{1}{2}n_1(n_1 + n_2 + 1)}{\sqrt{\frac{1}{12}n_1 n_2(n_1 + n_2 + 1)}} < -Z_{1-\alpha/2}.$$

One-tailed statistical test:
1. Null hypothesis: $H_0: \mu_1 = \mu_2$
2. Alternative hypothesis: $H_a: \mu_1 < \mu_2$ $(H_a: \mu_1 > \mu_2)$
3. Decision rule for an α-level test:
   (a) Exact test: Reject H_0 in favor of H_a if $T_1 - \frac{1}{2}n_1(n_1 + 1) < T_{\alpha}(n_1, n_2)$ [reject H_0 if favor of H_a if $T_1 - \frac{1}{2}n_1(n_1 + 1) > T_{1-\alpha}(n_1, n_2)$].
   (b) Large-sample test: Reject H_0 in favor of H_a if

$$\frac{T_1 - \frac{1}{2}n_1(n_1 + n_2 + 1)}{\sqrt{\frac{1}{12}n_1 n_2(n_1 + n_2 + 1)}} < -Z_{1-\alpha} \quad (> Z_{1-\alpha}).$$

Table 6.18. Worked Solution of Example 6.3.2.1 Using the Rank Sum Test Procedure

A. Data:

$$\text{Group } 1 = 6.5, 9.1, 8.4, 3.7$$

$$\text{Group } 2 = 14.5, 11.4, 16.4, 11.9, 10.3$$

B. Assumptions: The data represent two independent random samples from continuous populations differing at most in location.
C. Computations: The ranks of the data are:

Group 1		Group 2	
	Rank		Rank
6.5	2	14.5	8
9.1	4	11.4	6
8.4	3	16.4	9
3.7	1	11.9	7
		10.3	5
	$10 = T_1$		$35 = T_2$

D. One-tailed statistical test:
  1. Null hypothesis: H_0: $\mu_1 = \mu_2$
  2. Alternative hypothesis: H_a: $\mu_1 < \mu_2$
  3. Decision rule for 0.05 level test: Reject H_0 in favor of H_a if $T_1 - \frac{1}{2}(4)(5) < T_{0.05}(n_1, n_2)$.
E. Action taken: As $T_1 - 10 = 0$, it follows from Table 10 of the Appendix that H_0 should be rejected as $\Pr[T_1 - 10 = 0] = 0.0079$.

An alternative way to compute close approximations of Z in (6.20) and (6.21) is to compute the two-sample t statistic, as described in Table 6.5, based on the ranks of the data. The resulting t statistic closely approximates Z in (6.20) and (6.21) and, in fact, is considered slightly more accurate. For more details, refer to Iman (1976).

To illustrate the application of the large-sample procedure with many tied observations, we consider a data set presented in the *British Medical Journal* (Tyrer, 1978). (The data set is analyzed by a different method in the original paper.)

Example 6.3.2.2. In a study to assess the psychotropic-drug-prescribing patterns in general practice, 287 patients who were subsequently referred to a psychiatric outpatient clinic were studied. One aspect of the study

Table 6.19. Worked Solution of Example 6.3.2.2 Using the Rank Sum Procedure

---

A. Data: The data are:

Number of Drugs	0	1	2	3	4	Total
Men	35	46	27	4	3	115
Women	32	67	60	11	2	172

B. Assumptions: It is assumed that the data are two independent random samples from distributions with locations μ_1 and μ_2. Furthermore, the distributions are assumed to differ at most in their locations. Strictly speaking, we require that the underlying distributions are also continuous; however, this assumption is not absolutely crucial. In fact, as long as the data are on an ordinal scale and the number of tied observations for a given set of ranks does not approach the entire sample size, then the rank sum large-sample procedure may be followed.

C. Computations: If there were no ties, we would rank the 287 observations from 1 to 287. However, we see that there are numerous ties in the data. The relevant computations are summarized below:

Number of drugs	0	1	2	3	4
t_i = number of ties	67	113	87	15	5
Ranks tied for	1–67	68–180	181–267	268–282	283–287
Midrank	34	124	224	275	285

From this table and the previous one we see that

$$T_1 = 35(34) + 46(124) + 27(224) + 4(275) + 3(285) = 14{,}897,$$

$$T_2 = 32(34) + 67(124) + 60(224) + 11(275) + 2(285) = 26431$$

(*Continued*)

---

concerned the number of psychotropic drugs taken by men as compared to women. The following table summarizes the frequency distribution of number of psychotropic drugs being taken:

Number of Drugs	0	1	2	3	4	Total
Men	35	46	27	4	3	115
Women	32	67	60	11	2	172

The question of interest is whether the male and female frequency distribu-

Table 6.19. (*Continued*)

To check this computation, $T_1 + T_2$ should always equal $(n_1 + n_2)(n_1 + n_2 + 1)/2$. In this case, $n_1 = 115$ and $n_2 = 172$; hence, $(n_1 + n_2)(n_1 + n_2 + 1)/2 = 41,328$ while $T_1 + T_2 = 14,897 + 26,431 = 41,328$ as well. This equality will always hold whether we have tied observations or not. The computation in (6.21) requires various other quantities. Let us work with the denominator of (6.21) first:

$$\sum_{i=1}^{s} \left(t_i^3 - t_i \right) = 2,405,376,$$

$$\frac{n_1 n_2 \sum_{i=1}^{s} \left(t_i^3 - t_i \right)}{12(n_1 + n_2)(n_1 + n_2 - 1)} = 48,303.66,$$

$$\tfrac{1}{12} n_1 n_2 (n_1 + n_2 + 1) = 474,720,$$

$$\frac{n_1 n_2 (n_1 + n_2 + 1)}{12} - \frac{n_1 n_2 \sum_{i=1}^{s} \left(t_i^3 - t_i \right)}{12(n_1 + n_2)(n_1 + n_2 - 1)} = 426,416.34,$$

$$\tfrac{1}{2} n_1 (n_1 + n_2 + 1) = 16,560,$$

$$Z = \frac{14,897 - 16,560}{\sqrt{426,416.34}} = \frac{-1663}{653.01} = -2.55.$$

D. Two-tailed statistical test:
   1. Null hypothesis: H_0: $\mu_1 = \mu_2$
   2. Alternative hypothesis: H_a: $\mu_1 \neq \mu_2$
   3. Decision rule for 0.05 level test: Reject H_0 in favor of H_a if Z computed in step C is greater than $Z_{0.975}$ or less than $-Z_{0.975}$.
E. Action taken: From Table 4 of the Appendix, $Z_{0.975} = 1.96$, while the computed $Z = -2.55$; hence, the null hypothesis is rejected at the 5% level of significance. The P value for this result is $\Pr[Z < -2.55] + \Pr[Z > 2.55]$, since the test is two tailed. From Table 4 of the Appendix, $\Pr[Z > 2.55] = 0.0054$, and hence the P value is $2(0.0054) = 0.0108$.

---

tions are the same or are centered around the same number of psychotropic drugs being taken. Let us test this hypothesis at the 0.05 level of significance using the rank sum test procedure. This solution is outlined in Table 6.19.

The estimator of the location difference, $\mu_1 - \mu_2$, or treatment effect is developed along the same lines as the signed ranks estimator. For this procedure, we choose as an estimator $\tilde{d}$, the amount that the first sample's observations must be adjusted to make the two samples as consistent as possible with the null hypothesis. The procedure involves the following:

(i) compute all possible differences, $y_{1j_1} - y_{2j_2}$,

$$j_1 = 1, \ldots, n_1; \ j_2 = 1, 2, \ldots, n_2;$$

(ii) denote these ordered differences by $d_{(1)} < d_{(2)} < \cdots < d_{(n_1 n_2)}$.

The estimator of location difference is then defined by $\tilde{d}$, where: if $n_1 n_2$ is even, then

$$\tilde{d} = \frac{1}{2}\left[d_{(n_1 n_2/2)} + d_{(n_1 n_2/2 + 1)}\right], \tag{6.22}$$

while if $n_1 n_2$ is odd, then

$$\tilde{d} = d_{((n_1 n_2 + 1)/2)}. \tag{6.23}$$

In addition to the point estimator of $\mu_1 - \mu_2$ given by (6.22) and (6.23), a confidence interval should be reported with the results of the data analysis. It can be shown that

$$\Pr\left[\mu_1 - \mu_2 \le d_{(i)}\right] = \Pr\left[T_1 - \tfrac{1}{2}n_1(n_1 + 1) \le i - 1\right], \tag{6.24}$$

where the right-hand probability is determined under the null hypothesis (this probability can be determined from Table 10 of the Appendix). Thus, if

$$\alpha_1 = \Pr\left[\mu_1 - \mu_2 \le d_{(i)}\right], \quad 1 - \alpha_2 = \Pr\left[\mu_1 - \mu_2 \le d_{(j)}\right], \tag{6.25}$$

then the interval $[d_{(i+1)}, d_{(j)}]$ is a $(1 - \alpha_1 - \alpha_2)$ 100% confidence interval for $\mu_1 - \mu_2$.

Example 6.3.2.3. Returning to Example 6.3.2.1, let us consider the estimation of the location difference and a confidence interval for it. First, let us construct a table of differences; these are set out in Table 6.20 and ordered in Table 6.21.

The third column of Table 6.21 is determined directly from Table 10 of the Appendix. Since $n_1 n_2 = 20$, an even number, it follows from expression (6.22) that the estimator of location difference is $\tilde{d} = (d_{(10)} + d_{(11)})/2 =$

Table 6.20. All Possible Pairwise Differences for Example 6.3.2.1

Group 1	Group 2				
	10.3	11.4	11.9	14.5	16.4
3.7	6.6	7.7	8.2	10.8	12.7
6.5	3.8	4.9	5.4	8.0	9.9
8.4	1.9	3.0	3.5	6.1	8.0
9.1	1.2	2.3	2.8	5.4	7.3

Table 6.21. Ordered Differences for Example 6.3.2.1
and Associated Probabilities

i	$d_{(i)}$	$\Pr[\mu_1 - \mu_2 \le d_{(i)}] = \Pr[T_1 - \frac{1}{2}(n_1 + 1) \le i - 1]$
1	1.2	0.0079
2	1.9	0.0159
3	2.3	0.0317
4	2.8	0.0556
5	3.0	0.0952
6	3.5	0.1429
7	3.8	0.2063
8	4.9	0.2778
9	5.4	0.3651
10	5.4	0.4524
11	6.1	0.5476
12	6.6	0.6349
13	7.3	0.7222
14	7.7	0.7937
15	8.0	0.8571
16	8.0	0.9048
17	8.2	0.9444
18	9.9	0.9683
19	10.8	0.9841
20	12.7	0.9921

$(5.4 + 6.1)/2 = 5.75$. From Table 6.21, a two-sided confidence interval for $\mu_1 - \mu_2$, with confidence coefficient of 96.82%, is $[d_{(3)}, d_{(19)}]$. This follows since, from Table 6.21, we have $\Pr[\mu_1 - \mu_2 \le d_{(2)}] = \Pr[\mu_1 - \mu_2 < d_{(3)}] = 0.0159$ and $\Pr[\mu_1 - \mu_2 \le d_{(19)}] = 0.9841$. A one-sided 96.83% confidence interval is $[d_{(4)}, \infty]$. Thus, depending on one's need for a two-sided or a one-sided confidence interval, one could present either the two-sided 96.82% interval of $(2.3, 10.8)$ or the one-sided 96.83% confidence interval of $[2.8, \infty]$.

Table 6.22. Pairwise Differences for Example 6.3.2.2

Difference	Frequency
− 4	70 = (35)(2)
− 3	477 = (35)(11) + (46)(2)
− 2	2660 = (35)(60) + (46)(11) + (27)(2)
− 1	5410 = (35)(67) + (46)(60) + (27)(11) + (4)(2)
0	5872 = (35)(32) + (46)(67) + (27)(60) + (4)(11) + (3)(2)
1	3554 = (46)(32) + (27)(67) + (4)(60) + (3)(11)
2	1312 = (27)(32) + (4)(67) + (3)(60)
3	329 = (4)(32) + (3)(67)
4	96 = (3)(32)
	19,780 = (115)(172)

We once again see that the full range of inference is possible with the rank-sum-type test procedure.

For large n_1 and n_2, i and j in (6.25) may be approximated via the relationship (6.20). In particular, (6.24) is given by

$$\Pr\left[\mu_1 - \mu_2 \le d_{(i)}\right] = \Pr\left[T_1 - \tfrac{1}{2}n_1(n_1 + 1) \le i - 1\right]$$

$$\doteq \Pr\left[Z \le \frac{i - 1 - n_1 n_2/2}{\sqrt{n_1 n_2(n_1 + n_2 + 1)/12}}\right]. \quad (6.26)$$

Hence, the normal distribution may be used for placement of confidence intervals.

We now consider the computation of an estimator for the data of Example 6.3.2.2.

Example 6.3.2.4. Continuing with Example 6.3.2.2, we observe from Table 6.19 that the pairwise difference between a group 1 (male) response and a group 2 (female) response may only take the integer values between − 4 and + 4. In Table 6.22 we list the observed frequency of occurrence of each of these values.

There are an even number of differences, 19,780; hence, it follows from (6.22) that the estimator $\tilde{d} = \tfrac{1}{2}(d_{(9890)} + d_{(9891)}) = 0$. In a situation with as many ties as we have here, this estimator is not likely to be useful. A more informative estimator with such heavily tied data may be a weighted average difference determined from Table 6.22. In particular, denoting the weighted-average difference by d_w, we have the following: $d_w =$

$(19,780)^{-1}[(-4)(70) + (-3)(477) + (-2)(2660) + \cdots +4(96)] = -0.25$.
This value may be obtained directly from the data as well, in particular,
$d_w = (115)^{-1}[0(35) + 1(46) + \cdots +4(3)] - (172)^{-1}[0(32) + \cdots +4(2)] = 1.08 - 1.33 = -0.25$. Thus, for very heavily tied data in the form of a table
like Example 6.3.2.2, the estimator d_w may be preferable to the $\tilde{d}$ estimator.
An alternative way to summarize data like Example 6.3.2.2 is to perform an
analysis like that described in Table 6.19 and then report these results with
the entire table of raw data without attempting to estimate the location.

An additional point arises from this example: the question of "statistical"
versus "practical" significance. We see from the results of the rank sum test
that the location difference between males and females is highly statistically
significant ($P = 0.0108$). On the other hand, we find that the estimate of
absolute difference between the two is 0.25, which is, practically speaking,
quite small. Why, then, is the difference statistically significant? Here, we
are testing a hypothesis of absolute identity of two distributions. If sample
size is large enough, the *slightest* departure from the null hypothesis will be
detected even though the actual difference is very small in practical terms.
This, of course, is a result of the high power of test procedures with large
sample sizes. The conclusion is that a test procedure should generally be
accompanied by a corresponding set of estimates for the parameters being
compared. In this way, the magnitude of the differences may also be noted.
From the construction of statistical tests of hypotheses, an extremely large
sample size will usually result in the rejection of the null hypothesis, and
very small samples will nearly always result in the acceptance of the null
hypothesis. Therefore, only applying a statistical test procedure without
reporting estimates of the size of the effects is not recommended. The P
values and statistical significance are not sufficient by themselves; estimators of effects and confidence intervals with the tests provide for a more
comprehensive analysis.

Like the signed-rank test procedure, it is possible to determine the
sample size needed for the rank sum test. For the one-sided alternative
hypothesis that $\mu_1 - \mu_2 = \Delta > 0$ or the alternative hypothesis that $\mu_1 - \mu_2 = \Delta < 0$, and for normally distributed responses with common variance σ^2,
the number of observations n ($n = n_1 = n_2$) needed in each group for the
α-level rank sum test to have power $1 - \beta$ is

$$n = \frac{2\pi\sigma^2(Z_{1-\alpha} + Z_{1-\beta})^2}{3\Delta^2}.$$

Quantities $Z_{1-\alpha}$ and $Z_{1-\beta}$ are from Table 4 of the Appendix, and 2π is the
radian measure of the circle. For a two-sided alternative hypothesis, $Z_{1-\alpha}$

is replaced by $Z_{1-\alpha/2}$. Again note that this is $\pi/3$ times the sample size required for the two-sample t-test.

The sample size requirements for the rank sum test procedure depend on the underlying distribution of the responses. For distributions other than the normal, the reader may refer to Lehmann (1975, p. 74) for the determination of sample size.

6.4 SUMMARY

In the previous sections, inference procedures have been presented for data arising from a normal distribution and for nonnormal distributions. Naturally, one questions the comparative aspect of these test procedures. For example, in the matched-pairs design, either the paired t or signed-rank test could be appropriate to test the null hypothesis. If it is known a priori that data follow a normal distribution, the paired t-test should be applied. However, this information is not likely to be known beforehand, so it is possible that normal data could be analyzed by the signed-rank rather than the t-test. It turns out that very little information is lost in such a situation. In fact, using a widely accepted criterion of relative performance, called the asymptotic relative efficiency (a measure of relative power), the signed-rank test is 95.5% (i.e., $\pi/3 \times 100$) as efficient as the paired t-test for normally distributed data. Put another way, this says that the signed-rank test with 100 pairs of observations is equal in power to the paired t-test with 95.5 pairs of observations for *normally distributed data*! Thus, even in the situation in which the paired t-test is preferred, the signed-rank procedure compares quite favorably. For other underlying distributions the efficiency changes. The efficiency of the signed-rank test is never less than 86.4% of the paired t-test and exceeds 100% for many distributions. The same statements apply when comparing the rank sum and two-sample t-test procedures. It should be noted that if sample sizes are large, one may expect the significance level of the t-test to be accurate, even for nonnormal data.

There are numerous other nonparametric tests for comparing two continuous distributions. For further details on these tests, the texts by Conover (1971) and Lehmann (1975) may be consulted.

PROBLEMS

6.1. Five micrograms of a drug was injected into rats minutes after their blood pressures had been taken. After 30 min, their blood pressures were retaken. The data for the six animals are as follows:

Rat Number	Control Pressure	Drug Pressure
1	120	110
2	135	113
3	116	96
4	110	104
5	145	132
6	116	85

(a) Is there evidence at the 5% level of significance that the drug alters the blood pressure?

(b) Construct a 95% confidence interval for the mean difference.

(c) Construct a 99% confidence interval for the mean difference.

(d) Why is the 99% interval wider than the 95% interval?

6.2. Medical researchers at a leading University claim that their drug P-112 is superior to aspirin for relief of pain other than headache. Pharmacologists performed the following analgesic test: 20 mice were randomly assigned to receive either P-112 or aspirin (10 received P-112, 10 aspirin). After 20 mins, they were placed individually on a 55°C hot plate, and an observer recorded the time elapsed before they jumped. The latencies are as follows, in seconds:

Aspirin	P-112	Aspirin	P-112
6.7	5.9	3.2	15.5
3.8	6.0	7.6	4.2
5.2	5.2	7.4	14.0
4.2	6.8	3.1	4.7
5.3	14.7	4.2	4.7

A longer latency indicates greater pain relief.

(a) Use the two-sample t-test to test the hypothesis of equal latency times.

(b) Test the hypothesis of equal variances at $\alpha = 0.10$.

(c) Place a 90% confidence interval on the ratio of variances.

6.3. Vasoconstrictor responses to the intra-arterial injection of epinephrine were obtained in the perfused hindpaws of dogs. Responses were obtained before and 30 min after the administration of cocaine hydrochloride, 5 mg/kg i.m. Vasoconstriction was indicated by the increases in perfusion pressure.

Dog Number	Perfusion Pressure (mm Hg)	
	Precocaine	Postcocaine
1	40	78
2	24	36
3	6	6
4	28	24
5	64	110
6	24	64
7	8	20
8	44	40

(a) Use a nonparametric test to test the hypothesis of equal-response distributions pre- and postcocaine administration. Use $\alpha = 0.05$.

(b) Place a 90% confidence interval on μ_d.

(c) What is the signed-rank estimate of μ_d?

6.4. Drug A is a new agent that inhibits drug metabolism. In this study, pancreatic levels of CPH were obtained from rats receiving CPH alone and CPH plus drug A. Twenty rats were randomly divided into two groups. Group I received oral 22.5 mg/kg doses of CPH daily for eight days. In addition, they were given 20 mg/kg doses of drug A i.p. Group II received the same doses of CPH, but they were given i.p. doses of water equal in volume to the dose of drug A. Three hours after the eighth administration of CPH, all animals were sacrificed and their pancreas removed. The tissues were homogenized, extracted, and analyzed by gas chromatography for CPH.

mg CPH/g of Pancreas			
Group I, CPH + Drug A	Group II, CPH Only	Group I, CPH + Drug A	Group II, CPH Only
3.9	2.9	4.8	0.0
1.9	1.0	2.5	1.5
1.6	0.0	3.3	2.6
2.6	0.0	3.2	0.7
2.2	0.0		
3.0	2.1		

(a) Did drug A significantly alter the amount of CPH present in the pancreas? Use a nonparametric test to test against a two-sided alternative.

    (b) Place a 95% confidence interval on the difference between the groups' location.

6.5. Systolic blood pressures were recorded from normotensive and genetically hypertensive rats with the following results.

Systolic Blood Pressure (mm Hg)*	
Normotensive	Hypertensive
102	128
113	126
112	141
116	133
115	132
114	155
97	128
119	130
114	131
111	137
123	134
121	135
100	
112	
100	
116	
118	
109	
111	
114	
104	

*Each value represents the mean of
five determinations.

    (a) Are the two groups significantly different from each other?

    (b) Place a 99% confidence interval on the mean difference.

    (c) Assuming the pooled estimate of variance is a reasonable estimate of the population variance σ^2, what sample size per group is required to detect a mean difference of 5 mm Hg between the normotensive and hypertensive groups with 95% power? Use a one-sided alternative with $\alpha = 0.05$ and assume $n_1 = n_2$. What sample size is required to achieve 99% power?

6.6. The effects of propranolol on drinking behavior of ethanol-habituated rats were examined. A group of eight rats were allowed to drink from a 20% ethanol solution ad libitum for 10 days. The amount consumed by each animal during the last 10 hr before propranolol administration (10 mg/kg i.p.) and immediately after administration was recorded. The following results were obtained.

Rat Number	mL ETOH/hr	
	Before Drug	After Drug
1	0.86	0.25
2	*	0.11
3	1.26	0.50
4	1.05	*
5	0.64	0.35
6	0.34	0.45
7	0.79	0.67
8	0.60	*

*Indicates missing value.

Use an appropriate *t*-test to determine if propranolol significantly affects ethanol-drinking behavior in ethanol-habituated rats?

6.7.   Mice were pretreated with CPZ (20 mg/kg i.p.) or saline (10 mL/kg i.p.) 1 hr before determination of red blood cell 2, 3-DPG levels. The following data were obtained:

2, 3-DPG (μmol/g hemoglobin)

Saline	CPZ
24.3	29.3
22.4	26.4
26.2	27.2
23.5	26.5
29.7	28.6
	24.9

Is there sufficient evidence at the 0.05 significance level to conclude that CPZ increases 2, 3-DPG?

6.8.   This study was conducted to test the effect of ethanol on the retinal blood vessel dilation resulting from methanol administration. Methanol (1 g/kg) was given via a nasogastric tube to monkeys. The number of dilated retinal veins were counted from stereo photographs of the monkey's fundus. Two weeks later the experiment was repeated except that 30 min after the methanol dose, an oral dose of ethanol (1.4 g/kg) was also given orally. The following data resulted.

NUMBER OF DILATED VEINS

Monkey Number	Methanol Alone	Methanol and Ethanol
1	10	6
2	9	5
3	7	5
4	10	1
5	7	6
6	4	7
7	8	5
8	4	5
9	10	7

Test the equal means hypothesis at $\alpha = 0.05$.

REFERENCES

Bickel, P. J., and K. J. Doksum. (1981). An analysis of transformations revisited, *J. Am. Statist. Assoc.*, **76**, 296–311.

Box, G. E. P., and D. R. Cox. (1964). An analysis of transformations, *J. Roy. Statist. Soc.*, **B26**, 211–252.

Box, G. E. P., and D. R. Cox. (1982). An analysis of transformations revisited rebutted, *J. Am. Statist. Assoc.*, **77**, 209–210.

Cochran, W., and G. Cox. (1957). *Experimental Designs*, pp. 101–102, Wiley, New York.

Conover, W. J. (1971). *Practical Nonparametric Statistics*, Wiley, New York.

Iman, R. L. (1974). Use of a *t*-statistic as an approximation to the exact distribution of the Wilcoxon signed ranks test statistic. *Commun. Statist.*, **3**, 795–806.

Iman, R. L. (1976). An approximation to the exact distribution of the Wilcoxon–Mann–Whitney rank sum statistic. *Comm. Statist. Theory and Meth.*, **A5**, 587–598.

Lehmann, E. L. (1975). *Nonparametrics: Statistical Methods Based on Ranks*. Holden-Day, San Francisco.

Mann, H. B., and D. R. Whitney. (1947). On a test of whether one of two random variables is stochastically larger than the other, *Ann. Math. Statist.*, **18**, 50–60.

Satterthwaite, F. W. (1946). An approximate distribution of estimates of variance components, *Biometric Bulletin*, **2**, 110–114.

Tsuang, M., R. Woolson, and J. Simpson. (1980). The Iowa Structured Psychiatric Interview, *Acta Psychiat. Scand.* Suppl. 283, Vol. 62.

Tyrer, P. (1978). Drug treatment of psychiatric patients in general practice, *Br. Med. J.*, **2** (6143).

Wilcoxon, F. (1945). Individual comparisons by ranking methods, *Biometrics*, **1**, 80–83.

CHAPTER 7

Comparison of Two Groups: Chi-Square and Related Procedures

7.1 INTRODUCTION

In the previous chapter, we discussed group comparison procedures for numerical-scale data, that is, for interval-, ratio-, and ordinal-scale data. For example, the rank procedures require the data to be at least on an ordinal scale, while the t-test procedures require at least an interval scale. This chapter focuses on data that are categorized and may or may not be numerical; analysis of such data is called *categorical data analysis*. Examples of categorical response variables are marital status (categories of married, single, widowed, etc.), socioeconomic status, and other discrete variables. Moreover, a categorical variable may also be constructed from a continuous variable. For instance, we may know the length of psychiatric inpatient hospitalization for each of a group of psychotics; however, the data may be summarized in categories such as 0–6 months, 6–9 months, 9–12 months, and over 12 months. Hence, individual values are replaced by intervals, and the number of persons in each of these categories is totaled. Thus, categorical data may originate in a variety of ways, and the original response variate may be nominal, ordinal, ratio, or interval in scale.

This chapter continues the discussion of the two-group comparison problem introduced in Chapter 6. We distinguish, as we did in Chapter 6, the matched-pair design from the two-independent-samples design. Furthermore, we hold to the view that once a design is selected, the statistical analysis should conform to that design.

We shall see that large-sample statistical tests used for categorical data are usually based on the chi-square distribution, even though either the binomial, Poisson, or hypergeometric is the exact underlying model. We begin with the situation in which the response variate has two categories and then generalize the procedures to variables with more than two response categories.

7.2 CASE OF TWO RESPONSE CATEGORIES

The dichotomous response situation covers a wide range of applications. For example, in a study comparing incidence rates of psychoses among the relatives of a sample of manic-depressive probands to a group of schizophrenic probands, the response variable for each relative may be a dichotomous one: either the person has or does not have a psychosis. Similarly, in mortality studies, a mortality status of dead or alive is unquestionably a dichotomous response. As another example, for a clinical trial of two dosage schedules of an antidepressant for the treatment of major depressive disease, we might use the response as improved or not improved.

The goal of these studies is to compare the two rates or proportions. Let us first consider the matched-pair design and for convenience denote the two possible outcomes as 0 and 1.

7.2.1 McNemar's Chi-Square: A Test for Matched Pairs

The data for a matched-pair study may be characterized in the form of Table 7.1, where the response is either 0 or 1 for the ith member of pair j.

Each pair in the table falls into one and only one of the following four categories: (a) both members score a 0; (b) the group 1 member scores a 0, the group 2 member scores a 1; (c) the group 1 member scores a 1, the group 2 member scores a 0; and (d) both members score a 1. Thus, the data may be summarized in the form of Table 7.2.

Table 7.1. Typical Matched Pair Data for Dichotomous Response

Pair	Group 1	Group 2
1	1	0
2	1	1
3	0	0
$\vdots$	$\vdots$	$\vdots$
	0	1
	$\vdots$	$\vdots$
n	1	0

Table 7.2. Summary Data for Matched Pairs: Entry in Table Is Number of Pairs

		Group 1 0	Group 1 1	Total
Group 2	0	a	c	$a + c$
	1	b	d	$b + d$
		$a + b$	$c + d$	$a + b + c + d = n$

Note that the proportion of group 2 persons scoring a 1 is $(b + d)/n$, while the proportion of group 1 persons scoring a 1 is $(c + d)/n$. These two proportions differ if and only if b differs from c. It therefore follows that the sample evidence either for or against a null hypothesis of equal proportions lies in the numbers b and c since d is common to both proportions. Stated another way, the $a + d$ concordant pairs, the pairs in which both responses were the same, contribute nothing to a test of equal proportions, while the $b + c$ discordant pairs, the pairs in which both responses were different, contain the essential information. Intuitively, if b is close to c, we would not regard the two group proportions as different; if b is much greater than c, we would regard the second group's proportion as greater than that of the first group; while if b is a great deal less than c, we would regard the second group's proportion as less than that of the first group.

If we consider the total number of discordant pairs, $b + c$, as fixed, then one would expect these to be divided equally between the two discordant possibilities if the null hypothesis of equal proportions is true. Thus, the number of pairs b in which the group 1 member scores 0 while the group 2 member scores 1 may be viewed from a sampling point of view as a binomial random variable with parameter p equal to $\frac{1}{2}$ under the null hypothesis of equal proportions. Hence, a statistical test may be based on the observed value of $b + c$, the total number of discordant pairs, and b, the number of pairs in which the group 2 member scores a 1 while the group 1 member scores a 0. We outline the test in Table 7.3.

In Table 7.3, $B_{\alpha/2}(b + c, \frac{1}{2})$, $B_{1-\alpha/2}(b + c, \frac{1}{2})$, $B_{\alpha}(b + c, \frac{1}{2})$, and $B_{1-\alpha}$ $(b + c, \frac{1}{2})$ are obtained from the Table 2 of the Appendix (table of cumulative binomial probabilities). [$B_{\alpha}(n, p)$ is defined in the footnote to Table 2.] Expressions $Z_{1-\alpha}$ and $Z_{1-\alpha/2}$ are from Table 4 of the Appendix. The form of Z in Table 7.3 arises from the central limit theorem; in particular, for large $b + c$, recall that

$$\frac{b - (b + c)/2}{\sqrt{(b + c)(0.5)(0.5)}} = \frac{b - c}{\sqrt{b + c}}$$

Table 7.3. Outline of Matched Pairs Equal Proportions Test

A. Data: The data are as in Table 7.1 and summarized as in Table 7.2 with a, b, c, and d as indicated.
B. Assumptions: The pairs of observations are a random sample from a distribution in which the probability of a group 1 score of 1 is p_1 and is p_2 for group 2.
C. Computations:
   1. For the exact binomial test we need only b and $b + c$.
   2. For the large sample test $[(b + c) \geq 20]$ we also compute

$$Z = \frac{(b - c) - 1}{\sqrt{b + c}} \quad \text{if } b \geq c,$$

$$Z = \frac{(b - c) + 1}{\sqrt{b + c}} \quad \text{if } b < c.$$

D. Two-tailed statistical test:
   1. Null hypothesis: H_0: $p_1 = p_2$
   2. Alternative hypothesis: H_a: $p_1 \neq p_2$
   3. Decision rule for an α-level test: Reject H_0 if $b \leq B_{\alpha/2}(b + c, \frac{1}{2})$ or $b \geq B_{1-\alpha/2}(b + c, \frac{1}{2})$. For large samples, reject H_0 if Z in step C is greater than $Z_{1-\alpha/2}$ or less than $-Z_{1-\alpha/2}$.
One-tailed statistical test:
   1. Null hypothesis: H_0: $p_1 = p_2$
   2. Alternative hypothesis: H_a: $p_1 > p_2$ (H_a: $p_1 < p_2$)
   3. Decision rule for an α-level test: Reject H_0 if $b \leq B_\alpha(b + c, \frac{1}{2})$ $[b \geq B_{1-\alpha}(b + c, \frac{1}{2})]$. For large samples, reject H_0 if Z in C is less than $-Z_{1-\alpha}$ (is greater than $Z_{1-\alpha}$).

---

tends to be distributed like a normal random variable under the null hypothesis. It is customary to decrease the absolute value of $|b - c|$ by 1 as a "continuity correction." This is generally utilized for analyses of a single 2×2 table. This correction provides an adjustment for the fact that a continuous distribution (Z) is being used to approximate probabilities for a discrete distribution. We shall adopt this correction for analyses of 2×2 tables. For large values of $b + c$ the correction has little effect.

As the square of a standard normal variate is a chi-square random variable with one degree of freedom, it follows that the square of Z from Table 7.3, $(|b - c| - 1)^2/(b + c)$, is a chi-square variate with one degree of freedom. In this form, this test for matched pairs is called *McNemar's test*, named after the psychologist who proposed this procedure in 1947. McNemar's chi-square test procedure is formally described in Table 7.4.

Table 7.4. McNemar's Chi-Square Test for Correlated Proportions

---

A. Data: The data are as in Table 7.1 and summarized as in Table 7.2, with a, b, c, and d as indicated.
B. Assumptions: The pairs of observations are a random sample from a distribution in which the probability of a group 1 score of 1 is p_1 and is p_2 for group 2.
C. Computations: Let $\chi^2 = (|b - c| - 1)^2/(b + c)$
D. Two-tailed statistical test:
    1. Null hypothesis: H_0: $p_1 = p_2$
    2. Alternative hypothesis: H_a: $p_1 \neq p_2$
    3. Decision rule for an α-level test: Reject H_0 if $\chi^2 > \chi^2_{1-\alpha}(1)$.

The quantity $\chi^2_{1-\alpha}(1)$ is the $(1 - \alpha)$100th percentile of a chi-square with one degree of freedom; it is obtained from Table 6 of the Appendix. We note from Table 7.4 that McNemar's test is equivalent to the two-tailed large-sample Z test outlined in Table 7.3, and it is appropriate for large samples ($b + c \geq 20$). Two examples may help clarify the use of the various techniques for testing the null hypothesis of equal proportions.

Example 7.2.1.1. In a hypothetical clinical trial of an antidepressant drug, two dosage schedules were compared. Depressive patients were pair matched on the basis of sex, duration of illness, and socioeconomic status. One person in each pair was randomly assigned to treatment schedule 1 (high dose), the other to treatment schedule 2 (low dose). The response variable at the end of the trial was the psychiatrist's assessment of improvement, which was done blindly. The data are as follows:

		Treatment Group 1		
		Not Improved	Improved	
Treatment Group 2	Not Improved	8	40	48
	Improved	22	30	52
		30	70	100

The entry in the table is the number of pairs. Of this example, one could ask whether there is sufficient evidence at the 0.05 level of significance to reject the null hypothesis of equal-treatment efficacy in favor of two-sided alternatives.

In Table 7.5, Example 7.2.1.1 is analyzed with the large-sample test of Tables 7.3 and 7.4.

Table 7.5. Worked Solution of Example 7.2.1.1 Using McNemar's Chi-Square
Test Procedures

A. Data: The data are in the form of Table 7.2 with $a = 8$, $b = 22$, $c = 40$, and
   $d = 30$.
B. Assumptions: The pairs of observation are a random sample from a distribution
   in which the probability of improvement is p_1 (p_2) for group 1 (group 2).
C. Computations:

$$Z = \frac{22 - 40 + 1}{\sqrt{22 + 40}} = \frac{-17}{\sqrt{62}} = -2.16;$$

notice also that

$$Z^2 = \frac{(-17)^2}{62} = 4.66 = \chi^2 \quad (\text{McNemar's } \chi^2),$$

that is, Z^2 is identical to the McNemar chi square.
D. Two-tailed statistical test:
   1. Null hypothesis: H_0: $p_1 = p_2$
   2. Alternative hypothesis: H_a: $p_1 \neq p_2$
   3. Decision rule for a 0.05 level test: Reject H_0 in favor of H_a if Z computed
      in step C is greater than $Z_{0.975}$ or less than $-Z_{0.975}$. Equivalently, reject if χ^2
      is greater than $\chi^2_{0.95}(1)$.
E. Action taken: As $Z = -2.16$ and $-Z_{0.975} = -1.96$, we reject the null hypothesis and conclude that there is a treatment regimen difference. Also, since
   $\chi^2 = 4.66$ and $\chi^2_{0.95}(1) = 3.84$, the same conclusion is reached by the equivalent
   McNemar test.

In practice, we would either calculate the Z value or perform McNemar's
procedure, but not both, since they are equivalent.

This example provides further insight into the use of these statistical test
procedures to test the null hypothesis against a *two-sided alternative*. In
particular, the chi-square is a *one-tailed test*; yet it is directed at the
two-sided alternative. We see that the reason for this is that large negative
Z and large positive Z, when squared, become large positive chi-square
variates. That is, both tails of Z when squared go into the upper tail of χ^2
by the relation $\chi^2 = Z^2$. Hence, we see the reason for the one-tailed test
procedure for the chi-square distribution.

An approach to confidence interval estimation for this type of problem is
to place a confidence interval on the proportion $b/(b + c)$ of individuals

who improve on treatment 2 only among those persons in the discordant pairs. In this way, we focus in a given sample on the $b + c$ discordant pairs. This confidence interval (without continuity correction) is

$$\frac{b}{b+c} \pm Z_{1-\alpha/2} \sqrt{\frac{bc}{(b+c)^3}}. \qquad (7.1)$$

For example 7.2.1.1, a 95% confidence interval is $22/62 \pm 1.96$ $\sqrt{22(40)/(62)^3} = 0.35 \pm 0.12 = (0.23, 0.47)$. This is the same as saying that among those persons in the discordant pairs, those pairs where one and only one of the persons improved on treatment, we expect between 23 and 47% will improve on treatment 2. Naturally, the point estimate of the difference in proportions is $(b - c)/(b + c)$ and could be reported along with the tests and confidence intervals. A continuity correction may be used in (7.1) by adding $1/2(b + c)$ to $b/(b + c)$ if $b/(b + c) < .5$, or subtracting it if $b/(b + c) \geq .5$.

Example 7.2.1.2. In a small group of terminally ill persons, THC (cannabis) and morphine were compared for their analgesic properties. Each patient received one agent for three days followed by the other agent, with the order randomized. For each time period, the patients indicated if they felt the agent provided satisfactory pain relief. The data are:

		THC Pain Relief?		
	Pain Relief?	No	Yes	
Morphine	No	10	12	22
	Yes	8	10	18
		18	22	40

The entry in the tables is the number of pairs. Determine whether there is enough evidence at the 0.05 significance level to reject the hypothesis of equal analgesic effects.

The details of the solution are summarized in Table 7.6.

Application of the large-sample procedure to the data of Example 7.2.1.2 would result in $Z = [(8 - 12) + 1]/\sqrt{20} = -3/\sqrt{20} = -0.67$ for the Z value. At the 0.05 level of significance, $Z_{0.975}$ is 1.96; hence, the null hypothesis would not be rejected with this test, in agreement with the conclusion in Table 7.6.

Table 7.6. Worked Solution of Example 7.2.1.2 Using the Exact Binomial Matched Pairs Procedure

---

A. Data: The data are in the form of Table 7.2 with $a = 10$, $b = 8$, $c = 12$, and $d = 10$.
B. Assumptions: The pairs of observations are a random sample from a distribution in which the probability of pain relief is p_1 (p_2) for THC (morphine).
C. Computations: We have $b + c = 20$ and $b = 8$.
D. Two-tailed statistical test:
   1. Null hypothesis: H_0: $p_1 = p_2$
   2. Alternative hypothesis: H_a: $p_1 \neq p_2$
   3. Decision rule for 0.05 level test: Reject if $b \leq B_{0.025}(20, \frac{1}{2})$ or $b \geq B_{0.975}(20, \frac{1}{2})$.
E. Action taken: From step C, $b = 8$, and from Table 2 of the Appendix, $\Pr[b \leq 5] = 0.0207$ and $\Pr[b \geq 15] = 0.0207$; hence, since the observed b is 8 and is between 5 and 15, and the null hypothesis may not be rejected.

Sample size determination for these matched-pairs tests can be based on the exact binomial distribution or from the large-sample Z test. We consider only the large-sample situation and one-sided alternative hypotheses. In particular, denote by p_{12} the proportion of pairs in which the group 1 member improves but the group 2 member does not, while p_{21} is the proportion of pairs in which the group 1 member does not improve but the group 2 member does. The null hypothesis is $p = \frac{1}{2}$ versus $p > \frac{1}{2}$, where $p = p_{12}/(p_{12} + p_{21})$. For an α-level test to have power $1 - \beta$ for the alternative that $p = p^*$, the required number of *discordant pairs* $N = b + c$ is given by

$$N = \frac{\left(\sqrt{1/4}\, Z_{1-\alpha} + Z_{1-\beta} \sqrt{p^*(1 - p^*)} \right)^2}{(p^* - 1/2)^2}, \tag{7.2}$$

where $Z_{1-\alpha}$ and $Z_{1-\beta}$ are from Table 4 of the Appendix. Thus, in this situation, the investigator must estimate the number of pairs that will be discordant among the entire set of n pairs. If data from an earlier study are available to estimate p_{1+} and p_{+1}, the proportion of group 2 persons who improve and the proportion of group 1 persons who improve, respectively, then we can estimate the proportion of discordant pairs by $p_{1+}(1 - p_{+1}) + p_{+1}(1 - p_{1+})$. The total number ($n$) of pairs to be studied would be N from (7.2) divided by $p_{1+}(1 - p_{+1}) + p_{+1}(1 - p_{1+})$, that is, $n = N/[p_{1+}(1 - p_{+1}) + p_{+1}(1 - p_{1+})]$. For a two-sided alternative hypothesis, $Z_{1-\alpha}$ in (7.2) is replaced by $Z_{1-\alpha/2}$.

Example 7.2.1.3. A medical researcher plans to conduct a study of premature rupture of amniotic membrane (PROM) in order to determine if certain activities late in pregnancy predispose a mother to develop PROM. The study will be a pair-matched case-control design wherein each new PROM mother will be age–race–parity matched to a mother who did not develop PROM.

One major risk factor to be evaluated is coital activity within 4 weeks of delivery. Previous data suggest that 30% of mothers without PROM will have participated in coital activities during the last 4 weeks of their pregnancies. Suppose that the investigator would like to be able to detect a threefold ratio of p_{12} to p_{21} if it exists. That is, if $p_{12} = 3p_{21}$, then the investigator would like a good chance to be able to detect this relationship. Therefore, in the notation of (7.2), we would have

$$p^* = \frac{p_{12}}{p_{12} + p_{21}} = \frac{3p_{21}}{3p_{21} + p_{21}} = \frac{3}{4}.$$

If a two-tailed test at $\alpha = 0.05$ is to be performed and if a power of 0.85 is required to detect $p = \frac{3}{4}$, then using (7.2) the number of discordant pairs required is

$$N = \frac{\left(\sqrt{1/4}\,1.96 + 1.04\sqrt{(3/4)(1/4)}\,\right)^2}{(3/4 - 1/2)^2}$$

$$= 32.7 = 33.$$

In order to obtain 33 discordant pairs, we must determine the total number of pairs that must be studied. The best we can do is estimate this using the 30% exposure figure expected for the controls; in the notation for this problem, $p_{1+} = 0.30$. We also must compute p_{+1}, the proportion of the cases of PROM who are exposed. To estimate p_{+1}, we use the relationship

$$p_{+1} = \frac{p_{1+}R}{1 + p_{1+}(R - 1)},$$

where R is p_{12}/p_{21}, the R-fold increase we wish to detect; in this case, $R = 3$. The preceding formula for p_{+1} was derived by Schlesselman (1982) and assumes that cases and controls are independent of one another. While the assumption is probably tenuous at best, it is difficult to get any estimate of the total number of pairs required without introducing some assumption regarding the probability of a concordant pair's occurrence. The value of

p_{+1} is estimated to be $p_{+1} = 0.3(3)/[1 + (0.3)2] = 0.5625$; therefore, the proportion of discordant pairs is figured to be $p_{1+}(1 - p_{+1}) + p_{+1}(1 - p_{1+}) = 0.3(0.4375) + 0.5625(0.7) = 0.525$. Accordingly, we would propose studying $33/0.525 = 63$ pairs total, and it is expected that this will yield 33 discordant pairs.

7.2.2 Sign Test: A Test for Matched Pairs

A binomial-based test also applies in the situation where the response analyzed for each pair is simply the direction of the sign of the pairwise difference. For example, in Example 6.2.1.1, there are seven pairwise differences: 0.61, 0.64, 0.76, 0.45, 0.29, -0.11, and 0.12. If propranolol does not alter ethanol consumption, it may be argued that we expect one-half of

Table 7.7. Outline of the Sign Test for Matched Pairs

A. Data: The pairwise differences are as in Table 6.1, i.e., $d_1, \ldots, d_n$.
B. Assumptions: The scale of the observations is such that the direction or sign of each pairwise difference is meaningful. Furthermore, these pairwise differences are a random sample from an underlying continuous distribution with center (median) μ_d.
C. Computations:
   1. Discard all zero differences, let n denote the number that remain.
   2. Let T_+ denote the number of positive differences, T_- denote the number of negative differences ($T_+ = n - T_-$). If $n \geq 20$, then compute

$$Z = \frac{(T_+/n - 1/2) \pm 1/2n}{(1/\sqrt{4n})},$$

   where $+1/2n$ is used if $T_+/n < 1/2$ and $-1/2n$ is used if $T_+/n \geq 1/2$.
D. Two-tailed statistical test:
   1. Null hypothesis: H_0: $\mu_d = 0$
   2. Alternative hypothesis: H_a: $\mu_d \neq 0$
   3. Decision rule for an α-level test: Reject H_0 if $T_+ \leq B_{\alpha/2}(n, \frac{1}{2})$ or $T_+ \geq B_{1-\alpha/2}(n, \frac{1}{2})$. For large samples ($n \geq 20$), reject if $Z < -Z_{1-\alpha/2}$ or $Z > Z_{1-\alpha/2}$.
One-tailed statistical test:
   1. Null hypothesis: H_0: $\mu_d = 0$
   2. Alternative hypothesis: H_a: $\mu_d > 0$ (H_a: $\mu_d < 0$)
   3. Decision rule for an α-level test: Reject if $T_+ \geq B_{1-\alpha}(n, \frac{1}{2})$ [$T_+ \leq B_{\alpha}(n, \frac{1}{2})$]. For large samples, reject if $Z > Z_{1-\alpha}$ ($Z < -Z_{1-\alpha}$).

the pairwise differences to exceed zero and one-half to be less than zero. Thus, an alternative analysis to the t or signed-rank tests is to ignore the magnitude of each difference and only use the sign or the direction of each difference in forming a statistical test. Clearly, the binomial distribution may be used to construct such a test. This nonparametric test is called the *sign test*. The test procedure is identical to that described in Table 7.3. We present it again only to illustrate another example of the manner in which these binomial tests can be used. The procedure is outlined in Table 7.7.

In Table 7.7 the critical values of Z and $B(n, \frac{1}{2})$ are, respectively, obtained from Tables 4 and 2 in the Appendix. This large-sample test should only be used if $n \geq 20$. A $(1 - \alpha)100\%$ confidence interval for large samples is given by the expression (without continuity correction)

$$\frac{T_+}{n} \pm Z_{1-\alpha/2} \sqrt{\frac{T_+ T_-}{n^3}}. \tag{7.3}$$

An exact binomial confidence interval may be found in Conover (1971). The formal test procedure is in Table 7.7, and an example illustrating its use is detailed in Table 7.8.

It must be emphasized that although the sign test only requires knowledge of the direction (sign) of a difference, it may be applied to a set of continuous differences, in which case we merely discard the magnitudes of the differences. In this sense, the sign test is often viewed as a "quick and dirty" test procedure for the general matched-pair problem since it is very easy to perform relying only on the number of plus (or minus) differences. However, since information is lost by ignoring the magnitudes of the differences, the sign test would not be as powerful as a test such as the Wilcoxon signed-rank test, which makes use of the magnitudes.

This sign test is an alternative to the paired t and signed-rank tests discussed in Chapter 6. The sign test requires fewer assumptions and only requires data for which the direction of the difference is known. In this regard, the sign test applies to a much weaker scale of data. For completeness, we should point out that the sign test may be viewed (in large samples) as a chi-square test. If one squares the quantity Z in Table 7.7, then this can be used as single-degree-of-freedom chi-square statistic for testing the two-sided alternative hypothesis. The sign test is thus algebraically equivalent to McNemar's chi-square statistic.

Let us now turn to the problem of comparing two independent groups with a dichotomous response variable.

Table 7.8. Worked Solution for Example 6.2.1.1 Using the Sign Test

---

A. Data: The differences are 0.61, 0.64, 0.76, 0.45, 0.29, -11, and 0.12.
B. Assumptions: These differences constitute a random sample from a distribution with a median of μ_d.
C. Computations:
　1. $n = 7$.
　2. $T_+ = 6$, $T_- = 1$.
D. One-tailed statistical test:
　1. Null hypothesis: $H_0: \mu_d = 0$
　2. Alternative hypothesis: $H_a: \mu_d > 0$
　3. Decision rule for an 0.05 level test: Reject H_0 if $T_+ \geq B_{0.95}(7, \frac{1}{2})$.
E. Action taken: From Table 2 of the Appendix, $\Pr[T_+ \geq 7] = 0.0078$, $\Pr[T_+ \geq 6] = 0.0625$. Hence, at the 0.05 level of significance, the null hypothesis could not be rejected. It could be rejected, however, at the 0.0625 level. To apply the large sample test (not applicable to this case), the required critical value is 1.645 from Table 4 of the Appendix. Note that the computed

$$Z = \frac{6/7 - 1/2 - 1/2(7)}{1/\sqrt{4(7)}} = 1.51$$

would not reject H_0. Clearly, the exact test is the only appropriate one with an n of only 7.

7.2.3　Fisher's Exact Test: A Conditional Test for Two Independent Samples

The data for the two independent random samples consist of y_{ij}, where $y_{ij} = 0$ or 1 for the jth observation in group i. Typical data are described in Table 7.9.

A 2×2 table may be constructed to summarize these data, as in Table 7.10. This summary table is different from that for the matched-pairs design. The matched-pairs summary table (Table 7.2) could be presented in the form of Table 7.10, but such a presentation would be inappropriate since it would fail to show how the pairs responded.

If we denote by p_1 (p_2) the proportion of individuals in group 1 (2) who score a 1, then the main question is that of drawing an inference regarding the difference between p_1 and p_2. A widely known and frequently applied test was developed by Fisher (1935) and is called *Fisher's exact test*.

The rationale for the test procedure is as follows. Consider the null hypothesis that the two proportions p_1 and p_2 are equal and denote this

Table 7.9. Typical Dichotomous Response Data
for Two Independent Random Samples

Group 1	Group 2
1	0
0	0
1	1
0	1
0	.
0	.
.	0
.	
1	

Table 7.10. Summary Data for Dichotomous Response Data for Two
Independent Random Samples

Response	Group 1	Group 2	
1	a	c	$a + c$
0	b	d	$b + d$
	n_1	n_2	n

Note: $a + b = n_1$, $c + d = n_2$, $n_1 + n_2 = n$

common value by p. Under the hypothesis that $p_1 = p_2 = p$, we shall determine the probability distribution of a given the values $a + b$, $c + d$, $a + c$, and $b + d$. If $p_1 = p_2 = p$, then the probability that $a + c$ takes a certain value is binomial with n and p as parameters; therefore, under the null hypothesis,

$$\Pr[(a + c)|n, p] = \binom{n}{a + c} p^{a+c}(1 - p)^{n-(a+c)},$$

where $a + c$ can range from 0 to n. For group 1, the probability that a takes a certain value is also binomial with parameters $n_1 = a + b$ and p; therefore,

$$\Pr[a|(a + b), p] = \binom{a + b}{a} p^a (1 - p)^b.$$

Similarly, for group 2, we have

$$\Pr[c|(c + d), p] = \binom{(c + d)}{c} p^c (1 - p)^d.$$

Now the two groups are independent so their joint probability is the

Table 7.11. Fisher's Exact Test for Comparing Two Independent Random Samples

A. Data: The data y_{ij} are in the form of Table 7.9, as summarized in Table 7.10.
B. Assumptions: The two independent random samples arise from populations with probabilities of responding 1 equal to p_1 and p_2, respectively.
C. Computations: In order to test the hypothesis that $p_1 = p_2$, it is necessary to compute the probability of the observed table and of all tables more extreme than it. Under the null hypothesis, the probability of the observed table is

$$P_a = \left[\frac{(a+b+c+d)!a!b!c!d!}{(a+c)!(b+d)!(a+b)!(c+d)!} \right]^{-1}.$$

This is determined from the *hypergeometric* distribution. If we are interested in testing the hypotheses H_0: $p_1 = p_2$ vs. H_a: $p_1 < p_2$, then the next most extreme table is determined by keeping all the margins fixed and reducing a by 1 if possible. Thus, this table would be:

Response	Group 1	Group 2		
1	$a - 1$	$c + 1$	$a + c$	
0	$b + 1$	$d - 1$	$b + d$	
	$a + b$	$c + d$	$a + b + c + d = n$	

Hence its probability is

$$P_{a-1} = \left[\frac{(a+b+c+d)!(a-1)!(b+1)!(c+1)!(d-1)!}{(a+b)!(b+d)!(a+c)!(c+d)!} \right]^{-1}.$$

The next most extreme table is obtained by subtracting one more from $a - 1$ and so forth. The procedure stops when it is not possible to proceed further.

If we are interested in testing H_0: $p_1 = p_2$ vs. H_a: $p_1 > p_2$, then the next most extreme table to that observed is obtained by increasing a by 1; therefore, we have:

Response	Group 1	Group 2		
1	$a + 1$	$c - 1$	$a + c$	
0	$b - 1$	$d + 1$	$b + d$	
	$a + b$	$c + d$	$a + b + c + d = n$	

and

$$P_{a+1} = \left[\frac{(a+b+c+d)!(a+1)!(b-1)!(c-1)!(d+1)!}{(a+b)!(c+d)!(b+d)!(a+c)!} \right]^{-1}.$$

and so forth.
D. One-tailed statistical test:
  1. Null hypothesis: H_0: $p_1 = p_2$
  2. Alternative hypothesis: H_a: $p_1 < p_2$ (H_a: $p_1 > p_2$)
  3. Decision rule for an α-level test: Reject H_0 in favor of H_a if $P_a + P_{a-1} + \cdots \leq \alpha$ ($P_a + P_{a+1} + \cdots \leq \alpha$).

product

$$\left[\binom{a+b}{a}p^a(1-p)^b\right]\left[\binom{c+d}{c}p^c(1-p)^d\right].$$

The conditional probability of a and c given $a + c$ is obtained by taking this product and dividing by $\Pr[(a + c)|n, p]$, which yields

$$\Pr[a, c|(a + c), (a + b)] = \binom{a+b}{a}\binom{c+d}{c}\bigg/\binom{n}{a+c}, \quad (7.4)$$

since the terms involving p and $1 - p$ cancel. Note that a can range from 0 to the smaller of $a + c$ and $a + b$.

Expression (7.4) may be recognized as a hypergeometric probability (Chapter 4). To test H_0: $p_1 = p_2$, we can simply compute the probability for the observed table using (7.4) and then compute the probability for each table, which is more extreme than the observed under H_0. The sum of these probabilities would be the P value, and this test is called Fisher's exact test. It may be noted that (7.4) reduces to $(a + c)!(b + d)!(a + b)!(c + d)!/(a + b + c + d)!a!b!c!d!$.

The test is conditional on the observed set of marginal values, $a + c$, $b + d$, $a + b$, and $c + d$. In its usual form, Fisher's exact test is a one-sided test procedure, although it may be modified into a two-sided procedure. If $a + b = c + d$, then two-tailed probabilities may be obtained by doubling the corresponding one-tailed probabilities. On the other hand, if $a + b \neq c + d$, then doubling of the one-tailed probability is not correct, but direct enumeration of each tail is required. In Table 7.11, we outline the one-sided test procedure.

Two points should be made in connection with the preceding procedure. First, for a given observed table, the one-tailed probability may be obtained from Table 11 of the Appendix. Hence, it may not be necessary to carry out all of the computations described in step C. As stated above, for two-sided alternative hypotheses (i.e., H_a: $p_1 \neq p_2$) the one-tailed probability may be doubled provided $a + b = c + d$. In other situations, this may only be done by direct enumeration of each tail following the description given in Table 7.11.

A typical example of data that would be analyzed using the Fisher's exact test is presented in the following example.

Example 7.2.3.1. A psychiatric researcher, suspecting that suicidal thoughts or actions are more prevalent among depressed than manic patients, conducts a study of manic and depressive patients of comparable age and sex. During the course of their illnesses, 33 reports of suicidal thoughts or actions were noted: 14 occurred in the manic group of 20 while 19 occurred among the 20 depressed patients. Is this evidence sufficient to conclude that suicide tendencies are more likely to occur among depressive than among

Table 7.12. Worked Solution of Example 7.2.3.1 Using Fisher's Exact Test

A. Data: The data are of the form of Table 7.10 with $a = 19$, $b = 1$, $c = 14$, and $d = 6$.
B. Assumptions: The data represent two independent random samples with probability of suicide given by p_1 (p_2) for depressives (manics).
C. Computations: The probability of the observed table is

$$P_1 = \left(\frac{40!6!1!14!19!}{20!20!7!33!} \right)^{-1} = 0.0416$$

The only table more extreme is

		Depressive	Manic	
Attempted Suicide?	Yes	20	13	33
	No	0	7	7
		20	20	40

For this table, the probability is

$$P_0 = \left(\frac{40!7!0!13!20!}{20!20!7!33!} \right)^{-1} = 0.00416.$$

(Note: 0! is defined to be 1.)
D. One-tailed statistical test:
   1. Null hypothesis: H_0: $p_1 = p_2$
   2. Alternative hypothesis: H_a: $p_1 > p_2$
   3. Decision rule for a 0.05 level test: Reject H_0 if $P_0 + P_1$ from step C is less than or equal to 0.05.
E. Action taken: Since $P_0 + P_1 = 0.00416 + 0.04160 = 0.04576$ is less than 0.05, the hypothesis is rejected. Notice that the two-tailed probability, while not of interest here, would yield a P value of $2(0.04576) = 0.09152$.

---

manic patients? The data are as follows:

		Depressives	Manics	
Suicide Attempt?	Yes	19	14	33
	No	1	6	7
		20	20	40

The worked solution using Fisher's exact condition test follows in Table 7.12.

As noted, this test is a conditional test, and the probabilities are determined from the hypergeometric distribution. Specifically, the probability of the observed table is the probability of a given $a + b$ and $a + c$. More extreme tables are similarly computed by the variation of a with the margins $a + b$ and $a + c$ fixed. Thus, the test is a conditional test, conditional on the observed margins of the table.

It is clear from Table 7.11 that Fisher's exact test is not easy to conduct for large sample sizes; in fact, the tabular values of the test probabilities listed in Table 11 of the Appendix are only for a few select cases. Clearly, an approximation to this test procedure would be quite useful for larger samples.

For large n, a chi-square approximation may be used to approximate the two-tailed Fisher's exact test p value. In particular, it can be shown that

$$\frac{n[|ad - bc| - (n/2)]^2}{(a + b)(c + d)(a + c)(b + d)} \tag{7.5}$$

is an approximate chi-square variable with one degree of freedom for large n. Hence, to test H_0: $p_1 = p_2$ versus H_a: $p_1 \neq p_2$, the null hypothesis would be rejected if

$$\frac{n[|ad - bc| - (n/2)]^2}{(a + b)(c + d)(a + c)(b + d)} > \chi^2_{1-\alpha}(1).$$

Two points should be noted with regard to the use of this approximation. First, n should be sufficiently large such that

$$\frac{a + b}{n}(a + c) \geq 5, \qquad \frac{a + b}{n}(b + d) \geq 5,$$

$$\frac{c + d}{n}(a + c) \geq 5, \qquad \frac{c + d}{n}(b + d) \geq 5.$$

Second, the $-n/2$ portion of the numerator of (7.5) is the continuity correction. Recall from the previous section that this continuity correction is an adjustment to the statistic to correct for the fact that a continuous distribution (chi square) is being used to approximate the distribution of a discrete random variable (hypergeometric). While there is some controversy regarding the use of the continuity correction, the general consensus is that it should be used for analysis of a single 2×2 table.

We shall adopt the convention of using a continuity correction in all tests involving a comparison of two independent proportions. Some authors recommend use of continuity corrections for many other large-sample tests as well; however, our view is that their use is justified for 2×2 table problems, but not for other problems. The reader may wish to consult Fleiss (1981) or Conover (1971) for more discussion of the issues involved in continuity corrections and their use.

With regard to estimation of parameters for Fisher's exact test, one parameter often considered is the *odds ratio*. The odds ratio is defined by

$$\text{OR} = \frac{p_1(1 - p_2)}{p_2(1 - p_1)}. \tag{7.6}$$

This quantity is a measure of association between the two samples and the response. If the odds ratio is unity, then $p_1 = p_2$. Conversely, if $p_1 = p_2$, then $\text{OR} = 1$. For Example 7.2.3.1, the odds ratio estimate is $19(6)/1(14) = 8.14$, suggesting a strong association between diagnosis and suicidal thoughts or actions.

With regard to sample size requirements for Fisher's exact test, the tables of Haseman (1978) are useful. The sample sizes are summarized in Table 12 of the Appendix. This table provides sample size estimates per group for power probabilities of 0.5, 0.8, and 0.9 and for significance levels of 0.05 and 0.01 for one-tailed tests.

7.2.4 Chi-Square Test of Homogeneity for Two Independent Samples

The most straightforward approach to the estimation of p_1 and p_2 and their comparison is through the binomial distribution. Specifically, we know from Chapter 4 that a in Table 7.10 is distributed binomially with mean $n_1 p_1$ and variance $n_1 p_1(1 - p_1)$. Similarly, c is independently binomially distributed with mean $n_2 p_2$ and variance $n_2 p_2(1 - p_2)$. It follows from the central limit theorem that

$$Z = \frac{(\hat{p}_1 - \hat{p}_2) - (p_1 - p_2)}{\sqrt{\hat{p}_1(1 - \hat{p}_1)/n_1 + \hat{p}_2(1 - \hat{p}_2)/n_2}} \tag{7.7}$$

is an approximate standard normal random variable if n_1 and n_2 are both very large, where $\hat{p}_1 = a/n_1$ and $\hat{p}_2 = c/n_2$. Expression (7.7) is a useful result for placing confidence intervals on $p_1 - p_2$. For example, a continuity corrected $(1 - \alpha)$ 100% confidence interval for $p_1 - p_2$ is given by

$$\left[\left(\frac{a}{n_1} - \frac{c}{n_2} \right) \pm \frac{1}{2} \left(\frac{1}{n_1} + \frac{1}{n_2} \right) \right] \pm Z_{1-\alpha/2} \sqrt{\left[\frac{ab}{n_1^3} + \frac{cd}{n_2^3} \right]}, \tag{7.8}$$

where $\frac{1}{2}(1/n_1 + 1/n_2)$ is added if $a/n_1 - c/n_2$ is less than zero, and otherwise it is subtracted ($Z_{1-\alpha/2}$ is from Table 4 of the Appendix). In addition, a one-sided confidence interval is given by the interval

$$\left(\left[\left(\frac{a}{n_1} - \frac{c}{n_2}\right) \pm \frac{1}{2}\left(\frac{1}{n_1} + \frac{1}{n_2}\right)\right] - Z_{1-\alpha}\sqrt{\frac{ab}{n_1^3} + \frac{cd}{n_2^3}}, 1\right)$$

or   (7.9)

$$\left(-1, \left[\left(\frac{a}{n_1} - \frac{c}{n_2}\right) \pm \frac{1}{2}\left(\frac{1}{n_1} + \frac{1}{n_2}\right)\right] + Z_{1-\alpha}\sqrt{\frac{ab}{n_1^3} + \frac{cd}{n_2^3}}\right),$$

depending on the direction of interest to the investigator. All of the intervals (7.8) and (7.9) are $(1 - \alpha)$ 100% confidence intervals.

If there is interest in testing H_0: $p_1 = p_2$, then it is preferable to use the test statistic

$$Z = \frac{(a/n_1 - c/n_2)}{\sqrt{\hat{p}(1 - \hat{p})(1/n_1 + 1/n_2)}},$$ (7.10)

where $\hat{p} = (a + c)/n$ and is the pooled estimator of the common proportion p. For placement of confidence intervals on $p_1 - p_2$, we prefer the use of (7.7) in which the standard error of $\hat{p}_1 - \hat{p}_2$ is estimated by

$$s^*_{(\hat{p}_1 - \hat{p}_2)} = \sqrt{\frac{\hat{p}_1(1 - \hat{p}_1)}{n_1} + \frac{\hat{p}_2(1 - \hat{p}_2)}{n_2}}.$$

Note that (7.8) is equivalent to

$$\left[(\hat{p}_1 - \hat{p}_2) \pm \frac{1}{2}\left(\frac{1}{n_1} + \frac{1}{n_2}\right)\right] \pm Z_{1-\alpha/2}s^*_{(\hat{p}_1 - \hat{p}_2)}.$$

On the other hand, for testing the null hypothesis of equality of p_1 and p_2, the preferred estimator of the standard error of $\hat{p}_1 - \hat{p}_2$ is

$$s_{(\hat{p}_1 - \hat{p}_2)} = \sqrt{\hat{p}(1 - \hat{p})\left(\frac{1}{n_1} + \frac{1}{n_2}\right)},$$

where $\hat{p}$ is the pooled estimator of the *assumed* common proportion. This problem of different standard errors arises because the standard error of the difference of two binomial proportions depends on the values of p_1 and p_2. For testing the hypothesis of equality of p_1 and p_2, the assumed equality under H_0 should be used to estimate the standard error of $\hat{p}_1 - \hat{p}_2$, and this is done in (7.10). In contrast, when we place confidence intervals, we do not assume any relationship between p_1 and p_2, and consequently, the stan-

Table 7.13. Outline of Large-Sample Test for Two Independent Random Samples

A. Data: The data are as in Table 7.10.
B. Assumptions: The data are two independent random samples from populations with probabilities of score one given by p_1 and p_2, respectively. The sample sizes n_1 and n_2 are both assumed to be large.
C. Computations:
 1. Estimate the two proportions p_1 and p_2 by a/n_1 and c/n_2, respectively. Denote these by $\hat{p}_1$ and $\hat{p}_2$, respectively.
 2. Estimate the standard error of the difference between $\hat{p}_1 - \hat{p}_2$ under H_0: $p_1 = p_2$ by

$$s_{\hat{p}_1 - \hat{p}_2} = \sqrt{\hat{p}(1 - \hat{p})(1/n_1 + 1/n_2)},$$

 where $\hat{p} = (a + c)/(n_1 + n_2)$. $s_{\hat{p}_1 - \hat{p}_2}$ is the standard error computed under the hypothesis that $p_1 = p_2$.
 3. Compute

$$Z = \frac{(\hat{p}_1 - \hat{p}_2) \pm 1/2(1/n_1 + 1/n_2)}{s_{\hat{p}_1 - \hat{p}_2}},$$

 the continuity corrected Z test statistic [the continuity correction of $1/2$ $(1/n_1 + 1/n_2)$ is added if $\hat{p}_1 - \hat{p}_2$ is less than zero; otherwise it is subtracted].
 4. For two-tailed alternatives, one may use Z or the equivalent chi-square value $\chi^2 = Z^2$.
D. Two-tailed statistical test:
 1. Null hypothesis: H_0: $p_1 = p_2$
 2. Alternative hypothesis: H_a: $p_1 \neq p_2$
 3. Decision rule for an α-level test: Reject if Z is greater than $Z_{1-\alpha/2}$ or if Z is less than $-Z_{1-\alpha/2}$. Equivalently, reject if χ^2 is greater than $\chi^2_{1-\alpha}(1)$.
 One-tailed statistical test:
 1. Null hypothesis: H_0: $p_1 = p_2$
 2. Alternative hypothesis: H_a: $p_1 < p_2$ (H_a: $p_1 > p_2$)
 3. Decision rule for an α-level test: Reject H_0 if Z is less than $-Z_{1-\alpha}$ (reject H_0 if Z is greater than $Z_{1-\alpha}$).

dard error of $\hat{p}_1 - \hat{p}_2$ should be estimated in its most general form, namely with $s^*_{(\hat{p}_1 - \hat{p}_2)}$.

We now outline a large-sample test procedure for testing H_0: $p_1 = p_2$. This test is based on the statistic (7.10) with a continuity correction. The procedure in Table 7.13 may be employed to test H_0: $p_1 = p_2$.

In Table 7.13, $Z_{1-\alpha/2}$ and $Z_{1-\alpha}$ are from Table 4 of the Appendix, while $\chi^2_{1-\alpha}(1)$ is the upper $(1 - \alpha)$ 100 percentile of a chi square with one degree of freedom from Table 6 of the Appendix. Again, either a Z test or a χ^2 test may be performed for the two-sided alternatives: the tests are equivalent. In addition, the continuity correction may or may not be used; in our view, these corrections should be used for a 2×2 table.

If we do some simple algebra on Z^2 from Table 7.13, it follows that in terms of a, b, c, and d of Table 7.10,

$$\chi^2 = \frac{n(|ad - bc| - (n/2))^2}{(a + b)(a + c)(b + d)(c + d)}, \tag{7.11}$$

which is the most simple expression of the chi-square test statistic for a 2×2 table. Note that (7.11) is identical to (7.5). Consider the following example.

Example 7.2.4.1. In a historical prospective study of psychotic disorders, each person in a sample of 96 male schizophrenics and a sample of 94 female schizophrenics was classified on the basis of chronicity of illness during the 40-yr period of follow-up. Included in the classification scheme were the amounts of time spent in inpatient and outpatient care and the numbers of such contacts. Each person was then classified as being chronically ill if at least 75% of his follow-up time was spent in inpatient care or 90% of his follow-up time was spent in outpatient care. Additionally, the person was classified as chronically ill if he had at least one inpatient or one outpatient contact with a psychiatric care unit during each decade of the patient's follow-up. The data, gathered via a structured psychiatric interview, are summarized below:

		Males	Females
Chronically Ill?	Yes	19	33
	No	77	61
		96	94

At the 5% level of significance, test whether there is sufficient evidence to conclude that the illness rates are different between males and females.

Table 7.14. Worked Solution of Example 7.2.4.1

A. Data: The data are $a = 19$, $b = 77$, $c = 33$, $d = 61$, $n_1 = 96$, $n_2 = 94$, and $n = 190$.
B. Assumptions: The data are two independent random samples from populations in which p_1 and p_2 are proportions of persons who remain chronically ill among the males and the females, respectively.
C. Computations:

$$\hat{p}_1 = \frac{19}{96} = 0.1979$$

$$\hat{p}_2 = \frac{33}{94} = 0.3511$$

$$\hat{p} = \frac{19 + 33}{190} = 0.2737$$

$$s^*_{\hat{p}_1 - \hat{p}_2} = \sqrt{\frac{0.1979(0.8021)}{96} + \frac{0.3511(0.6489)}{94}} = 0.0639$$

$$s_{\hat{p}_1 - \hat{p}_2} = \sqrt{0.2737(0.7263)(1/96 + 1/94)} = 0.0647$$

$$Z = \frac{(0.1979 - 0.3511) + 1/2(1/96 + 1/94)}{0.0647} = -2.21$$

$$\chi^2 = \frac{190(|33(77) - 61(19)| - 95)^2}{96(94)(52)(138)} = 4.86 \doteq (2.21)^2$$

D. Two-tailed statistical test:
  1. Null hypothesis: H_0: $p_1 = p_2$
  2. Alternative hypothesis: H_a: $p_1 \neq p_2$
  3. Decision rule for a 0.05 level test: Reject H_0 if Z is less than $-Z_{0.975}$ or greater than $Z_{0.975}$. Equivalently, reject if χ^2 is greater than $\chi^2_{0.95}(1)$.
E. Action taken: From Table 4 of the Appendix, $-Z_{0.975} = -1.96$, while $Z = -2.21$; hence, the null hypothesis is rejected. [Equivalently, $\chi^2_{0.95}(1) = 3.84$, while $\chi^2 = 4.86$; hence, H_0 is rejected.] We conclude that the illness rates are not equal between the sexes.

This example involves substantial sample sizes, and it is therefore one in which the normal distribution (or chi-square) test would be reasonable to apply. In Table 7.14, the data are analyzed. For completeness, we include the confidence interval procedure as well.

A 95% confidence interval for $p_1 - p_2$ is given by

$$(0.1979 - 0.3511) + \tfrac{1}{2}\left(\tfrac{1}{96} + \tfrac{1}{94}\right) \pm (1.96)s^*_{\hat{p}_1 - \hat{p}_2} = -0.1427 \pm 0.1252$$

$$= (-0.2679, -0.0175).$$

It is difficult to give guidelines regarding "large" sample size. In general, with $\hat{p}$ the pooled value of the proportion, if $n_1\hat{p}$, $n_1(1 - \hat{p})$, $n_2\hat{p}$, and $n_2(1 - \hat{p})$ are all greater than 5, then the large-sample procedures should be accurate. If they are not all greater than 5, then Fisher's exact test may be applied for the purpose of testing hypotheses. These large-sample results arise from the central limit theorem, and it is known that the closer p_1 and p_2 are to $\tfrac{1}{2}$, the better that approximation is. As an illustration, in Example 7.2.4.1, $\hat{p}$ would be $(19 + 33)/190 = 52/190 = 0.27$, whence $1 - \hat{p} = 0.73$, and therefore $n_1\hat{p} = 96(0.27) = 25.9$, $n_1(1 - \hat{p}) = 96(0.73) = 70.1$, $n_2\hat{p} = 94(0.27) = 25.4$, and $n_2(1 - \hat{p}) = 94(0.73) = 68.6$. Thus, in this situation, all of the expected table entries are larger than 5, and the chi-square computations are appropriate using our criteria.

With regard to sample size requirements, we will consider the α-level test based on Z for the one-sided alternative that $p_1 > p_2$ and restrict consideration to equal sample sizes in the groups, that is, $n_1 = n_2$. The number, n, required in *each group* for the one-sided test to have size α and power $1 - \beta$ against the alternative that $p_1 - p_2 = \Delta$ is

$$n = \left[\frac{Z_{1-\beta}\sqrt{p_1(1 - p_1) + p_2(1 - p_2)} + Z_{1-\alpha}\sqrt{2\bar{p}(1 - \bar{p})}}{\Delta} \right]^2, \quad (7.12)$$

where $\bar{p} = (p_1 + p_2)/2$ and $Z_{1-\beta}$, $Z_{1-\alpha}$ are from Table 4 of the Appendix. For a two-sided alternative, $Z_{1-\alpha}$ is changed to $Z_{1-\alpha/2}$.

Example 7.2.4.2. Determine the sample size required for each sex in Example 7.2.4.1 if it is desired to test the equal-proportions hypothesis against the alternative that the male proportion chronically ill is 0.80 while the female proportion chronically ill is 0.75. Use $\alpha = 0.05$, $\beta = 0.1$, and the one-sided test.

In the notation of (7.12), we have $Z_{0.95} = 1.645$, $Z_{0.90} = 1.28$, $p_1 = 0.80$, $p_2 = 0.75$, $\bar{p} = 0.775$, and $\Delta = 0.05$. Substitution into (7.12) yields $n = 1192$ as the sample size for each group.

7.2.5 Comparison of Two Poisson Counts

Often count data are collected on large populations, and it is important to compare two groups. For example, suppose two Iowa counties of comparable population size and composition each report a specified number of colon cancer cases in a particular year. If one county reports 16 new cases while the other reports 34 new cases, what can be said about the differences between the two disease rates?

For this problem, it is reasonable to assume a Poisson model (see Chapter 4) for the number of colon cancer cases in each county. If we let Y_i be the observed number of cases in county i ($i = 1, 2$) and λ_i ($i = 1, 2$) be the mean of Y_i, then we are interested in testing H_0: $\lambda_1 = \lambda_2$.

Since we have assumed a priori that the counties are of equal population sizes and that the follow-up times are equal, then a simple test of H_0 may be formulated. If H_0 is true, then we would expect half of the total number of cases to be in the first group and half in the second group. Therefore, the number of cases in group 1 can be viewed as a binomial random variable with $n = Y_1 + Y_2$ and $p = \frac{1}{2}$ (under H_0). Thus, a test of H_0 is equivalent to our one-sample binomial test of H_0: $p = \frac{1}{2}$, which was described in Chapter 5. Hence, the test can be based on the exact binomial distribution, or if $Y_1 + Y_2 \geq 20$, it can be based on the standard normal distribution. For the two-sided alternative, the exact binomial rejection region is to reject H_0 at level α if

$$Y_1 \leq B_{\alpha/2}\left(Y_1 + Y_2, \tfrac{1}{2}\right) \quad \text{or} \quad Y_1 \geq B_{1-\alpha/2}\left(Y_1 + Y_2, \tfrac{1}{2}\right),$$

where $B_{\alpha/2}$ and $B_{1-\alpha/2}$ are from Table 2 of the Appendix. The standard normal large-sample test is based on the continuity-corrected statistic

$$Z = \frac{y_1/(y_1 + y_2) - 1/2 \pm 1/2(y_1 + y_2)}{\sqrt{1/4(y_1 + y_2)}} = \frac{(y_1 - y_2)}{\sqrt{y_1 + y_2}} \pm \frac{1}{\sqrt{y_1 + y_2}},$$

$$(7.13)$$

where $+1/2(y_1 + y_2)$ is used if $y_1 < y_2$ and $-1/2(y_1 + y_2)$ is used otherwise. The α-level rejection region for a two-tailed test is $Z > Z_{1-\alpha/2}$ or $Z < -Z_{1-\alpha/2}$.

Example 7.2.5.1. Consider the problem of comparing the colon cancer incidence rates in two counties for a 3-yr period. We assume that the population in the counties are of the same size and composition. We observe 16 cases in county 1 and 34 cases in county 2. Under the null hypothesis we expect half of the total of 50 cases $(16 + 34)$ to be from county 1. Let us use $\alpha = 0.05$ and construct both the exact binomial and the large-sample Z rejection regions. From Table 2 of the Appendix, with $n = 50$, $p = 0.50$, we find

$$B_{0.025}\left(50, \tfrac{1}{2}\right) = 17, \qquad B_{0.975}\left(50, \tfrac{1}{2}\right) = 33,$$

and since $16 \leq 17$, we would reject H_0. Notice that the exact size of this test is $0.01642 + 0.01642 = 0.03284$. For the large-sample test,

$$Z = \frac{(16/50 - 1/2) + 1/2(50)}{\sqrt{1/4(50)}} = -2.40$$

while $Z_{0.975} = 1.96$, $-Z_{0.975} = -1.96$. Hence, H_0 would be rejected with the large-sample approximate test, which is appropriate here since $Y_1 + Y_2 \geq 20$.

In many epidemiologic contexts, the two groups being compared may differ in population size and the amount of time exposed. For instance, suppose that the first county had twice the population size as the second county. Rather than expecting the number of cases to be equal under the null hypothesis, we would expect the first county to have twice as many cases. In this case, the null hypothesis of equal disease rates translates into H_0: $p = \tfrac{2}{3}$, that is, the fraction of the total cases that are in county 1 is $\tfrac{2}{3}$ since this county has twice the population.

In general, if the population-time (e.g., person-years of follow-up) in group 1 is PT_1 while the population-time is PT_2 for group 2, then under the hypothesis of equal disease rates $p = PT_1/(PT_1 + PT_2)$, where p is the proportion of the total number of cases expected to be from group 1. Thus, the null hypothesis is

$$H_0: p = \frac{PT_1}{(PT_1 + PT_2)} \qquad (= p_0, \text{ say}),$$

and the two-sided α-level exact binomial rejection region is

$$y_1 \leq B_{\alpha/2}(y_1 + y_2, p_0) \quad \text{or} \quad y_1 \geq B_{1-\alpha/2}(y_1 + y_2, p_0),$$

where $B_{\alpha/2}$ and $B_{1-\alpha/2}$ are from Table 2 of the Appendix. The large-sample test [if $(y_1 + y_2)p_0(1 - p_0) \geq 5$] is based on

$$Z = \frac{y_1/(y_1 + y_2) - p_0 \pm 1/2(y_1 + y_2)}{\sqrt{p_0(1 - p_0)/(y_1 + y_2)}},$$

rejecting for a two-sided alternative if $Z > Z_{1-\alpha/2}$ or $Z < -Z_{1-\alpha/2}$.

Example 7.2.5.2.   Suppose in Example 7.2.5.1 that county 2 has 3 times the population that county 1 has. Test the hypothesis of equal disease rates. We note that $PT_1/(PT_1 + PT_2) = 1/(1 + 3) = 1/4$; so under the null hypothesis of equal disease rates, we expect one-fourth of the cases to be in county 1 and three-fourths in county 2. From Table 2 of the Appendix, with $n = 50$, $p = 0.25$, we find

$$B_{0.025}(50, 0.25) = 6, \qquad B_{0.975}(50, 0.25) = 20,$$

and the exact α level is $0.01939 + 0.01392 = 0.03331$. Since $16 > 6$ and $16 < 20$, the null hypothesis is not rejected. Using the Z-test procedure, we compute

$$Z = \frac{(16/50 - 0.25) - 1/2(50)}{\sqrt{0.25(0.75)/50}} = 0.98;$$

and since $0.98 < 1.96$ and $0.98 > -1.96$, we cannot reject the null hypothesis.

Hence comparison of two Poisson distributions can be fairly easily done with the foregoing test procedures. Confidence intervals can also be generated for p using the one-sample binomial (and Z) procedures described in Chapter 5. Since $p = \lambda_1/(\lambda_1 + \lambda_2)$, it follows that the limits derived for p, say (p_L, p_u) for the lower and upper limits, may be transformed to obtain a confidence interval for λ_1/λ_2. In particular, since $\lambda_1/\lambda_2 = p/(1 - p)$, the lower limit for λ_1/λ_2 is $p_L/(1 - p_L)$ while the upper limit is $p_u/(1 - p_u)$. Hence, the techniques of Chapter 5 can be used to place a confidence interval on p, and then this interval may be transformed to one for λ_1/λ_2 as described above.

7.3   CASE OF MORE THAN TWO RESPONSE CATEGORIES

Thus far, we have only considered the situation where there are two response categories. However, in many situations, there are r ($r > 2$) categories of response for each individual. For example, in a study to contrast psychiatric incidence rates between two communities, the data were gathered in three categories of response: psychotic illness, psychiatric illness other than psychotic illness, and no psychiatric illness. In this situation, we may wish to know whether the distribution of diagnosis for one community differs from that of the other community. Again, the type of statistical estimation and testing procedures employed depend on whether the data are pair matched or are two independent random samples. Both instances are discussed below.

Table 7.15. Data Configuration for n Matched Pairs With r Response Categories[a]

		Group 1 Response Category			Total
		1	2	$\cdots\ r$	
Group 2 Response Category	1	a_{11}	a_{12}	$\cdots\ a_{1r}$	$a_{1.}$
	2	a_{21}	a_{22}	$\cdots\ a_{2r}$	$a_{2.}$
	$\vdots$	$\vdots$	$\vdots$	$\cdots\ \vdots$	$\vdots$
	r	a_{r1}	a_{r2}	$\cdots\ a_{rr}$	$a_{r.}$
	Total	$a_{.1}$	$a_{.2}$	$\cdots\ a_{.r}$	$a_{..} = n$

[a]Entries a_{ij} are the number of pairs.

7.3.1 Chi-Square Tests for Matched Samples

The data in this instance are in the form of Table 7.15.

One inference question is that of testing the hypothesis that $p_{1.} = p_{.1}$, $p_{2.} = p_{.2}$, $p_{3.} = p_{.3}, \ldots, p_{r.} = p_{.r}$, where $p_{i.}$ is the proportion of persons in group 2 who are in response category i and $p_{.j}$ is the proportion of persons in group 1 who are in response category j. The reader may note that for $r = 2$ the above table is identical to Table 7.2; thus, McNemar's test and

Table 7.16. Outline of Matched Pair Categorical Data Analysis with Three Response Categories

---

A. Data: The data are in the form of Table 7.15 with $r = 3$.

B. Assumptions: The data arise from a matched random sample with proportions $p_{.1}, p_{.2}, p_{.3}, (p_{1.}, p_{2.}, p_{3.})$ for categories 1, 2, and 3 for group 1 (group 2).

C. Computations:

$$\chi^2 = \frac{\bar{a}_{23}(a_{1.} - a_{.1})^2 + \bar{a}_{13}(a_{2.} - a_{.2})^2 + \bar{a}_{12}(a_{3.} - a_{.3})^2}{2(\bar{a}_{12}\bar{a}_{23} + \bar{a}_{12}\bar{a}_{13} + \bar{a}_{13}\bar{a}_{23})}$$

where $\bar{a}_{ij} = \frac{1}{2}(a_{ij} + a_{ji})$.

D. Two-sided alternative hypothesis:

1. Null hypothesis: H_0: $p_{1.} = p_{.1}, p_{2.} = p_{.2}, p_{3.} = p_{.3}$
2. Alternative hypothesis: H_a: $(p_{1.}, p_{2.}, p_{3.}) \neq (p_{.1}, p_{.2}, p_{.3})$
3. Decision rule for an α-level test: Reject if χ^2 in step C is greater than $\chi^2_{1-\alpha}(2)$.

---

the other inference procedures discussed in Section 7.2 may be applied. For the case of three responses (i.e., $r = 3$), the testing procedure is a little more complex but is still based on the chi-square distribution. It is described in Table 7.16.

This test is frequently called the *Stuart–Maxwell chi-square test* (Stuart, 1957; Maxwell, 1970). The statistic in step C of Table 7.16 is a form of the test statistic cited by Fleiss (1981) and due to Fleiss and Everitt (1971). Notice in Table 7.16 that the critical value in step D is that of a chi-square with two degrees of freedom, which may be obtained from Table 6 of the Appendix.

In some situations a table (3×3) like Table 7.15 may be collapsed into a 2×2 table by combining two categories of response into one. If this is done and a McNemar chi-square statistic is computed for the resulting table, then Fleiss (1981) recommends that the procedure outlined in Table 7.4 be followed with one exception: the resulting McNemar's chi square should be compared to a chi square with *two* degrees of freedom instead of the chi square with one degree of freedom. By using two degrees of freedom, the overall significance level for the Stuart–Maxwell test and the three possible McNemar tests (one for each 2×2 table) will be controlled.

Example 7.3.1.1.   In a study of the psychological and social effects on the wives of myocardial infarction patients, a semistructured interview was conducted and tape recorded on two occasions, 2 months after and 1 yr after the husband's infarction. One item that was rated was the wife's degree of anxiety or distress. The data are as follows:

		At Two Months Degree of Anxiety			
		None or Mild	Moderate	Severe	
	None or Mild	20	30	10	60
At One Year	Moderate	5	10	5	20
	Severe	5	5	10	20
		30	45	25	100

Determine whether there is sufficient evidence to conclude that the anxiety levels change from 2 months to 1 yr.

In Table 7.17, the solution to the example is outlined.

If it was of interest in Example 7.3.1.1 to compare the proportion of patients who had mild or no anxiety, the table could be collapsed into the

Table 7.17. Worked Solution to Example 7.3.1.1

A. Data: The data are in the form of Table 7.15 with $a_{11} = 20$, $a_{12} = 30$, $a_{13} = 10$, $a_{21} = 5$, $a_{22} = 10$, $a_{23} = 5$, $a_{31} = 5$, $a_{32} = 5$, $a_{33} = 10$.

B. Assumptions: The data are a matched random sample from a population with probability of mild, moderate, and severe given, respectively, by $p_{.1}, p_{.2}, p_{.3}$ ($p_{1.}, p_{2.}, p_{3.}$) at 2 months (1 yr).

C. Computations

$$\bar{a}_{12} = \frac{30 + 5}{2} = 17.5; \ a_{.1} = 30, \ a_{.2} = 45, \ a_{.3} = 25;$$

$$\bar{a}_{13} = \frac{10 + 5}{2} = 7.5; \ a_{1.} = 60, \ a_{2.} = 20, \ a_{3.} = 20;$$

$$\bar{a}_{23} = \frac{5 + 5}{2} = 5;$$

$$\chi^2 = \frac{5(60 - 30)^2 + 7.5(20 - 45)^2 + 17.5(20 - 25)^2}{2[5(17.5) + (17.5)(7.5) + (7.5)(5)]} = \frac{9625}{512.5} = 18.78.$$

D. Two-tailed statistical test:
1. Null hypothesis: H_0: $(p_{1.}, p_{2.}, p_{3.}) = (p_{.1}, p_{.2}, p_{.3})$
2. Alternative hypothesis: H_a: $(p_{1.}, p_{2.}, p_{3.}) \neq (p_{.1}, p_{.2}, p_{.3})$
3. Decision rule for a 0.05 level test: Reject H_0 in favor of H_a if χ^2 in step C is greater than $\chi^2_{0.95}(2)$.

E. Action taken: Since $\chi^2_{0.95}(2) = 5.99$ from Table 6 of the Appendix and we computed $\chi^2 = 18.78$ in step C, H_0 is rejected in favor of H_a. From Table 6 we also see that the P value for this result is less than 0.001.

---

following 2 × 2 table:

		Two Months Degree of Anxiety		
		Mild	Not Mild	
One Year	Mild	20	40	60
	Not Mild	10	30	40
		30	70	100

McNemar's chi square without continuity correction for this table is given by $\chi^2 = (40 - 10)^2/50 = 18.00$; with continuity correction, McNemar's chi square is $[(40 - 10) - 1]^2/50 = 16.82$. In either case, the value could be compared to $\chi^2_{0.95}(2) = 5.99$, and the hypothesis of equal proportions of patients who had mild or no anxiety would be rejected.

For the more general case in which $r > 3$, the test procedures require matrix algebra and are beyond the scope of this book. However, for completeness, we describe the procedure for reference purposes. The procedure is due to Maxwell (1970) and is cited by Everitt (1977).

For the $r \times r$ table as in Table 7.15, the chi-square test statistic for testing H_0: $(p_{1.}, p_{2.}, \ldots, p_{r.}) = (p_{.1}, p_{.2}, p_{.3}, \ldots, p_{.r})$ is

$$\chi^2 = f'V^{-1}f, \qquad (7.14)$$

where

$$f' = (a_{1.} - a_{.1}, a_{2.} - a_{.2}, \ldots, a_{r-1.} - a_{.r-1})$$

$$V = v_{ij}, \, i, \, j = 1, 2, \ldots, r - 1$$

$$v_{ij} = -(a_{ij} + a_{ji})$$

$$v_{ii} = a_{i.} + a_{.i} - 2a_{ii}$$

and V^{-1} is the matrix inverse of V. The statistic (7.14) may be compared to a chi-square distribution with $r - 1$ degrees of freedom in order to perform a test of H_0. Should this $r \times r$ table likewise be collapsed into various 2×2 tables by combining categories, the resulting McNemar chi-square statistics should be compared to a chi-square distribution with $r - 1$ degrees of freedom rather than one degree of freedom. By using $r - 1$ degrees of freedom, the overall significance level for the multiple tests will not exceed α.

The reader should refer to Forthofer and Lehnen (1981) for a fuller discussion of this general approach.

7.3.2 Chi-Square Tests for Two Independent Samples

For categorical data from two populations, each with more than two response categories, the form of the data for two independent random samples is given in Table 7.18.

The entry n_{ij} in Table 7.18 is the number of individuals in the jth response category from the ith group. The problem of major interest for data such as Table 7.18 is to test the hypothesis that the array of propor-

Table 7.18. Data Format for r Response Categories For Two Independent Random Samples

Response Category	Group 1	Group 2	
1	n_{11}	n_{21}	$n_{.1}$
2	n_{12}	n_{22}	$n_{.2}$
$\vdots$	$\vdots$	$\vdots$	$\vdots$
r	n_{1r}	n_{2r}	$n_{.r}$
	$n_{1.}$	$n_{2.}$	$n_{..}$

tions for group 1 is identical to that of group 2. The test procedure is once again the chi-square test. The basic principle in constructing the test is to compute an "expected number" of persons in each cell of Table 7.18 and compare these expected quantities to the observed n_{ij}. These expected quantities are computed under the assumption of the null hypothesis of equal group distributions. The test statistic is

$$\chi^2 = \sum_{i=1}^{2} \sum_{j=1}^{r} \frac{\left(n_{ij} - e_{ij}\right)^2}{e_{ij}}, \qquad (7.15)$$

where e_{ij} is the expected number of individuals in the (i, j)th cell of Table 7.18. Under the hypothesis that the proportions $(p_{11}, p_{12}, \ldots, p_{1r})$ for group 1 equal the proportions $(p_{21}, \ldots, p_{2r})$ for group 2, the quantities $e_{11}, \ldots, e_{2r}$ are easily determined. In particular, if $p_{11} = p_{21} = p_{.1}$ (say), then the expected number of persons in cell $(1, 1)$ is $n_{1.}p_{.1}$ and for cell $(2, 1)$ is $n_{2.}p_{.1}$. Similarly, for the jth response category, if $p_{1j} = p_{2j} = p_{.j}$, the expected number is $n_{i.}p_{.j}$. Hence, if we test the hypothesis

$$H_0: \quad \begin{pmatrix} p_{11} = p_{21} \\ p_{12} = p_{22} \\ \vdots \\ p_{1r} = p_{2r} \end{pmatrix} \qquad (7.16)$$

with the common values unspecified, it would seem appropriate to estimate e_{ij} by $n_{i.}(n_{.j}/n_{..})$ since $n_{.j}/n_{..}$ would be a logical estimator of the common value of p_{1j} and p_{2j}. Thus, for the null hypothesis (7.16), statistic (7.15) is

$$\chi^2 = \sum_{i=1}^{2} \sum_{j=1}^{r} \frac{\left(n_{ij} - n_{i.}n_{.j}/n_{..}\right)^2}{n_{i.}n_{.j}/n_{..}}. \qquad (7.17)$$

Table 7.19. Chi-Square Test Procedure for Two Independent Random Samples

A. Data: The data are of the form of Table 7.18.
B. Assumptions: The group 1 data are a random sample from a multinomial population with probabilities $p_{11}, p_{12}, \ldots, p_{1r}$, and the group 2 data are an independent random sample from a multinomial population with probabilities $p_{21}, p_{22}, \ldots, p_{2r}$.
C. Computations:
   1. Determine the expected number e_{ij} of observations for the (i, j)th cell. Under the null hypothesis, the quantity e_{ij} is determined by $e_{ij} = n_{i.}n_{.j}/n_{..}$.
   2. Compute

$$\chi^2 = \sum_{i=1}^{2} \sum_{j=1}^{r} \frac{(n_{ij} - e_{ij})^2}{e_{ij}} = \sum_{i=1}^{2} \sum_{j=1}^{r} \frac{(n_{ij} - n_{i.}n_{.j}/n_{..})^2}{(n_{i.}n_{.j}/n_{..})}$$

D. Two-tailed statistical test:
   1. Null hypothesis:

$$H_0: \begin{pmatrix} p_{11} \\ \vdots \\ p_{1r} \end{pmatrix} = \begin{pmatrix} p_{21} \\ \vdots \\ p_{2r} \end{pmatrix}$$

   2. Alternative hypothesis:

$$H_a: \begin{pmatrix} p_{11} \\ \vdots \\ p_{1r} \end{pmatrix} \neq \begin{pmatrix} p_{21} \\ \vdots \\ p_{2r} \end{pmatrix}$$

   3. Decision rule for an α-level test: Reject H_0 in favor of H_a if χ^2 in step C is greater than $\chi^2_{1-\alpha}(r - 1)$, a chi-square with $r - 1$ degrees of freedom.

Under the null hypothesis (7.16), expression (7.17) has a chi-square distribution with $r - 1$ degrees of freedom. We are now in a position to outline the chi-square test procedure for this problem (Table 7.19).

The quantity $\chi^2_{1-\alpha}(r - 1)$ is obtained from Table 6 of the Appendix. An example will illustrate the procedure.

Example 7.3.2.1. In a follow-up study, the effects of various life stresses on psychotic disorders were assessed. As part of this study, the number of major life stresses during a 40-yr follow-up period was determined for each of 174 schizophrenics and each of 214 patients with affective disorders. The data are as follows:

Number of Life Stresses in 40-yr period	Schizophrenics	Affective Disorders	Total
0	23	7	30
1	39	10	49
2	46	28	74
3	21	42	63
4	21	75	96
5	13	34	47
6	9	15	24
7	2	3	5
Total	174	214	388

Determine whether there is evidence of a difference between the two groups with respect to their numbers of life stresses.

We analyze these data in Table 7.20.

A $(1 - \alpha)$ 100% confidence interval for the difference between p_{1j} and p_{2j} is given by

$$\left(\frac{n_{1j}}{n_{1.}} - \frac{n_{2j}}{n_{2.}} \right) \pm \sqrt{\chi^2_{1-\alpha}(r-1)} \sqrt{\frac{n_{1j}(n_{1.} - n_{1j})}{n_{1.}^3} + \frac{n_{2j}(n_{2.} - n_{2j})}{n_{2.}^3}} ,$$

$$(7.18)$$

where $\chi^2_{1-\alpha}(r-1)$ is the $(1 - \alpha)$ 100th percentile of a chi-square distribution with $r - 1$ degrees of freedom. The degrees of freedom are $r - 1$ so that the overall confidence coefficient is $1 - \alpha$ for all confidence intervals of this form. All pairwise confidence intervals of interest for any j may be determined by the use of expression (7.18). Notice for $r > 2$ that (7.18) differs from (7.8) in that the critical value is $Z_{1-\alpha/2}$ for a dichotomous situation, while for r responses, it is $\sqrt{\chi^2_{1-\alpha}(r-1)}$. Notice that (7.18) is the same as (7.8) (apart from the continuity correction), if $r = 2$, since $Z^2_{1-\alpha} = \chi^2_{1-\alpha}(1)$ (use Tables 4 and 6 of the Appendix to verify this relation, e.g., $(1.96)^2 = 3.84$).

While the data in Example 7.3.2.1 may be analyzed with the chi-square test as we have done, it is also possible to analyze the data with the rank sum test described in Chapter 6 since the data is ordinal. Naturally, the version of the test with correction for ties should be used.

Table 7.20. Worked Solution of Example 7.3.2.1 Using Chi-Square Test Procedure

A. Data: The data are of the form of Table 7.18 with $n_{11} = 23$, $n_{12} = 39$, $n_{13} = 46$, $n_{14} = 21$, $n_{15} = 21$, $n_{16} = 13$, $n_{17} = 9$, $n_{18} = 2$, $n_{21} = 7$, $n_{22} = 10$, $n_{23} = 28$, $n_{24} = 42$, $n_{25} = 75$, $n_{26} = 34$, $n_{27} = 15$, $n_{28} = 3$.

B. Assumptions: The data are two independent and random multinomial samples with probability arrays given by

$$\begin{pmatrix} p_{11} \\ \vdots \\ p_{18} \end{pmatrix} \quad \text{and} \quad \begin{pmatrix} p_{21} \\ \vdots \\ p_{28} \end{pmatrix}$$

for groups 1 and 2, respectively.

C. Computations: In the following table we summarize the observed and expected numbers along with the contribution to the chi-square statistic.

	Schizophrenia			Affective Disorders		
j	n_{1j}	e_{1j}	$(n_{1j} - e_{1j})^2/e_{1j}$	n_{2j}	e_{2j}	$(n_{2j} - e_{2j})^2/e_{2j}$
1	23	13.45	6.78	7	16.55	5.51
2	39	21.97	13.19	10	27.03	10.73
3	46	33.19	4.95	28	40.81	4.02
4	21	28.25	1.86	42	34.75	1.51
5	21	43.05	11.30	75	52.95	9.18
6	13	21.08	3.10	34	25.92	2.52
7	9	10.76	0.29	15	13.24	0.23
8	2	2.24	0.03	3	2.75	0.02
	174	174	41.50	214	214	33.72

$$\chi^2 = 41.50 + 33.72 = 75.22$$

D. Two-tailed statistical test:
1. Null hypothesis: H_0: $p_{1j} = p_{2j}$ for $j = 1, 2, \ldots, 8$
2. Alternative hypothesis: H_a: $p_{1j} \neq p_{2j}$ for at least one j
3. Decision rule for a 0.05 level test: Reject H_0 in favor of H_a if χ^2 in step C is greater than $\chi^2_{0.95}(7)$.

E. Action taken: From Table 6 of the Appendix, $\chi^2_{0.95}(7) = 14.07$, while from step C $\chi^2 = 75.22$; hence, the null hypothesis is rejected.

7.4   SUMMARY

In this chapter, we have outlined a set of procedures that may be applied to categorical data. These techniques together with those outlined and studied in Chapter 6 provide a broad overview of the methods available for the comparison of two groups.

In a later chapter, we shall discuss again the chi-square procedure in connection with more complex problems. For further reading on this topic, the texts by Forthofer and Lehnen (1981), Fleiss (1981), and Conover (1971) may be consulted.

PROBLEMS

7.1. The exposure to asbestos among 189 workers with mesotheliomas and their age-matched controls is given in the following table (E = exposed; $\bar{E}$ = not exposed):

		Case $\bar{E}$	Case E	
Control	$\bar{E}$	123	43	166
	E	7	16	23
		130	59	189

Test the H_0 of equal exposure rates.

7.2. The smoking status among 51 persons with lung cancer and their matched unexposed controls is given in the next table (S = smoker; $\bar{S}$ = non-smoker):

		Cancer $\bar{S}$	Cancer S	
Control	$\bar{S}$	20	18	38
	S	6	7	13
		26	25	51

Test the hypothesis of equal smoking rates in the two groups.

7.3. From 12 persons treated on two occasions for recurrent headache, once with drug A and once with a relaxation method, 8 declared relief with drug A but not with the relaxation method and 4 found relief with the relaxation method but not with drug A. Test the hypothesis of equal effectiveness of the two treatments.

7.4. Fifty smokers began a short program to stop smoking. The program claims that at least 50% of those completing the program will have a decreased need to smoke. At the end, 22 declare a decreased need to smoke, and the rest felt an increased need to smoke. Using only this data, would you conclude the program has met its goal? Is this problem better addressed as a hypothesis testing or a confidence interval estimation problem?

7.5. Use of steroids (oral contraceptives) early in pregnancy was investigated in 165 mothers of children with some specific birth defects and in an independent sample of 165 mothers of normal children. In this last group, 10 mothers were exposed, and in the former group, 45 were exposed.

(a) Test the hypothesis that the proportion exposed is the same in the two groups.

(b) Place a 95% confidence interval on this difference in proportions.

	Birth Defects	No Birth Defects
Exposed	45	10
Not Exposed	120	155
	165	165

7.6. In an unmatched study of menopausal estrogen use and endometrial carcinoma, two independent samples of women are selected. One group is a sample of 230 women with newly diagnosed endometrial cancer, while the other group is a sample of 170 women free of the disease. All women were interviewed regarding their use of exogenous estrogen.

		Endometrial Cancer Yes	No	
Estrogen	User	80	20	100
	Non-user	150	150	300
		230	170	400

(a) Test the hypothesis of equal proportions using the chi-square test at $\alpha = 0.05$.

(b) Place a 95% confidence interval on the difference in the proportion using estrogen.

(c) Estimate the odds ratio and interpret.

7.7. A vaccine to prevent a certain type of influenza was tested in 400 persons. After 1 yr, the records of these people and those of another 400 untreated persons produced the following data:

	No Flu	Flu	Total
Treated	202	198	400
Not Treated	179	221	400

(a) On the basis of these data alone, would you conclude that the vaccine was producing some protection?

(b) Place a 99% confidence interval on the difference between the proportion.

7.8. A large series of patients with central retinal vein occlusion (CRVO) are divided in two primary diagnostic groups: 282 patients who have developed venous stasis retinopathy (VSR) and 78 patients who suffer hemorrhagic retinopathy (HR). The severity of the disease in each group is:

CRVO	Mild	Moderate	Marked	Total
VSR	89	142	51	282
HR	6	24	48	78

(a) Perform a test to compare the two groups.

(b) Using the dichotomous grouping of mild versus moderate or marked combined, determine if the proportion with mild severity differs between the two groups.

7.9. The results of aneurysm surgery 6 months after operation were assessed. For 108 patients with a preoperative level of consciousness defined as alert or drowsy (A) and for 83 patients that were stuporous or comatose (C), the resulting data are:

| | Six-Month Postoperative Assessment | | | |
Initial Consciousness Level	Good Recovery	Moderately Disabled	Severely Disabled	Death
A	67	19	7	15
C	9	12	19	43

Perform a test to compare these two groups of patients.

7.10. In a group of people in the 65–69 age range, the hypertension status, by sex, is the following.

Sex	Normotensive	Isolated Systolic Hypertension	Diastolic Hypertension
Males	172	91	43
Females	260	133	35

Is there a significant sex difference?

7.11. The number of new cases of coronary heart disease observed in 12 yr of follow-up in men, by age at first exam, is:

Age at First Exam	Number of New Cases	Person-Years
40–49	84	8376
50–62	149	7092

Is there sufficient evidence to conclude that the rates of disease are different in the two groups?

REFERENCES

Conover, W. J. (1971). *Practical Nonparametric Statistics*, Wiley, New York.

Cox, D. P. (1970). *Analysis of Binary Data*, Chapman & Hall, London.

Everitt, B. S. (1977). *The Analysis of Contingency Tables*, Chapman & Hall, London.

Fisher, R. A. (1935). The logic of inductive inference (with discussion), *J. Roy. Statist. Soc.*, **98**, 39–54.

Fleiss, J. L. (1981). *Statistical Methods for Rates and Proportions*, 2nd Ed., Wiley, New York.

Fleiss, J. L., and B. S. Everitt. (1971). Comparing the marginal totals of square contingency tables, *Br. J. Math. Statist. Psychol.*, **24**, 117–123.

Forthofer, R., and R. Lehnen. (1981). *Public Program Analysis*, Wadsworth, Belmont, CA.

Haseman, J. (1978). Exact sample sizes for use with the Fisher–Irwin test for 2 × 2 tables, *Biometrics*, **34**, 106–109.

McNemar, Q. (1947). Note on the sampling error of the difference between correlated proportions or percentages, *Psychometrika*, **12**, 153–157.

Maxwell, A. E. (1970). Comparing the classification of subjects by two independent judges, *Br. J. Statist. Psychol.*, **116**, 651–655.

Schlesselman, J. (1982). *Case-Control Studies*, Oxford University Press, Oxford.

Stuart, A. (1957). The comparison of frequencies in matched samples, *Br. J. Statist. Psychol.*, **110**, 29–32.

CHAPTER 8

Tests of Independence and Measures of Association for Two Random Variables

8.1 INTRODUCTION

The term *association* is widely used in scientific literature. Most readers would correctly assume that the term expresses a relationship between the two variables under consideration. In general, in order to study the association between two variables, a random sample is selected and the two variables are observed simultaneously for each person or thing. For example, upon review of a random sample of patients with affective disorders, a relationship might be observed between the age of onset of illness and the length of stay of the first inpatient hospitalization for each person. To study the association between these two variables requires at least two levels of analysis. The first stage of analysis is to decide whether the observed relationship between the two variables can be explained by their relationship to a third variable or a set of variables. If this is the case, then the third variable or set of variables should be included in that analysis. The second level of analysis is the purely statistical task of computing a measure of association and using it to draw an inference regarding the relationship between the two variables in the population.

Generally, the first stage of analysis is more difficult. It is possible to think of situations in which a secondary variable explains an association. For example, the rate of schizophrenia increases with decreasing socioeconomic class. In addition, race/ethnic groups are not evenly represented in all socioeconomic classes. If data are gathered that examine the relationship between the rate of schizophrenia as a function of race/ethnic group

—without the inclusion of socioeconomic class in the data collection—an association would likely be reported between race/ethnic group and the rate of disease. In this situation, the association is probably at least partly due to the fact that both variables are related to socioeconomic class. If the measure of association was computed between race/ethnic group and the rate of schizophrenia for persons of a given socioeconomic class, there probably would be less association between the two variables. In most situations, it is extraordinarily difficult to deal with this problem. A great deal of substantive knowledge is required to make appropriate assessments of secondary associations. Even with this knowledge it is imperative to bear in mind that a potential explanatory variable may not be observed or observable in a given study.

The second phase of analysis that we mentioned was the task of statistical analysis and inference. It is assumed that the first issue has been properly examined before proceeding to this phase of the analysis. The problems discussed in this chapter are the definition of measures of association, the estimation and the testing of hypotheses regarding these measures of association, and the choice of a measure of association. It will be assumed throughout that there are two random variables, X and Y, and that a random sample of pairs (X, Y) has been selected from a suitable population. The hypothesis of interest throughout this chapter is the hypothesis that the variables X and Y are independent, that is, there is no association of any type between X and Y. In a probability sense, the null hypothesis of independence says the following:

$$H_0: \Pr[X \le x, Y \le y] = \Pr[X \le x]\Pr[Y \le y] \qquad (8.1)$$

for all values of x and y.

If X and Y are both discrete variables, then (8.1) is equivalent to

$$H_0': \Pr[X = x, Y = y] = \Pr[X = x]\Pr[Y = y] \qquad (8.2)$$

for all values of x and y. Several examples may help clarify this concept.

Example 8.1.1. Suppose in a population consisting of 150 men and 450 women, 50 men have a characteristic while 100 men do not and 150 women have the characteristic and 300 women do not. Defining X as the sex of a person and Y as the characteristic of interest, it is clear that in this population we have:

	X = Male	X = Female	Total
Y = Yes	50	150	200
Y = No	100	300	400
Total	150	450	600

From the totals it is clear that

$$\Pr[X = \text{Male}] = \tfrac{150}{600} = \tfrac{1}{4},$$

$$\Pr[X = \text{Female}] = \tfrac{450}{600} = \tfrac{3}{4},$$

$$\Pr[Y = \text{Yes}] = \tfrac{200}{600} = \tfrac{1}{3},$$

$$\Pr[Y = \text{No}] = \tfrac{400}{600} = \tfrac{2}{3},$$

and that

$$\Pr[X = \text{Male}, Y = \text{Yes}] = \tfrac{50}{600} = \tfrac{1}{12},$$

$$\Pr[X = \text{Male}, Y = \text{No}] = \tfrac{100}{600} = \tfrac{2}{12},$$

$$\Pr[X = \text{Female}, Y = \text{Yes}] = \tfrac{150}{600} = \tfrac{3}{12},$$

$$\Pr[X = \text{Female}, Y = \text{No}] = \tfrac{300}{600} = \tfrac{6}{12}.$$

That the variables, sex and presence of the characteristic, are independent can be seen by observing that the above probabilities conform to expression (8.2). Thus, knowing the sex of a person does not alter our knowledge of the probability that a person has or does not have the characteristic Y.

Example 8.1.2. In a large population, 7% of the people have schizophrenia of 93% do not. Furthermore, 40% of the persons are in the lower socioeconomic class. The schizophrenic group is divided equally into the two social classes, that is, 3.5% of the population are both schizophrenic and in the lower social class, and 3.5% of the population are both schizophrenic and in the upper social class. The probabilities are then summarized as:

	Schizophrenic	Not Schizophrenic	Total
Lower Social Class	0.035	0.365	0.40
Upper Social Class	0.035	0.565	0.60
Total	0.07	0.93	

In this situation, the probability that a person is in the lower social class is related to our knowledge of the person's psychiatric diagnosis. Persons in the lower social class are more likely to have the schizophrenia diagnosis than those in the upper social class. In this case, the two variables of psychiatric diagnosis and social class are clearly dependent rather than independent variates, as can be seen by observing that these probabilities do not conform to Definition 3.2.3.1.

These two examples illustrate independence and dependence of two variables. The distinction can be made by simply observing the population data presented in the tables. Next, statistical procedures for studying dependence from sample data are presented.

8.2 PROCEDURES FOR NOMINAL, ORDINAL, INTERVAL, OR RATIO SCALES: CHI-SQUARE TEST OF INDEPENDENCE AND MEASURES OF ASSOCIATION

8.2.1 General $R \times C$ Tables

Frequently it is desirable to select a random sample from a population and observe two characteristics, X and Y, for each person. If X can only take R distinct values and Y can only take C distinct values, the data are frequently summarized into an $R \times C$ *contingency table* of the form of Table 8.1.

In Table 8.1, the entry N_{ij} is the number of persons in category i for X and j for Y. From (8.2), the variables X and Y are independent if and only if $\Pr[X = x_i, Y = y_j] = \Pr[X = x_i]\Pr[Y = y_j]$ for all values of x_i and y_j. Notice that we are not assuming anything about the scale of X or Y; they may be nominal or ordinal variables. Consider the following example:

Example 8.2.1.1. In a survey of a group of manic-depressive patients, 431 were selected for study, and two characteristics were recorded for each patient. One characteristic was whether the patient had experienced sleep difficulty in the past 6 months. There are four levels or categories for this variable: no sleep difficulty = y_1, early morning awakening = y_2, other

Table 8.1. Typical $R \times C$ Contingecy Table

		Y				
		y_1	y_2	$\cdots$	y_C	Total
	x_1	N_{11}	N_{12}	$\cdots$	N_{1C}	$N_{1.}$
	x_2	N_{21}	N_{22}	$\cdots$	N_{2C}	$N_{2.}$
X	$\vdots$	$\vdots$	$\vdots$	$\ddots$	$\vdots$	$\vdots$
	x_R	N_{R1}	N_{R2}	$\cdots$	N_{RC}	$N_{R.}$
Total		$N_{.1}$	$N_{.2}$	$\cdots$	$N_{.C}$	N

decreased sleep difficulty = y_3, and hypersomnia = y_4. Persons experiencing early morning awakening would be categorized into y_2 whether they had other decreased sleep difficulty or not. On the other hand, persons are classified into y_3 only if they have experienced decreased sleep difficulty at times other than in the early morning. The second characteristic that was measured for each person was one of dysphoria. There are three categories for this characteristic: x_1 = depressed only; x_2 = depressed in addition to being fearful, irritable, or worried; and x_3 = absence of depression. The data are as follows:

$$Y = \text{Sleep Difficulty}$$

		y_1	y_2	y_3	y_4	Total
	x_1	34	45	71	62	212
$X = $ Dysphoria	x_2	47	53	31	18	149
	x_3	15	22	14	19	70
Total		96	120	116	99	431

The principal question is whether the variables, sleep difficulty and dysphoria, are independent of one another or if they are associated with one another.

For the general $R \times C$ table, let

$p_{i.}$ = probability that an individual is in category x_i,

$p_{.j}$ = probability that an individual is in category y_j,

p_{ij} = probability that an individual is in category x_i and category y_j.

If X and Y are independent, then $p_{ij} = p_{i.}p_{.j}$, and the expected number of persons (out of N) in category (x_i, y_j) is $Np_{i.}p_{.j}$. Since $p_{i.}$ and $p_{.j}$ are unknown, we estimate them by $\hat{p}_{i.} = N_{i.}/N$ and $\hat{p}_{.j} = N_{.j}/N$, and thus the estimate of the expected number of persons in the (i, j)th cell of Table 8.1 is $E_{ij} = N(N_{i.}/N)(N_{.j}/N) = N_{i.}N_{.j}/N$. In order to test the hypothesis of independence, the chi-square distribution is used. The procedure is to simply compare the observed numbers to the expected numbers by computing

$$\sum_{i=1}^{R} \sum_{j=1}^{C} \frac{(N_{ij} - E_{ij})^2}{E_{ij}} = \chi^2.$$

Table 8.2. Outline of Chi-Square Test for Independence

A. Data: The data are as summarized in Table 8.1.

B. Assumptions: The data are a random sample of size N from the joint distribution of X and Y. In this population, we denote

$$p_{ij} = \Pr\left[X = x_i, Y = y_j \right],$$

$$p_{i.} = \Pr\left[X = x_i \right] \quad \text{and} \quad p_{.j} = \Pr\left[Y = y_j \right].$$

C. Computations:
   1. Compute the row and column totals $N_{i.}$ and $N_{.j}$ and the expected value of cell (i, j) by $E_{ij} = N_{i.} N_{.j}/N$.
   This is the expected value if X and Y are independent.
   2. Compute

$$\chi^2 = \sum_{i=1}^{R} \sum_{j=1}^{C} \frac{\left(N_{ij} - E_{ij} \right)^2}{E_{ij}}.$$

D. Statistical test:
   1. Null hypothesis: H_0: $p_{ij} = p_{i.} p_{.j}$ for all i, j (i.e., X and Y are independent).
   2. Alternative hypothesis: H_a: $p_{ij} \neq p_{i.} p_{.j}$ for some i, j (i.e., X and Y are dependent).
   3. Decision rule for an α-level test: Reject H_0 in favor of H_a if $\chi^2 > \chi^2_{1-\alpha}[(R-1)(C-1)]$.

This quantity χ^2 has a chi-square distribution with $(R-1)(C-1)$ degrees of freedom if the two variables are independent. Clearly, if χ^2 is large, this indicates that the observed and expected numbers differ greatly and the hypothesis of independence is untenable. More formally, the procedure may be summarized as in Table 8.2.

In Table 8.2, the critical value $\chi^2_{1-\alpha}[(R-1)(C-1)]$ is obtained from Table 6 of the Appendix. Notice also that in our presentation of the statistical test, no mention is made in Table 8.2 of one-sided or two-sided alternatives. This test procedure is a general procedure with the ability to detect the rather omnibus alternative specified in the second part of step D. An example may help clarify the test procedure. We return to Example 8.2.1.1 and test the hypothesis of independence (Table 8.3).

The preceding test procedure is a large-sample test, that is, it is assumed that the total sample size is large. In more precise terms, it is recommended that the chi-square procedure be used only if the minimum expected

Table 8.3. Worked Solution of Example 8.2.1.1 Using the Chi-Square Test of Independence

A. Data: The data are:

		Y = Sleep Difficulty				
		y_1	y_2	y_3	y_4	Total
	x_1	34	45	71	62	212
X = Dysphoria	x_2	47	53	31	18	149
	x_3	15	22	14	19	70
	Total	96	120	116	99	431

B. Assumptions: The data are a random sample of size 431 from the population of (X, Y).

C. Computations:

1. $N_{1.} = 212$, $N_{2.} = 149$, $N_{3.} = 70$, $N_{.1} = 96$, $N_{.2} = 120$, $N_{.3} = 116$, and $N_{.4} = 99$.

2. The expected values are then given as:

	y_1	y_2	y_3	y_4
x_1	47.2	59.0	57.1	48.7
x_2	33.2	41.5	40.1	34.2
x_3	15.6	19.5	18.8	16.1

where

$$E_{11} = \frac{(96)(212)}{431}, \quad E_{12} = \frac{(120)(212)}{431}, \ldots$$

3. To compute the test statistic we may proceed as follows:

		$N_{ij} - E_{ij}$	$(N_{ij} - E_{ij})^2$	$(N_{ij} - E_{ij})^2/E_{ij}$
x_1	y_1	−13.2	174.24	3.6915
	y_2	−14.0	196.00	3.3220
	y_3	13.9	193.21	3.3837
	y_4	13.3	176.89	3.6322
x_2	y_1	13.8	190.44	5.7361
	y_2	11.5	132.25	3.1867
	y_3	−9.1	82.81	2.0651
	y_4	−16.2	262.44	7.6737
x_3	y_1	−0.6	0.36	0.0231
	y_2	2.5	6.25	0.3205
	y_3	−4.8	23.04	1.2255
	y_4	2.9	8.41	0.5224
				$\chi^2 = 34.7825$

D. Statistical test:

1. Null hypothesis: H_0: $p_{ij} = p_{i.}p_{.j}$ for all i and j.
2. Alternative hypothesis: H_a: $p_{ij} \neq p_{i.}p_{.j}$ for some i and j.
3. Decision rule for a 0.05 level test: Reject H_0 if $\chi^2 > \chi^2_{0.95}(6)$.

E. Action taken: From step C, the computed value of the test statistic is 34.7825 while the critical value from Table 6 of the Appendix is $\chi^2_{0.95}(6) = 12.59$. Hence, at the 5% level of significance, the null hypothesis should be rejected, and we conclude that there is an association between the variables, dysphoria, and sleep difficulty.

number exceeds 1 and if the expected number exceeds 5 for 80% or more of the cells in the table. For a 2×2 contingency table, the minimum cell expected frequency should exceed 5.

In many situations, it is of interest to compute a measure of association for an $R \times C$ contingency table. The principal use of such a measure is to compare the degree of association in one table relative to another table of the same dimensions. One such measure of association is the statistic V introduced by Cramer (1946). If χ^2 is the computed value of the test statistic in Table 8.2, the statistic V is defined as

$$V = \left(\frac{\chi^2}{N \min\{R - 1, C - 1\}} \right)^{1/2}, \tag{8.3}$$

where the denominator is the product of N and the minimum of the two values, $R - 1$ or $C - 1$.

This statistic ranges between 0 and 1, with values closer to 1 indicating a higher degree of association. Once again, this statistic can be useful for comparing several tables of the same size. This measure of contingency does not require a particular scale for X and Y, that is, it may be used even for nominal data. For the data of Example 8.2.1.1, we had computed $X^2 = 34.7825$; therefore, $V = [34.7825/431(2)]^{1/2} = 0.2009$. The variance of V may be computed as σ_V^2, where this expression is defined by (11.3-9) in Bishop, Fienberg, and Holland (1975). The reader may refer to their text for further discussion of the use of V.

8.2.2　Odds Ratio and 2×2 Tables

For 2×2 tables, the most widely used measure of association is the odds ratio. With p_{ij} defined by $\Pr(X = x_i, Y = y_j)$, the probability distribution of X and Y can be summarized by the following table:

		Y	
		y_1	y_2
	x_1	p_{11}	p_{12}
X			
	x_2	p_{21}	p_{22}

The odds ratio, denoted OR, is defined as

$$\mathrm{OR} = p_{11} p_{22} / p_{12} p_{21} \tag{8.4}$$

If the variables X and Y are independent, the odds ratio is 1. It can take any value between 0 and $+\infty$. It is generally convenient to work with natural logarithms ($\log_e$) when dealing with the odds ratio. Hence, instead of expression (8.4), the parameter θ is used, where

$$\theta = \log_e OR = \log_e p_{11} - \log_e p_{12} - \log_e p_{21} + \log_e p_{22} \qquad (8.5)$$

is a measure of association for a 2×2 population contingency table. If X and Y are independent, then θ equals zero. Furthermore, if θ equals zero, X and Y are independent. Since p_{ij} is estimated by N_{ij}/N, the usual estimator of OR is $(N_{11}/N)(N_{22}/N)/(N_{12}/N)(N_{21}/N) = N_{11}N_{22}/N_{12}N_{21}$, and thus the usual estimator of θ is

$$\hat{\theta} = \log_e \widehat{OR} = \log_e \frac{N_{11}N_{22}}{N_{12}N_{21}}. \qquad (8.6)$$

The variance of $\hat{\theta}$ is estimated by

$$\hat{\sigma}_{\hat{\theta}}^2 = \frac{1}{N_{11}} + \frac{1}{N_{12}} + \frac{1}{N_{21}} + \frac{1}{N_{22}}, \qquad (8.7)$$

which is a good estimator if N is large. The estimator becomes less stable and unreliable if any of N_{11}, N_{12}, N_{21}, or N_{22} are close to zero.* A $(1 - \alpha)100\%$ confidence interval for the population log odds ratio θ is

$$\hat{\theta} \pm Z_{1-\alpha/2}\hat{\sigma}_{\hat{\theta}}, \qquad (8.8)$$

where $Z_{1-\alpha/2}$ is from Table 4 of the Appendix. A more extensive discussion of the odds ratio is given in Chapter 13. Let us consider a brief example.

Example 8.2.2.1. In a follow-up study of a sample of 264 persons with unipolar depressive illness, the sex and the number of subsequent inpatient hospitalizations were recorded. The summarized data are as follows:

$Y =$ Any Subsequent Hospitalizations?

		Yes	No	Total
	Male	48	75	123
$X =$ Sex				
	Female	32	109	141
	Total	80	184	264

Is there any evidence to suggest that the variables X and Y are associated?

---

*If any $N_{ij} = 0$, then 0.5 is added to each before computing (8.6) and (8.7).

In Example 8.2.2.1, it is evident that the chi-square test procedure may be used to test the hypothesis of independence. Alternatively, one can analyze these data by use of the odds ratio. In particular, one can estimate the logarithm of the odds ratio, place a $(1 - \alpha)100\%$ confidence interval on it, and if this interval fails to include the point zero, one concludes that there is an association between the two variables.

For the data of Example 8.2.2.1, the estimated odds ratio is $\widehat{OR}= (48)(109)/(32)(75) = 2.180$, its natural logarithm is 0.7793, the estimated variance of $\hat{\theta}$ is $\hat{\sigma}_{\hat{\theta}}^2 = \frac{1}{48} + \frac{1}{109} + \frac{1}{32} + \frac{1}{75} = 0.0746$, and the estimated standard error of $\hat{\theta}$ is given by $\hat{\sigma}_{\hat{\theta}} = \sqrt{0.0746} = 0.2731$. Since $Z_{0.975} = 1.96$, it follows that a 95% confidence interval for the population logarithm of the odds ratio is $0.7793 \pm (1.96)(0.2731) = (0.2440, 1.3146)$, and by taking anti-logarithms, it follows that the 95% confidence interval for the population odds ratio is given by $(e^{0.2440}, e^{1.3146}) = (1.2763, 3.7233)$. Notice that zero is not in the 95% confidence interval for the logarithm of the odds ratio, and 1 is not in the interval for the odds ratio; hence, at the 5% level of significance, the hypothesis of independence would be rejected. One concludes that the sex of the patient and the possibility of subsequent hospitalization are associated.

8.2.3   Measures and Tests of Agreement: Reliability—$R \times R$ Tables

One of the problems medical researchers encounter regularly is that of measuring the agreement between two observers This may develop when two observers rate or evaluate a group of persons independently.

Example 8.2.3.1. As an illustration, suppose that two cardiologists are asked to independently evaluate 200 electrocardiograms and to classify them into the three categories of normal, possible abnormality, and definite abnormality. For convenience, let us call the two cardiologists X and Y. Suppose that the results of the two cardiologists are as follows:

	Abnormality			
	Normal	Possible	Definite	Total
Cardiologists X	120	40	40	200
Cardiologist Y	100	60	40	200

This table is clearly not the best way to summarize the results since the table, as it stands, gives no indication of how the cardiologists compared in rating the same patient. Suppose that it is further known that the 200 patients were rated as in Table 8.4.

Table 8.4. Sample Electrocardiogram Diagnosis Data

| | | Cardiologist Y Abnormality | | | |
		Normal	Possible	Definite	Total
	Normal	90	30	0	120
Cardiologist X	Abnormality				
	Possible	0	20	20	40
	Definite	10	10	20	40
	Total	100	60	40	200

Is there evidence to conclude that the two cardiologists agree on their diagnosis?

In Example 8.2.3.1, we may postulate disagreement as the null hypothesis and some level of agreement as the alternative hypothesis. In this way, the hypothesis of disagreement is not discarded unless the observed data support the alternative of agreement rather convincingly. Several statistics are appropriate for this observer agreement problem. Before considering these, it is convenient to think of the general agreement problem in terms of Table 8.5.

Notationally, $p_{ij} = \Pr[X = i, Y = j]$, $p_{i.} = \Pr[X = i]$, and $p_{.j} = \Pr[X = j]$ are the joint and marginal probabilities in the population from which the sample in Table 8.5 is taken.

In the sample, several measures of observer agreement are easily computed. One such measure is simply the percentage of agreement. That is, $100\left[\sum_{i=1}^{R} N_{ii}/N\right]$. For the data of Table 8.4, this statistic is simply 65% $[= 100(90 + 20 + 20)/200]$. The problem with using this statistic is its interpretation. In particular, to what do we compare the 65%? About the

Table 8.5. General Structure for Observer Agreement Problem[a]

| | | Observer Y Rating | | | | |
		1	2	$\cdots$	R	Total
	1	N_{11}	N_{12}	$\cdots$	N_{1R}	$N_{1.}$
	2	N_{21}	N_{22}	$\cdots$	N_{2R}	$N_{2.}$
Observer X Rating	$\vdots$	$\vdots$	$\vdots$	$\ddots$	$\vdots$	$\vdots$
	R	N_{R1}	N_{R2}	$\cdots$	N_{RR}	$N_{R.}$
	Total	$N_{.1}$	$N_{.2}$	$\cdots$	$N_{.R}$	N

[a] Entry is the number of persons.

Table 8.6. Expected Cell Entries for Table 8.4 under the Hypothesis of Independence

		Normal	Cardiologist Y Abnormality Possible	Definite
Cardiologist X	Normal Abnormality	60	36	24
	Possible	20	12	8
	Definite	20	12	8

only situation in which percentage of agreement is a useful and informative number is when each cardiologist had rated the entire sample into one and the same diagnostic group. For example, if all 200 persons were diagnosed as normal by both cardiologists, this indicates that there is no variability in the patients with respect to diagnosis, and the only descriptive figure is the percentage of agreement.

Another measure that may incorrectly appear to be a measure of agreement is the chi-square statistic computed for the hypothesis of independence between the two cardiologists' ratings. Applying the test procedure of Table 8.2 to the data of Table 8.4, one obtains the set of expected cell entries in Table 8.6. Hence, the resulting 4 d.f. chi-square statistic is

$$109.67 = \left(\frac{(90 - 60)^2}{60} + \cdots + \frac{(20 - 8)^2}{8} \right).$$

This statistic is significant at the $p < 0.001$ level; hence, one concludes that there is an association between the two cardiologists' diagnostic ratings. Before we make any statements regarding the term *association* as it relates to *agreement*, let us suppose that the data of Table 8.4 were actually the data of Table 8.7.

Notice that in terms of number of agreements there are fewer in Table 8.7 (20) than in Table 8.4 (130). On the other hand, the marginal total columns are identical in the two tables, and thus the expected cell entries for Table 8.7 are also given by Table 8.6. Computing the four d.f. chi-square statistic for Table 8.7 results in a value of

$$133.33 = \frac{(20 - 60)^2}{60} + \cdots + \frac{(0 - 8)^2}{8},$$

Table 8.7. Alternative Data for Table 8.4

| | | Cardiologist Y Abnormality | | | |
		Normal	Possible	Definite	Total
	Normal	20	60	40	120
Cardiologist X	Abnormality				
	Possible	40	0	0	40
	Definite	40	0	0	40
	Total	100	60	40	200

an increase in the value of the chi-square meaning greater association! Thus, it is evident by this one example that the chi-square statistic for the test of independence will not do as a measure of agreement. The chi-square statistic measures all forms of association, including gross disagreement.

One statistic that is recommended for use as an indicator of observer agreement is the *kappa* statistic of Cohen (1960). This statistic is a chance-corrected measure of agreement and ranges up to 1, depending on the strength of agreement. If the statistic takes the value of zero, this indicates no agreement, negative values indicate disagreement, and positive values indicate agreement. Formally, the statistic is defined by

$$\hat{K} = \frac{\hat{p}_0 - \hat{p}_e}{1 - \hat{p}_e}, \tag{8.9}$$

where $\hat{p}_0$ is the observed proportion of agreement, that is, $\hat{p}_0 = \sum_{i=1}^{R} N_{ii}/N = \sum \hat{p}_{ii}$, and $\hat{p}_e$ is the expected proportion agreement if the two raters are rating independently of one another, that is, $\hat{p}_e = \sum_{i=1}^{R} N_{i.}N_{.i}/N^2 = \sum_{i=1}^{R} \hat{p}_{i.}\hat{p}_{.i}$. The quantity $\hat{p}_e$ is the expected agreement due to chance alone. The statistic $\hat{K}$ may range from $-\hat{p}_e/(1 - \hat{p}_e)$ to 1. It takes the value zero when the observed agreement is equal to the expected chance agreement. Clearly, the statistic $\hat{K}$ may be viewed as an estimator of the population quantity, $K = (p_0 - p_e)/(1 - p_e)$, where p_0 and p_e are corresponding population proportions.

The variance of $\hat{K}$ is estimated (Fleiss, 1981) by

$$\hat{\sigma}_{\hat{K}}^2 = \frac{1}{N(1 - \hat{p}_e)^2} \left[\hat{p}_e + \hat{p}_e^2 - \sum_{i=1}^{R} \hat{p}_{i.}\hat{p}_{.i}(\hat{p}_{i.} + \hat{p}_{.i}) \right], \tag{8.10}$$

and the standard error of $\hat{K}$ is estimated by the square root of expression

(8.10). To test the hypothesis of no observer agreement while adjusting for chance agreement, the statistic

$$Z = \hat{K}/\hat{\sigma}_{\hat{K}} \tag{8.11}$$

may be compared to the standard normal distribution values of $Z_{1-\alpha/2}$ and $-Z_{1-\alpha/2}$ for a two-tailed test.

Returning to the example of Table 8.4, we see $\hat{p}_0$ is equal to 0.65 while the expected chance agreement is 0.40, as computed from Table 8.6. The standard error of $\hat{K}$ is

$$\hat{\sigma}_{\hat{K}} = \left(1/200(0.6)^2\right)^{1/2}$$

$$\times \left\{0.4 + (0.4)^2 - [0.3(1.10) + 0.06(0.5) + 0.04(0.4)]\right\}^{1/2}$$

$$= 0.05 \text{ and } \hat{K} = 0.417;$$

therefore, expression (8.11) is $8.34 = 0.417/0.05$, and there is basis for rejecting the hypothesis of no agreement, since $8.34 > 1.96$.

There are various extensions of this procedure. One extension is the weighted kappa, in which coefficients or weights are used to express the relative importance of various types of disagreement. For example, for the data of Table 8.4, a disagreement on a diagnosis of possible or definite abnormality may not be regarded as serious as a disagreement in which one cardiologist diagnoses a patient as possible or definite abnormality, and the other cardiologist diagnoses the patient in the normal category. If w_{ij} is a "weight" that expresses the degree of seriousness in cardiologist X classifying a patient into category i while cardiologist Y classifies the patient into category j, a weighted kappa, $\hat{K}_w$, may be constructed. The main difficult in applying the weighted kappa lies in the determination of, and the justification for, a set of weights. The reader is referred to Fleiss (1981) and Landis and Koch (1977) for further details on the construction of the weighted kappa statistic.

Another extension of the kappa statistic is in the direction of measuring agreement among more than two raters, say K raters. Strictly speaking, this problem is one of measuring association among K, rather than two, random variables and does not fit into the description of this chapter. However, to properly complete the agreement discussion, we shall discuss this problem in the following optional section.

8.2.4 Measures of Agreement among K Raters

This section continues the development of the preceding section by extending the agreement statistics to the case of measures of agreement among more than two raters. The statistics and presentation in this section are indebted to Fleiss (1971). The type of situation where this measure is necessary appears in Table 8.8, in which 27 patients with a particular retinopathy had the severity of their retinopathy rated by four ophthalmologists. From Table 8.8, it is evident that all four ophthalmologists rated the second person with a mild retinopathy, while for the first person three of the ophthalmologists agreed on a rating of moderate, and the other classified the retinopathy as mild.

To treat the general problem, the following notation is useful:

N = total number of persons classified,

K = number of raters per person,

R = number of categories possible,

n_{ij} = number of ophthalmologists who rate person i into category j.

For the data of Table 8.8, $N = 27$, $K = 4$, $R = 3$, and $n_{11} = 1$, $n_{12} = 3$, $n_{13} = 0$, $n_{21} = 4$, $n_{22} = 0, \ldots, n_{27,1} = 3$, $n_{27,2} = 0$, $n_{27,3} = 1$, are the values of these quantities for this particular problem. It is useful to compute the proportion of all classifications that fall into group j. This quantity, denoted $\hat{p}_j$, is

$$\hat{p}_j = \frac{1}{NK} \sum_{i=1}^{N} n_{ij} \tag{8.12}$$

for $j = 1, 2, \ldots, R$. These figures are summarized in the bottom line of Table 8.8. We note that with K raters there are $\binom{K}{2} = K(K-1)/2$ possible rater pairs. Furthermore, the two raters in each of these pairs may agree or disagree on their classifications. Thus, for each person, there are $K(K-1)/2$ possible opportunities for agreement or disagreement among the pairs of ophthalmologists. Clearly, for person i, the actual number of agreements among pairs of ophthalmologists is given by

$$\left[\frac{n_{i1}(n_{i1}-1)}{2} + \frac{n_{i2}(n_{i2}-1)}{2} + \cdots + \frac{n_{iR}(n_{iR}-1)}{2} \right] = \sum_{j=1}^{R} \frac{n_{ij}(n_{ij}-1)}{2}.$$

$$\uparrow \qquad\qquad\quad \uparrow \qquad\qquad\qquad\quad \uparrow$$

Number of pairs   Number of pairs   Number of pairs $\tag{8.13}$
agreeing on   agreeing on   agreeing on
category 1   category 2   category R

$$= \binom{n_{i1}}{2} \qquad = \binom{n_{i2}}{2} \qquad\qquad = \binom{n_{iR}}{2}$$

Table 8.8. Disease Severity Rating of 27 Patients by Four Ophthalmologists Per Person[a]

| | Category | | |
| | Mild | Moderate | Severe |
Patient	($j = 1$)	($j = 2$)	($j = 3$)
1	1	3	—
2	4	—	—
3	1	—	3
4	—	3	1
5	—	—	4
6	—	2	2
7	2	—	2
8	3	—	1
9	3	1	—
10	—	1	3
11	1	—	3
12	4	—	—
13	—	1	3
14	—	4	—
15	3	—	1
16	1	1	2
17	—	1	3
18	1	3	—
19	—	—	4
20	1	2	1
21	4	—	—
22	1	3	—
23	—	3	1
24	—	—	4
25	2	2	—
26	—	4	—
27	3	—	1
	35	34	39
$\hat{p}_j$	0.324	0.315	0.361

$\hat{p}_j$ = proportion of all classifications assigned to category j.
[a]Entry is the number of ophthalmologists assigning a particular severity.

The proportion of pairs agreeing for person i is therefore given by

$$\hat{p}_i = \frac{\sum_{j=1}^{R} n_{ij}(n_{ij}-1)/2}{K(K-1)/2} = \sum_{j=1}^{R} \frac{n_{ij}(n_{ij}-1)}{K(K-1)}. \qquad (8.14)$$

The overall agreement may be determined by computing the mean of (8.14) for the N persons; that is,

$$\bar{p} = \frac{\sum_{i=1}^{N} \hat{p}_i}{N} = \frac{1}{NK(K-1)}\left[\left(\sum_{i=1}^{N}\sum_{j=1}^{R} n_{ij}^2\right) - NK\right]. \qquad (8.15)$$

From Table 8.8, $\hat{p} = [1/27(4)(3)][304 - (27)(4)] = 0.6049$; that is, on the basis of these data, we would estimate that two ophthalmologists would agree on the classification of a randomly selected patient approximately 60% of the time.

It can be shown that the expected chance agreement is given by squaring each term at the foot of Table 8.8 and summing; that is, the expected chance agreement is estimated by $\bar{p}_e$, where

$$\bar{p}_e = \sum_{j=1}^{R} \hat{p}_j^2. \qquad (8.16)$$

The *generalized kappa statistic* is then defined as follows:

$$\hat{K}_G = \frac{\bar{p} - \bar{p}_e}{1 - \bar{p}_e}, \qquad (8.17)$$

with a variance estimated by

$$\hat{\sigma}_{\hat{K}_G} = \frac{2}{NK(K-1)}\frac{\sum_{j=1}^{R}\hat{p}_j^2 - (2K-3)\left(\sum_{j=1}^{R}\hat{p}_j^2\right)^2 + 2(K-2)\sum_{j=1}^{R}\hat{p}_j^3}{\left(1 - \sum_{j=1}^{R}\hat{p}_j^2\right)^2}. \qquad (8.18)$$

Once again, a test may be conducted by utilizing the result that

$$Z = \hat{K}_G / \hat{\sigma}_{\hat{K}_G} \qquad (8.19)$$

is a standard normal variate.

For the data of Table 8.8, it is clear that

$$\bar{p}_e = (0.324)^2 + (0.315)^2 + (0.361)^2 = 0.3345,$$

$$\hat{K}_G = (0.6049 - 0.3345)/(1 - 0.3345) = 0.4063,$$

$$\hat{\sigma}^2_{\hat{K}_G} = \frac{2}{27(4)(3)} \frac{0.3345 - 5(0.1119) + 2(2)(0.1123)}{(1 - 0.3345)^2} = 0.0031248,$$

$$\hat{\sigma}_{\hat{K}_G} = \sqrt{0.0031248} = 0.0559,$$

$$Z = 0.406/0.056 = 7.25.$$

Comparing 7.25 to the standard normal distribution, it is noted that 7.25 yields an infinitesimal P value ($p < 0.0001$ from Table 4 of the Appendix), which means the generalized kappa statistic shows significant agreement.

We now turn our attention again to the case of two random variables.

8.3   PROCEDURES FOR ORDINAL, INTERVAL, OR RATIO SCALES: KENDALL'S TAU AND SPEARMAN'S RANK CORRELATION COEFFICIENT

8.3.1 Order Association: Kendall's Tau

The previous section made no assumption at all regarding the scale of the variable; that is, the methods of analysis are valid for nominal-, ordinal-, interval-, or ratio-scale data. If one has data on two ordinal-scale variables, these procedures are obviously applicable; for example, a chi-square test as described in Table 8.2 may be applied to test for association. On the other hand, if there is an ordering of categories for each variable (i.e., X and Y), it is clear that this ordering is not accounted for in the analysis of the previous section. This raises the issue of construction of procedures, which will use the ordering of the variables. To generalize, the measures of *order association* for ordinal data are more efficient for order relationships between X and Y than those described in the previous section. We now proceed to a discussion of some measures of order association between two variables X and Y where both X and Y are at least ordinal in scale. This discussion is due largely to Quade (1971, 1986).

Two observations (X_1, Y_1) and (X_2, Y_2) are *concordant* if they are in the same order with respect to each variable—that is, if $X_1 < X_2$ and $Y_1 < Y_2$ or $X_1 > X_2$ and $Y_1 > Y_2$. They are *discordant* if they are in the reverse ordering for X and Y—if $X_1 < X_2$ and $Y_1 > Y_2$ or $X_1 > X_2$ and $Y_1 < Y_2$. The observations are *tied* if $X_1 = X_2$ or $Y_1 = Y_2$ or both. If the two observations are plotted on an XY plot, the observations are concordant if the line joining the two points has a positive slope. The observations are discordant if the line joining the two points has a negative slope, and otherwise they are tied.

The variables X and Y are said to have a *positive order association* (*negative order association*) if a randomly chosen pair (X_1, Y_1) and (X_2, Y_2) are more likely to be concordant (discordant) than discordant (concordant). There is no order association if the pair is equally likely to be concordant or discordant. Thus, if the variables X and Y are independent, then there is no order association. However, if there is no order association, the variables may be dependent, although not in the order association fashion.

Denote the probabilities of concordance, discordance, and ties by p_C, p_D, and p_T, respectively. There are numerous measures of order association. The term *Kendall's tau*, after Kendall (1938), usually refers to such measures; τ_b designates Kendall's rank correlation coefficient in the statistical literature. The following are measures of order association:

$$\tau_a = p_C - p_D,$$

$$\tau_b = (p_C - p_D)\big/\sqrt{(1 - p_X)(1 - p_Y)}, \qquad (8.20)$$

$$\tau_d = (p_C - p_D)\big/(p_C + p_D),$$

where p_X and p_Y are the probabilities of a tie on X or on Y, respectively. The three indices differ in how they treat the tied observations: τ_a is an unconditional index of order association while τ_d (introduced and called *gamma* by Goodman and Kruskal, 1954) is a conditional index, and τ_b treats the ties differently than τ_d.

Given a random sample of observations $(X_1, Y_1), \ldots, (X_N, Y_N)$, we know that there are $\binom{N}{2} = N(N-1)/2$ distinct ways to choose two pairs (X_i, Y_i)

and (X_j, Y_j). Let

n_C = number of concordant pairs among the $N(N - 1)/2$,

n_D = number of discordant pairs among the $N(N - 1)/2$,

n_T = number of tied pairs among the $N(N - 1)/2$, (8.21)

n_X = number of tied X's pairs,

n_Y = number of tied Y's pairs,

$n = N(N - 1)/2$.

Then reasonable estimates for p_C, p_D, p_X, and p_Y are n_C/n, n_D/n, n_X/n, and n_Y/n, respectively. Following Quade (1971), it is reasonable to estimate the quantities for expression (8.20) by t_a, t_b, and t_d, where

$$t_a = \frac{n_C - n_D}{n},$$

$$t_b = (n_C - n_D)/\sqrt{(n - n_X)(n - n_Y)},$$ (8.22)

$$t_d = (n_C - n_D)/(n_C + n_D).$$

As an illustration of the computation of the indices, suppose we have five depressive patients; the ages of onset of their illness and the lengths of their first inpatient hospitalization are known. The data are in Table 8.9.

The second patient is tied (on Y) with the third and discordant with the fourth, the third patient is discordant with the fourth, and the fourth patient is tied (on X) with the fifth. The remaining pairs are all concordant. Thus, of the $10 = \binom{5}{2}$ pairs, there are $n_C = 6$ concordant pairs, $n_D = 2$ discordant pairs, and $n_T = 2$ tied pairs. The sample suggests a positive

Table 8.9. Age of Onset of Illness and Length of Hospitalization for Depressed Patients ($N = 5$)

	Patient				
	1	2	3	4	5
X = Age (years)	44	34	40	26	26
Y = Length (weeks)	13	3	3	11	2

order association; we have

$$t_a = \frac{6 - 2}{10} = 0.4, \qquad t_d = \frac{6 - 2}{6 + 2} = 0.5,$$

$$t_b = \frac{6 - 2}{\sqrt{(10 - 1)(10 - 1)}} = 0.4444.$$

In order to use these quantities to make an inference regarding the population quantities τ_a, τ_b, and τ_d, the standard errors are useful.

To determine these standard errors requires some further notation. Again following Quade (1971), for the pair (X_i, Y_i), let C_i, D_i, and T_i denote the number of observations that are respectively concordant, discordant, and tied with (X_i, Y_i). Clearly, for each $i = 1, 2, \ldots, N$, it is true that $C_i + D_i + T_i = N - 1$; also, it is easy to show that

$$\sum_{i=1}^{N} C_i = 2n_C,$$

$$\sum_{i=1}^{N} D_i = 2n_D, \tag{8.23}$$

$$\sum_{i=1}^{N} T_i = 2n_T.$$

Then the standard errors for t_a, t_b, and t_d are given, respectively, by

$$s_a = \frac{2\sqrt{N\sum_{i=1}^{N}(C_i - D_i)^2 - \left[\sum_{i=1}^{N}(C_i - D_i)\right]^2}}{N(N - 1)\sqrt{N - 1}},$$

$$s_b = \frac{n}{\sqrt{n - n_X}\sqrt{n - n_Y}} s_a, \tag{8.24}$$

$$s_d = \frac{n}{n_C + n_D} s_a,$$

where n, n_X, n_Y, n_C, and n_D are given by expression (8.21). For large samples ($N \geq 20$) the standard normal distribution may be used to test hypotheses regarding τ_a, τ_b, or τ_d by referencing t_a/s_a, t_b/s_b, or t_d/s_d to the standard normal distribution. The quantities t_a/s_a and t_d/s_d are always equal; however, one may prefer working with one statistic rather

Table 8.10. Outline of Test for Order Association Using Kendall's Tau
(Large Sample Test)

A. Data: A random sample is selected from a bivariate population of (X, Y), where the scales of X and Y are at least ordinal. The data are denoted by $(X_1, Y_1), (X_2, Y_2), \ldots, (X_N, Y_N)$.

B. Assumptions: Both X and Y are at least ordinal in their scales, and N is at least 20.

C. Computations:

1. Let

$$n = N(N - 1)/2$$

$$C_i = \text{number of pairs concordant with } (X_i, Y_i)$$

$$D_i = \text{number of pairs discordant with } (X_i, Y_i)$$

$$T_i = \text{number of pairs tied with } (X_i, Y_i)$$

$$n_{X_i} = \text{number of pairs with the } X\text{'s tied with } X_i$$

$$n_{Y_i} = \text{number of pairs with the } Y\text{'s tied with } Y_i$$

2. Perform the following computations:

$\dfrac{(X, Y)}{(X_1 Y_1)}$,	$\dfrac{C_i}{C_1}$,	$\dfrac{D_i}{D_1}$,	$\dfrac{T_i}{T_1}$,	$\dfrac{C_i - D_i}{C_1 - D_1}$,
$\vdots$	$\vdots$	$\vdots$	$\vdots$	$\vdots$
(X_N, Y_N),	$\dfrac{C_N}{\sum_{i=1}^{N} C_i}$,	$\dfrac{T_N}{\sum_{i=1}^{N} D_i}$,	$\dfrac{T_N}{\sum_{i=1}^{N} T_i}$,	$\dfrac{C_N - D_N}{\sum_{i=1}^{N}(C_i - D_i)}$,

$\dfrac{(C_i - D_i)^2}{(C_1 - D_1)^2}$,	$\dfrac{n_{X_i}}{n_{X_1}}$,	$\dfrac{n_{Y_i}}{n_{Y_1}}$
$\vdots$	$\vdots$	$\vdots$
$\dfrac{(C_N - D_N)^2}{\sum_{i=1}^{N}(C_i - D_i)^2}$,	$\dfrac{n_{X_N}}{\sum_{i=1}^{N} n_{X_i}}$,	$\dfrac{n_{Y_N}}{\sum_{i=1}^{N} n_{y_i}}$

The remaining computations depend on whether the data analyst is interested in τ_a, τ_b, or τ_d. For completeness, we present the computations for all three.

Table 8.10. Continued.

3. From step 2 and from the notation of (8.21) and (8.23), we see that

$$n_X = \tfrac{1}{2}\left(\Sigma_{i=1}^N n_{X_i}\right), \qquad n_Y = \tfrac{1}{2}\left(\Sigma_{i=1}^N n_{Y_i}\right)$$

$$n_C = \tfrac{1}{2}\left(\Sigma_{i=1}^N C_i\right), \qquad n_D = \tfrac{1}{2}\left(\Sigma_{i=1}^N D_i\right) \qquad (8.26)$$

$$n_T = \tfrac{1}{2}\left(\Sigma_{i=1}^N T_i\right)$$

4. As a result,

$$t_a = \frac{n_C - n_D}{n}, \qquad s_a = \frac{2\sqrt{N\Sigma_{i=1}^N(C_i - D_i)^2 - \left[\Sigma_{i=1}^N(C_i - D_i)\right]^2}}{N(N-1)\sqrt{N-1}},$$

$$t_b = \frac{n_C - n_D}{\sqrt{(n - n_X)(n - n_Y)}}, \qquad s_b = \frac{n}{\sqrt{(n - n_X)(n - n_Y)}} s_a, \qquad (8.27)$$

$$t_d = \frac{(n_C - n_D)}{(n_C + n_D)}, \qquad s_d = \frac{n}{n_C + n_D} s_a.$$

5. If there are no X nor Y ties, then there is only one t, i.e., $t_a = t_b = t_d$. The computations are more straightforward without tied pairs.

Two-tailed statistical test:

1. Null hypothesis: H_0: $\tau_a = 0$ ($\tau_b = 0$ or $\tau_d = 0$)
2. Alternative hypothesis: H_a: $\tau_a \neq 0$ ($\tau_b \neq 0$ or $\tau_d \neq 0$)
3. Decision rule for an α-level test: Reject H_0 in favor of H_a if t_a/s_a (t_b/s_b or t_d/s_d) $> Z_{1-\alpha/2}$ or t_a/s_a (t_b/s_b or t_d/s_d) $< -Z_{1-\alpha/2}$.

One-tailed statistical test:

1. Null hypothesis: H_0: $\tau_a = 0$ ($\tau_b = 0$ or $\tau_d = 0$)
2. Alternative hypothesis: H_a: $\tau_a > 0$ ($\tau_a < 0$) $\tau_b > 0$ [($\tau_b < 0$) or $\tau_d > 0$ ($\tau_d < 0$)].
3. Decision rule for an α-level test: Reject H_0 in favor of H_a if t_a/s_a (t_b/s_b or t_d/s_d) $> Z_{1-\alpha}$ ($< -Z_{1-\alpha}$).

than the other. The $(1 - \alpha)$ 100% confidence intervals for τ_a, τ_b, and τ_d are

$$t_a \pm Z_{1-\alpha/2}s_a \quad \text{for } \tau_a,$$

$$t_b \pm Z_{1-\alpha/2}s_b \quad \text{for } \tau_b, \qquad (8.25)$$

$$t_d \pm Z_{1-\alpha/2}s_d \quad \text{for } \tau_d,$$

respectively, where $Z_{1-\alpha/2}$ is from Table 4 of the Appendix. Notice from (8.22) that if neither the X's nor the Y's have any ties, then the indices t_a, t_b, and t_d are equal. In addition, their standard errors are equal in the absence of both X and Y ties. We summarize the test procedures for both one- and two-sided alternative hypotheses in Table 8.10

The quantities $Z_{1-\alpha/2}$ and $Z_{1-\alpha}$ are obtained from Table 4 of the Appendix. The above testing procedure serves for large samples.

As an example of the procedure consider the following example, in which there are 25 persons selected from an ophthalmology clinic, and the age and the intraocular pressure (right eye) are recorded.

Denoting the age by X and the intraocular pressure by Y, the 25 observations are given in the first two columns of Table 8.11. Note that for ease in computing the concordant, discordant, and tied pairs, the data are ordered from the smallest X to the largest X. The data concordances, discordances, and ties are as listed in the table.

From Table 8.11 and by using the relationships in expression (8.26), one obtains $n_X = 7$, $n_Y = 31$, $n_C = 219$, $n_D = 43$, and $n_T = 38$; also note that $n = 25(25 - 1)/2 = 300$ and $n_C + n_D + n_T = 300$, as it should. Hence, we have a check on the arithmetic. By using expression (8.27), we note that

$$t_a = \frac{219 - 43}{300} = 0.5867,$$

$$t_b = \frac{219 - 43}{\sqrt{300 - 7}\sqrt{300 - 31}} = 0.6269,$$

$$t_d = \frac{219 - 43}{219 + 43} = 0.6718,$$

and

$$s_a = \frac{2\sqrt{25(5204) - (352)^2}}{25(24)\sqrt{24}} = 0.05356,$$

$$s_b = \frac{(300)(0.05356)}{\sqrt{300 - 7}\sqrt{300 - 31}} = 0.05722,$$

$$s_d = \frac{(300)(0.05356)}{219 + 43} = 0.06132.$$

The Z statistics for testing the hypothesis of no order association between

Table 8.11. Data on Age (X) and Intraocular Pressure (Y) for 25
Ophthalmologic Patients

Observation i	X_i	Y_i	C_i	D_i	T_i	$C_i - D_i$	$(C_i - D_i)^2$	n_{X_i}	n_{Y_i}
1	35	15	23	0	1	23	529	0	1
2	40	17	20	3	1	17	289	0	1
3	41	16	21	2	1	19	361	0	1
4	44	18	19	3	2	16	256	0	2
5	45	15	20	3	1	17	289	0	1
6	48	19	15	4	5	11	121	0	5
7	50	19	15	2	7	13	169	2	5
8	50	18	18	2	4	16	256	2	2
9	50	17	18	3	3	15	225	2	1
10	52	16	17	6	1	11	121	0	1
11	54	19	18	1	5	17	289	0	5
12	55	18	17	3	4	14	196	2	2
13	55	21	14	6	4	8	64	2	2
14	55	20	16	3	5	13	169	2	3
15	57	19	17	2	5	15	225	0	5
16	58	20	18	3	3	15	225	0	3
17	59	19	16	3	5	13	169	0	5
18	60	23	17	5	2	12	144	1	1
19	60	19	15	3	6	12	144	1	5
20	61	22	19	5	0	14	196	0	0
21	63	23	19	4	1	15	225	0	1
22	65	21	17	5	2	12	144	0	2
23	67	20	16	5	3	11	121	0	3
24	71	21	18	4	2	14	196	0	2
25	77	20	15	6	3	9	81	0	3
Total			438	86	76	352	5204	14	62

age and intraocular pressure are

$$Z_a = t_a/s_a = 0.5867/0.05356 = 10.96,$$

$$Z_b = t_b/s_b = 0.6269/0.05722 = 10.96,$$

$$Z_d = t_d/s_d = 0.6718/0.06132 = 10.96.$$

A one-sided P value from Table 4 of the Appendix is $P < 0.0001$. Thus, at
the 0.01% level of significance, the null hypothesis of no order association
would be rejected in favor of a positive order association between the two
variables.

In the next sections, two additional measures of association are considered.

8.3.2 Spearman Rank Correlation Coefficient

One of the most widely known measures of correlation is the rank correlation coefficient, which owes its name to Spearman (1904). This measure is used widely due to its simplicity and ease of computation. Essentially, only the ranks of the X's among themselves and the ranks of the Y's among themselves are required for its computation. Intuitively speaking, if the X rank and the Y rank for each pair of (X, Y) tend to be close together, then there appears to be a positive association among the rank orders of the X's and Y's. Conversely, if the rank of X and the rank of Y tend to be far apart so that a reverse ordering of X's appears to be associated with the Y's, then there is a negative rank order relationship. If there is absolutely no rank order relationship between the X's and the Y's, then the ranks of the Y's for a given ranking of the X's will appear to be a random assignment of the rankings. To clarify these comments, suppose the data gathered for a study consist of the data on patients 1, 2, and 5 of Table 8.9, that is, $(X, Y) = (44, 13), (34, 3), (26, 2)$. The ranks of the X's are 3, 2, and 1, respectively, for 44, 34, and 26. Similarly, the ranks of the Y's are 3, 2, and 1, respectively, for 13, 3, and 2. Hence, replacing the three pairs by their ranks we have $(3, 3)$, $(2, 2)$, and $(1, 1)$. The X ranks are in perfect alignment with the Y ranks, and hence we have a perfect positive rank order relationship. If the original pairs had been $(X, Y) = (44, 2)$, $(34, 3)$, and $(26, 13)$, then the respective rank pairs would be $(3, 1)$, $(2, 2)$, and $(1, 3)$, a perfect reverse ordering of the Y ranks with the X ranks. This would be regarded as a negative rank order relationship between X and Y. Naturally, a sample of size 3 is too small to draw any general conclusions regarding the population rank order relationship.

The *Spearman rank correlation coefficient* is defined as follows:

$$r_S = \frac{\sum_{i=1}^{N}(R_i - \bar{R})(S_i - \bar{S})}{\sqrt{\sum_{i=1}^{N}(R_i - \bar{R})^2 \sum_{i=1}^{N}(S_i - \bar{S})^2}}, \qquad (8.28)$$

where for a random sample of size N, $(X_1, Y_1), \ldots, (X_N, Y_N)$ are from a bivariate population and R_i is the rank of X_i among $X_1, \ldots, X_N$, and S_i is the rank of Y_i among $Y_1, \ldots, Y_N$, $\bar{R} = \sum_{i=1}^{N} R_i / N$, and $\bar{S} = \sum_{i=1}^{N} S_i / N$. We see from notation (8.28) that r_S is indeed measuring the strength of the rank

Table 8.12. Behavior Ratings for 20 Hyperactive Children

Child	In School	At Home	R_i	S_i	$S_i - R_i$	$(S_i - R_1)^2$
1	89	88	20	18	-2	4
2	64	71	15	14	-1	1
3	46	54	7	10	$+3$	9
4	59	45	12	5	-7	49
5	72	76	16	15	-1	1
6	30	40	2	2	0	0
7	79	83	18	17	-1	1
8	60	53	13	9	-4	16
9	56	46	10	6	-4	16
10	88	92	19	20	$+1$	1
11	40	60	6	11	$+5$	25
12	36	44	4	4	0	0
13	34	39	3	1	-2	4
14	78	81	17	16	-1	1
15	54	61	9	12	$+3$	9
16	39	48	5	7	$+2$	4
17	58	90	11	19	$+8$	64
18	29	50	1	8	$+7$	49
19	48	43	8	3	-5	25
20	61	68	14	13	-1	1
			$\overline{210}$	$\overline{210}$		$\sum_{i=1}^{N} D_i^2 = 280$

order relationship. If we let $D_i = S_i - R_i$, then it can be shown that

$$r_S = 1 - \frac{6\sum_{i=1}^{N} D_i^2}{N^3 - N}. \tag{8.29}$$

As a brief illustrative example, suppose that data were gathered on 20 hyperactive youths receiving treatment. A behavior rating is developed for purposes of both in-school and at-home evaluation of each child. The rating scale ranges in both cases between 0 and 100, with 100 being saintly behavior. The question of interest is one of determining if there is an association between the behavior at the two places. The data are as in Table 8.12.

Thus, $\overline{R} = \frac{210}{20} = 10.5$, and $\overline{S} = \frac{210}{20} = 10.5$, that is, they are equal. In fact, in general $\overline{R} = \overline{S} = (N + 1)/2$. Using formula (8.29), one finds that $r_S = 1 - 6(280)/[(20)^3 - 20] = 0.7895$. This strongly suggests a positive rank order relationship between X and Y. In order to determine if the correlation differs significantly from zero, we introduce a test procedure based on the t distribution. The formula for this test statistic is

$$t = \frac{r_S\sqrt{N-2}}{\sqrt{1-r_S^2}}, \tag{8.30}$$

which has an approximate t distribution with $N-2$ degrees of freedom when the null hypothesis of no association is true (Conover, 1980).

In reference to the use of assumptions, the Spearman rank correlation procedure assumes that the pairs (X_i, Y_i), $i = 1, \ldots, N$, are a random sample from a population of (X, Y), where X and Y are at least ordinal in scale; these are the same assumptions that were made for using Kendall's tau. While Spearman's rank correlation coefficient is easier to compute than Kendall's tau, Kendall's tau is easier to interpret and approaches the normal distribution more quickly than Spearman's rank correlation coefficient under the null hypothesis of independence (Conover, 1980).

For the data of Table 8.12, we have from expression (8.30) $t = 0.7895\sqrt{20-2}/\sqrt{1-(0.7895)^2} = 5.46$, which yields $P < 0.0001$ when compared with the $t(18)$ distribution. Hence, there is strong evidence to support a positive rank order association between X and Y (behavior at school and at home).

8.4 PROCEDURES FOR INTERVAL OR RATIO SCALES

8.4.1 Pearson Product Moment Correlation Coefficient

Our final correlation coefficient is perhaps the most widely used, and it also is the one first introduced into the statistical literature. If the two variables X and Y have a joint normal (i.e., bivariate normal) distribution, then their joint probability distribution function is given by Figure 8.1. There is a parameter in the population that reflects the tendency for the X's and Y's to be close to a straight line. This parameter is the linear correlation coefficient and is denoted by ρ. It is a population measure of the strength of a linear relationship. For a random sample $(X_1, Y_1), \ldots, (X_N, Y_N)$ from this bivariate normal distribution, the usual estimator for ρ is r, where

$$r = \frac{\sum_{i=1}^{N}(X_i - \overline{X})(Y_i - \overline{Y})}{\sqrt{\sum_{i=1}^{N}(X_i - \overline{X})^2 \sum_{i=1}^{N}(Y_i - \overline{Y})^2}}. \tag{8.31}$$

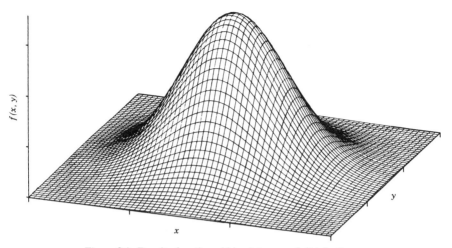

Figure 8.1. Density function of bivariate normal distribution.

This statistic, first introduced by Pearson (1900), is called the Pearson product moment correlation coefficient. If there is a perfect linear relationship between X and Y, that is, X and Y are always on a straight line, then $r = +1$ or $r = -1$ depending on whether the relationship is direct or inverse—if X and Y increase together or if an increase in X is associated with a decrease in Y, respectively. In estimator (8.31), $\overline{X}$ and $\overline{Y}$ are the usual sample means of X and Y. If $r = 0$ in (8.31), then there is no linear relationship. Figure 8.2 represents scatter plots (diagrams of the joint distribution of X and Y) for various sample correlation coefficients.

From the standpoint of statistical inference, if (X, Y) are bivariate normally distributed, then the quantity

$$t = r \frac{\sqrt{N - 2}}{\sqrt{1 - r^2}} \tag{8.32}$$

has a t distribution with $N - 2$ d.f. Thus, to test the hypothesis, for example, that $\rho = 0$, the statistic (8.32) may be computed and tested in the usual way for a one- or two-sided alternative.

The statistic (8.32) has a symmetric distribution only when the null hypothesis $\rho = 0$ is true. For other types of null hypotheses, the distribution is skewed, and a normal approximation to this distribution is not feasible.

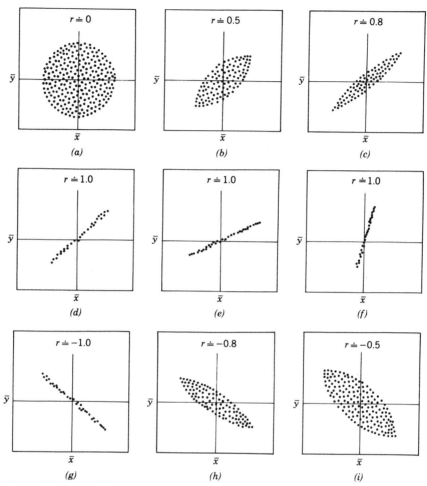

Figure 8.2. Scatter diagrams for different correlation coefficients: (a) $r \doteq 0$; (b) $r \doteq 0.5$; (c) $r \doteq 0.8$; (d–f) $r \doteq 1.0$; (g) $r \doteq -1.0$; (h) $r \doteq -0.8$; (i) $r \doteq -0.5$.

This problem can be solved using Fisher's Z transformation defined as

$$Q = \frac{1}{2}\log_e \frac{1 + r}{1 - r}.$$

The statistic Q has approximately the normal distribution with mean $(1/2)\log_e[(1 + \rho)/(1 - \rho)]$ and variance $1/(N - 3)$ when N is 20 or bigger. Thus, to test the null hypothesis H_0: $\rho = \rho_0 \neq 0$, the test statistic with an approximately standard normal distribution under H_0 is

$$Z = \left[\frac{1}{2}\log_e\frac{1+r}{1-r} - \frac{1}{2}\log_e\frac{1+\rho_0}{1-\rho_0}\right]\bigg/(1/\sqrt{N-3}) \qquad (8.33)$$

(Snedecor and Cochran, 1980).

Example 8.4.1.1. Twenty-five patients in an ophthalmologic clinic register the following values of intraocular pressure and age:

Subject	1	2	3	4	5	6	7	8	9	10	11	12	13	14
Age	35	40	41	44	45	48	50	50	50	52	54	55	55	55
IOP	15	17	16	18	15	19	19	18	17	16	19	18	21	20

Subject	15	16	17	18	19	20	21	22	23	24	25
Age	57	58	59	60	60	61	63	65	67	71	77
IOP	19	20	19	23	19	22	23	24	23	24	22

From expression (8.31), we have a Pearson correlation $r = +0.84482$. Now, as an example to test H_0: $\rho = \rho_0 = 0.75$, we have, from expression (8.33),

$$Z = \left[\frac{1}{2}\log_e\frac{1+0.84482}{1-0.84482} - \frac{1}{2}\log_e\frac{1+0.75}{1-0.75}\right]\bigg/(1/\sqrt{25-3}) = 1.242,$$

and from Table 4 of the Appendix, the corresponding one-tailed P value is 0.11, that is, there is no evidence to reject H_0.

It is evident by comparing (8.28) and (8.31) that the Spearman and Pearson correlation have a comparable form: the Spearman correlation is simply the Pearson correlation based upon the ranks of the data. The Spearman is appropriate for any ordinal or continuous data, while the Pearson is particularly appropriate for normally distributed data. Clearly, if there are a few extreme observations in the sample, the Spearman correlation will generally be less influenced by them.

8.4.2 Comparison of Two-Product-Moment Correlation Coefficients

When two independent estimators of the Pearson correlation are obtained, it may be of interest to know whether they are estimates of the same population coefficient ρ. Fisher's Z transformation defined in the above paragraph can be applied to each of the two sample correlation coefficients. Let r_1 be the sample correlation obtained with a sample of size n_1, and let

r_2 be the sample correlation from an independent sample of size n_2. Then $Q_1 = \frac{1}{2}\log_e[(1 + r_1)/(1 - r_1)]$ and $Q_2 = \frac{1}{2}\log_e[(1 + r_2)/(1 - r_2)]$ each have an approximate normal distribution, and thus under the null hypothesis, $Q_1 - Q_2$ has a normal distribution with zero mean and variance $1/(n_1 - 3) + 1/(n_2 - 3)$; hence, a standardized normal distribution can be used to test the proposed null hypothesis.

Example 8.4.2.1. A researcher observes two correlation coefficients in two independent samples. If $r_1 = 0.871$ with $n_1 = 70$ and $r_2 = 0.742$ with $n_2 = 55$, then the transformed values are

$$Q_1 = \frac{1}{2}\log_e\frac{1 + 0.871}{1 - 0.871} = 1.3372 \quad \text{and} \quad Q_2 = \frac{1}{2}\log_e\frac{1 + 0.742}{1 - 0.742} = 0.9549.$$

Then $Q_1 - Q_2 = 0.3823$, and the variance is $\frac{1}{67} + \frac{1}{52} = 0.034156$; the statistical test is $0.3823/\sqrt{0.034156} = 2.0685$, and according to Table 4 of the Appendix, the P value is 0.02, that is, there is evidence to reject the null hypothesis of equal population correlation coefficients.

8.5 SUMMARY

In the preceding sections, we have considered a rather broad set of procedures to measure the association between two random variables. In the next chapter, we treat a somewhat related problem of fitting statistical models to express one variable as a function of another.

Several statistical software packages can solve the procedures presented in this chapter. For example, in SAS, the procedure CORR will compute the Pearson product moment correlation, the Spearman rank order correlation, and Kendall's tau-b (Sall, 1985). These statistics are also computed in the program P4F of the BMDP statistical package (Dixon, 1983).

PROBLEMS

8.1. A prospective study was conducted in 894 diseased eyes with various types of retinal vein occlusion (RVO): venous stasis retinopathy (VSR), hemorrhagic retinopathy (HR), hemi-VSR, hemi-HR, major branch retinal vein occlusion (BRVO), and macular BRVO. The classification of these eyes with respect to the severity of the disease at first visit is presented in the following table. Test the hypothesis of no association between the variables by following the procedure in Table 8.2. Compute Cramer's V statistic.

Disease	Severity			
	Mild	Moderate	Marked	Totals
VSR	107	168	72	347
HR	10	35	63	108
Hemi-VSR	27	35	22	84
Hemi-HR	9	5	21	35
Major-BRVO	64	34	130	228
Macular BRVO	79	2	11	92
Totals	296	279	319	894

8.2. Determine if the classifications of disease and sex are independent by using the chi-square test on the following data for 828 patients.

Disease	Sex		
	Female	Male	Totals
VSR	133	187	320
HR	39	63	102
Hemi-VSR	42	35	77
Hemi = HR	11	22	33
Major BRVO	110	95	205
Macular BRVO	33	58	91
Totals	368	460	828

8.3. From a survey of the smoking habits of female patients, the following data are summarized:

		Smoker	Nonsmoker
Respiratory	Yes	198	12
Problems?	No	259	37

(a) Estimate the odds ratio.

(b) Obtain a 95% confidence interval for the logarithm of the population odds ratio.

(c) Obtain the 95% confidence interval for the population odds ratio.

8.4. In a large hospital, premature births and drinking behavior of the mother are recorded. For a given year the data are:

		Alcohol Consumption	
		Heavy	Light or none
Birth	Premature	12	97
	Normal	19	268

Answer the same questions as in Problem 8.3.

8.5. A cross-classification of the presence/absence of corneal scars for 400 study subjects was done by two ophthalmologists. The data are:

		Ophthalmologist 2	
		Absent	Present
Ophthalmologist 1	Absent	380	4
	Present	6	10

To study the strength of agreement between the two examining ophthalmologists,

(a) obtain an estimator for kappa,

(b) obtain an estimator of the standard error of kappa, and

(c) test the hypothesis of no agreement.

8.6. Given the following distribution of spouse pairs by years of education of husband and wife, from a cohort of 1698 spouse pairs, estimate and test for concordance among the pairs by using an appropriate statistic.

Husband's Education	Wife's Education			
	College Graduate	H.S. Graduate[a] Graduate	Less than H.S. Graduate	Totals
College graduate	296	478	14	788
H.S. graduate	108	604	60	772
Less than H.S. graduate	8	95	35	138
Totals	412	1177	109	1698

Source: L. Suarez and E. Barrett-Connor. (1984). Is an educated wife hazardous to your health? *Am. J. Epidemiol.*, **119**, 244–249.
[a] H.S. = high school.

8.7. An investigation of coding by seven nosologists of the deaths in hypertensive participants in a prospective epidemiologic study gives the following results after using the death certificates of 35 decedents:

	Category for Primary Cause of Death				
Decedent	Arteriosclerotic Disease	Cerebrovascular	Other Heart Disease	Renal Disease	Other
1	1	—	5	1	—
2	—	—	—	—	7
3	1	—	5	1	—
4	—	3	—	4	—
5	4	—	—	—	3
6	—	5	—	2	—
7	1	—	5	—	1
8	—	3	—	—	4
9	2	—	3	2	—
10	—	1	—	6	—
11	—	—	—	—	7
12	—	1	2	4	—
13	—	2	—	5	—
14	6	1	—	—	—
15	4	—	—	1	2
16	—	—	3	4	—
17	1	2	1	3	—
18	6	1	—	—	—
19	—	—	1	6	—
20	5	—	2	—	—
21	3	—	—	—	4
22	—	—	2	5	—
23	—	6	—	—	1
24	5	—	1	1	—
25	7	—	—	—	—
26	—	1	6	—	—
27	1	—	1	5	—
28	—	2	—	—	5
29	—	7	—	—	—
30	—	—	1	2	4
31	—	6	—	1	—
32	5	—	2	—	—
33	—	—	1	6	—
34	—	—	6	—	1
35	—	—	—	7	—

To study the level of agreement among the seven nosologists, compute

(a) the proportion of pairs agreeing on diagnoses for each person, $\hat{p}_i$;

(b) the proportion of overall agreement, $\bar{p}$;

(c) the expected chance agreement, $\bar{p}_e$;

(d) the generalized kappa statistic;

(e) the variance of the generalized kappa statistic, and

(f) a test statistic and draw conclusions.

8.8. (a) Compute the measures of order association τ_a, τ_b, and τ_d for the data in Example 8.4.1.1.

(b) Obtain 95% confidence intervals for the calculated Kendall's tau in part (a) and draw conclusions.

8.9. Using the Pearson product moment correlation coefficients in the table, test the corresponding null hypotheses then test the hypothesis of equal correlations.

r	n	H_0
0.37	190	$\rho = 0$
0.48	165	$\rho = 0.60$

8.10. Test if the following sample correlations from independent samples have the same population correlation:

Sample	r	n
I	0.76	19
II	0.61	20

REFERENCES

Bishop, Y. M. M., S. E. Fienberg, and P. W. Holland. (1975). *Discrete Multivariate Analysis: Theory and Practice*. MIT Press, Cambridge, MA.

Cohen, J. (1960). A coefficient of agreement for nominal scales, *Educ. Psychol. Meas.*, **20**, 37–46.

Conover, W. J. (1980). *Practical Nonparametric Statistics*, 2nd ed., Wiley, New York.

Cramer, H. (1946). *Mathematical Methods of Statistics*, Princeton University Press, Princeton, NJ.

Dixon, W. J. (1983). *BMDP Statistical Software*, University of Berkeley Press, Berkeley, CA.

Fleiss, J. L. (1971). Measuring nominal scale agreement among many raters, *Psychol. Bull.*, **76**, 378–382.

Fleiss, J. L. (1981). *Statistical Methods for Rates and Proportions*, 2nd ed., Wiley, New York.

Goodman, L. A. and W. H. Kruskal. (1954). Measures of association for cross-classifications, *JASA*, **49**, 723–764.

Kendall, M. G. (1938). A new measure of rank correlation, *Biometrika*, **30**, 81–93.

Kleinbaum, D. G. and L. L. Kupper. (1978). *Applied Regression Analysis and Other Multivariable Methods*, Duxbury North Scituate, MA.

Landis, J. R., and G. G. Koch. (1977). The measurement of observer agreement for categorical data, *Biometrics*, **33**, 159–174.

Pearson, K. (1900). On the criterion that a given system of deviations from the probable in the case of a correlated system of variables is such that it can reasonably be supposed to have arisen from random sampling, *Philosoph. Magazine*, **50**, 157–175.

Quade, D. (1971). Order Association. Class Lecture Notes, University of North Carolina.

Quade, D. (1986). Personal communication.

Sall, J. (1985). *SAS User's Guide*, SAS Institute, Cary, NC.

Snedecor, G. W. and W. G. Cochran. (1980). *Statistical Methods*, Iowa State University Press, Iowa.

Spearman, C. (1904). The proof and measurement of association between two things, *American Journal of Psychology*, **15**, 72–101.

CHAPTER 9

Least-Squares Regression Methods: Predicting One Variable from Another

9.1 INTRODUCTION

Most medical researchers involved in the study of pharmacological agents for therapeutic or other purposes are familiar with the problems of evaluating the relationship between dosage and response, that is, the relationship that expresses a particular response (e.g., degree of pain relief) as a mathematical function of the dose of the drug. One way of designing such investigations is to choose several doses of the drug and then select several experimental units to be studied at each dose. For instance, a study determining the effects of various doses of propranolol on the ethanol consumption of alcohol-habituated rats might randomly divide 15 rats into three groups of 5 each. The first group of 5 might receive 2.5 mg/kg, the second 5 mg/kg, while the third group might receive 10 mg/kg. To continue this hypothetical illustration, let us assume that the response variable is the number of milliliters of ethanol consumed per hour during the 10-hr time period following propranolol administration. The data from this study appear in Table 9.1.

The data from Table 9.1 are plotted in Figure 9.1 such that the ethanol consumption is a function of the common logarithm of the dose. From Figure 9.1, it appears that the mean ethanol consumption is increasing in a linear fashion with the $\log_{10}$ dose. It would seem that a reasonable *model* for the data is

$$\mu_{Y|X} = \beta_0 + \beta_1 X, \tag{9.1}$$

Table 9.1. Ethanol Consumption of 15 Rats Receiving Propranolol

Dose (mg/kg)	Log$_{10}$ Dose (mg/kg)	Ethanol (mL/h)
2.5	0.4	0.08, 0.12, 0.15, 0.20, 0.24,
5.0	0.7	0.28, 0.34, 0.36, 0.38, 0.46,
10.0	1.0	0.52, 0.56, 0.62, 0.65, 0.72

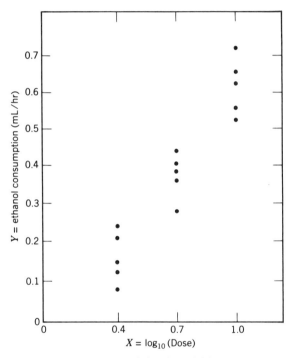

Figure 9.1. Plot of data from Table 9.1.

where $\mu_{Y|X}$ is the mean value of Y, the ethanol consumption, for a given value of X, the logarithm of the dose. The parameters, β_0 and β_1,—the Y intercept and slope, respectively—are unknown. If we are able to estimate them, we would have an estimated functional relationship between the mean of the random variable Y and the *independent* variable X. Model (9.1) is a statistical relationship rather than a pure mathematical relationship; this function relates a parameter for a random variable to another variable that can be either random or nonrandom. The situation of this hypothetical example is characteristic of the general class of practical problems where certain values of a nonrandom variable (X) are selected for study and a random variable (Y) is studied at each of these selected (X) values. An important aspect of this problem that differentiates it from the problems of the previous chapter is the fact that X is not a random variable, while it was a random variable in correlation problems. However, if X is random and one is interested in modeling Y given X, then the methods of this chapter still apply, but then it must be remembered that the analysis is a conditional analysis on X.

Expressions like (9.1), termed *regression* equations, give the relationship between the mean of a random variable (Y) and a given value of the variable X. The most general form of a regression equation is

$$\mu_{Y|X} = f(X), \tag{9.2}$$

that is, $\mu_{Y|X}$ is some function of X. Expression (9.1) recognized a particular model: the *linear regression* situation. The inference drawn from Equation (9.2) involves the estimation of unknown parameters and testing hypotheses regarding them. So, for example, in Equation (9.1), the main inference entails the estimation of β_0 and β_1 and testing hypotheses regarding them. For the most part, we shall restrict attention in this chapter to model (9.1), though many other regression models exist. Draper and Smith (1966) and Kleinbaum and Kupper (1978) provide a comprehensive treatment of various nonlinear regression problems.

The term *regression* was historically introduced by Francis Galton (1886). While studying the relationship between the heights of fathers and their sons, he noted that the mean height of sons of very tall men tended to be less extreme than their fathers' heights, and the mean height of sons of very short men tended to be less extreme than their fathers' heights. Galton termed this phenomenon *regression toward mediocrity*. The term *regression* remains to this day.

In the next section, we discuss a procedure for estimating β_0 and β_1 for model (9.1).

9.2 PRINCIPLE OF LEAST SQUARES

It is clear from Fig. 9.1 that no one straight line passes through all 15 points. In view of this, we seek the line that best "fits" the data of Figure 9.1. Therefore, it is necessary to specify the criteria used in determining the best fitting line. One criterion is the *least-squares principle*.

In advance of a definition, let us specify the assumptions regarding the data necessary to the operation of the principle. At this point, assume that there are N pairs of (X, Y), denoted $(X_1, Y_1), \ldots, (X_N, Y_N)$, and that the X's are fixed quantities while the Y's are random variables. Furthermore, we shall assume for the time being that the variance of each Y_i is the same regardless of the X_i value. This latter assumption instructs us to treat each Y_i equally in the statistical analysis; there are situations in which this assumption is not tenable (see Section 9.6). The final assumption is that the Equation (9.1) is the appropriate model for expressing the relationship between the mean of Y given X. To summarize, the three assumptions are as follows.

(a) The X's are measured without error. The X's are fixed or the analysis is viewed as conditional on the given observed values of X.

(b) The variance of Y at each X is $\sigma^2_{Y|X}$ and is the same for all values of X, that is, $\sigma^2_{Y|X} = \sigma^2$. $\hspace{2cm}$ (9.3)

(c) The mean of Y at each X is $\mu_{Y|X}$ and is given by the linear equation $\mu_{Y|X} = \beta_0 + \beta_1 X$.

By whatever method, estimates of β_0 and β_1 are computed, and the predicted mean of Y at X_i is given by

$$\hat{Y}_i = \hat{\beta}_0 + \hat{\beta}_1 X_i, \hspace{2cm} (9.4)$$

where $\hat{\beta}_0$ and $\hat{\beta}_1$ are the estimators of β_0 and β_1. The line $\hat{Y} = \hat{\beta}_0 + \hat{\beta}_1 X$ is called the estimated regression line or the *fitted regression line*. If $\hat{\beta}_0$ and $\hat{\beta}$ are "good" estimators of β_0 and β_1, then one would naturally expect Y_1 to be close to $\hat{Y}_1$, Y_2 to be close to $\hat{Y}_2$, and so forth. If they are not close, then one might wonder if the best estimators of β_0 and β_1 have been chosen. The *least-squares principle* means that the choice of the estimators β_0 and β_1 should decrease the sum of the squared distances between the Y_i's and the $\hat{Y}_i$'s to the smallest value possible for the entire set of data; that is, the least-squares principles states that $\hat{\beta}_0$ and $\hat{\beta}_1$ should be chosen so that

$$\sum_{i=1}^{N} \left[Y_i - \left(\hat{\beta}_0 + \hat{\beta}_1 X_i \right) \right]^2 \hspace{2cm} (9.5)$$

is a minimum. By applying differential calculus, the minimum of (9.5) yields the least-squares estimates of β_0 and β_1 to be

$$\hat{\beta}_1 = \frac{\sum_{i=1}^{N} \left(X_i - \overline{X} \right) \left(Y_i - \overline{Y} \right)}{\sum_{i=1}^{N} \left(X_i - \overline{X} \right)^2}, \hspace{2cm} (9.6a)$$

and

$$\hat{\beta}_0 = \overline{Y} - \hat{\beta}_1 \overline{X}, \tag{9.6b}$$

where $\overline{X} = \sum_{i=1}^{N} X_i/N$ and $\overline{Y} = \sum_{i=1}^{N} Y_i/N$. A simple computing formula for $\hat{\beta}_1$ is

$$\hat{\beta}_1 = \frac{\sum_{i=1}^{N} X_i Y_i - \left(\sum_{i=1}^{N} X_i\right)\left(\sum_{i=1}^{N} Y_i\right)/N}{\sum_{i=1}^{N} X_i^2 - \left(\sum_{i=1}^{N} X_i\right)^2/N}. \tag{9.7}$$

Hence, the estimator for the mean of Y at X_i is given by

$$\hat{Y}_i = \hat{\beta}_0 + \hat{\beta}_1 X_i, \tag{9.8}$$

where $\hat{\beta}_0$ and $\hat{\beta}_1$ are as in (9.6). An estimator for the variance Y at X is given by

$$\hat{\sigma}_{Y|X}^2 = \frac{\sum_{i=1}^{N}\left(Y_i - \hat{Y}_i\right)^2}{N-2}, \tag{9.9}$$

where $\hat{Y}_i$ is from (9.8). The divisor $N-2$ appears rather than $N-1$ in (9.9) since two parameter estimators, $\hat{\beta}_0$ and $\hat{\beta}_1$, determine $\hat{Y}_i$. To estimate the variances of $\hat{\beta}_0$ and $\hat{\beta}_1$, apply the following equations:

$$\hat{\sigma}_{\hat{\beta}_0}^2 = \hat{\sigma}_{Y|X}^2 \left[\frac{1}{N} + \frac{\overline{X}^2}{\sum_{i=1}^{N}\left(X_i - \overline{X}\right)^2}\right] \quad \text{and} \quad \hat{\sigma}_{\hat{\beta}_1}^2 = \hat{\sigma}_{Y|X}^2 \left[\frac{1}{\sum_{i=1}^{N}\left(X_i - \overline{X}\right)^2}\right], \tag{9.10}$$

respectively, where $\hat{\sigma}_{Y|X}^2$ is given by (9.9).

9.3   TESTING HYPOTHESES AND PLACING CONFIDENCE INTERVALS FOR NORMALLY DISTRIBUTED Y

The least squares estimation scheme from the previous section requires only the set of assumptions in (9.3) for its validity; thus, no assumption has yet been made regarding the distribution of Y. However, in order to test hypotheses and place confidence intervals, the additional assumption that Y has a normal distribution is required. The set of assumptions can be graphically portrayed such as occurs in Figure 9.2, where there is a normal distribution of Y's for each value of X. If this is the case, then the

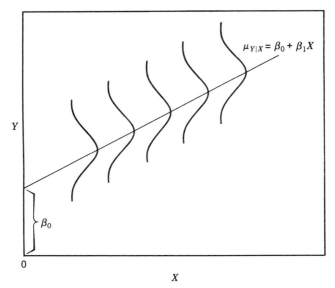

Figure 9.2. Graphical display of assumptions for normal theory linear regression problem.

following results are available:

$$\frac{\hat{\beta}_1 - \beta_1}{\hat{\sigma}_{\beta_1}} = t(N - 2), \qquad (9.11)$$

$$\frac{\hat{\beta}_0 - \beta_0}{\hat{\sigma}_{\beta_0}} = t(N - 2), \qquad (9.12)$$

that is, both (9.11) and (9.12) are distributed as a t variable with $N - 2$ degrees of freedom. As a consequence, $(1 - \alpha)100\%$ confidence intervals for β_0 and β_1 are

$$\hat{\beta}_0 \pm t_{1-\alpha/2}(N - 2)\hat{\sigma}_{\beta_0} \qquad (9.13)$$

and

$$\hat{\beta}_1 \pm t_{1-\alpha/2}(N - 2)\hat{\sigma}_{\beta_1}, \qquad (9.14)$$

respectively; $t_{1-\alpha/2}(N - 2)$ is found in Table 5 of the Appendix. In an analogous manner, a $(1 - \alpha)100\%$ confidence interval for $\mu_{Y|X}$ at $x = X_0$, a specific value, is given by

$$\left(\hat{\beta}_0 + \hat{\beta}_1 X_0\right) \pm t_{1-\alpha/2}(N - 2)\hat{\sigma}_{Y|X}\left[\frac{1}{N} + \frac{(X_0 - \overline{X})^2}{\Sigma_{i=1}^{N}(X_i - \overline{X})^2}\right]^{1/2}, \qquad (9.15)$$

since the estimated standard error of $\hat{\beta}_0 + \hat{\beta}_1 X_0$ may be shown to be

$$\hat{\sigma}_{Y|X} \left[\frac{1}{N} + \frac{(X_0 - \bar{X})^2}{\sum_{i=1}^{N}(X_i - \bar{X})^2} \right]^{1/2}. \tag{9.16}$$

Furthermore, in Equation (9.1), no regression relationship exists between Y and X if $\beta_1 = 0$. In Table 9.2 is a test procedure for the testing of the hypothesis that $\beta_1 = 0$.

Table 9.2. Outline of Procedure for Testing $\beta_1 = 0$ in Model (9.1)

A. Data: (X_i, Y_i), $i = 1, 2, \ldots, N$.
B. Assumptions:
   1. The X's are measured without error, and the X's are fixed or the analysis is viewed as conditional on the given observed values of X.
   2. The variance of Y at each X is $\sigma^2_{Y|X}$ and does not depend on X, i.e., $\sigma^2_{Y|X} = \sigma^2$.
   3. The mean of Y at X is denoted by $\mu_{Y|X}$ and is given by $\mu_{Y|X} = \beta_0 + \beta_1 X$.
   4. The distribution of Y at each X is a normal distribution.
C. Computations:

   1. $\hat{\beta}_1 = \dfrac{\sum_{i=1}^{N} X_i Y_i - \left(\sum_{i=1}^{N} X_i\right)\left(\sum_{i=1}^{N} Y_i\right)/N}{\sum_{i=1}^{N} X_i^2 - \left(\sum_{i=1}^{N} X_i\right)^2 / N}$,

   2. $\hat{\beta}_0 = \bar{Y} - \hat{\beta}_1 \bar{X}$,

   3. $\hat{\sigma}^2_{Y|X} = \dfrac{\sum_{i=1}^{N}(Y_i - \hat{Y}_i)^2}{N - 2}$,

   4. $\hat{\sigma}_{\hat{\beta}_1} = \hat{\sigma}_{Y|X} \left[\dfrac{1}{\sum_{i=1}^{N}(X_i - \bar{X})^2} \right]^{1/2}$, and

   5. $t = \hat{\beta}_1 / \hat{\sigma}_{\hat{\beta}_1}$.
D. Two-tailed statistical test:
   1. Null hypothesis: H_0: $\beta_1 = 0$
   2. Alternative hypothesis: H_a: $\beta_1 \neq 0$
   3. Decision rule for an α-level test: Reject H_0 in favor of H_a if $t > t_{1-\alpha/2}$ $(N - 2)$ or $t < -t_{1-\alpha/2}(N - 2)$.
   One-tailed statistical test:
   1. Null hypothesis: H_0: $\beta_1 = 0$
   2. Alternative hypothesis: H_a: $\beta_1 > 0$ $(\beta_1 <)$
   3. Decision rule for an α-level test: Reject H_0 in favor of H_a if $t > t_{1-\alpha}$ $(N - 2)$ $[t < -t_{1-\alpha}(N - 2)]$.

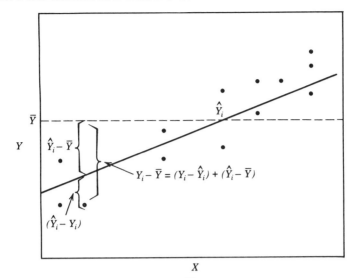

Figure 9.3. Partition of $Y_i - \bar{Y}$ into two component parts.

In Table 9.2, the values $t_{1-\alpha/2}(N-2)$ and $t_{1-\alpha}(N-2)$ are from Table 5 of the Appendix.

The statistical analysis for the linear regression problem also leads to an interesting partition of the sum of squares of the variable Y. We recall that the sum of squares for a variable is given by

$$\sum_{i=1}^{N}\left(Y_i - \bar{Y}\right)^2, \quad \text{where } \bar{Y} = \frac{\sum_{i=1}^{N}Y_i}{N}. \tag{9.17}$$

If the fitted regression line is given by $\hat{Y}_i = \hat{\beta}_0 + \hat{\beta}_1 X_i$, then each deviation in (9.17) may be written as

$$\left(Y_i - \bar{Y}\right) = \left(Y_i - \hat{Y}_i\right) + \left(\hat{Y}_i - \bar{Y}\right). \tag{9.18}$$

In this formula, the total deviation equals the deviation of the observation about the fitted line plus the deviation of the fitted line about the grand mean. Figure 9.3 illustrates this relationship. By squaring (9.18) and summing on i, the identity

$$\sum_{i=1}^{N}\left(Y_i - \bar{Y}\right)^2 = \sum_{i=1}^{N}\left(Y_i - \hat{Y}_i\right)^2 + \sum_{i=1}^{N}\left(\hat{Y}_i - \bar{Y}\right)^2 \tag{9.19}$$

Table 9.3. Analysis of Variance for Linear Regression Analysis[a]

Source	d.f.	SS	MS	F
Regression	1	$\text{SSR} = \sum_{i=1}^{N} (\hat{Y}_i - \bar{Y})^2$	$\text{MSR} = \text{SSR/d.f.}$	MSR/MSE
Error	$N - 2$	$\text{SSE} = \sum_{i=1}^{N} (Y_i - \hat{Y}_i)^2$	$\text{MSE} = \text{SSE/d.f.}$	
Total	$N - 1$	$\text{SST} = \sum_{i=1}^{N} (Y_i - \bar{Y})^2$		

[a]Abbreviations: d.f. is number of degrees of freedom; SS is sum of squares; MS is mean square, equal to SS/d.f.

can be derived; that is, the total sum of squares of Y involves the sum of two terms. The first term is the sum of squares due to the variability of the observations about the fitted line (sum of squares *error*) while the second term is the variability of the fitted line about the grand mean (sum of squares *due to regression*). As the left side of (9.19) has $N - 1$ d.f. while the term $\sum_{i=1}^{N}(Y_i - \hat{Y}_i)^2$ has $N - 2$ d.f., it follows that the term $\sum_{i=1}^{N}(\hat{Y}_i - \bar{Y})^2$ has 1 d.f. These relationships form the table of variability of Y, denoted ANOVA, for "analysis of variance," which is given in Table 9.3.

Computationally, the sums of squares in Table 9.3 are more easily determined via the formulas

$$\text{SST} = \sum_{i=1}^{N} \left(Y_i - \bar{Y} \right)^2 = \sum_{i=1}^{N} Y_i^2 - \frac{\left(\sum_{i=1}^{N} Y_i \right)^2}{N},$$

$$\text{SSR} = \sum_{i=1}^{N} \left(\hat{Y}_i - \bar{Y} \right)^2 = \hat{\beta}_1 \left[\sum_{i=1}^{N} X_i Y_i - \frac{\left(\sum_{i=1}^{N} X_i \right)\left(\sum_{i=1}^{N} Y_i \right)}{N} \right], \quad (9.20)$$

$$\text{SSE} = \text{SST} - \text{SSR}.$$

The quantity SSR is the amount of the total sum of squares accounted for by the linear regression.

A useful measure of the importance of the variable X is to consider the *coefficient of determination* R^2, where

$$R^2 = \text{SSR/SST}; \quad (9.21)$$

this figure ranges from 0 to 1 and is closer to 1 if X is a good linear predictor of Y. Thus, the coefficient of determination is the proportion of the Y variability accounted for by the regression analysis.

We note also that the analysis of variance table (Table 9.3) may be carried one additional step. The ratio of the two mean squares, MSR/MSE, has utility as another test statistic for the two-sided alternative hypothesis, H_a: $\beta_1 \neq 0$, of Table 9.2. Note that MSE is equal to $\hat{\sigma}^2_{Y|X}$, and thus MSE estimates $\sigma^2_{Y|X}$. Under H_0: $\beta_1 = 0$, MSR also estimates $\sigma^2_{Y|X}$, but under H_a: $\beta_1 \neq 0$, MSR estimates a quantity larger than $\sigma^2_{Y|X}$. Furthermore, it can be shown that the statistic MSR/MSE follows an F distribution with 1 and $N - 2$ degrees of freedom under H_0: $\beta_1 = 0$. Since under H_a: $\beta_1 \neq 0$, the ratio tends to be larger, then to test H_0: $\beta_1 = 0$ versus H_a: $\beta_1 \neq 0$, the statistic MSR/MSE is compared to $F_{1-\alpha}(1, N - 2)$. If MSR/MSE $>$ $F_{1-\alpha}(1, N - 2)$, where $F_{1-\alpha}(1, N - 2)$ is taken from Table 7 of the Appendix, then the null hypothesis is rejected in favor of H_a at the α level of significance. (Note that this test procedure is similar to the earlier discussion of the chi-square distribution, in which we noted that a one-tailed test arises for a two-sided alternative hypothesis.) It may be of interest to the reader that the ratio MSR/MSE is equal to t^2, where t is computed in Table 9.2. Hence, the two test procedures are, as they should be, equivalent.

Let us now return to the data of Table 9.1 pictured in Figure 9.1. The computations are:

$$\sum_{i=1}^{N} X_i = 0.40 + 0.40 + \cdots + 0.40 + 0.70 + \cdots$$

$$+ 0.70 + 1.00 + \cdots + 1.00 = 10.5,$$

$$\sum_{i=1}^{N} Y_i = 0.08 + 0.12 + \cdots + 0.65 + 0.72 = 5.68,$$

$$\sum_{i=1}^{N} X_i^2 = (0.4)^2 + \cdots + (0.4)^2 + (0.7)^2 + \cdots$$

$$+ (0.7)^2 + (1.0)^2 + \cdots + (1.0)^2 = 8.25,$$

$$\sum_{i=1}^{N} Y_i^2 = (0.08)^2 + (0.12)^2 + \cdots + (0.65)^2 + (0.72)^2 = 2.7298,$$

$$\sum_{i=1}^{N} X_i Y_i = (0.4)(0.08) + \cdots + (0.4)(0.24) + (0.7)(0.28) + \cdots$$

$$+ (0.7)(0.46) + 1(0.52) + \cdots + 1(0.72) = 4.66.$$

Hence, we have

$$\overline{X} = \frac{10.5}{15} = 0.7, \qquad \overline{Y} = \frac{5.68}{15} = 0.38,$$

$$\sum_{i=1}^{N} X_i^2 - \frac{\left(\sum_{i=1}^{N} X_i\right)^2}{N} = 8.25 - \frac{(10.5)^2}{15} = 0.9,$$

$$\text{SST} = \sum_{i=1}^{N} Y_i^2 - \frac{\left(\sum_{i=1}^{N} Y_i\right)^2}{N} = 2.7298 - \frac{(5.68)^2}{15} = 0.5790,$$

$$\sum_{i=1}^{N} X_i Y_i - \frac{\left(\sum_{i=1}^{N} X_i\right)\left(\sum_{i=1}^{N} Y_i\right)}{N} = 4.66 - \frac{(10.5)(5.68)}{15} = 0.684.$$

Therefore,

$$\hat{\beta}_1 = \frac{0.684}{0.9} = 0.76,$$

$$\hat{\beta}_0 = 0.38 - (0.76)(0.7) = -0.15, \tag{9.22}$$

$$\hat{Y}_i = -0.15 + 0.76 X_i.$$

The sum of squares due to regression is SSR = $(0.76)(0.684) = 0.5198$, and the SSE is SSE = $0.5790 - 0.5198 = 0.0592$. The analysis-of-variance table is therefore given by the following:

ANOVA

Source	df	SS	MS	F
Due to regression	1	0.5198	0.5198	113.00
Error	13	0.0592	0.0046	
Total	14	0.5790		

From Table 7 of the Appendix, we find that $F_{0.99}(1, 13) = 9.07$; thus, the F statistic is highly significant, and we conclude that $\beta_1 \neq 0$. As $t_{0.975}(13) = 2.16$, we find 95% confidence intervals for β_0 and β_1 quite directly. First, one notes that

$$\hat{\sigma}_{\beta_1} = \{0.0046\}^{1/2} \left(\frac{1}{0.9}\right)^{1/2} = 0.0715,$$

Table 9.4. Observed Values, Predicted Values, Residual and Standard Error Estimate of $\hat{Y}_i$*

i	X_i	Y_i	$\hat{Y}_i$	$(Y_i - \hat{Y}_i)$	$\hat{\sigma}_{Y\mid X}\left[\dfrac{1}{N} + \dfrac{(X_0 - \overline{X})^2}{\Sigma_{i=1}^{N}(X_i - \overline{X})^2}\right]^{1/2}$
1	0.4	0.08	0.15	−0.07	0.0277
2	0.4	0.12	0.15	−0.03	0.0277
3	0.4	0.15	0.15	0	0.0277
4	0.4	0.20	0.15	0.05	0.0277
5	0.4	0.24	0.15	+0.09	0.0277
6	0.7	0.28	0.38	−0.10	0.0175
7	0.7	0.34	0.38	−0.04	0.0175
8	0.7	0.36	0.38	−0.02	0.0175
9	0.7	0.38	0.38	0	0.0175
10	0.7	0.46	0.38	+0.08	0.0175
11	1.0	0.52	0.61	−0.09	0.0277
12	1.0	0.56	0.61	−0.05	0.0277
13	1.0	0.62	0.61	+0.01	0.0277
14	1.0	0.65	0.61	+0.04	0.0277
15	1.0	0.72	0.61	+0.11	0.0277

*$\hat{Y}_i = -0.15 + 0.76 X_i$; $\hat{\sigma}_{Y\mid X} = \{0.0046\}^{1/2}$; $\Sigma_{i=1}^{N}(X_i - \overline{X})^2 = 0.9$.

and

$$\hat{\sigma}_{\beta_0} = \{0.0046\}^{1/2}\left\{\frac{1}{15} + \frac{(0.7)^2}{0.9}\right\}^{1/2} = 0.0530.$$

Hence, 95% confidence intervals for β_1 and β_0 are, respectively, $(0.76) \pm (2.16)(0.0715) = (0.61, 0.91)$ and $-0.15 \pm (2.16)(0.0530) = (-0.26, -0.04)$.

These intervals are interpreted in the usual way. They may also be used for testing hypotheses. For example, since 0 is not in the 95% confidence interval for β_1, one concludes that the 5% level test for two-sided alternatives would conclude that $\beta_1 \neq 0$. In order to use the fitted regression Equation (9.22), let us evaluate the equation for each value of x in the ethanol consumption problem. Table 9.4 lists the predicted values, the observed values, their difference, and the estimated standard error (9.16) of $\hat{Y}_i$.

In Figure 9.4, the regression line $(\hat{Y})$ is plotted as a function of X. It is fairly clear that the line fits the data well. From the analysis-of-variance table, we readily compute $R^2 = 0.5198/0.5790 = 0.898$; that is, 89.8% of

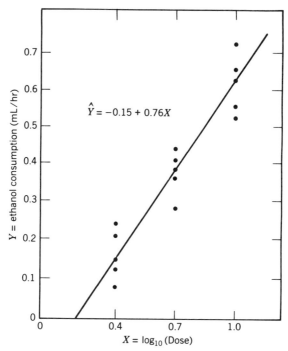

Figure 9.4. Plot of least-squares linear regression line for ethanol consumption data..

the total variability in Y is accounted for by X. This, of course, means that X is a fairly good predictor variable for Y for this data set. If N is small, however, the quantity R^2 may not be a particularly reliable indicator of the strength of the relationship in the population. Thus, R^2 should be considered a good estimator of the true proportion of the total variability explained only if N is rather large, say at least 20. Since $N = 15$ for this data set, the R^2 estimate should be interpreted with caution.

Another important issue that arises in analyzing data for a linear regression is the question of lack of fit of the linear regression model. In the next section this issue is discussed.

9.4 LACK OF FIT OF LINEAR REGRESSION MODEL

Earlier in this chapter it was mentioned that a full account of regression analysis is provided in the text of Draper and Smith (1966) or Kleinbaum and Kupper (1978). In this section, the problem of lack of fit of the linear regression model is presented, that is, a procedure for arriving at a yes or no decision regarding the hypothesis that the linear regression is an appropriate model for the data.

The proposed procedure is discussed for the data in Table 9.1. Recall that the regression model describes the mean value of Y as a function of X. In Table 9.1, for instance, there were several Y values for each X value, which makes it reasonable to compute the mean Y value for each distinct X value. The mean values of Y in our example are 0.158, 0.364, and 0.614; the X values ($\log_{10}$ dose) are 0.4, 0.7, and 1.0, respectively. At each X value, there exists a true random error. The "true" error sum of squares at the three distinct X values can be calculated in the following way.

X Value	"True" Error Sum of Squares
$X = 0.4$	$(0.08 - 0.158)^2 + (0.12 - 0.158)^2 + (0.15 - 0.158)^2$ $+ (0.2 - 0.158)^2 + (0.24 - 0.158)^2 = 0.01608$
$X = 0.7$	$(0.28 - 0.364)^2 + (0.34 - 0.364)^2 + (0.36 - 0.364)^2$ $+ (0.38 - 0.364)^2 + (0.46 - 0.364)^2 = 0.01712$
$X = 1.0$	$(0.52 - 0.614)^2 + (0.56 - 0.614)^2 + (0.62 - 0.614)^2$ $+ (0.65 - 0.614)^2 + (0.72 - 0.614)^2 = 0.02432$

The total "true" error sum of squares is thus given by $(0.01608) + (0.01712) + (0.02432) = 0.0575$, with 12 d.f. as each of the three groups contributes four degrees of freedom.

This sum of squares reflects the inherent random variability of each set of Y values about their mean. What remains on subtracting this sum of squares from the original error sum of squares is a lack-of-fit sum of squares. Essentially, this means the original sum of squares due to error has been partitioned into a pure-error sum of squares plus a lack-of-fit sum of squares. We may then consider a summary table for these data (Table 9.5).

The lack-of-fit mean square measures the deficit of the Y means in matching the fitted regression line; hence, it is a measure of nonlinearity.

Table 9.5. Analysis of Variance for Data of Table 9.1 with Lack-of-Fit Component

Source		d.f.		SS		MS	F
Due to regression		1			0.5198	0.5198	
Error $\{$ Lack of fit		13 $\{$	1	0.0592 $\{$	0.0017	0.0017	0.35
Pure error			12		0.0575	0.00479	
Total		14			0.5790		

Table 9.6. Procedure for Testing Fit of Linear Regression Model

A. Data:
1. There are k distinct values of X denoted $X_1, \ldots, X_k$.
2. At X_i there are $n_i (> 1)$ values of Y denoted $Y_{i1}, \ldots, Y_{in_i}$.

B. Assumptions:
1. The X_i are fixed and measured without error.
2. The mean of Y at X is $\mu_{Y|X} = \beta_0 + \beta_1 X$.
3. The variance of Y at X is $\sigma^2_{Y|X}$ and $\sigma^2_{Y|X} = \sigma^2$.
4. The distribution of Y is normal for each X.
5. $Y_{i1}, \ldots, Y_{in_i}$ is a random sample.

C. Computations:

1. $$\hat{\beta}_1 = \frac{\left[\sum_{i=1}^{k}\sum_{j=1}^{n_i} X_i Y_{ij} - \left(\sum_{i=1}^{k}\sum_{j=1}^{n_i} X_i \right)\left(\sum_{i=1}^{k}\sum_{j=1}^{n_i} Y_{ij} \right) / \sum_{i=1}^{k} n_i \right]}{\left[\sum_{i=1}^{k}\sum_{j=1}^{n_i} X_i^2 - \left(\sum_{i=1}^{k}\sum_{j=1}^{n_i} X_i \right)^2 / \sum_{i=1}^{k} n_i \right]}.$$

2. $$\text{SSR} = \hat{\beta}_1 \left[\sum_{i=1}^{k}\sum_{j=1}^{n_i} X_i Y_{ij} - \frac{\left(\sum_{i=1}^{k}\sum_{j=1}^{n_i} X_i \right)\left(\sum_{i=1}^{k}\sum_{j=1}^{n_i} Y_{ij} \right)}{\sum_{i=1}^{k} n_i} \right].$$

3. $$\text{SST} = \sum_{i=1}^{k}\sum_{j=1}^{n_i} Y_{ij}^2 - \frac{\left(\sum_{i=1}^{k}\sum_{j=1}^{n_i} Y_{ij} \right)^2}{\sum_{i=1}^{k} n_i}.$$

4. $\text{SSE} = \text{SST} - \text{SSR}$.

5. $$\text{SSPE} = \sum_{i=1}^{k}\sum_{j=1}^{n_i} Y_{ij}^2 - \sum_{i=1}^{k} \frac{\left(\sum_{j=1}^{n_i} Y_{ij} \right)^2}{n_i}.$$

6. $\text{SSLF} = \text{SSE} - \text{SSPE}$.

ANOVA

Source		d.f.	SS	MS	F
Due to regression		1	SSR		
Error	Lack of fit	$k - 2$	SSE $\begin{cases} \text{SSLF} \\ \text{SSPE} \end{cases}$	MSLF	MSLF/MSPE
	Pure error	$\sum_{i=1}^{k} (n_i - 1)$		MSPE	
Total		$\left(\sum_{i=1}^{k} n_i \right) - 1$	SST		

D. Test for lack of fit:
1. Null hypothesis: H_0: $\mu_{Y|X}$ is linear in X
2. Alternative hypothesis: H_a: $\mu_{Y|X}$ is nonlinear in X
3. Decision for an α-level test: Reject H_0 in favor of H_a if MSLF/MSPE $> F_{1-\alpha}(k - 2, \sum_{i=1}^{k}(n_i - 1))$.

294

To determine if the lack of fit is significant, compare the lack-of-fit mean square to the pure-error mean square. The ratio of these two mean squares follows an F distribution with 1 and 12 d.f. if the linear regression model is appropriate. Thus, large values of F indicate a lack of fit. For this example, the ratio is 0.35, while the critical value at the 0.05 level is $F_{0.95}(1, 12) = 4.75$; hence, there is no evidence for a lack of fit; that is, the linear regression model provides an adequate description of the data.

This procedure more generally follows the arrangement given in Table 9.6.

The critical value of F, $F_{1-\alpha}(k - 2, \Sigma_{i=1}^{k}(n_i - 1))$, is determined from Table 7 of the Appendix.

To test the goodness of fit of the linear relationship using the procedure in Table 9.6, it is necessary to have multiple Y values for at least one of the X_i values. Ideally, there should be replicates at each X_i.

Two additional comments about the test for the linearity of the model may be appropriate. First, this test does not intend to "prove" that the regression relationship is linear. It is only designed to decide whether the linear model provides an adequate description of the data—there could be other models that are also adequate. Second, it should be remembered that an association, such as a linear relationship, between two variables does not necessarily imply a causal relationship.

If the linear model is not adequate, then the data may be analyzed with polynomial or other nonlinear regression procedures. These procedures are not discussed in this text. The reader may refer to Kleinbaum and Kupper (1978) for a more complete presentation of these procedures.

Finally, if there are no Y replicates for any of the X's, then the only procedure to examine lack of fit or nonlinearity is to perform a regression analysis that includes linear and nonlinear X terms. Again, the reader may refer to Kleinbaum and Kupper (1978).

In the next section, we examine the linear regression problem for the case in which the Y's are to be related to several different X variables. Following this, we return to the simple linear regression problem in which the Y's may not have the same variances.

9.5   MULTIPLE LINEAR REGRESSION

Thus far we have been considering the model $\mu_{Y|X} = \beta_0 + \beta_1 X$; this is called the simple linear regression model because Y is regressed on only one independent variable X. However, we could also consider the model $\mu_{Y|X_1, X_2, \ldots, X_k} = \beta_0 + \beta_1 X_1 + \beta_2 X_2 + \cdots + \beta_k X_k$, where there are k independent variables. For example, for $k = 2$, we could have $Y =$ systolic blood pressure, X_1 = age, and X_2 = weight, and our model could be $\mu_{Y|X_1, X_2} = \beta_0 + \beta_1 X_1 + \beta_2 X_2$. Note that simple linear regression is the special case of multiple linear regression when $k = 1$.

There are several reasons for fitting a multiple linear regression model instead of a simple linear regression model:

1. The multiple regression model will often provide a significantly better prediction model since more factors (i.e., independent variables) are taken into account.

2. It is possible to determine if a variable is useful for predicting Y when other variables are included in the model. For example, in the model referred to above, where blood pressure was regressed on age and weight, we can determine if age is useful for predicting systolic blood pressure given that weight is also included in the model and thus, in effect, control for weight. Hence, multiple linear regression is an alternative to matching since variables can be controlled for by including them in the model and then testing if the independent variable of interest is still useful.

3. Several models can be fitted and the best model ('best' will depend on the criteria) can be chosen.

The general data layout for the multiple linear regression model is given in the following table:

Y	X_1	X_2	$\cdots$	X_k
Y_1	X_{11}	X_{21}	$\cdots$	X_{k1}
Y_2	X_{12}	X_{22}	$\cdots$	X_{k2}
Y_3	X_{13}	X_{23}	$\cdots$	X_{k3}
$\vdots$	$\vdots$	$\vdots$		$\vdots$
Y_N	X_{1N}	X_{2N}	$\cdots$	X_{kN}

Least-squares estimates $\hat{\beta}_0, \hat{\beta}_1, \ldots, \hat{\beta}_k$ will be such that $\sum_{i=1}^{N}(Y_i - \hat{Y}_i)^2$ is minimized, where $\hat{Y}_i = \hat{\beta}_0 + \hat{\beta}_1 X_{1i} + \cdots + \hat{\beta}_k X_{ki}$. The fitted regression model is then $\hat{Y} = \hat{\beta}_0 + \hat{\beta}_1 X_1 + \cdots + \hat{\beta}_k X_k$. (In the multiple linear regression situation with $k > 2$, the fitted model will be a k-dimensional hyperplane, while for the simple linear regression situation, the fitted model is a straight line.) Although formulas for computing these estimates will not be discussed, almost every regression computer program will automatically print them out. What is important to note is that the least-squares estimates, as in the simple linear case, minimize the sum of the squared deviations from the sample points to the fitted model.

Table 9.7. Analysis of Variance for Multiple Linear Regression Analysis

Source	d.f.[a]	SS	MS	F
Regression	k	$SSR = \sum_{i=1}^{N} (\hat{Y}_i - \overline{Y})^2$	$MSR = SSR/d.f.$	MSR/MSE
Error	$N - k - 1$	$SSE = \sum_{i=1}^{N} (Y_i - \hat{Y}_i)^2$	$MSE = SSE/d.f.$	
Total	$N - 1$	$SST = \sum_{i=1}^{N} (Y_i - \overline{Y})^2$		

[a] The term k is the number of independent variables.

The analysis of variance for the multiple linear regression model is given in Table 9.7. This table is similar to Table 9.3 except that the degrees of freedom depend on k, the number of independent variables.

The coefficient of multiple determination, denoted by R^2, is defined by $R^2 = SSR/SST$, analogous to the simple linear regression situation, and again is the proportion of the Y variability accounted for by the fitted model.

There are two sets of hypotheses of interest. If $\beta_1 = \beta_2 = \cdots = \beta_k = 0$, then none of the independent variables are useful for predicting Y; that is, the model as a whole is not useful. Thus, we are interested in testing H_0: $\beta_1 = \beta_2 = \cdots = \beta_k = 0$ (model not useful) against H_a: $\beta_j \neq 0$ for some $j = 1, 2, \ldots, k$ (model is useful). If the test of the model's usefulness is significant, then we would like to know if a particular variable, say X_j, is useful in the model; that is, if $\beta_j \neq 0$. Thus, we are interested in testing H_0: $\beta_j = 0$ (X_j is not useful in the model) versus H_a: $\beta_j \neq 0$ (X_j is useful in the model).

If it is assumed that the variance of Y for a given set of X values, $\sigma^2_{Y|X_1, X_2, \ldots, X_k}$, is constant and also that the Y_i's are normally distributed and independent, then the following results can be proved.

1. MSE estimates $\sigma^2_{Y|X_1, X_2, \ldots, X_k}$, that is, $MSE = \hat{\sigma}^2_{Y|X_1, X_2, \ldots, X_k}$; while MSR estimates $\sigma^2_{Y|X_1, \ldots, X_k}$ if $\beta_1 = \beta_2 = \cdots = \beta_k = 0$ and estimates a quantity larger than $\sigma^2_{Y|X_1, \ldots, X_k}$ if $\beta_j = 0$ for some $j = 1, 2, \ldots, k$. Also, the F ratio, $F = MRS/MSE$, has an $F(k, N - k - 1)$ distribution if $\beta_1 = \beta_2 = \cdots = \beta_k = 0$. Thus, to test H_0: $\beta_1 = \beta_2 = \cdots = \beta_k = 0$ versus H_a: $\beta_j \neq 0$ for some $j = 1, 2, \ldots, k$, the null hypothesis is rejected if $F = MSR/MSE > F_{1-\alpha}(k, N - k - 1)$.

2. For $j = 0, 1, \ldots, k$, $(\hat{\beta}_j - \beta_j)/\hat{\sigma}_{\hat{\beta}_j}$ has a $t(N - k - 1)$ distribution. Thus, to test H_0: $\beta_j = 0$ against H_a: $\beta_j \neq 0$, the null hypothesis is rejected if $t = \hat{\beta}_j/\hat{\sigma}_{\hat{\beta}_j} > t_{1-\alpha/2}(N - k - 1)$ or if $t < -t_{1-\alpha/2}$ $(N - k - 1)$. A $(1 - \alpha)100\%$ confidence interval for β_j is $\hat{\beta}_j \pm t_{1-\alpha/2}$ $(N - k - 1)\hat{\sigma}_{\hat{\beta}_j}$.

Example 9.5.1. A researcher is interested in studying the effect that age and weight have on systolic blood pressure. The data for a hypothetical sample of 30 subjects is given in Table 9.8.

Table 9.8. Age, Weight, and Systolic Blood Pressure in Hypothetical Sample

Age	Weight	Systolic Blood Pressure
14	94	97
12	95	100
16	104	100
13	107	106
11	108	119
21	116	111
17	117	106
15	117	117
17	122	111
20	124	126
21	125	115
17	125	118
23	125	124
12	128	126
16	128	116
15	129	131
19	134	125
24	134	125
24	136	128
12	137	130
23	137	138
23	138	131
20	139	129
13	141	127
18	141	131
18	143	126
19	150	142
24	171	165
25	172	157
22	172	163

Table 9.9. Regression Analysis, Systolic Blood Pressure Regressed on Age

		ANOVA			
Source	d.f.	SS	MS	F	P
Regression	1	2495.65	2495.65	12.32	0.0015
Error	28	5671.02	202.54		
Total	29	8166.67			

	Parameter Estimates			
Variable	Estimate	SE*	t	P
Intercept	85.22	11.53	7.39	.0001
Age	2.18	.62	3.51	.0015

*SE = standard errors of parameter estimates.

Table 9.10. Regression Analysis, Systolic Blood Pressure Regressed on Weight

		ANOVA			
Source	d.f.	SS	MS	F	P
Regression	1	7368.09	7368.09	258.3	0.0001
Error	28	798.58	28.52		
Total	29	8166.67			

	Parameter Estimates			
Variable	Estimate	SE*	t	P
Intercept	19.25	6.63	2.90	0.0071
Weight	0.809	0.050	16.18	0.0001

*SE = standard errors of parameter estimates.

The researcher fits three regression models: (1) blood pressure is regressed on age; (2) blood pressure is regressed on weight; and (3) blood pressure is regressed on age and weight. The analyses of variance and parameter estimates, as they might appear on a regression program, are shown in Tables 9.9–9.11.

Table 9.9 shows the results for blood pressure regressed on age. There is a significant linear relationship between age and blood pressure since the P value based upon either the F statistic or the t statistic is 0.0015. Similarly, from Table 9.10, which shows the results of blood pressure regressed on weight, we would conclude that there is a significant linear relationship between weight and blood pressure, since the P value for both the F-test and the t-test is 0.0001.

Table 9.11 shows the results for blood pressure regressed on age and weight. Since the P value for the F statistic is 0.0001, we would conclude

Table 9.11. Regression Analysis, Systolic Blood Pressure Regressed on Age
and Weight

| | | ANOVA | | | |
Source	d.f.	SS	MS	F	P
Regression	2	7370.28	3685.13	124.9	0.0001
Error	27	796.39	29.50		
Total	29	8166.67			
		Parameter Estimates			
Variable		Estimate	SE*	t	P
Intercept		19.353	6.755	2.865	0.0080
Age		−0.080	0.294	−0.272	0.7876
Weight		0.819	0.063	13.000	0.0001

*SE = standard errors of parameter estimates.

that the model is useful. Since the P value for the t statistic corresponding
to age is 0.7876, we would conclude that age is not useful in this model.
Similarly, we would conclude that weight is useful in this model since the P
value for its t statistic is 0.0001. Thus, although there is a linear relationship
between blood pressure and age and between blood pressure and weight, we
see that weight is the more important predictive variable since the model
with both weight and age is statistically no better than the model with just
weight.

If there are two or more insignificant t values when a multiple linear
regression model is fitted, this does not imply that all of the variables with
the insignificant t values are not useful as a group in the model. It only
means that each of these variables is not useful individually given that the
other variables are in the model. For instance, suppose a model with the
five independent variables $X_1, X_2, \ldots, X_5$ is fitted, and it turns out that
the t statistics for X_2 and X_5 are both insignificant. This means that X_2 is
not needed in the model given that X_1, X_3, X_4, and X_5 are in the model. It
also means that X_5 is not needed in the model given that X_1, X_2, X_3, and
X_4 are in the model. It does not mean that X_2 and X_5 are together not
useful in the model. The reader is referred to Kleinbaum and Kupper
(1978) for more discussion of this topic.

9.6 WEIGHTED LEAST SQUARES

For the data $(X_i, Y_1), \ldots, (X_N, Y_N)$, there may be reason to conclude that
the variance of Y_i depends on the X_i. In place of the assumptions in

expression (9.3), we assume the following new set of suppositions:

(a) The X_i's are fixed and measured without error.
(b) The variance of Y at X_i is

$$\sigma_{Y|X}^2 = 1/w_i. \tag{9.23}$$

(c) The mean of Y at X is

$$\mu_{Y|X} = \beta_0 + \beta_1 X_i.$$

In this situation, $\hat{\beta}_0$ and $\hat{\beta}_1$ are chosen such that

$$\sum_{i=1}^{n} \left[Y_i - \left(\hat{\beta}_0 + \hat{\beta}_1 X_i \right) \right]^2 w_i \tag{9.24}$$

is minimized. These are then called the *weighted* least-squares estimates of β_0 and β_1. The estimates on solving (9.24) are

$$\hat{\beta}_1 = \frac{\sum_{i=1}^{N} w_i \left(X_i - \overline{X} \right) \left(Y_i - \overline{Y} \right)}{\sum_{i=1}^{N} w_i \left(X_i - \overline{X} \right)^2}, \tag{9.25}$$

$$\hat{\beta}_0 = \overline{Y} - \hat{\beta}_1 \overline{X},$$

where

$$\overline{X} = \frac{\sum_{i=1}^{N} w_i X_i}{\sum_{i=1}^{N} w_i}, \qquad \overline{Y} = \frac{\sum_{i=1}^{N} w_i Y_i}{\sum_{i=1}^{N} w_i}.$$

The fitted regression is then $\hat{Y} = \hat{\beta}_0 + \hat{\beta}_1 X$.

Weighted least-squares estimation has many areas of potential application. One very useful application is related to categorical data problems involving rates. We discuss this problem in the next section.

9.7 LOGISTIC REGRESSION ANALYSIS OF RATES

The previous section introduced the weighted least-squares regression analysis. We expand and apply those results in this section to a rather practical problem involving rates. To fix ideas, let us consider the following illustra-

Table 9.12. Results of Treatment with a MAOI by Age of Patient

Age of Admission	Number Improved	Number Not Improved	Total
28–32	3	24	27
32–36	3	18	21
36–40	6	26	32
40–44	6	13	19
44–48	11	15	26
48–52	12	13	25
52–56	10	10	20
56–60	12	11	23
60–64	12	5	17

tion. In a clinical trial of several drugs used for the treatment of depression, it was of interest to study the treatment success rates as a function of the admission age of the patient. Treatment success was evaluated by comparing each patient with the pre- and posttreatment Hamilton (1960, 1967) rating scale for depression. After the standard treatment of six weeks with a monoamine oxidase inhibitor (MAOI), the data in Table 9.12 are obtained.

In this example, we suppose that it is of interest to express the improvement rates as a function of the admission age of the patient. Therefore, the age of admission properly constitutes the X variable, with values corresponding to the midpoints of the various age intervals. Hence, we have $X_1 = 30$, $X_2 = 34$, $X_3 = 38, \ldots, X_9 = 62$. Conversely, the dependent variable Y is the proportion of improved patients. Clearly, $Y_1 = \frac{3}{27} = 0.1111$, $Y_2 = \frac{3}{21} = 0.1429$, $Y_3 = 0.1875$, $Y_4 = 0.3158$, $Y_5 = 0.4231$, $Y_6 = 0.48$, $Y_7 = 0.50$, $Y_8 = 0.5217$, and $Y_9 = 0.7059$. Because the quantities Y_i are proportions, their variances may be determined from the binomial distribution. That is, we should assume that $n_{i.}Y_i$ has a binomial distribution with mean $p_i n_{i.}$ and variance $n_{i.}p_i(1 - p_i)$, where $n_{i.}$ is the total number of patients studied in age group i. If one models the mean p_i of Y_i as a linear function of X_i, it is necessary to place restrictions on the estimation and testing schemes to avoid the possibility of obtaining predicted values outside of the interval from 0 to 1. One model that ensures this is the *logistic model*. It states that the logarithm (base e) of the odds, $p_i/(1 - p_i)$, is a linear function of X_i, that is,

$$\log_e \frac{p_i}{1 - p_i} = \beta_0 + \beta_1 X_i \tag{9.26}$$

or that

$$p_i = \frac{e^{\alpha + \beta X_i}}{1 + e^{\alpha + \beta X_i}}. \tag{9.27}$$

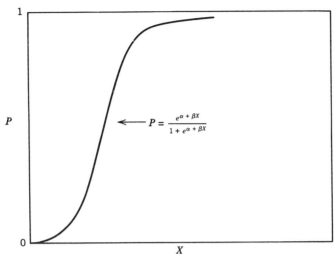

Figure 9.5. The logistic model (9.27).

Graphically, expression (9.27) is an S-shaped curve starting at 0 and approaching 1, as shown in Figure 9.5. Consider, for example, the data in Table 9.12 in the layout in Table 9.13. The "logit" of the ith sample proportion is

$$\log_e \frac{n_{i1}}{n_{i2}}. \tag{9.28}$$

The estimated variance of (9.28) is

$$\frac{1}{n_{i1}} + \frac{1}{n_{i2}}. \tag{9.29}$$

If we let $Y_i = \log_e(n_{i1}/n_{i2})$, then the weighted least-squares analysis applies directly to these data by setting the variance of Y at X_i [$1/w_i$ in

Table 9.13. Typical Data Layout for Regression Analysis of Rates

i	X_i	Number Improved	Number Not Improved	Total
1	X_1	n_{11}	n_{12}	$n_{1.}$
2	X_2	n_{21}	n_{22}	$n_{2.}$
3	X_3	n_{31}	n_{32}	$n_{3.}$
$\vdots$	$\vdots$	$\vdots$	$\vdots$	$\vdots$
k	X_k	n_{k1}	n_{k2}	$n_{k.}$

(9.23)] equal to $1/n_{i1} + 1/n_{i2}$; that is, $w_i = (1/n_{i1} + 1/n_{i2})^{-1}$. Strictly speaking, these weights are the estimated weights since the actual variances are estimated by (9.29), and the population variances are unknown. We shall use the estimated weights as if they were the true weights. For large samples, such a procedure is acceptable (Grizzle, Starmer, and Koch, 1969). Hence, the weighted least-squares estimates for β_0 and β_1 are, for the logistic regression model, given by the following:

$$\hat{\beta}_1 = \frac{\sum_{i=1}^{k}(1/n_{i1} + 1/n_{i2})^{-1}(X_i - \bar{X})(Y_i - \bar{Y})}{\sum_{i=1}^{k}(1/n_{i1} + 1/n_{i2})^{-1}(X_i - \bar{X})^2},$$

$$\hat{\beta}_0 = \bar{Y} - \hat{\beta}_1\bar{X}, \tag{9.30}$$

where

$$Y_i = \log_e\frac{n_{i1}}{n_{i1}},$$

$$\bar{X} = \frac{\sum_{i=1}^{k}(1/n_{i1} + 1/n_{i2})^{-1}X_i}{\sum_{i=1}^{k}(1/n_{i1} + 1/n_{i2})^{-1}},$$

$$\bar{Y} = \frac{\sum_{i=1}^{k}(1/n_{i1} + 1/n_{i2})^{-1}\log_e(n_{i1}/n_{i2})}{\sum_{i=1}^{k}(1/n_{i1} + 1/n_{i2})^{-1}}.$$

The variance of $\hat{\beta}_1$ is estimated by $\hat{\sigma}_{\beta_1}^2$, where

$$\hat{\sigma}_{\beta_1}^2 = \left[\sum_{i=1}^{k}\left(\frac{1}{n_{i1}} + \frac{1}{n_{i2}}\right)^{-1}(X_i - \bar{X})^2\right]^{-1}, \tag{9.31}$$

and that of $\hat{\beta}_0$ is estimated by $\hat{\sigma}_{\beta_0}^2$, where

$$\hat{\sigma}_{\beta_0}^2 = \left[\left(\sum_{i=1}^{k}\left(\frac{1}{n_{i1}} + \frac{1}{n_{i2}}\right)^{-1}\right)^{-1} + \frac{\bar{X}^2}{\sum_{i=1}^{k}(1/n_{i1} + 1/n_{i2})^{-1}(X_i - \bar{X})^2}\right]. \tag{9.32}$$

The quantity SSE is given by

$$SSE = \sum_{i=1}^{k}\left(\frac{1}{n_{i1}} + \frac{1}{n_{i2}}\right)^{-1}Y_i^2 - \bar{Y}^2\left[\sum_{i=1}^{k}\left(\frac{1}{n_{i1}} + \frac{1}{n_{i1}}\right)^{-1}\right]$$

$$- \hat{\beta}_1^2\left[\sum_{i=1}^{k}\left(\frac{1}{n_{i1}} + \frac{1}{n_{i2}}\right)^{-1}(X_i - \bar{X})^2\right]. \tag{9.33}$$

Table 9.14. Summary Computations for Linear Regression Analyses of Logistic Response for Data of Table 9.12

(1) i	(2) X_i	(3) n_{i1}	(4) n_{i2}	(5) $Y_i = \log_e(n_{i1}/n_{i2})$	(6) $(1/n_{i1} + 1/n_{i2})^{-1}$	(7) $(2)*(6)$	(8) $(5)*(6)$	(9) $(6)*X_i^2$	(10) $(6)*Y_i^2$
1	30	3	24	−2.0794	2.6667	80.0000	−5.5451	2400.0300	11.5306
2	34	3	18	−1.7918	2.5714	87.4276	−4.6074	2972.5384	8.2556
3	38	6	26	−1.4663	4.8750	185.2500	−7.1482	7039.5000	10.4814
4	42	6	13	−0.7732	4.1053	172.4226	−3.1742	7241.7492	2.4543
5	46	11	15	−0.3102	6.3462	291.9252	−1.9686	13428.5592	0.6107
6	50	12	13	−0.0800	6.2400	312.0000	−0.4992	15600.0000	0.0399
7	54	10	10	0.0000	5.0000	270.0000	0.0000	14580.0000	0.0000
8	58	12	11	0.0870	5.7391	332.8678	0.4993	19306.3324	0.0434
9	62	12	5	0.8755	3.5294	218.8228	3.0899	13567.0136	2.7053
Total					41.0731	1950.7160	−19.3535	96135.7228	36.1212

This quantity may be used to test the goodness of fit of the linear logistic model. The quantity SSE has a chi-square distribution with $k - 2$ degrees of freedom. If SSE is greater than $\chi^2_{1-\alpha}(k - 2)$, this indicates that the linear model for the logits [i.e., the linear model $Y_i = \beta_0 + \beta_1 X_i$, where $Y_i = \log_e(n_{i1}/n_{i2})$] does not fit well and that nonlinear models should be considered. In Table 9.14, we present the summary computations for the data in Table 9.12.

Essentially, all of the relevant summary statistics may be determined from the figures in Table 9.14. In particular, we find

$$X = \frac{1950.7160}{41.0731} = 47.49376, \qquad \overline{Y} = \frac{-19.3535}{41.0731} = -0.4712,$$

$$\sum_{i=1}^{k}\left(\frac{1}{n_{i1}} + \frac{1}{n_{i2}}\right)^{-1}(X_i - \overline{X})^2$$

$$= \sum_{i=1}^{k}\left(\frac{1}{n_{i1}} + \frac{1}{n_{i2}}\right)^{-1}X_i^2 - \frac{\left[\sum_{i=1}^{k}(1/n_{i1} + 1/n_{i2})^{-1}X_i\right]^2}{\sum_{i=1}^{k}(1/n_{i1} + 1/n_{i2})^{-1}}$$

$$= 96,135.7228 - \frac{(1950.7160)^2}{41.0731} = 3488.8831,$$

$$\sum_{i=1}^{k}\left(\frac{1}{n_{i1}} + \frac{1}{n_{i2}}\right)^{-1}(Y_i - \overline{Y})^2$$

$$= \sum_{i=1}^{k}\left(\frac{1}{n_{i1}} + \frac{1}{n_{i2}}\right)^{-1}Y_i^2 - \frac{\left[\sum_{i=1}^{k}(1/n_{i1} + 1/n_{i2})^{-1}Y_i\right]^2}{\sum_{i=1}^{k}(1/n_{i1} + 1/n_{i2})^{-1}}$$

$$= 36.1212 - \frac{(-19.3535)^2}{41.0731} = 27.0019,$$

$$\sum_{i=1}^{k}\left(\frac{1}{n_{i1}} + \frac{1}{n_{i2}}\right)^{-1}(X_i - \overline{X})(Y_i - \overline{Y})$$

$$= \sum_{i=1}^{k}\left(\frac{1}{n_{i1}} + \frac{1}{n_{i2}}\right)^{-1}X_iY_i$$

$$- \frac{\left[\sum_{i=1}^{k}(1/n_{i1} + 1/n_{i2})^{-1}X_i\right]\left[\sum_{i=1}^{k}(1/n_{i1} + 1/n_{i2})^{-1}Y_i\right]}{\sum_{i=1}^{k}(1/n_{i1} + 1/n_{i2})^{-1}}$$

$$= -622.9303 - \frac{(1950.7160)(-19.3535)}{41.0731} = 296.2402,$$

as $\sum_{i=1}^{k}(1/n_{i1} + 1/n_{i2})^{-1}X_iY_i = (80.00)(-2.0794) + \cdots + (218.8228)(0.8755) = -622.9303$. Hence, it follows from (9.30) and (9.31) that

$$\hat{\beta}_1 = \frac{296.2402}{3488.8831} = 0.0849,$$

$$\hat{\beta}_0 = -0.4712 - (0.0849)(47.4938) = -4.5035,$$

$$\hat{\sigma}_{\hat{\beta}_1}^2 = (3488.8831)^{-1} = 0.00029 \quad (\hat{\sigma}_{\hat{\beta}_1} = 0.01703),$$

$$\hat{\sigma}_{\hat{\beta}_0}^2 = (41.0731)^{-1} + (47.4938)^2(3488.8831)^{-1} = 0.6709 \quad (\hat{\sigma}_{\hat{\beta}_0} = 0.8191),$$

and

$$SSE = 27.0019 - (0.0849)^2(3488.8831) = 1.8540.$$

The regression is, therefore, given by $\hat{Y}_i = -4.5035 + 0.0849X_i$.

The logits are graphically plotted in Figure 9.6 as a function of X with the fitted regression line sketched in. To test the hypothesis that the linear

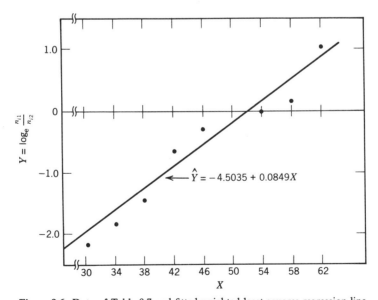

Figure 9.6. Data of Table 9.7 and fitted weighted least-squares regression line.

model for the logits is an adequate fit to the data, compare the statistic SSE to the chi-square distribution with $k - 2 = 7$ d.f. From Table 6 of the Appendix, we find $\chi^2_{0.95}(7) = 14.07$, while we computed SSE to be 1.8540; hence, at the 5% level of significance, we find no evidence of nonlinearity. Even being more liberal with the type I error rate, we note from Table 6 of the Appendix that $\chi^2_{0.90}(7) = 12.02$ and $\chi^2_{0.75}(7) = 9.04$. Hence, even at the very high level of 25%, we find no evidence of a nonlinear relationship as $1.8540 < 9.04$.

Having convinced ourselves that there is no need to explore nonlinear relationships, the next question is to decide if the coefficient $\hat{\beta}_1$ is significantly different from zero. This is decided by constructing the ratio $\hat{\beta}_1/\hat{\sigma}_{\hat{\beta}_1}$ and comparing it to the standard normal distribution. As $\hat{\beta}_1/\hat{\sigma}_{\hat{\beta}_1} = 0.0849/0.017 = 4.994$, and $Z_{0.975} = 1.96$, we would conclude, at the 5% level of significance, that the slope differs from zero; that is, there is a significant linear relationship between the logit and the admission age. A $(1 - \alpha)100\%$ confidence interval for β_1 is

$$\hat{\beta}_1 \pm Z_{1-\alpha/2}\hat{\sigma}_{\hat{\beta}_1}, \tag{9.34}$$

where $Z_{1-\alpha/2}$ is found in Table 4 of the Appendix. In addition, a $(1 - \alpha)100\%$ confidence interval for the mean logit of p at a particular value of X, say, $X = X_0$, may also be determined. This $(1 - \alpha)100\%$ confidence interval is given by

$$\left(\hat{\beta}_0 + \hat{\beta}_1 X_0\right) \pm Z_{1-\alpha/2}\hat{\sigma}_{(\hat{\beta}_0 + \hat{\beta}_1 X_0)}, \tag{9.35}$$

where $Z_{1-\alpha/2}$ is from Table 4 of the Appendix, $\hat{\beta}_0$ and $\hat{\beta}_1$ are given by (9.30), and $\hat{\sigma}_{(\hat{\beta}_0 + \hat{\beta}_1 X_0)}$ is the estimated standard deviation of the predicted logit at X_0. In particular, we have

$$\hat{\sigma}_{(\hat{\beta}_0 + \hat{\beta}_1 X_0)}$$

$$= \left\{ \frac{1}{\left[\sum_{i=1}^{k}(1/n_{i1} + 1/n_{i1})^{-1}\right]} + \frac{\left(X_0 - \bar{X}\right)^2}{\sum_{i=1}^{k}(1/n_{i1} + 1/n_{i2})^{-1}\left(X_i - \bar{X}\right)^2} \right\}^{1/2} .$$

$$\tag{9.36}$$

The confidence interval (9.35), for $\log[p/(1 - p)]$ at $X = X_0$, may be inverted into one for p itself by the relationship (9.27). Specifically, if the

Table 9.15. Predicted Logits and Proportions for Data of Table 9.12[a]

					95% Confidence Interval[b]			
					For Logit		For p	
					Lower	Upper	Lower	Upper
i	X_i	Y_i	$\hat{Y}_i$	$\hat{p}_i$	$\hat{\sigma}_{\hat{Y}_i}$	Limit	Limit	Limit	Limit
1	30	-2.0794	-1.9565	0.1238	0.3348	-2.6127	-1.3003	0.0683	0.2141
2	34	-1.7918	-1.6169	0.1656	0.2767	-2.1592	-1.0746	0.1035	0.2545
3	38	-1.4663	-1.2773	0.2180	0.2240	-1.7163	-0.8383	0.1523	0.3019
4	42	-0.7732	-0.9377	0.2814	0.1816	-1.2936	-0.5818	0.2152	0.3586
5	46	-0.3102	-0.5981	0.3548	0.1580	-0.9078	-0.2884	0.2874	0.4284
6	50	-0.0800	-0.2585	0.4357	0.1617	-0.5754	$+0.0584$	0.3599	0.5146
7	54	0.0000	0.0811	0.5203	0.1909	-0.2931	$+0.4553$	0.4272	0.6119
8	58	0.0870	0.4207	0.6037	0.2366	-0.0430	$+0.8844$	0.4892	0.7077
9	62	0.8755	0.7603	0.6814	0.2909	$+0.1901$	$+1.3305$	0.5474	0.7909

[a] $\hat{Y}_i = -4.5035 + 0.0849 X_i$; $\hat{p}_i$ is expression (9.38), $\hat{\sigma}_{\hat{Y}_i}$ is expression (9.36).
[b] Using Equation (9.37).

confidence interval at (9.35) is denoted by $(l_{\text{lower}}, l_{\text{upper}})$, then the corresponding interval for the proportion at $X = X_0$ is

$$\left(\frac{e^{l_{\text{lower}}}}{1 + e^{l_{\text{lower}}}}, \frac{e^{l_{\text{upper}}}}{1 + e^{l_{\text{upper}}}} \right). \qquad (9.37)$$

Clearly, the point estimate of p at X_0 is similarly given by

$$\hat{p} = \frac{e^{\hat{\beta}_0 + \hat{\beta}_1 X_0}}{1 + e^{\hat{\beta}_0 + \hat{\beta}_1 X_0}}. \qquad (9.38)$$

For the data of Table 9.12, we compute the predicted logits, the corresponding proportion, and the standard error of the predicted logit in Table 9.15.

The table points out that the standard error of Y_i is larger at the extremes of X's than in the middle of the X values.

An additional comment on this type of analysis is also in order. If an occasional n_{ij} in Table 9.13 is zero, then the weights are undefined. In this situation, the user may replace the zero n_{ij} by $\frac{1}{2}$ and follow the analysis procedure as usual. This suggestion is based on the comments of Grizzle et al. (1969, p. 491).

With reference to the entire statistical analysis, whose basis is the logistic regression model, the procedure should be undertaken only if the sample sizes are all fairly large and most of the sample proportions are not close to 0 or 1. Forthofer and Lehnen (1981) recommend that the preceding weighted least-squares analyses not be done if any of the expected counts in the table are less than 5. This guideline may be somewhat conservative. In general, if the expected proportions range from 0.2 to 0.8, the preceding would produce reliable results.

The reader should also be aware that procedures do exist for the estimation of the logistic parameters using iterative techniques. The most common iterative procedures are those arising from maximum-likelihood estimation. These procedures are not dependent on all $n_{ij} > 0$; however, iteration is required to solve the resulting estimation equations. The text of Bishop, Fienberg, and Holland (1975) discusses these alternative methods of analyses for this class of inference problems.

9.8 SUMMARY

This chapter has discussed various procedures for fitting regression models. We have based the discussion almost entirely on the principle of least squares. This class of procedures, while generally applicable to biological data, may not be appropriate if there are extreme observations. In this situation, various nonparametric regression schemes should be considered. The text of Hollander and Wolfe (1973) discusses various alternatives for these problems.

There are other possible models for the multiple regression problem. One model is the polynomial regression model. A second-order polynomial to relate, for example, systolic blood pressure (Y) to age (X) can be expressed as $\mu_{Y|X, X^2} = \beta_0 + \beta_1 X + \beta_2 X^2$. This model is the simplest linear model beyond the straight-line regression model. The interested reader can consult Kleinbaum and Kupper (1978).

Weighted least squares and logistic regression analysis can both be extended to include the situation of more than one independent variable. The interested reader can refer to Forthofer and Lehnen (1981).

There are several computational procedures to perform the regression analyses of this chapter. SAS has the REG procedure for many regression models, and for logistic regression the procedure is LOGIST. This latter program appears in SUGI Supplemental Library (Sall, 1982, 1983). BMDP [Dixon (1983)] has a special chapter that covers many types of regression models. The program P1R can be used for the regression models of this chapter. For logistic regression, the specific program is PLR.

PROBLEMS

9.1. To establish if the increase in ammonia concentration in blood is constant during storage at 4°C, samples of blood were stored varying lengths of time and the ammonia concentration determined. Data giving the ammonia concentration for whole-blood samples stored various lengths of time are presented in the following table.

Days Storage	Whole Blood (NH_3-N μg/100 mL)	Days Storage	Whole Blood (NH_3-N μg/100 mL)
0	128	5	214
1	167	20	685
3	244	21	770
4	185	21	930
5	194	21	620

Source: P. W. Spear, M. Sass, and J. J. Cincotti. (1956). Ammonia levels in transfused blood, *J. Lab. Clin. Med.*, **48**, 702–707.

The determination of the NH_3 concentration of the blood on 0 day was made from 1 to 2 hr after shedding but may, for ease in analysis, be assumed to be made at time 0 day.

Graph the data, and by inspection, determine if the relationship between NH_3 concentration and time can be approximated by a straight line. What are the least-squares estimates of the intercept and slope? Is there sufficient evidence to conclude that the ammonia concentration does increase during storage? What is the estimate of the rate of increase of ammonia concentration and its 95% confidence interval?

The ammonia level in freshly drawn blood has been found to be near zero and hence suggests that the level in circulating blood may be zero. Does this result and suggestion fit with the fitted straight line? How do you explain this discordance? Does it limit the use of the fitted line?

9.2. The systolic blood pressure (SBP) in 36 women in the age interval 20–82 years is given below:

Age	30	25	55	47	27	21	30	27	31
SBP	105	110	112	116	117	119	120	112	122
Age	34	35	47	20	52	55	48	52	47
SBP	123	125	122	119	129	132	134	136	140
Age	40	48	60	38	54	59	63	60	62
SBP	142	142	143	145	145	151	159	160	163
Age	63	45	38	72	67	81	44	82	60
SBP	168	160	170	170	171	171	172	205	180

Produce a scatter diagram for this data, and determine if a straight-line regression model of SBP (Y) on Age (X) is reasonable. Obtain

(a) the least-squares estimators of β_0 and β_1;

(b) the estimator of the variance of Y at X, $\sigma_{Y|X}^2$;

(c) the estimators of the variances of $\hat{\beta}_0$ and $\hat{\beta}_1$;

(d) confidence intervals for β_0 and β_1;

(e) confidence interval for the mean of Y at $X = 24$ years;

(f) the ANOVA table and R^2, the coefficient of determination; and

(g) conclusions from the above analysis.

9.3. Obtain the ANOVA table for the linear regression of the weight on age for the 17 children below. Check if the straight-line model is adequate.

Age (months)	.2	.2	.2	1.5	1.5	1.5
Weight (kg)	3.0	2.5	2.7	4.7	4.7	5.2
Age (months)	6	6	12	12	15	24
Weight (kg)	7.7	8.0	9	8.6	10.1	12
Age (months)	36	48	48	60	60	
Weight (kg)	14.1	15.2	15.1	18	17	

9.4. The observed physiologic response Y to a drug dose X is observed in six rats. The data are:

X	2.6	3.1	4.2	6.5	8.0	9.3
Y	1.2	2.3	3.4	4.1	3.0	1.8

(a) Draw a scatter diagram for this data.

(b) Obtain the least-squares estimators of β_0 and β_1.

(c) Obtain the coefficient of determination R^2.

(d) Test the null hypothesis $H_0: \beta_1 = 0$.

(e) Draw conclusions from the above analysis.

9.5. The following table presents the prevalence of retinopathy in diabetic patients according to the duration of diabetes, for each sex:

Duration (yr)	Females Midpoint	With Retinopathy	Total
0–1	0.5	4	25 (16%)
1–3	2	15	50 (30%)
4–6	5	14	40 (35%)
7–9	8	22	55 (40%)
10–12	11	18	36 (50%)

Duration (yr)	Males Midpoint	With Retinopathy	Total
0–1	0.5	8	50 (16%)
1–3	2	9	36 (25%)
4–6	5	26	65 (40%)
7–9	8	15	28 (55%)
10–12	11	13	19 (70%)

Use the logistic regression model to analyze this data for each sex. Use the midpoints for the values of the independent variable. What conclusion would you draw from these analyses?

REFERENCES

Bishop, Y. M. M., S. E. Fienberg, and P. W. Holland. (1975). *Discrete Multivariate Analysis: Theory and Practice*, MIT Press, Cambridge, MA.

Dixon, W. J. (1983). *BMDP Statistical Software*, University of California Press, Berkeley, CA.

Draper, N., and H. Smith. (1966). *Applied Regression Analysis*, Wiley, New York.

Forthofer, R. N., and R. G. Lehnen. (1981). *Public Program Analysis*, Lifetime Learning Publications, CA.

Galton, Francis (1886). Family likeness in stature, *Proceedings of Royal Society of London*, **40**, 42–63.

Grizzle, J. E., C. F. Starmer, and G. G. Koch. (1969). Analysis of categorical data for linear models, *Biometrics*, **25**, 489–504.

Hamilton, M. (1960). A rating scale for depression. *Journal of Neurology, Neurosurgery and Psychiatry*. **23**, 56–62.

Hamilton, M. (1967). Development of a rating scale for primary depressive illness. *British Journal of Social and Clinical Psychology*. **6**: 278–296.

Hollander, M., and D. A. Wolfe. (1973). *Nonparametric Statistical Methods*, Wiley, New York.

Kleinbaum, D. G., and L. L. Kupper. (1978). *Applied Regression Analysis and Other Multivariate Methods*, Duxbury, MA.

Sall, J. P. (1982). *SAS User's Guide: Statistics*, SAS Institute, Cary, NC.

Sall, J. P. (1983). *SUGI Supplemental Library, User's Guide*, SAS Institute, Cary, NC.

CHAPTER 10

Comparing More Than Two Groups of Observations: Analysis of Variance for Comparing Groups

10.1 INTRODUCTION

In Chapter 6, we introduce a variety of statistical procedures for comparing two groups of individuals. Essentially, the methods in that chapter were of two distinct types: statistical methods for normally distributed data and methods for general ratio–interval scale data. These procedures were termed *t*-tests and rank tests; the latter tests used rank-ordered relationships among the observations, while the former used the actual numerical values. In this chapter, *t*-test procedures are generalized for comparing more than two groups. The general situation in which this procedure applies is when there are *g* distinct groups with a sample of observations for each. For example, in a clinical trial of various pharmacological treatments for nonpsychotic depression (Young et al., 1979), five treatments ($g = 5$) were compared. They were as follows: (1) trimipramine plus placebo; (2) phenelzine plus placebo; (3) isocarboxazid; (4) phenelzine plus trimipramine; and (5) isocarboxazid plus trimipramine. The 135 patients in their sample were assigned randomly into the five treatment groups with the result that 25, 25, 34, 26, and 25 patients were assigned to treatment 1, 2, 3, 4, and 5, respectively. They rated each patient for severity of depression using a six-point scale at the end of the treatment period of six weeks. One goal in this study was to compare the five treatment groups with respect to the six-week depression scores. Of primary interest was whether an overall difference existed between the treatment groups with respect to the depres-

314

sion score at six weeks. Specifically, it was advantageous to discover which particular pairs of treatments were different with respect to their depression scores. Clearly, in addition to these questions of determining if the treatment groups were different in response, there was also the question of estimating the magnitude of the differences. Thus, similar to Chapter 6, there are questions of testing hypotheses as well as estimating the magnitude of the differences.

In this example, the fact that randomization was used to assign patients to treatment groups introduces the important element of unbiasedness in the comparability of the five treatment groups. Any differences between treatment groups with respect to the depression scores are not likely to be a reflection of a treatment assignment bias because neither patients nor doctors controlled the assignment of individuals to a treatment group. In contrast, in observational studies, the absence of randomization in the study design admits to the possibility of a bias, even though statistical comparisons may still be made between the treatment groups. For example, in a population survey to study differences between occupational groups with respect to the levels of daily alcohol consumption, the persons are self-selected or otherwise selected nonrandomly into the occupational groups. Because randomization was not used, statistical differences in alcohol consumption between these groups may be a consequence of their occupation, a consequence of heavy drinkers preferentially entering certain occupational groups, both, or neither.

The explanation for the differences could be better clarified through the use of *poststratification*. Poststratification is simply the process of dividing the sample (after the data have been collected) into various groups according to different influences on the response variable and the classification variable. In this example, people could be grouped into their preemployment drinking habits. Then comparisons would be made between the occupational groups within each stratum.

In any event, the problem of comparing a multiple number of groups may arise in experimental or nonexperimental studies. The methods discussed in this chapter, like those of the other chapters, may be applied to both types of studies. The interpretation of the results may generally be expected to be more difficult for nonexperimental studies, however.

As we may recall, two basic statistical designs were presented in Chapter 6. One was an independent sample design while the other was a matched-pair design. Essentially these two designs differ on the basis of their stratification. For two independent samples, there is no stratification, the only classification variable being the group membership variable. For matched-pair designs, people are classified not only on the basis of the treatment group membership but also on the basis of their pair membership. In such designs, people are first classified into matched pairs; in each pair, one member belongs (or will belong) to group A and the other member to group B. Within pairs, people differ only with regard to the group membership of interest, but people from different pairs differ with respect to matching or pairing characteristics as well. The goal of this design is to remove the variability due to the matching variable from the analysis. In this way, the amount of variation in the remaining data is smaller than it would otherwise be, thus permitting a better opportunity to look at the group difference of interest. To see this point more clearly, let us consider the following example.

Example 10.1.1. A group of 16 depressed patients were entered into a clinical trial of two different treatment regimens on a particular tricyclic antidepressant. For convenience, the treatment regimens were denoted by group 1 and group 2. Immediately prior to commencement of treatment and five weeks posttreatment, each person was evaluated blindly by a psychiatrist using a rating scale for depression. The data for statistical analysis was each person's posttreatment minus pretreatment depression score. As the persons chosen for the study varied with respect to their age, sex, and length of illness, a matched-pair design was used for the study. After creating eight matched pairs, one person in each pair was selected at random to receive treatment regimen 1; the other received regimen 2. The data are as follows:

	Depression Score		
Pair Number	Group 1	Group 2	Difference
1	-38	-30	-8
2	2	4	-2
3	-14	0	-14
4	-40	-42	2
5	-8	$+10$	-18
6	-20	$+2$	-22
7	-8	-8	0
8	20	42	-22

Is there evidence of a difference in treatment efficacy on the basis of these data?

In order to solve this problem, the procedure of Table 6.2 may be applied directly, assuming normality. Following Table 6.2, we obtain the pairwise differences of -8, -2, -14, 2, -18, -22, 0, and -22 for pairs 1–8. In the notation of Table 6.2, we find $\bar{d} = -10.5$, $s_{\bar{d}} = 3.48$, and a seven-degrees-of-freedom paired t statistic of -3.017 ($p < 0.05$). Of particular note is the result that the estimated standard error for the mean difference is 3.48. This number is a reflection of the amount of chance or uncontrolled variation that must be used as a benchmark in assessing the sample mean difference. In order to assess the effect that pairing had on this analysis, let us suppose the 16 patients were not paired but were assigned completely at random to the two groups, the only restriction being that we have 8 patients per group. Strictly speaking, we should not perform a two-sample t-test on the data, of Example 10.1.1, as the samples are not independent. However, for purposes of illustrating the effect that pairing has apparently made, let us ignore the pairing and treat the data as if there were two independent samples. If we do this, then we note from the data that the difference in sample means is again -10.5, since the group 1 mean is -13.25, while the group 2 mean is -2.75. On the other hand, following the two-sample t procedure in Table 6.5, the estimated standard error of the difference in sample means is $s_{\bar{y}_1 - \bar{y}_2} = 11.44$ with a 14-degrees-of-freedom t statistic of -0.92.

This example clearly illustrates the effect that pairing can have on a problem. The variability that is unaccounted for is 11.44 if the data were from an unpaired design, while it is 3.48 for the paired design. We must emphasize that in practice it is not valid to do a two-sample t-test on paired data; we do it here only to illustrate a point. We are creating a hypothetical situation by saying that we assume that the data values would be the same as in Example 10.1.1 if the data were unpaired. Another interesting feature of this analysis is to notice the effect that the degrees of freedom play in these competing designs. In particular, we observe that the paired design has one-half the degrees of freedom that the two-independent-samples design has. In effect, there is more information with which to estimate the uncontrolled variability in the independent samples' design. Thus, we pay a price for pairing in terms of degrees of freedom. This simply leads to the conclusion that one should not match on unimportant variables. If one does, the reduction in degrees of freedom is not offset by a comparable reduction in the unexplained variability.

The same general principles apply to the multiple-group testing and comparison problems. For example, in order to compare the $g = 5$ treatments in the antidepressant clinical trial mentioned earlier, one possible design is the one the researchers apparently used. In particular, assign treatments completely at random with no restrictions, apart from a possible sample size restriction for each group. Such an experimental design is, therefore, termed the *completely random design* (CRD). The CRD is the multiple group generalization of the two-independent-samples design.

An alternative design is the *randomized complete block design* (RCBD). This design is the multiple group generalization of the paired-data design. Essentially, patients are grouped into *blocks* of g persons per block; within a block the patients are homogeneous or similar with regard to a set of blocking or stratifying characteristics. For example, they may be the same age, sex, and social class. Having determined such blocks, the g treatments are then assigned at random within each block. The assignment is performed in such a way that each treatment appears once and only once in each block. Thus, the complete set of treatments is represented in each block. As the treatments are also assigned randomly, the design is therefore called the randomized complete block design. There are many other designs that impose restrictions on the randomization scheme; the RCBD is the simplest one, however.

One design, more complicated but of particular value in psychiatric research, is the *incomplete block design*. In this design the complete set of treatments does not appear in each block. This design is useful in studies of rater agreement. If a group of interviewers is to be used in a study, a test of their overall and pairwise agreement must be conducted in order to certify the interviewers. In such observer agreement studies, it may neither be feasible nor sensible to have all of the raters interview each patient. This is especially so if the number of raters (g) is large, say, greater than 5. In such cases, it is possibly more reasonable to have each patient interviewed, at most, three times. In order to design a proper study for this agreement question, unless there is some a priori reason for studying some interviewers more intensely than others, all possible pairs of interviewers should appear together an equal number of times, and each interviewer should conduct the same number of interviews. Incomplete block (patients are the blocks in this context) designs with such properties are called *balanced incomplete block designs* (BIBD). A catalog of such designs is found in Cochran and Cox's text (1957) on experimental designs. The design and the statistical analysis of such designs can be complex and is beyond the scope of the present text. If such a design is contemplated, an investigator should discuss the situation in advance with a statistician since the analysis for such studies can become complicated if the study is not properly designed.

We have focused on statistical designs that employ randomization, that is, experimental studies. If an observational study is performed that gives rise to data in the general form of the CRD (RCBD or other designs), then the statistical analysis appropriate for this design may be applied. As noted previously, the interpretation of the results may require greater caution because of the lack of randomization. Nevertheless, with care, the techniques described in the subsequent sections may be applied to experimental or observational studies.

10.2 WHY SPECIAL TECHNIQUES FOR MULTIPLE-GROUP COMPARISONS?

The emphasis on special techniques for comparing more than two groups may seem puzzling. On the surface, it seems quite reasonable to perform the two group tests of Chapter 6 for all possible pairs of the g groups. For example, in the earlier discussion of the clinical trial of the five treatments for nonpsychotic depression, why not simply do a two-sample t (or Wilcoxon rank sum) test for each of the 10 possible pairs of comparisons, that is, 1 versus 2, 1 versus 3, ..., 4 versus 5? One problem with such an approach is the sheer computational effort that would be required. While this point makes such an approach unattractive, it is not reason enough to rule out the approach, especially since computers are able to do the required arithmetic. One of the main difficulties with this approach is the problem of specifying and adequately controlling the type I error rate for the entire set of comparisons. To elucidate this point, suppose that there is no real difference between the five treatment groups. Formally, the null hypothesis is that the depression score distribution is the same for each of the five treatment groups. Suppose that a data analyst compares treatment 1 to treatment 2 with a two-sample t-test and compares treatment 4 to treatment 5 with a two-sample t-test. What is the probability that either or both tests reject the null hypothesis when the null hypothesis is true? Clearly, if each of the two-sample t-tests is performed at the 0.05 level, then owing to the independence of the two tests, the probability that both tests correctly accept the null hypothesis is $(0.95)^2$. Therefore, the probability that at least one of the two t-tests falsely rejects the null hypothesis is $1 - (0.95)^2$, which is 0.0975. Thus, the significance for the two pairwise tests is considerably above the conventional 0.05. To assess the significance for the set of all 10 possible comparisons, each done at the 0.05 level separately, the computations are more cumbersome owing to the dependence of the tests. It can be shown, however, that if the tests are independent, then the actual significance level is $1 - (0.95)^{10}$, which is 0.40. That is, if 10 independent pairwise comparisons are performed at the 0.05 significance level, then the probability that at least one will be declared significant under the null hypothesis is 0.40. In general, the error rate for such

Table 10.1. Data Layout for Completely Random Design

Group 1	Group 2	$\cdots$	Group g
y_{11}	y_{21}	$\cdots$	y_{g1}
y_{12}	y_{22}	$\cdots$	y_{g2}
$\vdots$	$\vdots$		$\vdots$
y_{1n_1}	y_{2n_2}	$\cdots$	y_{gn_g}

procedures is $1 - (1 - \alpha)^k$, where $k = \binom{g}{2} = g(g - 1)/2$. Hence, there is a clear need for a statistical test procedure that will permit a global comparison of g groups while keeping the error rate at a prescribed level. The various statistical procedures in this chapter permit such a comparison.

10.3 ANALYSIS OF VARIANCE FOR COMPLETELY RANDOM DESIGNS

10.3.1 General Aspects of Problem

The basic data layout for the CRD is as given in Table 10.1. The entry y_{ij} is the jth observation (replicate) in group i ($i = 1, 2, \ldots, g$; $j = 1, 2, \ldots, n_i$).

In this section, we consider statistical inferences that can be made regarding these g groups for response variables that follow a normal distribution. It is also assumed that these g samples are random samples from their respective populations and that the g samples are independent of one another. The statistical procedure in this chapter is the major procedure used in practice for comparing means of g groups. The name of the procedure is the *analysis of variance*. The process of comparing the g population means usually involves three steps:

1. the analysis of variance, which is simply the arithmetic process of partitioning the total sample variation of the y's into recognized sources of variability;
2. the F-test, which is the formal statistical test for judging whether the sample means are significantly different; and
3. a multiple comparison procedure, whereby various pairs and/or combinations of groups are compared to one another.

The assumptions we are making for the data of Table 10.1 are the following:

1. The g samples are independent random samples. This assumption is ensured by randomized assignment of treatments for experimental studies; in some observational studies it is simply assumed.
2. The observations in group i (for each $i = 1, 2, \ldots, g$) are a random sample from a normal probability distribution with mean μ_i and variance σ_i^2.
3. The g population variances, $\sigma_1^2, \ldots, \sigma_g^2$, are all equal to a common variance σ^2.

Assumptions 1–3 are straightforward generalizations of the two-sample t procedure assumptions given in Section 6.2.2. The second and third assumptions are equivalent to the statement that observation y from the ith group has the normal probability density function

$$f(y) = \frac{1}{\sigma\sqrt{2\pi}} \exp\left(-\frac{(y - \mu_i)^2}{2\sigma^2} \right), \qquad -\infty < y < \infty. \qquad (10.1)$$

Another more succinct manner of expressing assumptions 1–3 is in a *linear additive model*. This approach has the value of generalizaing to more complicated study designs. The *linear additive model* for assumptions 1–3 is

$$y_{ij} = \mu_i + e_{ij}, \qquad (10.2)$$

where μ_i is the mean for the ith group, and the e_{ij}'s are independent random sampling error variables that have a normal distribution with mean zero and variance σ^2. Model (10.2) says that each observation has a mean value in the population from which it was selected, and it has an error term that reflects the random uncontrolled variability of the sampling process. A little reflection on model (10.2) should convince us that there are situations where we expect such a model to be reasonable, but there are others in which the model is a naive oversimplification of the data. For completeness, we should also indicate that model (10.2) is sometimes written in its "treatment (or group) effects" form. In particular, since for any constant value μ we can write $\mu_i = \mu + (\mu_i - \mu)$, it is sometimes useful to write model (10.2) in the form

$$y_{ij} = \mu + \tau_i + e_{ij}, \qquad (10.3)$$

where the ith treatment, or group, effect is $\tau_i = \mu_i - \mu$. Clearly, if we choose μ to be the mean of the μ_i, that is, $\mu = \sum_{i=1}^{g}\mu_i/g$, then it is evident that $\sum_{i=1}^{g}\tau_i = \sum_{i=1}^{g}(\mu_i - \mu) = 0$. That is, model (10.3) imposes an arithmetic restriction on the parameters in the model. Rather than focusing too intensely on the various possible values of μ, it is better for us to simply note that models (10.2) and (10.3) are equivalent, and (10.3) is written in a *treatment effects* form.

Our main interest is to make a statistical inference regarding the g population means. Therefore, we discuss procedures for testing

$$H_0: \mu_1 = \mu_2 = \cdots = \mu_g \quad \text{versus} \quad H_a: \text{the means are not all equal} \quad (10.4)$$

and procedures for estimating the various treatment group differences.

In order to better understand the various procedures we shall be using, it is helpful if we study first the case in which the g sample sizes are equal, that is, $n_1 = n_2 = n_3 = \cdots = n_g = n$.

10.3.2 Equal Sample Sizes

10.3.2.1 Analysis of Variance

If $n = n_1 = n_2 = \cdots = n_g$, then the data of Table 10.1 may be written in the form of Table 10.2. In Table 10.2, y_{i+} is the sum of the observations in group i while $\bar{y}_{i+}$ is its sample mean; therefore, $y_{i+} = \sum_{j=1}^{n}y_{ij}$ and $\bar{y}_{i+} = y_{i+}/n$. Similarly, the grand total and grand mean are $y_{++} = \sum_{i=1}^{g}y_{i+} = \sum_{i=1}^{g}\sum_{j=1}^{n}y_{ij}$ and $\bar{y}_{++} = y_{++}/gn$, respectively. In order to derive a test for H_0 in expression (10.4), let us consider what we know about the data of Table 10.2 under assumptions 1–3. Also, since we wish to make an inference regarding the g population means $\mu_1, \ldots, \mu_g$, it certainly is reasonable to consider the corresponding sample means $\bar{y}_{1+}, \ldots, \bar{y}_{g+}$. Proceeding with the development, the distribution of $\bar{y}_{i+}$ is normal with mean

Table 10.2. Data Layout for Completely Random Design with Equal Sample Sizes

	Group 1	Group 2	$\cdots$	Group g	
	y_{11}	y_{21}	$\cdots$	y_{g1}	
	$\vdots$	$\vdots$		$\vdots$	
	y_{1n}	y_{2n}	$\cdots$	y_{gn}	
Total	y_{1+}	y_{2+}	$\cdots$	y_{g+}	y_{++}
Mean	$\bar{y}_{1+}$	$\bar{y}_{2+}$	$\cdots$	$\bar{y}_{g+}$	$\bar{y}_{++}$

μ_i and variance σ^2/n. This fact follows directly from Section 4.7. Furthermore, the sample means $\bar{y}_{i+}$ are independent of one another since the g random samples were independent. Under the null hypothesis, one has $\mu_1 = \mu_2 = \cdots \mu_g = \mu$; thus, when the null hypothesis is true, each $\bar{y}_{i+}$ has the same mean and variance. The independence of $\bar{y}_{1+}, \ldots, \bar{y}_{g+}$ coupled with the null hypothesis translates into the following statement:

$\bar{y}_{1+}, \ldots, \bar{y}_{g+}$ is a random sample from a normal population with

mean μ and variance σ^2/n when the null hypothesis is true.   (10.5)

Using statement (10.5), it is clear that an estimator of μ is $\bar{y}_{++}$, where $\bar{y}_{++} = \sum_{i=1}^{g} \bar{y}_{i+}/g$, while an estimator of σ^2/n is $\sum_{i=1}^{g}(\bar{y}_{i+} - \bar{y}_{++})^2/(g - 1)$. Therefore, multiplication by n results in an estimator of σ^2 of the form $n\sum_{i=1}^{g}(\bar{y}_{i+} - \bar{y}_{++})^2/(g - 1)$. Since this estimator is based on the differences between the group means, this variability is termed *between-group mean variability*, and we denote this estimator of σ^2 by $\hat{\sigma}_B^2$; thus one has

$$\hat{\sigma}_B^2 = \frac{n\sum_{i=1}^{g}(\bar{y}_{i+} - \bar{y}_{++})^2}{g - 1}. \tag{10.6}$$

Notice that this estimator of σ^2 is based on the variability of the g "observations" $\bar{y}_{1+}, \ldots, \bar{y}_{g+}$; it has therefore $g - 1$ degrees of freedom associated with it. Furthermore, estimator (10.6) is a proper and valid estimator of σ^2 only if the null hypothesis is true. If the null hypothesis is not true, then it can be shown that the quantity (10.6) estimates σ^2 plus a positive term that reflects the magnitude of the difference between the g group means. Specifically, it can be shown that the mean value of (10.6) in repeated random sampling is

$$\sigma^2 + n \sum_{i=1}^{g} (\mu_i - \mu)^2/(g - 1), \quad \text{where} \quad \mu = \sum_{i=1}^{g} \mu_i/g. \tag{10.7}$$

An alternative estimator of σ^2 is obtainable by pooling the within-group variability in precisely the same manner we did in the two-sample t procedure (Chapter 6). Thus, generalizing expression (6.4) to g groups and denoting the estimator by $\hat{\sigma}_w^2$, one has

$$\hat{\sigma}_w^2 = \frac{(n - 1)s_1^2 + (n - 1)s_2^2 + \cdots + (n - 1)s_g^2}{(n - 1) + (n - 1) + \cdots + (n - 1)}, \tag{10.8}$$

where $s_i^2 = \sum_{j=1}^{n}(y_{ij} - \bar{y}_{i+})^2/(n-1)$. Clearly, estimator (10.8) can be written in the alternative form

$$\hat{\sigma}_w^2 = \sum_{i=1}^{g} \sum_{j=1}^{n} (y_{ij} - \bar{y}_{i+})^2/g(n-1). \tag{10.9}$$

This estimator is a valid and proper estimator of σ^2 regardless of which hypothesis, the null hypothesis or its alternative, is true. As the estimator is based on the variability *within* groups, it seems reasonable that this property of being a valid estimator of σ^2 should be the case since its computation does not depend on the difference in group means. Notice that the estimator is based on $g(n-1)$ degrees of freedom.

It is now quite straightforward to propose a test of H_0. As it can be shown that the estimators $\hat{\sigma}_B^2$ and $\hat{\sigma}_w^2$ are independent of each other and since both are estimating σ^2 under the null hypothesis, it is appropriate to consider the ratio $\hat{\sigma}_B^2/\hat{\sigma}_w^2$. From Section 4.8, it is evident that this ratio has an F distribution with $g-1$ and $g(n-1)$ as its two-degree-of-freedom parameters. Since this ratio is expected to be close to 1 under the null hypothesis, while it is expected to be greater than 1 under the alternative hypothesis (because, under H_a, $\hat{\sigma}_B^2$ estimates (10.7) while $\hat{\sigma}_w^2$ estimates σ^2), large values of $\hat{\sigma}_B^2/\hat{\sigma}_w^2$ lead to rejecting the null hypothesis. Thus, one would reject H_0 if $\hat{\sigma}_B^2/\hat{\sigma}_w^2$ exceeded $F_{1-\alpha}(g-1, g(n-1))$, the $100(1-\alpha)$th percentile of an $F(g-1, g(n-1))$ distribution obtained from Table 7 of the Appendix. Thus, a test for the means is based on a variance ratio.

This entire development may be approached from a somewhat different point of view. In particular, the total sum of squares for the data of Table 10.2 may be written as

$$\text{SST} = \sum_{i=1}^{g} \sum_{j=1}^{n} (y_{ij} - \bar{y}_{++})^2, \tag{10.10}$$

which is the total variability about the overall mean, $\bar{y}_{++}$. This sum of squares is based on $gn-1$ d.f. If one rewrites this sum of squares, by adding and subtracting $\bar{y}_{i+}$, inside the square as

$$\text{SST} = \sum_{i=1}^{g} \sum_{j=1}^{n} \left[(y_{ij} - \bar{y}_{i+}) + (\bar{y}_{i+} - \bar{y}_{++})\right]^2 \tag{10.11}$$

and performs the necessary algebra in squaring and summing the above

Table 10.3. Analysis of Variance for Data of Table 10.2

Source (of Variation)	d.f.	SS	MS	F
Between groups	$g - 1$	$SSB = \sum_{i=1}^{g} n(\bar{y}_{i+} - \bar{y}_{++})^2$	$\hat{\sigma}_B^2 = \dfrac{\sum_{i=1}^{g} n(\bar{y}_{i+} - \bar{y}_{++})^2}{g - 1}$	$\dfrac{\hat{\sigma}_B^2}{\hat{\sigma}_w^2}$
Within groups (error)	$g(n - 1)$	$SSW = \sum_{i=1}^{g} \sum_{j=1}^{n} (y_{ij} - \bar{y}_{i+})^2$	$\hat{\sigma}_w^2 = \dfrac{\sum_{i=1}^{g}\sum_{j=1}^{n}(y_{ij} - \bar{y}_{i+})^2}{g(n - 1)}$	
Total	$gn - 1$	$SST = \sum_{i=1}^{g} \sum_{j=1}^{n} (y_{ij} - \bar{y}_{++})^2$		

terms, it can be shown that

$$SST = \sum_{i=1}^{g} \sum_{j=1}^{n} (y_{ij} - \bar{y}_{i+})^2 + \sum_{i=1}^{g} n(\bar{y}_{i+} - \bar{y}_{++})^2. \qquad (10.12)$$

That is, the total sum of squares (10.10) can be partitioned into two components, a within-group component and a between-group component. As these components are the respective numerators of $\hat{\sigma}_w^2$ and $\hat{\sigma}_B^2$, their respective degrees of freedom are $g(n - 1)$ and $g - 1$. This entire process of partitioning a total sum of squares into recognized sources of variation is called the *analysis of variance*. We see that the resulting partition leads directly to our F ratio for testing hypotheses. The summary analysis-of-variance table is presented in Table 10.3.

Notice that the sum of squares (SS) and the degrees of freedom (d.f.) both partition into additive components. One further comment is required before illustrating these methods. Computational formulas for the SS in Table 10.3 greatly simplify the arithmetic. The formulas are

$$SSB = \sum_{i=1}^{g} \frac{y_{i+}^2}{n} - \frac{y_{++}^2}{gn},$$

$$SST = \sum_{i=1}^{g} \sum_{j=1}^{n} y_{ij}^2 - \frac{y_{++}^2}{gn}, \qquad (10.13)$$

$$SSW = SST - SSB.$$

Table 10.4. Outline of F-test for Equal-Means Hypothesis for Comparing g Groups with n Observations Per Group

---

A. Data: y_{ij}, $i = 1, 2, \ldots, g$; $j = 1, 2, \ldots, n$ from Table 10.2.

B. Assumptions: Stated by assumptions 1–3 in Section 10.3.1.

C. Computations: Compute the analysis of variance table as in Table 10.3 using formulas (10.13) for the computations. Compute $F = \hat{\sigma}_B^2 / \hat{\sigma}_w^2$.

D. Statistical test:
    1. Null Hypothesis: $H_0: \mu_1 = \mu_2 = \cdots = \mu_g$.
    2. Alternative hypothesis: H_a: The means are not all equal.
    3. Decision rule for an α-level test: Reject H_0 in favor of H_a if F computed in step C is greater than $F_{1-\alpha}(g - 1, g(n - 1))$, where this value is taken from Table 7 of the Appendix.

Substitution of (10.13) into Table 10.3 adds to the ease of computation. The entire procedure for testing the equal-means hypothesis for the data of Table 10.2 may now be summarized (Table 10.4).

An illustration may help to clarify the procedures in Table 10.4.

Example 10.3.2.1.1. Twenty rats were assigned to five treatment groups of equal size on a completely random basis. The five treatment groups were:

    A: Phenobarbital (75 mg/kg) daily for 3 days.
    B: Chlortetracycline (low dose) daily for 5 days.
    C: Chlortetracycline (med-dose) daily for 5 days.
    D: Chlortetracycline (high dose) daily for 5 days.
    E: Saline control.

Twenty-four hours after the last pretreatment, hexobarbital (60 mg/kg) was administered i.p., and the sleeping time for each animal was measured in minutes. The following data were obtained:

Sleeping Time, 30 min

A	B	C	D	E
10	12	9	14	10
4	10	4	9	6
6	13	4	10	8
4	7	5	11	4

At the 5% significance level, is there a difference between the five groups with respect to the sleeping times?

Let us assume that assumptions 1–3 (Section 10.3.1) hold for these data, and therefore we shall use the analysis-of-variance (ANOVA) F-test to test the hypothesis in question. The worked solution is outlined in Table 10.5.

In a problem like the preceding example, to conclude that there are differences between the groups is not a completely satisfying endpoint for the analysis. The next step in such analyses is to compare the various groups or particular sets of groups in which we are interested. Such procedures for comparing various groups are called *multiple-comparison procedures*. These are discussed in the following section.

10.3.2.2 Multiple Comparisons

There are a variety of statistical procedures for the comparison of means in an analysis-of-variance setting. These procedures differ primarily in the types of comparisons of interest. One procedure permits a comparison of all pairs of means, another permits the comparison of all $g - 1$ of the means to a specific mean, another procedure is appropriate for any pairwise comparison selected in advance of the data analysis, while another procedure is valid for all linear combinations of the means.

The procedures also differ in the manner in which they control the type I error rate. There are two such methods discussed in this book: procedures that control the error rate on a per comparison basis and those that control the error rate on a per experiment basis. A test procedure is said to control the error rate at an α level if the probability that the test rejects the null hypothesis falsely is α. If a multiple-comparison procedure controls the error rate at α for each comparison separately while paying no attention to the error rate for other comparisons that are planned, the error rate is said to be on a *per-comparison* basis. This method of controlling the error rate is acceptable for group comparisons that are planned at the start of the experiment. One such procedure is called the *least significant difference* and is based on the t distribution.

A procedure is said to control the error rate on a *per-experiment* or *experimentwise* basis if the error rate is controlled at a fixed level α for all comparisons as a group jointly. In other words, if it is of interest to require that all of the comparisons made have a joint probability of being correct at $1 - \alpha$, then a per-experiment method should be used to control the error rate. With such methods of controlling the error rate, the data analyst specifies a set of comparisons that are of interest and then selects an appropriate multiple-comparison procedure that controls the type I error for the set of comparisons simultaneously at α.

Several experimentwise procedures are particularly noteworthy. *Dunnett's procedure* (1964) is a multiple-comparison procedure for comparing $g - 1$ of the groups to one other group. For example, in Example

Table 10.5. Worked Solution of Example 10.3.2.1 Using Analysis-of-Variance F-Test

A. Data:

$$\begin{array}{ll}
\text{Group } A \text{ observations:} & 10,4,6,4 \\
\text{Group } B \text{ observations:} & 12,10,13,7 \\
\text{Group } C \text{ observations:} & 9,4,4,5 \\
\text{Group } D \text{ observations:} & 14,9,10,11 \\
\text{Group } E \text{ observations:} & 10,6,8,4
\end{array}$$

B. Assumptions: The distribution of sleeping times is normally distributed for each of the five groups and the variances are equal. The five samples constitute independent random samples.

C. Computations:

$$\begin{array}{ll}
y_{1+} = 24 & \bar{y}_{1+} = 6 \\
y_{2+} = 42 & \bar{y}_{2+} = 10.5 \\
y_{3+} = 22 & \bar{y}_{3+} = 5.5 \\
y_{4+} = 44 & \bar{y}_{4+} = 11 \\
y_{5+} = 28 & \bar{y}_{5+} = 7 \\
y_{++} = 160 & \bar{y}_{++} = 8
\end{array}$$

$$\text{SST} = 10^2 + 4^2 + \cdots + 8^2 + 4^2 - \frac{(160)^2}{20} = 202$$

$$\text{SSB} = \frac{24^2}{4} + \cdots + \frac{28^2}{4} - \frac{(160)^2}{20} = 106$$

$$\text{SSW} = 202 - 106 = 96$$

ANOVA

Source	d.f.	SS	MS	F
Between groups	4	106	26.5	4.14
Within groups	15	96	6.4	
Total	19	202		

D. Statistical test:
   1. Null hypothesis: H_0: $\mu_1 = \mu_2 = \mu_3 = \mu_4 = \mu_5$.
   2. Alternative hypothesis: H_a: Means are not all equal.
   3. Decision rule for a 0.05 level test: Reject if $F > F_{0.95}(4, 15)$.
E. Action taken: From Table 7 of the Appendix, $F_{0.95}(4, 15) = 3.06$, while the computed F in step C is 4.14; hence, the null hypothesis is rejected at the 0.05 level. There is a statistically significant difference in the sleeping times of the five groups.

10.3.2.1.1, it may be logical to compare all means to group E, the control group. In this manner, statements could be made regarding all test treatments as compared to the control group. Another experimentwise multiple-comparison procedure is *Tukey's procedure* (1953). This procedure permits the comparison of all possible pairs of means. This procedure controls the error rate for $\binom{g}{2}$ comparisons, while Dunnett's controls the error rate for only $g - 1$ comparisons. It is easier to find a difference between the control group and another group with Dunnett's (as compared to Tukey's) procedure since there are fewer comparisons for which the error rate is controlled. Another multiple-comparison procedure is *Scheffé's procedure* (1953). This experimentwise multiple-comparison procedure permits any possible linear comparison of the means. For example, in Example 10.3.2.1.1, it may be, of interest to compare the mean response of groups A and B together versus the mean of groups C and D together. Scheffé's procedure is so flexible that this or any other *linear comparison* (also called linear contrast) may be made. This procedure is more conservative than Tukey's since the type I error rate is controlled for a wider class of comparisons.

For exploratory data analysis, involving comparisons suggested by the data, Scheffé's or Tukey's procedure should be applied. It is an inappropriate use of statistics to apply a procedure like the *least significant difference* to comparisons suggested by the data. Exploring data in order to find differences is many times an important aspect of the data analysis. Improperly used statistical comparisons can easily turn up false leads. Investigators involved in exploratory statistical analyses with multiple numbers of groups should regard Tukey's, Scheffé's, or Dunnett's procedure as the "normal" multiple-comparison procedures to use.

10.3.2.2.1 Least Significant Difference (lsd)

This procedure should only be applied to one or two comparisons that are planned comparisons. It may not be applied to comparisons suggested by the data. The procedure controls the error rate on a *per-comparison* basis. The least significant difference is defined by the identity

$$\text{lsd}(\alpha) = t_{1-\alpha/2}[g(n-1)]\sqrt{\hat{\sigma}_w^2\left(\frac{2}{n}\right)}, \tag{10.14}$$

where $\text{lsd}(\alpha)$ is the least significant difference at level α, $t_{1-\alpha/2}[g(n-1)]$ is from Table 5 of the Appendix, $\hat{\sigma}_w^2$ is from the analysis of variance in Table 10.3; notice that $\sqrt{\hat{\sigma}_w^2(2/n)}$ is the standard error for a difference between two group means. Thus, for convenience, let us denote this standard error by $s_{\bar{d}}$, that is, let

$$s_{\bar{d}} = \sqrt{\hat{\sigma}_w^2 \left(\frac{2}{n}\right)}. \tag{10.15}$$

It is useful to recall that a two-sample t-test for comparing two means, $\bar{X}_A$ and $\bar{X}_B$, would have the form $(\bar{X}_A - \bar{X}_B)/s_{\bar{d}}$; rejection of the null hypothesis in favor of two-sided alternatives occurs if

$$|(\bar{X}_A - \bar{X}_B)/s_{\bar{d}}| > t_{1-\alpha/2}(\text{d.f.}), \tag{10.16}$$

where d.f. is the number of degrees of freedom of $s_{\bar{d}}$. By multiplying both sides of expression (10.16) by $s_{\bar{d}}$, it follows that, in order for a difference between two means to be declared statistically significant at the α level, it must be at least as large as $t_{1-\alpha/2}(\text{d.f.})s_{\bar{d}}$. This is the least significant difference.

The procedure is applied by computing (10.16) and then comparing the absolute difference of the pair of means of interest. If the absolute difference exceeds formula (10.14), the difference is declared significant at the α level.

In Table 10.6 the least-significant-difference procedure is summarized.

Example 10.3.2.2.1.1.   Suppose in Example 10.3.2.1.1 that the investigators are particularly interested in comparing group A to group B, and *this comparison was planned before seeing any of the results.* Using the least significant difference, is there evidence of a difference between these two groups at the 5% level of significance?

Table 10.6. Outline of Least-Significant-Difference Multiple-Comparison Procedure

---

A. Data: y_{ij}, $i = 1, 2, \ldots, g$; $j = 1, 2, \ldots, n$, from Table 10.2.
B. Assumptions: Stated by assumptions 1–3 in Section 10.3.1, and it is also assumed that there are one or two comparisons between the g groups that were planned a priori and are not chosen on the basis of the results.
C. Computations: Determine $\hat{\sigma}_w^2$ from the analysis of variance (Table 10.3). Compute $s_{\bar{d}} = \sqrt{\hat{\sigma}_w^2 (2/n)}$ and determine $t_{1-\alpha/2}[g(n-1)]$ from Table 5 of the Appendix. Compute $\text{lsd}(\alpha) = (s_{\bar{d}})t_{1-\alpha/2}[g(n-1)]$, and for the pair of means of interest, $\bar{y}_{A+}$ and $\bar{y}_{B+}$, compute $|\bar{y}_{A+} - \bar{y}_{B+}|$.
D. Two-tailed statistical test:
   1. Null hypothesis: $H_0: \mu_A = \mu_B$
   2. Alternative hypothesis: $H_a: \mu_A \neq \mu_B$
   3. Decision rule for an α-level test: Reject H_0 in favor of H_a if $|\bar{y}_{A+} - \bar{y}_{B+}| > \text{lsd}(\alpha)$.

From Table 10.5, $\hat{\sigma}_w^2 = 6.4$; hence, $s_{\bar{d}} = 1.79$ as $n = 4$. From Table 5 of the Appendix, $t_{0.975}(15) = 2.131$; hence, $\text{lsd}(0.05) = (1.79)(2.131) = 3.814$.

The actual difference between groups A and B in mean sleeping times is -4.5. As 4.5 exceeds 3.814, the two groups are declared significantly different at the 0.05 level.

As a final comment, it may be noted that the least-significant-difference procedure can be applied independently of the result of the F-test from the analysis of variance. In particular, the outcome of the F-test in no way comprises the appropriateness of applying the least-significant-difference method.

10.3.2.2.2 Dunnett's Procedure

To compare all means to a control group, Dunnett's procedure (1964) for multiple comparisons may be applied. It is like the least significant difference in that only one value is computed for comparison to the various group mean differences. This procedure permits one-sided or two-sided comparisons and confidence intervals that are easily obtained. In Table 13 of the Appendix, the one-sided and two-sided critical values of Dunnett's statistic are tabulated for significance levels of 0.05 and 0.01 and for values of g from 2 to 10. In addition, the degrees of freedom in the "within-groups" term of the analysis of variance tables is referred to as "error d.f." in Table 13 of the Appendix. In Table 10.7, Dunnett's procedure is summarized. For convenience, let group g be the control group in the remainder of this section.

The $(1 - \alpha)$ 100% confidence intervals for the pairwise "treatment"-control difference in means are given by

$$(\bar{y}_{i+} - \bar{y}_{g+}) \pm C_{1-\alpha}(p, \text{error d.f.})s_{\bar{d}} \qquad (10.17)$$

for each $i = 1, 2, \ldots, g - 1$, and where $C_{1-\alpha}(p, \text{error d.f.})$ is from the two-sided part of Table 13 of the Appendix with $p = g - 1$ and error d.f. $= g(n - 1)$. The intervals (10.17) are two-sided confidence intervals. One-sided $(1 - \alpha)$100% confidence intervals may be obtained via

$$\left[(\bar{y}_{i+} - \bar{y}_{g+}) - C_{1-\alpha}(p, \text{error d.f.})s_{\bar{d}}, \infty\right] \qquad (10.18)$$

or

$$\left[-\infty, (\bar{y}_{i+} - \bar{y}_{g+}) + C_{1-\alpha}(p, \text{error d.f.})s_{\bar{d}}\right], \qquad (10.19)$$

depending on the direction of interest, where $C_{1-\alpha}(p, \text{error d.f.})$ is from the one-sided part of Table 13 of the Appendix with $p = g - 1$ and error d.f. $= g(n - 1)$.

Table 10.7. Outline of Dunnett's Procedure for Comparing All Means to a Control Group

---

A. Data: y_{ij}, $i = 1, 2, \ldots, g$; $j = 1, 2, \ldots, n$, from Table 10.2.

B. Assumptions: Stated by assumptions 1–3 (Section 10.3.1); it is also assumed that one of the g groups is designated in advance of data collection as the control group to which all others will be compared. Without loss of generality, let the last group, g, be the control group.

C. Computations: Determine $s_{\bar{d}}$ by $s_{\bar{d}} = \sqrt{\hat{\sigma}_w^2(2/n)}$, where $\hat{\sigma}_w^2$ is obtained from the analysis of variance (Table 10.3). From Table 13 of the Appendix, determine for significance level α the critical value $C_{1-\alpha}(p, \text{error d.f.})$, where $p = g - 1$, error d.f. $= g(n - 1)$, and $\alpha = 0.05$ or 0.01. Compute $D_{1-\alpha} = C_{1-\alpha}(p, \text{error d.f.})s_{\bar{d}}$.

D. Two-tailed statistical test:
   1. Null hypothesis: H_0: $\mu_1 = \mu_g$; $\mu_2 = \mu_g$; $\ldots$; $\mu_{g-1} = \mu_g$.
   2. Alternative hypothesis: H_a: At least one of the means $\mu_1, \ldots, \mu_{g-1}$ is not equal to μ_g.
   3. Decision rule for an α-level test: Determine $C_{1-\alpha}(p, \text{error d.f.})$ from the two-sided part of Table 13 of the Appendix. If, for any $i = 1, \ldots, g - 1$, $|\bar{y}_{g+} - \bar{y}_{i+}| > D_{1-\alpha}$, then conclude that $\mu_g \neq \mu_i$ at the α level of significance.
   One-tailed statistical test:
   1. Null hypothesis: H_0: $\mu_1 = \mu_g, \ldots, \mu_{g-1} = \mu_g$
   2. Alternative hypothesis: H_a: $\mu_g > \mu_1$ or $\mu_g > \mu_{g-1}$ (H_a: $\mu_g < \mu_1$ or $\mu_g < \mu_{g-1}$)
   3. Decision rule for an α-level test: Obtain $C_{1-\alpha}(p, \text{error d.f.})$ from the one-sided part of Table 13 of the Appendix. If, for any $i = 1, \ldots, g - 1$, $\bar{y}_{g+} - \bar{y}_{i+} > D_{1-\alpha}(\bar{y}_{g+} - \bar{y}_{i+} < D_{1-\alpha})$, then conclude $\mu_g > \mu_i(\mu_g < \mu_i)$ at the α level of significance.

These intervals [(10.17), (10.18), and (10.19)] are *simultaneous* $(1 - \alpha)100\%$ *confidence intervals* in the sense that $1 - \alpha$ of the sets of $g - 1$ intervals computed using these formulas will include all $g - 1$ of the mean differences. The content of this statement is quite different from the pairwise confidence interval in which $1 - \alpha$ of the individual intervals include the *one* difference of the pairwise comparison. Naturally, intervals of the form of (10.17) are wider than comparable two-sample t intervals.

Example 10.3.2.2.2.1. In Example 10.3.2.1.1, suppose the investigators are interested in determining if any of the groups A, B, C, or D is different from group E. Perform Dunnett's two-sided procedure at $\alpha = 0.05$. Previously, $s_{\bar{d}}$ was computed as 1.79. From the two-sided part of Table 13 of the Appendix, we find $C_{0.95}(4, 15) = 2.79$; hence, the critical value of the test is $D_{0.95} = (2.79)(1.79) = 5$. The sample means from Table 10.5 are 6, 10.5, 5.5,

11, and 7. Comparing each of 6, 10.5, 5.5, and 11 to 7, we note that none of the differences exceeds 5 ($D_{0.95} = 5$); thus, one could not conclude that the four treatment groups A, B, C and D differ from the control group E. The reader may also verify that 95% simultaneous confidence intervals for the various treatment control differences are as follows [using expression (10.17)]:

Group A, control: $(-6, 4)$

Group B, control: $(-1.5, 8.5)$

Group C, control: $(-6.5, 3.5)$

Group D, control: $(-1, 9)$

Notice that all four intervals include the point zero. This must be the case since the value of zero indicates the null hypothesis of no difference, and our hypotheses tests must coincide with the corresponding confidence intervals.

10.3.2.2.3 Tukey's Procedure

In some problems, an investigator is unable to restrict the set of planned comparisons at the start of the study and may therefore be interested in all possible comparisons of the g means. *Tukey's procedure* permits such numerous comparisons and controls the error rate for the experiment as a unit, that is, a per-experiment error rate, The procedure is a two-sided procedure, and it does permit estimation via confidence intervals. Table 10.8 summarizes this procedure.

Table 10.8. Outline of Tukey's Procedure for Making All Pairs of Comparisons

---

A. Data: y_{ij}, $i = 1, 2, \ldots, g$; $j = 1, 2, \ldots, n$, from Table 10.2.

B. Assumptions: Stated by assumptions 1–3 (Section 10.3.1).

C. Computations: Determine $Q_\alpha(p, \text{error d.f.})$ from Table 14 of the Appendix (table of studentized range critical values), where α is 0.05 or 0.01, $p = g$, and error d.f. $= g(n - 1)$. From the analysis of variance (Table 10.3), determine $\hat{\sigma}_w^2$; then compute $(s_{\bar{y}}) = \sqrt{\hat{\sigma}_w^2(1/n)}$ and then compute $T_\alpha = s_{\bar{y}} Q_\alpha(p, \text{error d.f.})$.

D. Two-tailed statistical test

   1. Null hypothesis: H_0: $\mu_1 = \mu_2, \ldots, \mu_{g-1} = \mu_g$

   2. Alternative hypothesis: H_a: $\mu_1 \neq \mu_2$ or $\mu_1 \neq \mu_3$ or $\ldots$ or $\mu_{g-1} \neq \mu_g$

   3. Decision rule for an α-level test: If for any pair of groups A and B we find $|\bar{y}_{A+} - \bar{y}_{B+}| > T_\alpha$, then these two groups are said to be statistically significantly different at the α level.

Confidence intervals (two-sided) with confidence coefficient $(1 - \alpha)$ are easily obtained via

$$(\bar{y}_{i+} - \bar{y}_{k+}) \pm T_\alpha \qquad (10.20)$$

for all $i \neq k = 1, 2, \ldots, g$. These $\binom{g}{2} = g(g - 1)/2$ confidence intervals are simultaneous $(1 - \alpha)100\%$ confidence intervals. note in particular the simplicity of the computations in (10.20).

Example 10.3.2.2.3.1.   Suppose in Example 10.3.2.1.1 that the investigators are unable to focus attention on a particular set of planned comparisons at the start of the study. Assuming that all pairwise comparisons are of interest, peform Tukey's procedure and also place 95% simultaneous confidence intervals on all pairs of differences.

From previous expressions, we note that $s_{\bar{y}} = 1.26$. From Table 14 of the Appendix, $Q_{0.05}(5, 15) = 4.37$; hence, $T_{0.05} = (4.37)(1.26) = 5.51$. Let us now summarize the set of possible pairs of differences and confidence intervals (10.20) as below:

Comparison Group–Group	Mean Difference	95% Confidence Interval
$A-B$	-4.5	$(-10.01, 1.01)$
$A-C$	0.5	$(-5.01, 6.01)$
$A-D$	-5	$(-10.51, +0.51)$
$A-E$	-1	$(-6.51, 4.51)$
$B-C$	5	$(-0.51, 10.51)$
$B-D$	-0.5	$(-6.01, 5.01)$
$B-E$	3.5	$(-2.01, 9.01)$
$C-D$	-5.5	$(-11.01, 0.01)$
$C-E$	-1.5	$(-7.01, 4.01)$
$D-E$	4	$(-1.51, 9.51)$

Note that none of the pairwise differences exceeds 5.51 in absolute magnitude; however, the C versus D comparison is very close to significance. The confidence intervals should be reported since they describe the magnitude of the differences. One should also notice that the 95% confidence limit for each pairwise difference also includes zero.

An interesting question arises in comparing the results of the analysis-of-variance F-test with the results of Tukey's procedure. The F-test was statistically significant, but Tukey's procedure fails to declare any pairwise comparison of the groups significant. Why the apparent contradiction? In actual fact, the F-test from the analysis of variance is a more powerful and sensitive test procedure. The F-test not only compares the various pairs of means, it seeks to find differences that may be of a more complex form. For example, in the data of Example 10.3.2.1.1, Tukey's procedure is unable to declare the -5.5 as significant because each mean is only based on four observations. On the other hand, the analysis-of-variance F-test is accounting for any linear combination of the means that might lead to a significant difference. For example, the combination mean of groups A and C is 5.75, while that of groups B and D is 10.75, a difference of 5 min. More importantly, each of these means would be based on eight rather than four observations, that is, double the sample size. The analysis-of-variance F-test recognizes such situations and tells us through its significance that there is some comparison of these groups means that is not explainable by chance alone. Thus, although its significance does say that the groups are not a homogeneous set, this does not imply that at least one pairwise comparison of the groups will be significant. This point seems paradoxical since the F value can be significant while the pairwise comparisons may not be. The reasons are the following: (1) the Tukey procedure generates only all pairwise comparisons and (2) the F-test inspects the group comparisons for the most sensitive linear comparisons (contrasts) of the groups.

The next multiple-comparison procedure, the Scheffé procedure, is a direct extension of the F-test for the analysis of variance. If the F-test in the analysis of variance is significant, the Scheffé multiple-comparison procedure guarantees that at least one linear comparison of the groups will be declared significant.

10.3.2.2.4   Scheffé's Procedure
Scheffé's procedure is an experimentwise multiple-comparison procedure that permits the data analyst to make any linear comparison of the set of means. The procedure also permits the computation of a simultaneous confidence interval for any linear comparison. In addition, the procedure has the following guarantees:

1. If the analysis-of-variance F-test is not significant at level α, then Scheffé's procedure will declare all possible linear comparisons of groups to be nonsignificant at level α.
2. If the analysis-of-variance F-test is significant at level α, then Scheffé's procedure guarantees that there is at least one linear contrast of the g

Table 10.9. Outline of Scheffé's Multiple-Comparison Procedure

---

A. Data: y_{ij}, $i = 1, 2, \ldots, g$; $j = 1, 2, \ldots, n$, from Table 10.2.

B. Assumptions: Stated by assumptions 1–3 (Section 10.3.1); the constants $C_1, \ldots, C_g$ satisfy $\Sigma_{i=1}^{g} C_i = 0$.

C. Computations: Determine $\hat{\sigma}_w^2$ from the analysis of variance (Table 10.3); let $s^2 = \hat{\sigma}_w^2$. For the particular set of constants $C_1, \ldots, C_g$, compute the interval (10.21), where $F_{1-\alpha}(g - 1, g(n - 1))$ is from Table 7 of the Appendix:

$$\sum_{i=1}^{g} C_i \bar{y}_{i+} \pm s\sqrt{(g - 1) F_{1-\alpha}(g - 1, g(n - 1))\left(\Sigma_{i=1}^{g} C_i^2/n\right)}. \quad (10.21)$$

D. Two-tailed statistical test:
  1. Null hypothesis: $H_0: \Sigma_{i=1}^{g} C_i \mu_i = 0$
  2. Alternative hypothesis: $H_a: \Sigma_{i=1}^{g} C_i \mu_i \neq 0$
  3. Decision rule for an α-level test: If zero is in the interval (10.21), do not reject H_0; otherwise reject H_0.

---

group means that will be declared significant using Scheffé's procedure at level α.

Before explaining the procedure, we have the following definition:

Definition 10.3.2.2.4.1. A *linear contrast* of a set of means $\bar{y}_{1+}, \ldots, \bar{y}_{g+}$ is a linear function of the means, that is, a function of the form $C_1 \bar{y}_{1+} + C_2 \bar{y}_{2+} + \cdots + C_g \bar{y}_{g+}$, such that the coefficients $C_1, C_2, \ldots, C_t$ sum to zero.

Notationally, a linear contrast is $\Sigma_{i=1}^{g} C_i \bar{y}_{i+}$ such that $\Sigma_{i=1}^{g} C_i = 0$. It is evident that a contrast is the measure of a type of difference between the sample means. For example, if $C_1 = 1, C_2 = -1, C_3 = \cdots = C_g = 0$, then the resulting contrast is the simple comparison of groups 1 and 2, that is, $\bar{y}_{1+} - \bar{y}_{2+}$.

The analysis-of-variance F-test is really inspecting the data for any values of $C_1, \ldots, C_g$ satisfying $\Sigma_{i=1}^{g} C_i = 0$, that lead to large values of the resulting contrasts. That is why, when the F-test is significant, there are linear contrasts of the means that are significantly different from zero. In Table 10.9, Scheffé's procedure is outlined.

The interval in (10.21) is $(1 - \alpha)100\%$ simultaneous confidence interval for the linear contrast $\Sigma_{i=1}^{g} C_i \mu_i$.

As mentioned earlier, if the F-test analysis of variance is significant at level α, then there is at least one set of coefficients $C_1, C_2, \ldots, C_g$ that will lead to rejection of the null hypothesis in Table 10.9 when using this procedure.

Example 10.3.2.2.4.1. Suppose in Example 10.3.2.1.1 that the investigators wished to allow themselves the latitude to compare any linear function of the group means. Hence, Scheffé's procedure should be employed for purposes of the multiple comparisons. Place 95% simultaneous confidence limits on the following two linear contrasts: contrast $(1) = \mu_1 + \mu_3 - \mu_2 - \mu_4$, and contrast $(2) = \mu_3 - \mu_4$. From Table 10.5, we have $s^2 = 6.4$; $\bar{y}_{1+} = 6$, $\bar{y}_{2+} = 10.5$, $\bar{y}_{3+} = 5.5$, $\bar{y}_{4+} = 11$, and $\bar{y}_{5+} = 7$; $n = 4$; and $g = 5$. Also from Table 7 of the Appendix, $F_{0.95}(4, 15) = 3.06$.

Hence, the computations for contrast 1 are $\sum_{i=1}^{5} C_i \bar{y}_{1+} = -10$ and $s\sqrt{(g-1)(3.06)(4/n)} = 8.85$ with the 95% confidence interval given by $-10 \pm 8.85 = (-18.85, -1.14)$. Accordingly, there is a significant difference between the mean of the first and third groups and the mean of the second and fourth groups, as zero is not in the 95% confidence interval. The computations for contrast 2 yield $\sum_{i=1}^{g} C_i \bar{y}_{i+} = -5.5$ and $s\sqrt{4(3.06)(2/n)} = 6.26$ with 95% confidence interval given by $(-11.76, 0.76)$; hence, there is no significant difference between the third and fourth groups.

Scheffé's procedure is more conservative than Tukey's, since it is controlling the error rate for all possible linear comparisons among the group means. Nevertheless, for the data analyst who is scanning the data for whatever might "turn up," this procedure is useful since it controls the error rate at the desired level. The statistical analyst who employs this procedure need not worry about the so-called multiple-comparison problem since adequate error control is built into the procedure. That confidence intervals are so easily produced further enhances this method's attractiveness.

10.3.2.2.5 Bonferroni's Procedure

Suppose we want to make, say, k comparisons with a confidence coefficient of *at least* $1 - \alpha$. *Bonferroni's procedure* requires that each comparison be made at the $1 - \alpha/k$ confidence level; this procedure will guarantee a simultaneous confidence level of at least $1 - \alpha$.

This procedure is very general; it will work in most situations. It tends to be a conservative procedure, especially if many comparisons are made; that is, the true confidence level tends to be greater than $1 - \alpha$. It would most often be used when a few comparisons are to be made and none of the previously mentioned procedures are appropriate. To make k comparisons using Bonferroni's procedure, follow the least-significant-difference procedure with α replaced by α/k.

10.3.3 Unequal Sample Sizes

If sample sizes are not necessarily equal in the completely random design, the general data layout is of the form of Table 10.10.

Table 10.10. Data Layout for Completely Random Design with Unequal Sample Sizes

	Group 1	Group 2	$\cdots$	Group g	
	y_{11}	y_{21}	$\cdots$	y_{g1}	
	$\vdots$	$\vdots$		$\vdots$	
	y_{1n_1}	y_{2n_2}	$\cdots$	y_{gn_g}	
Total	y_{1+}	y_{2+}	$\cdots$	y_{g+}	y_{++}
Mean	$\bar{y}_{1+}$	$\bar{y}_{2+}$	$\cdots$	$\bar{y}_{g+}$	$\bar{y}_{++}$

Table 10.10 yields the following computations:

$$y_{i+} = \sum_{j=1}^{n_i} y_{ij} \quad \text{and} \quad \bar{y}_{i+} = \sum_{j=1}^{n_i} y_{ij} \Big/ n_i,$$

$$y_{++} = \sum_{i=1}^{g} \sum_{j=1}^{n_i} y_{ij} \quad \text{and} \quad \bar{y}_{++} = y_{++}/N,$$

where $N = \sum_{i=1}^{g} n_i$. In principle, the data of Table 10.2 are a special case of Table 10.10 so that we may expect the procedures of the previous section to apply here as well. This is, in fact, true. Virtually all of the methods of the previous section are easily adapted to permit inferences for the means $\mu_1, \ldots, \mu_g$ of groups $1, \ldots, g$. Since the development for many of the procedures follows closely that of the previous section, we primarily focus on the results in this section rather than repeat the same arguments.

10.3.3.1 Analysis of Variance
The assumptions for the data of Table 10.10 are as stated in assumptions 1–3 (Section 10.3.1). As before, the main interest is in testing hypotheses (10.4) and estimating various group differences.

From a definitional standpoint, the analysis of variance is given in Table 10.11.

Computational formulas for the sums of squares in Table 10.11 are given by

$$\text{SSB} = \sum_{i=1}^{g} \frac{y_{i+}^2}{n_i} - \frac{y_{++}^2}{N},$$

$$\text{SST} = \sum_{i=1}^{g} \sum_{j=1}^{n_i} y_{ij}^2 - \frac{y_{++}^2}{N}, \tag{10.22}$$

$$\text{SSW} = \text{SST} - \text{SSB}.$$

Table 10.11. Analysis of Variance for Data of Table 10.10

Source	d.f.	SS	MS	F
Between groups	$g - 1$	$\sum_{i=1}^{g} n_i(\bar{y}_{i+} - \bar{y}_{++})^2 = \text{SSB}$	$\hat{\sigma}_B^2 = \dfrac{\text{SSB}}{g - 1}$	$\dfrac{\hat{\sigma}_B^2}{\hat{\sigma}_w^2}$
Within groups	$N - g$	$\sum_{i=1}^{g} \sum_{j=1}^{n_i} (y_{ij} - \bar{y}_{i+})^2 = \text{SSW}$	$\hat{\sigma}_w^2 = \dfrac{\text{SSW}}{N - g}$	
Total	$N - 1$	$\sum_{i=1}^{g} \sum_{j=1}^{n_i} (y_{ij} - \bar{y}_{++})^2 = \text{SST}$		

Notice that in Table 10.11 the degrees of freedom between groups is $g - 1$, as it should be, since g means are being compared. In addition, the within-group degrees of freedom consists of $(n_1 - 1) + (n_2 - 1) + \cdots + (n_g - 1)$, which is $N - g$. The terms $\hat{\sigma}_B^2$ and $\hat{\sigma}_w^2$ have exactly the same interpretation as before, namely, the between-groups and within-groups estimators of the variance σ^2 when H_0 is true. If H_0 is false, then $\hat{\sigma}_B^2$ is an estimator of $\sigma^2 + \sum_{i=1}^{g} n_i(\mu_i - \mu)^2/(g - 1)$, while $\hat{\sigma}_w^2$ is an estimator of σ^2 both under H_0 and the alternative hypothesis. The ratio $\hat{\sigma}_B^2/\hat{\sigma}_w^2$ is therefore expected to be close to 1 if H_0 is true; otherwise, it is expected to be greater than 1. We summarize the overall test procedure in Table 10.12.

An illustration may be useful to clarify the nature of the computations and the test procedure.

Example 10.3.3.1.1. Nineteen patients requiring pain relief on a continuing basis volunteered to participate in a study to determine if the amount of

Table 10.12. Outline of F-Test for Equal-Means Hypothesis for Comparing g Groups with n_i Observations in ith Group ($i = 1, 2, \ldots, g$)

A. Data: y_{ij}, $i = 1, 2, \ldots, g$; $j = 1, 2, \ldots, n_i$, from Table 10.10; Let $N = n_1 + n_2 + \cdots + n_g$.

B. Assumptions: Stated by assumptions 1–3 (Section 10.3.1).

C. Computations: Compute the analysis of variance (as in Table 10.11) using formulas (10.22) for the computations. Compute $F = \hat{\sigma}_B^2/\hat{\sigma}_w^2$.

D. Statistical test:

   1. Null hypothesis: H_0: $\mu_1 = \cdots = \mu_g$.

   2. Alternative hypothesis: H_a: The means are not all equal.

   3. Decision rule for an α-level test: Reject H_0 in favor of H_a if F computed in step C is greater than $F_{1-\alpha}(g - 1, N - g)$, where this value is taken from Table 7 of the Appendix.

plasma-free morphine (6 hr posttreatment) varies with the mode of morphine administration. The patients were assigned completely at random to one of four groups. The groups and resulting sample sizes are:

Groups	Mode of Administration	Number of Patients
1	Intravenously	6
2	Intramuscularly	4
3	Subcutaneously	5
4	Orally	4

The following results for plasma-free levels occurred 6 hr after taking equal amounts of the drug:

	Group 1	Group 2	Group 3	Group 4
	12	12	9	12
	10	16	7	8
	7	15	6	8
	8	9	11	10
	9	—	7	—
	14	—	—	—
Total (y_{i+})	60	52	40	38
Mean ($\bar{y}_{i+}$)	10	13	8	9.5

At the 5% level of significance, is there sufficient evidence to conclude that the level of plasma-free morphine 6 hr postadministration varies by the mode of administration?

Let us assume that assumptions 1–3 (Section 10.3.1) hold and test the hypothesis that $\mu_1 = \mu_2 = \mu_3 = \mu_4$ using the procedures of Table 10.12. The worked solution is outlined in Table 10.13.

In the next section, we discuss the issue of multiple comparisons for data in which there are an unequal number of observations per group.

10.3.3.2 Multiple Comparisons

The issues regarding type I error rates apply to all multiple-group comparison problems; hence, the points discussed in Section 10.3.2.2 should be borne in mind. When the sample sizes are not equal in the comparison groups, the immediately applicable procedures of those discussed are the least-significant-difference, Scheffé, and Bonferroni procedures.

The least significant difference may be applied to one or two planned comparisons. Essentially, the procedure is a two-sample t-test. Thus, for

Table 10.13. Worked Solution of Example 10.3.3.1.1 Using Analysis-of-Variance
F-Test

A. Data:

$$\text{Group 1 observations: } 12, 10, 7, 8, 9, 14$$

$$\text{Group 2 observations: } 12, 16, 15, 9$$

$$\text{Group 3 observations: } 9, 7, 6, 11, 7$$

$$\text{Group 4 observations: } 12, 8, 8, 10$$

B. Assumptons: The distribution of the plasma-free levels of morphine follow a normal distribution for each of the four groups and the variances are equal. The four samples constitute independent random samples.
C. Computations:

$$y_{1+} = 60 \qquad \bar{y}_{1+} = 10$$

$$y_{2+} = 52 \qquad \bar{y}_{2+} = 13$$

$$y_{3+} = 40 \qquad \bar{y}_{3+} = 8$$

$$y_{4+} = 38 \qquad \bar{y}_{4+} = 9.5$$

$$y_{++} = 190 \qquad \bar{y}_{++} = 10.0$$

$$\text{SST} = 12^2 + 10^2 + \cdots + 10^2 - \frac{(190)^2}{19} = 148$$

$$\text{SSB} = \frac{(60)^2}{6} + \frac{(52)^2}{4} + \frac{(40)^2}{5} + \frac{(38)^2}{4} - \frac{(190)^2}{19} = 57$$

$$\text{SSW} = 148 - 57 = 91$$

ANOVA

Source	d.f.	S	MS	F
Between groups	3	57	19	3.13
Within groups	15	91	6.07	
Total	18	148		

D. Statistical test:
1. Null hypothesis: H_0: $\mu_1 = \mu_2 = \mu_3 = \mu_4$.
2. Alternative hypothesis: H_a: The means are not all equal.
3. Decision rule for a 0.05 level test: Reject if $F > F_{0.95}(3, 15)$.
E. Action taken: From Table 7 of the Appendix, $F_{0.95}(3, 15) = 3.29$, while the computed F in step C is 3.13; therefore, the null hypothesis would not be rejected.

one or two planned comparisons, the t-test may be applied for purposes of assessing the significance of the difference. The quantity

$$\text{lsd}(\alpha) = t_{1-\alpha/2}(N - g)\hat{\sigma}_w\sqrt{\frac{1}{n_i} + \frac{1}{n_{i'}}} \qquad (10.23)$$

is computed, where $t_{1-\alpha/2}(N - g)$ is from Table 5 of the Appendix, $\hat{\sigma}_w$ is from the analysis-of-variance table, n_i and $n_{i'}$ are the sample sizes for the ith and i'th groups being compared. The test procedure is now applied as described in Table 10.6.

Example 10.3.3.2.1. Suppose in Example 10.3.3.1.1 that the investigator was especially interested in the comparison of the intravenous and oral routes of administration. Using the least significant difference, is there evidence of a difference between these two routes of morphine administration at the 5% significance level? From Table 5 of the Appendix, $t_{0.975}(15)$ = 2.131, while from Table 10.13, $\hat{\sigma}_w^2 = 6.07$, $\bar{y}_{1+} = 10$, $\bar{y}_{4+} = 9.5$, $n_1 = 6$, and $n_4 = 4$. Hence, the mean difference is 0.5, while the least significant difference is computed as $(2.131)(\sqrt{6.07})(\sqrt{\frac{1}{6} + \frac{1}{4}}) = 3.39$. As 0.5 does not exceed the least significant difference of 3.39, there is no evidence to conclude that there is a difference between these two routes of administration.

Scheffé's procedure is easily adapted to accommodate unequal sample sizes. His procedure permits the comparison of linear functions of the means. For any linear contrast $\sum_{i=1}^{g}(C_i\bar{y}_{i+}$, where $\sum_{i=1}^{g}C_i = 0$, Scheffé's $(1 - \alpha)100\%$ confidence intervals for $\sum_{i=1}^{g}C_i\mu_i$ are given by

$$\sum_{i=1}^{g} C_i\bar{y}_{i+} \pm \hat{\sigma}_w\sqrt{(g - 1)F_{1-\alpha}((g - 1), N - g)\sum_{i=1}^{g}\frac{C_i^2}{n_i}}, \qquad (10.24)$$

where $F_{1-\alpha}((g - 1), N - g)$ is from Table 7 of the Appendix. The intervals given by (10.24) are simultaneous confidence intervals for all contrasts of the form $\sum_{i=1}^{g}C_i\mu_i$. The intervals are used and interpreted in the same fashion described in Table 10.9.

Example 10.3.3.2.2. Suppose in Example 10.3.3.1.1 that the investigators wish to place a 95% confidence interval on the difference of the mean response of the first three groups minus the mean of the fourth group using Scheffé's procedure. Clearly, $C_1 = C_2 = C_3 = \frac{1}{3}$, and $C_4 = -1$ is one set of contrast coefficients that measures this difference. From Table 10.13, we have $\hat{\sigma}_w = \sqrt{6.07} = 2.46$, $\frac{1}{3}\bar{y}_{1+} + \frac{1}{3}\bar{y}_{2+} + \frac{1}{3}\bar{y}_{3+} - \bar{y}_{4+} = 0.83$, and $g = 4$. As

$F_{0.95}(3, 15) = 3.29$ and $\sum_{i=1}^{4}(C_i^2/n_i) = 0.3185$, it follows that

$$\hat{\sigma}_w\sqrt{(g-1)F_{1-\alpha}(g-1, N-g)\left[\sum_{i=1}^{g}\frac{C_i^2}{n_i}\right]} = 4.37,$$

and the 95% confidence interval is $(-3.54, 5.20)$.

Note that in Example 10.3.3.2.2 the 95% confidence interval includes zero.

While data analysts often find Scheffé's procedure adequate in the unequal sample size situation, there have been discussions in the statistical literature regarding modifications of Tukey's procedure for unequal sample sizes.

Kramer (1956) proposed an extension of Tukey's procedure to test all pairwise comparisons of the g group means. This procedure is to simply perform Tukey's procedure with the n in Table 10.8 replaced by the harmonic mean of the sample sizes for the two groups being compared. Hence, to compare groups i and i', the $(1 - \alpha)100\%$ confidence interval for $\mu_i - \mu_{i'}$ is

$$(\bar{y}_{i+} - \bar{y}_{i'+}) \pm Q_\alpha(g, N-g)\hat{\sigma}_w\left[\frac{1}{2}\left(\frac{1}{n_i} + \frac{1}{n_{i'}}\right)\right]^{1/2}. \qquad (10.25)$$

In (10.25), $\hat{\sigma}_w$ is the square root of the mean square within groups in Table 10.11. This procedure is sometimes called the *Tukey–Kramer procedure*.

Example 10.3.3.2.3. For the morphine plasma data of Example 10.3.3.1.1, it is of interest to generate tests of all pairwise comparisons using (10.25). Using $\alpha = 0.05$, $Q_{0.05}(4, 15) = 4.08$, the following simultaneous confidence intervals are obtained:

Group vs. Group		$\bar{y}_{i+} - \bar{y}_{i'+}$	$Q_{0.05}(4, 15)\hat{\sigma}_w$ $[(1/n_i + 1/n_{i'})/2]^{1/2}$	95% Confidence Interval
1	2	$10 - 13 = -3$	4.588	$-7.588, 1.588$
1	3	$10 - 8 = 2$	4.304	$-2.304, 6.304$
1	4	$10 - 9.5 = 0.5$	4.588	$-4.088, 5.088$
2	3	$13 - 8 = 5$	4.768	$0.232, 9.768$
2	4	$13 - 9.5 = 3.5$	5.026	$-1.526, 8.526$
3	4	$8 - 9.5 = -1.5$	4.768	$-6.268, 3.268$

The conclusion from this table is that the means of groups 2 (mean = 13.0) and 3 (mean = 8.0) are significantly different.

This procedure is the recommended procedure for all pairwise comparisons in the one-way analysis of variance with unequal sample sizes. Dunnett (1980) has shown that the procedure performs quite well compared to its competitors. An excellent account of these studies and the competing procedures is given in Stoline (1981).

For the simultaneous estimation of all pairwise differences of means, the Tukey procedure for the case of equal sample sizes and the Tukey–Kramer procedure for unequal sample sizes are recommended (under the assumption that $\sigma_1^2 = \cdots = \sigma_g^2$, as stated in the original assumptions).

Extensions of Dunnett's procedure for comparison of all means to a control have also been proposed for the unbalanced design; however, these procedures are based on the multivariate t distribution and are not discussed further here. The reader may refer to Miller (1977) for a further account of this.

Bonferroni's procedure can be used for k comparisons by following the least-significant-difference procedure with α replaced by α/k. Again, this procedure would be most useful when a few comparisons, planned in advance, are to be made and none of the other procedures are applicable.

10.3.4 Analysis with Subsamples

Suppose in Example 10.3.2.1.1 that the investigators actually studied each animal on two separate occasions. Furthermore, assume that those two separate measurements for each animal may be regarded as an independent replication of the same experiment. Hence, in this type of experiment, the linear additive model (10.3) perhaps should be revised to read

$$y_{ijk} = \mu + \tau_i + e_{ij} + \delta_{ijk} \quad \text{for } i = 1, \ldots, g;$$

$$j = 1, 2, \ldots, n; \ k = 1, 2, \ldots, r, \tag{10.26}$$

where μ is the grand mean, τ_i is the group effect for the ith group, e_{ij} is the random effect associated with animal-to-animal variability, while δ_{ijk} is the random effect of the replicate measurements made on the jth animal in group i. In this case, the number of replications is $r = 2$. The animal-to-animal source of variability and the replicate variability are assumed to act independently of one another. The basic data may be summarized in the form of Table 10.14.

Table 10.14. Data Layout for Completely Random Design with Subsamples

Experimental Unit	Group 1				...	Group g		
	Replicate					Replicate		
	1	2	...	r	...	1	2	...	r
1	y_{111}	y_{112}	...	y_{11r}	...	y_{g11}	y_{g12}	...	y_{g1r}
2	y_{121}	y_{122}	...	y_{12r}	...				
$\vdots$	$\vdots$	$\vdots$		$\vdots$		$\vdots$	$\vdots$		$\vdots$
n	y_{1n1}	y_{1n2}	...	y_{1nr}	...	y_{gn1}	y_{gn2}	...	y_{gnr}

Denoting the various group, animal, and grand totals by

$$y_{i++} = \sum_{j=1}^{n} \sum_{k=1}^{r} y_{ijk} \quad \text{for } i = 1, 2, \ldots, g,$$

$$y_{ij+} = \sum_{k=1}^{r} y_{ijk} \quad \text{for } i = 1, 2, \ldots, g; \; j = 1, 2, \ldots, n, \quad (10.27)$$

$$y_{+++} = \sum_{i=1}^{g} \sum_{j=1}^{n} \sum_{k=1}^{r} y_{ijk},$$

then the total sum of squares may be written as

$$\text{SST} = \sum_{i=1}^{g} \sum_{j=1}^{n} \sum_{k=1}^{r} y_{ijk}^2 - \frac{y_{+++}^2}{gnr}. \quad (10.28)$$

Also, Equation (10.28) may be partitioned into three components, namely, SSB with $g - 1$, SSE with $g(n - 1)$, and SSR with $gn(r - 1)$ degrees of freedom. These are the between-group variability, the experimental unit variability within groups, and the replicate variability. In the notation of Table 10.14, they are computed by

$$\text{SSB} = \sum_{i=1}^{g} \frac{y_{i++}^2}{nr} - \frac{y_{+++}^2}{gnr},$$

$$\text{SSS} = \sum_{i=1}^{g} \sum_{j=1}^{n} \frac{y_{ij+}^2}{r} - \frac{y_{+++}^2}{gnr},$$

$$\text{SSE} = \text{SSS} - \text{SSB},$$

$$\text{SSR} = \text{SST} - \text{SSS}. \quad (10.29)$$

Table 10.15. Analysis of Variance for CRD with Subsampling[a]

Source	d.f.	SS	MS	F
Between groups	$g - 1$	SSB	$MSB = \dfrac{SSB}{g - 1}$	$\dfrac{MSB}{MSE}$
Experimental units within groups	$g(n - 1)$	SSE	$MSE = \dfrac{SSE}{g(n - 1)}$	$\dfrac{MSE}{MSR}$
Replicates on experimental units	$gn(r - 1)$	SSR	$MSR = \dfrac{SSR}{gn(r - 1)}$	
Total	$gnr - 1$	SST		

[a]SST is defined by (10.28); SSB, SSE, SSR by (10.29).

The sums of squares and degrees of freedom may then be summarized as in Table 10.15.

The F ratios in Table 10.15 may be used to test hypotheses of interest. In particular, in order to test

$$H_0: \mu_1 = \mu_2 = \cdots = \mu_g \quad \text{versus} \quad H_a: \text{Not all } \mu_i \text{ equal,} \quad (10.30)$$

the F ratio MSB/MSE may be compared to $F_{1-\alpha}(g - 1, g(n - 1))$. If it exceeds this value, the null hypothesis would be rejected at the α level of significance. In order to determine if the experimental unit variability is greater than the replicate variability, the quantity MSE/MSR may be compared to $F_{1-\alpha}(g(n - 1), gn(r - 1))$. One ordinarily expects this quantity to be significant, as the experimental units are generally more variable than the measurement or sampling variability.

Example 10.3.4.1. Suppose the data of Example 10.3.2.1.1 were as follows:

Group A		Group B		Group C		Group D		Group E	
1, 2	Total	1, 2	Total	1, 2	Total	1, 2	Total	1, 2	Total
8, 12	20	10, 14	24	2, 16	18	12, 16	28	9, 11	20
1, 7	8	9, 11	20	2, 6	8	8, 10	18	5, 7	12
3, 9	12	12, 14	26	2, 6	8	10, 10	20	7, 9	16
6, 2	8	4, 10	14	4, 6	10	11, 11	22	3, 5	8
y_{i++}	48		84		44		88		56
$\bar{y}_{i++}$	6		10.5		5.5		11		7

Test the equal-group-means hypothesis at $\alpha = 0.05$. Clearly, we have

$$y_{+++} = 320, \qquad \bar{y}_{+++} = 8,$$

$$\text{SST} = 8^2 + \cdots + 5^2 - \frac{(320)^2}{40} = 620,$$

$$\text{SSS} = \frac{20^2 + \cdots + 8^2}{2} - \frac{(320)^2}{40} = 404,$$

$$\text{SSB} = \frac{48^2 + \cdots + 56^2}{8} - \frac{(320)^2}{40} = 212,$$

$$\text{SSR} = 620 - 404 = 216,$$
$$\text{SSE} = 404 - 212 = 192.$$

Hence,

ANALYSIS OF VARIANCE

Source	d.f.	SS	MS	F
Between groups	4	212	53.0	4.14
Experimental units in groups	15	192	12.8	1.19
Replicates in experimental units	20	216	10.8	
Total	39	620		

Therefore, since $F_{0.95}(4, 15) = 3.06$, it follows that there is a significant difference between the group means at the 5% level. As $F_{0.95}(15, 20) = 2.20$, the indication is that the replicate error and experimental unit error are of the same order of magnitude. This is typically not the case.

The methods of the section are particularly useful in situations in which duplicate or triplicate measurements are made of a response variable.

10.4 ANALYSIS OF VARIANCE FOR RANDOMIZED COMPLETE BLOCK DESIGNS

10.4.1 General Aspects of Problem

The basic data layout of the randomized complete block design is as described in Table 10.16. The basic design consists of grouping individuals into blocks and then assigning treatments at random within each block. The

Table 10.16. Data Layout for Randomized Complete Block Design Group

Block	Group 1	Group 2	$\cdots$	g	Total	Mean
1	y_{11}	y_{21}	$\cdots$	y_{g1}	y_{+1}	$\bar{y}_{+1}$
2	y_{12}	y_{22}	$\cdots$	y_{g2}	y_{+2}	$\bar{y}_{+2}$
$\vdots$	$\vdots$	$\vdots$		$\vdots$	$\vdots$	$\vdots$
n	y_{1n}	y_{2n}	$\cdots$	y_{gn}	y_{+n}	$\bar{y}_{+n}$
Total	y_{1+}	y_{2+}	$\cdots$	y_{g+}	y_{++}	$\bar{y}_{++}$
Mean	$\bar{y}_{1+}$	$\bar{y}_{2+}$	$\cdots$	$\bar{y}_{g+}$		

main requirement is that each treatment appears exactly once in each block, although, this can be relaxed for more complex designs not discussed here.

This design is the matched-pairs design in the case in which $g = 2$. Like the matched-pair design, the main purpose of the design is to remove the block-to-block variability from the unexplained variability. The total sum of squares for Table 10.16 is given by

$$\text{SST} = \sum_{i=1}^{g} \sum_{j=1}^{n} (y_{ij} - \bar{y}_{++})^2. \tag{10.31}$$

Furthermore, it may be demonstrated that

$$\sum_{i=1}^{g} \sum_{j=1}^{n} (y_{ij} - \bar{y}_{++})^2 = \sum_{i=1}^{g} n(\bar{y}_{i+} - \bar{y}_{++})^2 + \sum_{j=1}^{n} g(\bar{y}_{+j} - \bar{y}_{++})^2$$

$$+ \sum_{i=1}^{g} \sum_{j=1}^{n} (y_{ij} - \bar{y}_{i+} - \bar{y}_{+j} + \bar{y}_{++})^2,$$

that is, the total sum of squares may be additively partitioned into a sum of squares for groups, a sum of square for blocks, and a sum-of-squares residual (or unexplained). These sums of squares measure the heterogeneity of various aspects of the data. The sum of squares for groups is a measure of the failure of the group means to be the same, the sum of squares for blocks is a measure of the failure of the block means to be the same, while the residual sum of squares may be viewed as a measure of the failure of the group differences to be the same for all blocks. A *linear additive model* for the y_{ij} may be written as

$$y_{ij} = \mu + \tau_i + \beta_j + e_{ij}, \tag{10.32}$$

where μ is the grand mean, τ_i is the effect due to the ith group, β_j is the effect due to the jth block, and e_{ij} is the random error.

In order to proceed with the analysis, we require the following assumptions for the data of Table 10.16.

1. The data in Table 10.16 conform to model (10.32).   (10.33)
2. The e_{ij}'s in (10.32) are independently normally distributed with mean zero and variance σ^2. (Randomization ensures the independence of the e_{ij}'s; normality and equality of variance are assumed.)

10.4.2   Analysis of Variance

It is generally of interest to draw an inference regarding the group mean differences; hence for model (10.32) the hypotheses are stated as

$$H_0: \tau_1 = \cdots = \tau_g \quad \text{versus} \quad H_a: \text{Groups not all equal.} \tag{10.34}$$

Computationally, the various sums of squares are best computed by the formulas

$$\text{SST} = \sum_{i=1}^{g} \sum_{j=1}^{n} y_{ij}^2 - \frac{y_{++}^2}{gn} \quad \text{(total)};$$

$$\text{SSB} = \sum_{i=1}^{g} \frac{y_{i+}^2}{n} - \frac{y_{++}^2}{ng} \quad \text{(between groups)};$$

$$\text{SSBL} = \sum_{j=1}^{n} \frac{y_{+j}^2}{g} - \frac{y_{++}^2}{ng} \quad \text{(between block means)};$$

$$\text{SSE} = \text{SST} - \text{SSB} - \text{SSBL} \ (\text{residual or error}). \tag{10.35}$$

Their respective degrees of freedom are $gn - 1$, $g - 1$, $n - 1$, and $(g - 1)(n - 1)$. We summarize the analysis-of-variance F-test procedure in Table 10.17.

Example 10.4.2.1.   A comparative study of four methods of treating hyperactive boys was undertaken. Sixteen boys were chosen for the study and were first grouped on the basis of several factors, including age, length of illness, and severity of illness. The four treatments, A, B, C, and D, were then randomly assigned to one of the four boys in each block. The boys were rated by their school teachers using a structured schedule for assessment of hyperactivity. The resulting hyperactivity scores at the end of the treatment period are:

		Treatments			
Block	A	B	C	D	Total
1	41	61	62	43	207
2	48	68	62	48	226
3	53	70	66	53	242
4	56	72	70	52	250
Total	198	271	260	196	925
Mean	49.5	67.7	65.0	49.0	

The hyperactivity scores are scaled from 1 to 100, ranging from no evidence of hyperactivity to severe hyperactivity. Is there evidence at $\alpha = 0.05$ to conclude that the methods of treatment differ?

Following the procedures of Table 10.17, one readily obtains the following:

$$SST = 41^2 + \cdots + 52^2 - \frac{(925)^2}{16} = 1492.4375,$$

$$SSB = \frac{198^2 + \cdots + 196^2}{4} - \frac{(925)^2}{16} = 1188.6875,$$

$$SSBL = \frac{207^2 + \cdots + 250^2}{4} - \frac{(925)^2}{16} = 270.6875,$$

$$SSE = 33.0625.$$

Hence, the analysis-of-variance table that results is:

ANALYSIS OF VARIANCE

Source	d.f.	SS	MS	F
Between groups	3	1188.6875	396.229	107.86
Between blocks	3	270.6875	90.229	
Residual	9	33.0625	3.6736	
Total	15	1492.4375		

From Table 7 of the Appendix, one obtains $F_{0.95}(3, 9) = 3.86$; hence, there is a highly significant difference in the treatment methods.

10.4.3 Multiple Comparisons

The multiple-comparison procedures discussed in Section 10.3.2.2 may be applied as indicated there with one exception. The exception is that the

Table 10.17. Outline of F-Test for Equal-Means Hypothesis for Randomized Complete Block Design

A. Data: y_{ij}, $i = 1, 2, \ldots, g$; $j = 1, \ldots, n$, from Table 10.16.
B. Assumptions: Stated by (10.33).
C. Computations: Using formulas (10.35), compute the following analysis-of-variance table:

Analysis of Variance

Source	d.f.	SS	MS	F
Between groups	$g - 1$	SSB	$\text{MSB} = \dfrac{\text{SSB}}{g-1}$	$\dfrac{\text{MSB}}{\text{MSE}}$
Between blocks	$n - 1$	SSBL	$\text{MSBL} = \dfrac{\text{SSBL}}{n-1}$	
Residual or error	$(g-1)(n-1)$	SSE	$\text{MSE} = \dfrac{\text{SSE}}{(g-1)(n-1)}$	
Total	$gn - 1$	SST		

D. Statistical test:
   1. Null hypothesis: H_0: $\tau_1 = \cdots = \tau_g$.
   2. Alternative hypothesis: H_a: Not all equal.
   3. Decision rule for an α-level test: Reject H_0 in favor of H_a if F in step C exceeds $F_{1-\alpha}(g - 1, (g - 1)(n - 1))$.

error term, s^2, is MSE from Table 10.17 with degrees of freedom given by $(g - 1)(n - 1)$. For convenience, the revised procedures are written below with $s = \sqrt{\text{MSE}}$:

$$\text{lsd}(\alpha) = s\sqrt{2/n}\, t_{1-\alpha/2}[(g - 1)(n - 1)] \quad \text{(least significant difference)};$$

$$(10.36)$$

$$D_{1-\alpha} = s\sqrt{2/n}\, C_{1-\alpha}(g - 1, (g - 1)(n - 1)) \quad \text{(Dunnett's procedure)};$$

$$(10.37)$$

$$T_\alpha = s\sqrt{1/n}\, Q_\alpha(g, (g - 1)(n - 1)) \quad \text{(Tukey's procedure)}; \quad (10.38)$$

$$\sum_{i=1}^{g} C_i \bar{y}_{i+} \pm s\sqrt{(g - 1) F_{1-\alpha}(g - 1, (g - 1)(n - 1)) \left[\sum_{i=1}^{g} \frac{C_i^2}{n} \right]}$$

$$\text{(Scheffé's procedure)}. \quad (10.39)$$

The procedures are otherwise used and interpreted in the same manner as described in Section 10.3.2.2.

Applying Tukey's procedure, for example, to the data of Example 10.4.2.1 yields $T_{0.05} = (4.42)\sqrt{3.673}\sqrt{\frac{1}{4}} = 4.24$. The pairwise absolute mean differences are $A - B = 18.2^*$, $A - C = 15.5^*$, $A - D = 0.5$, $B - C = 2.7$, $B - D = 18.7^*$ and $C - D = 16.0^*$, with the significant ones denoted by asterisks.

10.4.4 A Word about Assumptions

With the CRD, the homogeneity of variance can be checked by examining the within-group variances. With the RCBD, it is a little more difficult to detect departures from the homogeneity of errors assumption. One possible guideline is to inspect the MSBL term. If it is very highly significant when compared to the MSE, this may indicate departures from homogeneity.

Strictly speaking, the analysis-of-variance techniques are justified when the assumptions of independence, normality, and equal variance hold. However, mild departures from these assumptions still produce reliable results. This property of the analysis of variance is called robustness. The normality assumption does not need to hold exactly provided the sample size is large, at least 20 observations per population. The assumption of variance homogeneity is most important for the correct analysis of the data. In case of heterogeneity of the variance, the data might be transformed using the square root, the natural logarithm, or some other mathematical function to obtain variance homogeneous data. This transformation can also improve the normality of data.

Another option to analyze the data is to use nonparametric methods, as presented in Chapter 11. Special attention should also be given to the way the observations are generated to assure independence of the data. If successive observations tend to be correlated, then special techniques should be used to perform the analysis. The reader may refer to Neter, Wasserman, and Kutner (1985) for a further account of this topic.

10.5 SAMPLE SIZE CONSIDERATIONS

We only discuss the problem of sample size determination for the completely random design with an equal n per group. Often, one is interested in determining sample size requirements for each treatment group. Since σ^2, the underlying common variance, is usually unknown, the common procedure for sample size determination is to specify the mean difference of

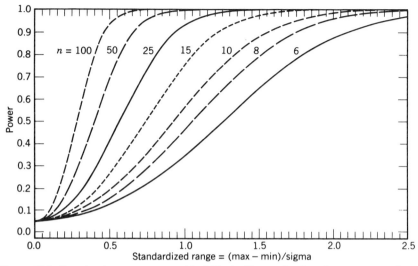

Figure 10.1. Sample sizes per group with 0.05 significance level and two groups (from Kastenbaum et al., 1970, by permission of authors and publishers).

interest in standard deviation units. Kastenbaum, Hoel, and Bowman (1970) have generated tables for such situations and have expressed these as a function of the maximum minus minimum mean difference in standard deviation units. This difference is termed the *standardized range* in Figures 10.1–10.5. These figures correspond to tests at the 0.05 significance level, and have been computer generated from the formulae of Kastenbaum et al. (1979). Each curve on the figures indicate the number of experimental units per treatment group. Figure 10.1 corresponds to the sample size figure referred to in Chapter 6 when discussing sample size requirements for the two-sample *t*-test. Several examples will illustrate the use of these figures.

Example 10.5.1. For a study to compare the systolic blood pressure (SBP) of two groups of patients according to treatment, it is necessary to define the corresponding sample size to be able to detect a difference assuming the SBP means for the two populations are $\mu_1 = 110$ and $\mu_2 = 130$.

From other studies in systolic blood pressure, it is known that the population variance for patients given the same treatment is $\sigma^2 = 400$. Then the number of patients to be assigned to each group to detect a difference with power equal to 0.75 and $\alpha = 0.05$ can be read from Figure 10.1, with a standardized range of $(130 - 110)/20 = 1.0$. The recommended sample sizes are between the $n = 15$ and $n = 10$ curves. Hence, $n_1 = 13$ and $n_2 = 13$ are approximate sample sizes.

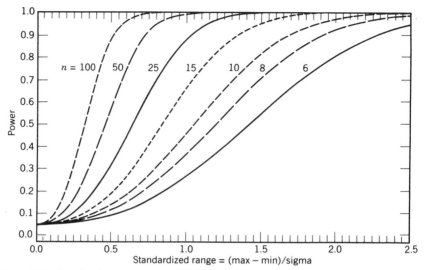

Figure 10.2. Sample sizes per group with 0.05 significance level and three groups (from Kastenbaum et al., 1970, by permission of authors and publishers).

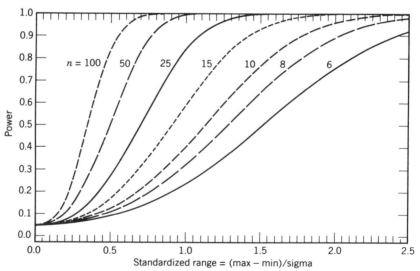

Figure 10.3. Sample sizes per group with 0.05 significance level and four groups (from Kastenbaum et al., 1970, by permission of authors and publishers).

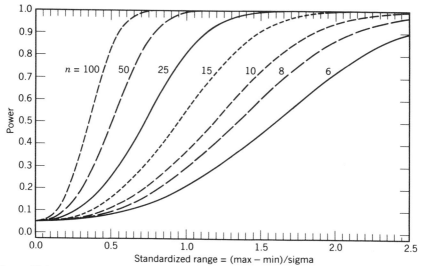

Figure 10.4. Sample sizes per group with 0.05 significance level and five groups (from Kastenbaum et al., 1970, by permission of authors and publishers).

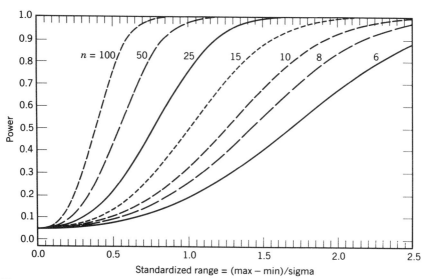

Figure 10.5. Sample sizes per group with 0.05 significance level and six groups (from Kastenbaum et al., 1970, by permission of authors and publishers).

355

Example 10.5.2. If in the former example the investigator has available only six subjects per treatment, then it is interesting to find the power available to detect a difference ($\alpha = 0.05$) given the same parametric values. The standardized range is 1.0 as before. Then, from Figure 10.1, reading the power value in the vertical axis corresponding to the $n = 6$ curve and to a standardized range equal to 1 gives 0.37 approximately as the power available to find a significant difference.

Example 10.5.3. From a pilot study it is known that the mean values of four treatment groups are $\mu_1 = 100$, $\mu_2 = 94$, $\mu_3 = 110$, and $\mu_4 = 105$, with a common variance $\sigma^2 = 225$. Now it is required to determine the group sample sizes to be able to detect a difference among the four group means with a 0.85 power and $\alpha = 0.05$. The value of the standardized range is (max-min)$/\sigma = (110 - 94)/15 = 1.07$; then, using Figure 10.3, with power equal to 0.85, we find that the group sample size is between the curves $n = 25$ and $n = 15$. A conservative approach could be to take $n_1 = n_2 = n_3 = n_4 = 25$.

Example 10.5.4. If in Example 10.5.3 there are only 15 patients available per treatment group, then we can evaluate the power attained with these sample sizes. Reading the curve $n = 15$ in Figure 10.3, we have that for a standardized range equal to 1.06 the power to reject the null hypothesis H_0: $\mu_1 = \mu_2 = \mu_3 = \mu_4$ is approximately 0.69.

10.6 GRAPHICAL DISPLAY OF MEANS

Often it is useful to plot means and measures of variability for each treatment group. One alternative is to plot $\bar{x} \pm$ s.e., where s.e. is the standard error of $\bar{x}$. Consider the following hypothetical example.

Example 10.6.1. The change in volume of an original meal left in the stomach of nine healthy dogs treated with six different drugs results in the mean values and standard errors given in Table 10.18. The analysis of variance for this randomized complete block design yielded an MSE $= 144$ with 40 degrees of freedom $[(6 - 1)(9 - 1)]$.

Applying Tukey's procedure to this data, with $s = 12$, $Q_{0.05}(6, 40) = 4.23$ and $T_{0.05} = 12\sqrt{\frac{1}{9}}(4.23) = 16.92$, gives the following results: all the pairwise comparisons are significant, except the differences between treatments 1 and 5, 2 and 5, 2 and 6, and 3 and 4. The one-standard-error intervals are

Table 10.18. Mean and Standard Errors (s.e.) by Treatment Group

	Treatment Group					
	1	2	3	4	5	6
n	9	9	9	9	9	9
$\bar{x}$	123	141	55	50	129	148
s.e.	3.5	4.6	3.8	4.4	4.3	3.4

(119.5–126.5), (136.4–145.6), (51.2–58.8), (45.6–54.4), (124.7–133.3), and (144.6–151.4), respectively. The plot of these intervals is presented in Figure 10.6.

We note that the intervals for treatments 2 and 5 do not overlap while according to Tukey's procedure these treatments are not significantly different. Thus, to have consistency between similar means and interval overlaps and also to guarantee that significantly different means have intervals that do not overlap, it is necessary to use a simultaneous measure of variability

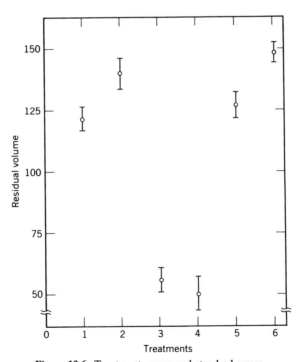

Figure 10.6. Treatment means and standard errors.

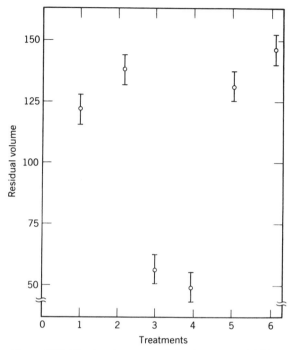

Figure 10.7. Treatment means and simultaneous variability.

for the means. One solution is to use intervals based on those resulting from Tukey's procedure, that is,

$$\bar{x} \pm \tfrac{1}{2}Q_\alpha(g, g(n - 1))s\sqrt{1/n}, \qquad (10.40)$$

where $s = \sqrt{MSE}$, n is the number of observations in each mean, and Q is the α percent critical value of the studentized range statistic from Table 14 of the Appendix. Applying expression (10.40) with $Q = 4.23$, $s = 12$, and $n = 9$ to the means in Table 10.18, we obtain the treatment group intervals (114.54–131.46), (132.54–149.46), (46.54–63.46), (41.54–58.46), (120.54–137.46), and (139.54–156.46), as shown in Figure 10.7.

Thus, if the analyst wants to plot means with "error bars," in which nonoverlapping bars correspond to significant differences, then intervals of the form of (10.40) can be used. On the other hand, if it is of interest to plot $\bar{x} \pm$ s.e., the analyst should be aware that nonoverlapping intervals do not imply that the means are different. If such an interpretation is to be required of the graph, then intervals based on the appropriate multiple-comparison procedure should be plotted (Andrews et al., 1980).

10.7 SUMMARY

The analyses described in this chapter provide a fairly broad set of statistical techniques for the comparison of g means. Of the assumptions made in the chapter, by far the most important is that of homogeneity of variance. If this assumption is not met, then it is advisable to apply one of the variance-equalizing transformations discussed in Chapter 6. The analysis-of-variance and the multiple-comparison procedures are somewhat sensitive to deviations from the assumption of equal variance.

While the analysis of variance is a fundamental statistical procedure for the partition of a total sum of squares into recognized sources of variation, the situations considered in this chapter represent the simplest applications of the procedure. The technique extends to more complex experimental designs, and a full account of these extensions is presented in Cochran and Cox (1957). For unbalanced designs, the more general approach to the comparison of means is based on the general linear regression model (see Kleinbaum and Kupper, 1978), from which the analysis of variance is obtained as a special case. The interested reader may also consult Neter et al. (1985) for further details.

The multiple-comparison methods presented in this chapter are recommended, and most of them are included in statistical software like SAS and BMDP. Dunnett's procedure is useful to compare several treatments with a control but requires equal sample sizes to use the critical values in Table 13 of the Appendix. For pairwise comparisons, Tukey's procedure produces narrower confidence intervals than the competing procedure of Scheffé. This last method is the most appropriate to explore the data using contrasts defined after examining the data. Since Scheffé's method covers all the possible comparisons of the means, it assures a minimum confidence coefficient of at least $1 - \alpha$. The least-significant-difference procedure should be used only for one or two planned comparisons. For a few comparisons for which none of the procedures apply, Bonferroni's procedure can be used. Further discussion of multiple comparisons is found in Miller (1981, 1977).

Computational procedures to generate analysis of experimental design models are included in many statistical packages. Procedures like ANOVA and GLM of SAS can be used for the type of models presented in this chapter. More advanced techniques are included in these programs, allowing, for example, for the presence of different treatment effects per block in a RCBD. This is called treatment-by-block interaction. When this interaction is large, the main treatment effects cannot be evaluated simply because those effects will depend on the block effect. A data transformation may remove such interaction.

In the BMDP statistical package, there are also several programs to analyze numerically the ANOVA and multiple-comparison problems.

PROBLEMS

10.1. The measure of the percentage of fat content in hens under four different types of diet—is given in the following table.

ID	Control Diet	ID	Diet I	ID	Diet II	ID	Diet III
1	13.6	7	12.9	13	23.0	19	12.3
2	22.9	8	22.7	14	23.3	20	22.4
3	13.5	9	22.6	15	23.1	21	22.5
4	13.7	10	12.5	16	13.2	22	12.5
5	23.4	11	12.7	17	12.9	23	22.6
6	23.5	12	12.4	18	23.2	24	12.2

(a) Perform an analysis of variance of this data.

(b) Use Dunnett's procedure to compare the diets with the control group.

10.2. Three groups of 10 young volunteers each were observed in a study to assess the number of errors made during a simple arithmetic task while working under different levels of noise. The results of the study are shown in the next table.

ID	Continuous Low Noise	ID	Continuous Intermediate Noise	ID	Intermittent Intermediate Noise
10	4	20	9	30	8
11	3	21	10	31	14
12	5	22	8	32	10
13	3	23	9	33	16
14	2	24	11	34	9
15	4	25	6	35	12
16	3	26	8	36	15
17	3	27	10	37	14
18	6	28	10	38	18
19	4	29	7	39	16

(a) Perform multiple comparisons of the means of these three groups using Tukey's procedure for an overall α value of 0.05; comment on the results observed.

(b) Suggest another design to assess the effect of noise—continuous and intermittent—on the response variable.

10.3. In a trial to test a new anti-inflammatory drug (X) at four doses versus a certain aspirin dose and a placebo, the same number of rheumatoid arthritis patients are randomly allocated to these six treatment groups for a period of time. Due to several reasons, the number of patients that completed the trial in each group are not equal. A pooled index used to measure the treatment effectiveness to improve the symptoms is given in the next table.

Placebo	Aspirin (20 mg)	Dose 1 X(10 mg)	Dose 2 X(15 mg)	Dose 3 X(20 mg)	Dose 4 X(25 mg)
6.2	17.1	5.2	16.4	35.2	41.8
5.8	26.6	5.3	17.9	30.4	45.2
9.5	21.8	6.9	18.3	37.2	43.2
10.2	26.1	5.8	19.5	29.5	46.5
8.3	25.4	6.6	16.9	34.6	41.7
7.9	19.8	—	17.5	31.9	
9.2	21.5	—	19.1		
11.6	23.5	—	18.8		
8.9	24.8	—	17.1		
—	23.5				
—	25.7				

(a) Obtain an analysis-of-variance table.

(b) Compare the means of the treatment groups using the Tukey–Kramer procedure; comment on the results.

10.4. Monkeys with induced high blood pressure due to a surgical procedure in their kidneys were randomly allocated to one of four antihypertensive drugs. The changes in systolic blood pressure are indicated in the table; unequal sample sizes resulted due to surgical failure (change = before–after drug).

Drug 1	Drug 2	Drug 3	Drug 4
15	6	28	19
19	7	30	18
12	10	24	16
21	7	25	21
16	10	29	23
20		28	20
13			18
			17

(a) Obtain an analysis-of-variance table.

(b) Use the Tukey–Kramer procedure for pairwise comparisons.

10.5. Seven patients with moderate hypertension who had learned to measure their own blood pressure with a sphygmomanometer and a stethoscope entered a pilot study to evaluate their blood pressure at home in the mornings and evenings for 10 days. Measures were made while lying, then after 2 min standing. The mean values of the observed systolic blood pressure (SBP) are:

Subject	Morning Lying	Morning Standing	Evening Lying	Evening Standing
1	143	148	152	157
2	144	149	151	152
3	141	153	155	155
4	135	141	149	156
5	153	157	163	165
6	152	139	165	168
7	159	157	162	166

Use the Tukey and least-significant-difference procedures to study the effect of time of day for each position of the subject on their measure of SBP.

10.6. To measure the strength of the trunk flexor muscle, the time was measured in seconds for 40 boys and 40 girls aged 3–6 years while doing three types of exercises. The test score means are:

	Boys			Girls		
Age	Exercise 1	Exercise 2	Exercise 3	Exercise 1	Exercise 2	Exercise 3
3	18.8	25.2	33.5	16.4	27.9	31.2
4	20.2	27.3	39.6	24.1	30.1	37.3
5	27.2	19.4	42.4	32.9	34.2	44.3
6	30.3	29.5	49.6	35.5	35.5	47.8

Compare exercises within sex using Scheffé's method.

REFERENCES

Andrews, H. P., R. D. Snee, and M. H. Sarner. (1980). Graphical display of means, *Am. Statist.*, **34**, 195–199.

Cochran, W. G., and G. M. Cox. (1957). *Experimental Design*, Wiley, New York.

Dunnett, C. W. (1964). New tables for multiple comparisons with a control, *Biometrics*, **20**, 482–491.

Dunnett, C. W. (1980). Pairwise multiple comparisons in the homogeneous variance, unequal sample size case, *JASA*, **75**, 789–795.

Kastenbaum, M., D. G. Hoel, and K. O. Bowman, (1970). Sample size requirements: One-way analysis of variance, *Biometrika*, **57**, 421–430.

Kleinbaum, D. G., and L. L. Kupper, (1978). *Applied Regression Analysis and Other Multivariable Methods*, Duxbury, North Scituate MA.

Kramer, C. Y. (1956). Extension of multiple range tests to group means with unequal numbers of replications, *Biometrics*, **12**, 307–310.

Miller, R. G. (1977). Developments in multiple comparisons: 1966–1976, *JASA*, **72**, 779–788.

Miller, R. G. (1981). *Simultaneous Statistical Inference*, Springer-Verlag, New York.

Neter, J., W. Wasserman, M. H. Kutner, (1985). *Applied Linear Statistical Models*, 2nd ed. Irwin, Homewood, ILL.

Scheffé, H. (1953). A method for judging all contrasts in the analysis of variance, *Biometrika*, **40**, 87–104.

Stoline, M. R. (1981). The status of multiple comparisons: Simultaneous estimation of all pairwise comparisons in one-way ANOVA designs, *Am. Statist.*, **35**, 134–141.

Tukey, J. W. (1953). *The problem of multiple comparisons*, Department of Mathematics, Princeton University, (manuscript).

Young, J. P. R., M. H. Lader, and W. C. Hughes (1979). Controlled trial of trimipramine, monoamine oxidase inhibitors, and combined treatment in depressed outpatients, *Br. Med. J.*, **6201**(2), 1315–1317.

Comparing More Than Two Groups of Observations: Rank Analysis of Variance for Group Comparisons

11.1 INTRODUCTION

The previous chapter discussed statistical inference procedures for the situation in which data followed a normal distribution. In many cases, the assumption of normality may not be safely made; thus, this chapter introduces nonparametric techniques for comparing several groups. It is assumed that the data are continuous or at least can be ranked. These procedures are multiple-group generalizations of the rank tests discussed in Chapter 6.

As in Chapter 10, the completely random design and the randomized complete block designs are discussed in Chapter 11. The general design assumptions and comments regarding multiple comparisons, which were raised in Chapter 10, also apply in this chapter. All tests in Chapter 11 are large-sample tests, meaning that the tests require large sample sizes for their validity.

11.2 RANK ANALYSIS OF VARIANCE FOR COMPLETELY RANDOM DESIGNS

11.2.1 General Aspects of Problem

The basic data layout for the completely random design (CRD) is given in Table 11.1. The entry y_{ij} is the jth observation or replicate in group i ($i = 1, 2, \ldots, g$; $j = 1, \ldots, n_i$).

Table 11.1. Data Layout for Completely Random Design

Group 1	Group 2	$\cdots$	Group g
y_{11}	y_{21}	$\cdots$	y_{g1}
$\vdots$	$\vdots$		$\vdots$
y_{1n_1}	y_{2n_2}	$\cdots$	y_{gn_g}

Following the general line of reasoning of Chapter 10, it is assumed that the *linear additive model* for y_{ij} is

$$y_{ij} = \mu_i + e_{ij}, \tag{11.1}$$

where μ_i is the mean for the ith group, while e_{ij} is a random error that comes from some distribution with a zero mean and variance σ^2. Furthermore, the e_{ij} are independently distributed. The distribution of each e_{ij} (hence y_{ij}) is also assumed to be a continuous distribution, but we do not require it to be the normal distribution. As in the preceding chapter, we assume that the observations in the g groups are distributed independently of one another, a condition that is met by completely random assignment of individuals to groups.

The main inference question is whether the g groups differ in the responses, y, that they produce. To this end, the problem may be formulated in the context of model (11.1):

$$H_0: \mu_1 = \cdots = \mu_g \quad \text{versus} \quad H_a: \text{Not all equal.} \tag{11.2}$$

Without further assumptions on the y_{ij}'s, such as normality, a good procedure is to use the rank order of the observations. Referring to Section 6.3.2, the Wilcoxon–Mann–Whitney rank sum test arose by considering the ranks of the observations in the two groups. This procedure is generalized here to the case of g groups. The ranking procedure is quite straightforward. The smallest observation in the g groups receives the rank of 1, the next largest receives the rank of 2, and so on, until finally the largest observation receives the rank of N where $N = n_1 + n_2 + \cdots + n_g$. These ranks replace the original observations of Table 11.1; subsequent analysis will use these ranks. Thus, the ranks of the data of Table 11.1 may be summarized in tabular form as in Table 11.2.

In Table 11.2, R_{ij} is the rank of observation y_{ij} among the entire set of N observations. The total quantities in the table are defined by

$$R_{i+} = \sum_{j=1}^{n_i} R_{ij}, \qquad R_{++} = \sum_{i=1}^{g} R_{i+}, \tag{11.3}$$

Table 11.2. Ranks of Data of Table 11.1

	Group 1	Group 2	$\cdots$	Group g	
	R_{11}	R_{21}	$\cdots$	R_{g1}	
	$\vdots$	$\vdots$		$\vdots$	
	R_{1n_1}	R_{2n_2}	$\cdots$	R_{gn_g}	
Total	R_{1+}	R_{2+}	$\cdots$	R_{g+}	R_{++}
Mean	$\bar{R}_{1+}$	$\bar{R}_{2+}$	$\cdots$	$\bar{R}_{g+}$	$\bar{R}_{++}$

while

$$\bar{R}_{i+} = R_{i+}/n_i, \qquad \bar{R}_{++} = R_{++}/N. \tag{11.4}$$

Under the null hypothesis, each of $N!/n_1! \cdots !n_g!$ possible assignments of ranks to the observations is equally likely; thus, for each of these assignments, it is possible to compute some measure of difference between the groups. One measure of distance that seems reasonable is to compare the $\bar{R}_{i+}$. Intuitively, if the null hypothesis is true, one would expect these g mean ranks to be close to one another. One measure of distance between these mean ranks is the Kruskal–Wallis (1952) statistic.

11.2.2 Kruskal–Wallis Test

The *Kruskal–Wallis test* statistic for H_0 is a measure of difference between the mean ranks. It is quite like the between-group sum of squares (SSB) of the last chapter. The following statistic is the one proposed by Kruskal and Wallis (1952):

$$K = \frac{12}{N(N+1)} \sum_{i=1}^{g} n_i (\bar{R}_{i+} - \bar{R}_{++})^2. \tag{11.5}$$

Strictly speaking, the null-hypothesis sampling distribution of K depends on the configuration of sample sizes $(n_1, \ldots, n_g)$; thus, exact tables are generally available for various special cases, for example, $g = 3$ or $n_1 = n_2 = \cdots = n_g = n$. Such tables may be found in specialized texts on nonparametric methods such as Hollander and Wolfe (1973). Fortunately, there is a large-sample approximation to K. In particular, under the null hypothesis, the sampling distribution of K is approximately a chi-square with $g - 1$ d.f. This approximation is a good approximation if N is large and the smallest n_i is not too small (each at least 5).

If there are tied observations, the midrank procedure of Chapter 6 is recommended. For example, if the three observations 13.1, 13.1, and 13.1 were scheduled to receive the ranks of 5, 6, and 7, dependent on whether they were distinct rather than equal, the midrank procedure would assign the rank of 6 [$= (5 + 6 + 7)/3$] to each one. Evaluating K proceeds in the manner defined in statistic (11.5). However, rather than using K as the test statistic, it is recommended that the tie-corrected version, K_T, be used:

$$K_T = \frac{K}{1 - \left(\sum_{l=1}^{r} (S_l^3 - S_l)/(N^3 - N) \right)}, \qquad (11.6)$$

where r is the number of tied categories with S_1 in the first category, S_2 in the second, and so forth. If there are no ties, then $K = K_T$. The Kruskal–Wallis test procedure is summarized in Table 11.3.

Table 11.3. Outline of Kruskal–Wallis Test for Comparing g Groups

---

A. Data: y_{ij}, $i = 1, 2, \ldots, g$; $j = 1, 2, \ldots, n_i$, from Table 11.1.

B. Assumptions: y_{ij} conforms to the model (11.1) where the e_{ij} are independently and identically distributed with zero mean and variance σ^2. The distribution of e_{ij} is further assumed to be a continuous distribution. The independence of the e_{ij} (and therefore y_{ij}) is ensured by the completely random assignment of individuals to groups. All $n_i \geq 5$.

C. Computations:
   1. Rank the y_{ij} from smallest to largest using midranks for tied observations.
   2. Denoting the ranks and means of the ranks as in Table 11.2, compute the statistics

$$K = \frac{12}{N(N + 1)} \sum_{i=1}^{g} n_i (\overline{R}_{i+} - \overline{R}_{++})^2,$$

or if there are ties, compute

$$K_T = \frac{K}{1 - \left(\sum_{l=1}^{r} (S_l^3 - S_l)/(N^3 - N) \right)},$$

where S_1 is the number of ties in the first tied category, S_2 is the number of ties in the second tied category, and so forth.

D. Statistical test:
   1. Null hypothesis: H_0: $\mu_1 = \mu_2 = \cdots = \mu_g$.
   2. Alternative hypothesis: H_a: Not all equal.
   3. Decision rule for an α-level test: Reject H_0 if K_T (or K if no ties) exceeds $\chi_{1-\alpha}^2(g - 1)$ where $\chi_{1-\alpha}^2(g - 1)$ is from Table 6 of the Appendix.

For small sample sizes, the reader should compare K to exact critical values in Hollander and Wolfe (1973).

An illustration may help to clarify the test procedure.

Example 11.2.2.1. Consider a situation in which the behavioral effects of chlorpromazine on amphetamine-treated pigeons were observed. Suppose that three distinct doses of chlorpromazine were studied. Calling these doses low, middle, and high, 29 pigeons were assigned at random to one of four groups: namely, amphetamine, amphetamine plus low dose of chlorpromazine, amphetamine plus middle dose of chlorpromazine, and amphetamine plus high dose of chlorpromazine. The resulting data are as follows:

NUMBER OF PECKS PER UNIT OF TIME

Amphetamine	Amphetamine Plus Low Dose	Amphetamine Plus Middle Dose	Amphetamine Plus High Dose
14.10	11.00	9.65	10.53
10.75	9.73	10.05	10.71
9.41	11.31	11.75	11.43
10.65	13.89	11.06	8.99
11.49	12.10	10.51	9.02
13.55	10.31	—	10.22
11.11	11.86	—	13.03
13.49	—	—	10.49
—	—	—	11.34

At the 5% level of significance, is there any evidence to conclude that there is a difference between the four groups?

In Table 11.4, the data of this example are analyzed via the Kruskal–Wallis procedure.

It should be observed that there is a simple computational form for the statistic K. Using the notation of Table 11.2, the form is

$$K = \left(\frac{12}{N(N+1)} \sum_{1=1} \frac{R_{i+}^2}{n_i} \right) - 3(N+1), \qquad (11.7)$$

which is the computational form of expression (11.5).

Table 11.4. Worked Solution of Example 11.2.2.1 Using the Kruskal–Wallis Test

A. Data:
  Group 1: 14.10, 10.75, 9.41, 10.65, 11.49, 13.55, 11.11, 13.49
  Group 2: 11.00, 9.73, 11.31, 13.89, 12.10, 10.31, 11.86
  Group 3: 9.65, 10.05, 11.75, 11.06, 10.51
  Group 4: 10.53, 10.71, 11.43, 8.99, 9.02, 10.22, 13.03, 10.49, 11.34
B. Assumptions: The data represent four independent samples from continuous
  populations differing at most in their locations.
C. Computations: The ranks of the data are as follows:

Group 1	Group 2	Group 3	Group 4
29	15	4	11
14	5	6	13
3	18	22	20
12	28	16	1
21	24	10	2
27	8	58	7
17	23		25
26	121		9
149			19
			107

Totals:

$R_{1+} = 149$ $R_{2+} = 121$ $R_{3+} = 58$ $R_{4+} = 107$ $R_{++} = 435$

Means:

$\bar{R}_{1+} = 18.63$ $\bar{R}_{2+} = 17.29$ $\bar{R}_{3+} = 11.60$ $\bar{R}_{4+} = 11.89$ $\bar{R}_{++} = 15$

As $N = 29$, it follows that

$$K = \frac{12}{29(30)}\left[8(18.63 - 15)^2 + 7(17.29 - 15)^2\right.$$

$$\left. + 5(11.60 - 15)^2 + 9(11.89 - 15)^2\right]$$

$$= 3.96 = K_T,$$

as there are no ties.
D. Statistical test:
  1. Null hypothesis: $H_0: \mu_1 = \mu_2 = \mu_3 = \mu_4$.
  2. Alternative hypothesis: H_a: Not all equal.
  3. Decision rule for a 0.05 level test: Reject H_0 in favor of H_a if $K > \chi^2_{0.95}(3)$.
E. Action taken: As $\chi^2_{0.95}(3) = 7.81$ and $K = 3.96$, there is not sufficient evidence
  to reject H_0 at the 5% level.

11.2.3 Multiple Comparisons

Recall that the analysis-of-variance procedures of Chapter 10 were frequently followed by a multiple-comparison procedure whereby various pairwise comparisons among the g groups are made. There are comparable procedures for the rank test procedure as well.

Once again we resort, however, to large-sample approximations with one exception. The one exception is the planned-comparison situation. In this case, the error rate is to be controlled on a per-comparison basis similar to the least significant difference. Thus, for example, if before collecting the data, the researcher planned to compare one group against another, then it is perfectly legitimate to compare these two groups with the Wilcoxon–Mann–Whitney rank sum test of Chapter 6. Consequently, the error rate stated for that test would apply only to that particular comparison and no others. This type of procedure may be used only for one or two comparisons planned at the start of the study. The comments made in Chapter 10 regarding the least significant difference would apply here as well.

In most comparisons of g groups, the data analyst is probably interested in comparing all possible pairs of means or comparing all means to a single, say, control, mean. Two such procedures are discussed next.

11.2.3.1 Procedure for All Pairwise Comparisons

Dunn (1964) proposed a large-sample procedure that controls the error rate on an experimentwise basis. It may be applied for comparison of all $g(g-1)/2$ possible pairs of comparisons. The procedure is to take the mean ranks of Table 11.2, $\overline{R}_{1+}, \ldots, \overline{R}_{g+}$, and for any pair of groups, say group c and d, compute the quantity

$$Z_{cd} = \frac{\overline{R}_{c+} - \overline{R}_{d+}}{\sqrt{[N(N+1)/12](1/n_c + 1/n_d)}}. \tag{11.8}$$

In order to control the experimentwise error rate at level α, the values $Z_{1-\alpha/g(g-1)}$ and $-Z_{1-\alpha/g(g-1)}$, are determined from Table 4 of the Appendix and one concludes that $\mu_c \neq \mu_d$ if Z_{cd} is outside that interval. This procedure may be applied to all pairwise comparisons, and the error rate will be no greater than α for the entire set jointly. This procedure tends to be quite conservative; that is, usually the error rate will be much less than α, in which case the confidence intervals will be wider than necessary to have an error rate of exactly α. This procedure is an application of Bonferroni's procedure discussed in Section 10.3.2.2.5 and is summarized in Table 11.5. Let us apply this procedure to the data of Example 11.2.2.1.

Table 11.5. Outline of Procedure for All Pairwise Comparisons

A. Data: y_{ij}, $i = 1, \ldots, g$; $j = 1, \ldots, n_i$, from Table 11.1.
B. Assumptions: Same as those for Table 11.3.
C. Computations:
   1. Take the quantities $n_1, \ldots, n_g$, $\overline{R}_{1+}, \ldots, \overline{R}_{g+}$, and $N = \sum_{i=1}^{g} n_i$ from Table 11.2.
   2. For all possible pairs of means [there are $g(g - 1)/2$], compute

$$Z_{cd} = \frac{\overline{R}_{c+} - \overline{R}_{d+}}{\sqrt{[N(N+1)/12](1/n_c + 1/n_d)}}$$

D. Two-tailed statistical test:
   1. Null hypothesis: H_0: $\mu_c = \mu_d$ for all pairs (c, d).
   2. Alternative hypothesis: H_a: $\mu_c \neq \mu_d$ for at least one pair (c, d).
   3. Decision rule for α-level test: If $|Z_{cd}| \geq Z_{1-\alpha/g(g-1)}$, then reject H_0 in favor of H_a.

Example 11.2.3.1.1. Suppose in Example 11.2.2.1 that the investigators were interested in all possible pairwise comparisons among the groups. Perform the procedure at the 0.05 level. Recall that:

	Group 1	Group 2	Group 3	Group 4
n_i	8	7	5	9
$\overline{R}_{i+}$	18.63	17.29	11.60	11.89

The relevant computations for the pairwise comparisons are the following:

Group	Comparison, versus	Group	$\overline{R}_{c+} - \overline{R}_{d+}$	$(1/n_c + 1/n_d)$	Z_{cd}
1		2	1.34	0.268	0.30
1		3	7.03	0.325	1.45
1		4	6.74	0.236	1.63
2		3	5.69	0.343	1.14
2		4	5.40	0.254	1.26
3		4	-0.29	0.311	-0.06

From Table 4 of the Appendix, we find $Z_{0.996} = 2.65$, ($[1 - 0.05/4(3)] = 0.996$). As none of the Z_{cd} exceeds 2.65 or is less than -2.65, none of the pairwise differences may be declared significantly different from zero.

In the next section, a multiple-comparison procedure is discussed for the problem of comparing $g - 1$ of the groups to a single group.

Table 11.6. Procedure for Comparing All Means to a Control

A. Data: y_{ij}, $i = 1, \ldots, g$; $j = 1, \ldots, n_i$, from Table 11.1.
B. Assumptions: Same as those for Table 11.3.
C. Computations:
   1. Take the quantities $n_1, \ldots, n_g$, $\overline{R}_{1+}, \ldots, \overline{R}_{g+}$, and $N = \Sigma_{i=1}^{g} n_i$ from Table 11.2.
   2. Denote the "control" group mean by $\overline{R}_{1+}$. i.e., the first group.
   3. For all comparisons to group 1, compute

$$Z_{1d} = \frac{\overline{R}_{1+} - \overline{R}_{d+}}{\sqrt{[N(N+1)/12](1/n_1 + 1/n_d)}} \qquad d = 2, \ldots, g.$$

D. Two-tailed statistical test:
   1. Null hypothesis: H_0: $\mu_1 = \mu_d$ for each $d = 2, \ldots, g$.
   2. Alternative hypothesis: H_a: $\mu_1 \neq \mu_d$ for some d.
   3. Decision rule for an α-level test: If $|Z_{1d}| > Z_{1-\alpha/2(g-1)}$, then reject H_0 in favor of H_a.
   The critical value of $Z_{1-\alpha/2(g-1)}$ is taken from Table 4 of the Appendix.

11.2.3.2 Procedure for All Treatment Comparisons to a Control

This procedure may be regarded as an analogue to Dunnett's procedure insofar as a single group is to be contrasted to all of the remaining groups. Furthermore, the error rate is controlled on an experimentwise basis. The procedure is summarized in Table 11.6. We now apply this procedure to the data of Example 11.2.2.1.

Example 11.2.3.2.1. Suppose in Example 11.2.2.1 that the investigators were interested in all comparisons to group 1, the group with no chloropromazine. Perform the procedure at the 0.05 level. Recall that:

	Group 1	Group 2	Group 3	Group 4
n_i	8	7	5	9
$\overline{R}_{i+}$	18.63	17.29	11.60	11.89

The relevant computations for the various comparisons are as follows:

Group	Comparison versus Group (d)	$\overline{R}_{1+} - \overline{R}_{d+}$	$1/n_1 + 1/n_d$	Z_{1d}
1	2	1.34	0.268	0.30
1	3	7.03	0.325	1.45
1	4	6.74	0.236	1.63

Table 11.7. Data Layout for Randomized Complete Block Design

Block	Group 1	$\cdots$	Group g
1	y_{11}	$\cdots$	y_{g1}
$\vdots$	y_{12}	$\cdots$	y_{g2}
	$\vdots$		$\vdots$
n	y_{1n}	$\cdots$	y_{gn}

From Table 4 of the Appendix, we find $Z_{0.992} \doteq 2.40$, $[(1 - 0.05/6) = 0.992]$. As none of the Z_{1d} exceeds 2.40 or is less than -2.40, we cannot declare any difference as being significant at the 0.05 level.

With regard to estimation of a pairwise difference $\mu_c - \mu_d$ for any two groups c and d, it is suggested that the pairwise estimator be determined via expressions (6.22) and (6.23). This estimator is useful to report in addition to the significance test results.

It should be noted that other procedures for multiple comparisons are also possible [the reader may refer to Miller (1981), Lehmann (1975), and Hollander and Wolfe (1973) for a discussion of these alternatives].

11.3 RANK ANALYSIS OF VARIANCE FOR RANDOMIZED COMPLETE BLOCK DESIGNS

11.3.1 General Aspects of Problem

The basic layout for the randomized complete block design is in Table 11.7. The basic design consists of grouping individuals into blocks and then assigning treatments at random within each block. The essential requirement is that each treatment appears exactly once in each block.

As noted in the previous chapter, this design is the generalization of the matched-pairs design to the case of g groups. It is further assumed that a *linear additive model* for the data is given by

$$y_{ij} = \mu + \tau_i + \beta_j + e_{ij}, \tag{11.9}$$

where μ is the grand mean, τ_i is the effect due to the ith group, β_j is the effect due to the jth block, and e_{ij} is the random error. Our key assumptions regarding the data of Table 11.7 are as follows:

1. The data in Table 11.7 conform to model (11.9).
2. The e_{ij} in (11.9) are independently and identically distributed with zero mean and variance σ^2. Note that randomization ensures the independence of the e_{ij}, while the equal variance condition must be assumed.
3. The e_{ij} come from a continuous distribution.

The main inference question is that of testing the hypothesis

$$H_0: \tau_1 = \cdots = \tau_g \quad \text{versus} \quad H_a: \text{Not all equal.} \qquad (11.10)$$

The test procedure we discuss in this chapter is based on the ranking of the g observations in each block from 1 to g. This is done for each block separately. Under the null hypothesis, the $g!$ assignments of ranks are equally likely. Thus, across the n blocks, the $(g!)^n$ possible assignments of intrablock ranks are equally likely.

11.3.2 Friedman's Test

Conceivably, a test statistic may be the sum of the ranks received for group 1, then the sum for group 2, and so on. Under the null hypothesis, these g rank sums should be close to one another. A test statistic that compares these g sums is the *Friedman* test (1937).

The basic ranks for the data of Table 11.7 are summarized in Table 11.8.

In Table 11.8, R_{ij} is the rank of y_{ij} among the observations in block j. The quantities R_{i+} and $\overline{R}_{i+}$ are defined by

$$R_{i+} = \sum_{j=1}^{n} R_{ij}, \qquad \overline{R}_{i+} = R_{i+}/n. \qquad (11.11)$$

Table 11.8. Intrablock Ranks for Data of Table 11.7

	Block	Group 1	$\cdots$	Group g
	1	R_{11}	$\cdots$	R_{g1}
	$\vdots$	$\vdots$		$\vdots$
	n	R_{1n}	$\cdots$	R_{gn}
Total		R_{1+}	$\cdots$	R_{g+}
Mean		$\overline{R}_{1+}$	$\cdots$	$\overline{R}_{g+}$

The Friedman test statistic is defined in terms of Table 11.8 by

$$Q = \frac{12n}{g(g+1)} \sum_{i=1}^{g} \left(\overline{R}_{i+} - \overline{R}_{++} \right)^2, \tag{11.12}$$

where $\overline{R}_{++} = (g+1)/2$.

The rationale for the test is that if the statistic (11.12) is large, this indicates that the g groups may be different. For large values of n, the statistic Q has a chi-square distribution with $g - 1$ degrees of freedom. Computationally, the statistic (11.12) is most easily computed via

$$Q = \frac{12}{ng(g+1)} \left(\sum_{i=1}^{g} R_{i+}^2 \right) - 3n(g+1). \tag{11.13}$$

Table 11.9. Outline of Friedman Test for Comparing g Groups (Randomized Complete Block Design)

A. Data: y_{ij}, $i = 1, \ldots, g$; $j = 1, 2, \ldots, n$, from Table 11.7.

B. Assumptions: Stated by assumptions 1–3 (Section 11.3.1) and $n \geq 15$.

C. Computations:
   1. Rank the y_{ij} from smallest to largest in each block individually using midranks for tied observations.
   2. Denote the ranks as in Table 11.8.
   3. Compute

   $$Q = \frac{12}{ng(g+1)} \left(\sum_{i=1}^{g} R_{i+}^2 \right) - 3n(g+1),$$

   or if there are ties, compute

   $$Q_T = \frac{Q}{1 - \sum_{j=1}^{n}\sum_{i=1}^{s_j}\left(S_{ij}^3 - S_{ij} \right) \Big/ ng(g^2 - 1)},$$

   where S_{1j} is the number of observations in the first tied group of block $j, \ldots, S_{s_j j}$ is the number of observations in the s_jth tied group of block j.

D. Statistical test:
   1. Null hypothesis: H_0: $\tau_1 = \cdots = \tau_g$.
   2. Alternative hypothesis: H_a: τ_i not all equal.
   3. Decision rule for an α-level test: Reject H_0 in favor of H_a if Q (or if ties Q_T) is greater than $\chi^2_{1-\alpha}(g-1)$ where $\chi^2_{1-\alpha}(g-1)$ is from Table 6 of the Appendix.

If there are tied observations within a block, then midranks should be used. If there are any ties, then the statistic for testing H_0 is Q_T, where

$$Q_T = \frac{Q}{1 - \sum_{j=1}^{n}\sum_{i=1}^{s_j}\left(S_{ij}^3 - S_{ij}\right)\big/ng(g^2 - 1)} \tag{11.14}$$

and S_{ij} equals the number of observations in the first tied group in block $j, \ldots, S_{s_j j}$ equals the number of observations in the s_jth tied group in block j.

The Friedman test procedure is summarized in Table 11.9.

For small sample sizes ($n < 15$), the exact tables of Hollander and Wolfe (1973) or Lehmann (1975) should be consulted. We illustrate the procedure in Table 11.9 with an example. Strictly speaking, the sample size in Example 11.3.2.1 is too small to justify use of the chi-square tables. We do so for illustration only.

Example 11.3.2.1. For the hyperactivity scores data of Example 10.4.2.1, test with Friedman's statistic the hypothesis that the four treatments are equally effective at $\alpha = 0.05$. The solution is outlined in Table 11.10.

11.3.3 Multiple Comparisons

Recall that the analysis-of-variance test for the randomized complete block design was followed by various pairwise multiple comparisons. As it was in that situation, if there are one or two planned comparisons at the start of the study, then these may be done with the error rate controlled on a per-comparison basis. Since Friedman's test may be regarded as an extension of the sign test, the appropriate pairwise comparison procedure would be the sign test applied to the pairwise differences. For example, if in the preceding worked illustration it was of a priori interest to compare the first and second treatment groups, then the pairwise sign test would involve the four differences, $-20, -20, -17,$ and -16. The test procedure would then be the sign test applied to these differences.

Generally, if one is interested in making more than just one or two planned comparisons, then procedures are required that control the error rate on an experimentwise basis. We now discuss two such procedures, which are described in greater detail in Hollander and Wolfe (1973).

11.3.3.1 All Pairwise Comparisons

It is assumed in this section and in Section 11.3.3.2 that n, the number of blocks, is rather large and that it is of interest to perform all pairwise comparisons. The procedure is described in Table 11.11.

Table 11.10. Worked Solution to Example 11.3.2.1 (10.4.2.1) Using
Friedman's Procedure

A. Data: The hyperactivity scores are:

	Treatment Group			
Block	A	B	C	D
1	41	61	62	43
2	48	68	62	48
3	53	70	66	53
4	56	72	70	52

B. Assumptions: Stated by assumptions 1–3 (Section 11.3.1).
C. Computations: The corresponding intrablock ranks are given by:

	Treatment Group			
Block	A	B	C	D
1	1	3	4	2
2	1.5	4	3	1.5
3	1.5	4	3	1.5
4	2	4	3	1
Total (R_{i+})	6	15	13	6
Mean ($\bar{R}_{i+}$)	1.5	3.75	3.25	1.5

The statistic Q is therefore

$$Q = \frac{12}{(4)(4)(5)}(6^2 + 15^2 + 13^2 + 6^2) - 3(4)(5) = 9.9.$$

Furthermore, as there are two observations which are tied in block 2, it follows
that $S_{12} = 2, s_2 = 1$. Similarly, for block 3, there are two ties; hence,
$S_{13} = 2, s_3 = 1$. As a consequence,

$$Q_T = \frac{9.9}{1 - 12/(4)(4)(15)} = \frac{9.9}{0.95} = 10.42.$$

D. Statistical test:
  1. Null hypothesis: H_0: $\tau_1 = \tau_2 = \tau_3 = \tau_4$.
  2. Alternative hypothesis: H_a: Not all equal.
  3. Decision rule for 0.05 level test: Reject H_0 in favor of H_a if Q_T exceeds
     $\chi^2_{0.95}(3)$.
E. Action taken: From Table 6 of the Appendix, we find $\chi^2_{0.95}(3) = 7.81$, while
   Q_T is 10.51: hence, the null hypothesis is rejected, and we conclude that there is
   a difference between the four treatment groups.

377

Table 11.11. Procedure for all Pairwise Comparisons Following Friedman's Test

---

A. Data: y_{ij}, $i = 1, \ldots, g$; $j = 1, \ldots, n$ from Table 11.7.
B. Assumptions: Stated by assumptions 1–3 (Section 11.3.1) and $n \geq 15$.
C. Computations:
    1. Rank the y_{ij} from smallest to largest in each individual block using midranks for tied observations.
    2. Denote the ranks as in Table 11.8.
    3. For each pair of groups c and d, compute

$$Z_{cd} = \frac{\left| \overline{R}_{c+} - \overline{R}_{d+} \right|}{\sqrt{g(g+1)/12n}}$$

D. Two-tailed statistical test:
    1. Null hypothesis: H_0: $\tau_c = \tau_d$
    2. Alternative hypothesis: H_a: $\tau_c \neq \tau_d$
    3. Decision rule for an α-level test: Reject H_0 in favor of H_a if Z_{cd} exceeds $QP_{1-\alpha}(g)$, where $QP_{1-\alpha}(g)$ is from Table 15 of the Appendix.

As an illustration of the above procedure, let us consider the data of Example 10.4.2.1 once again. As before, the sample sizes are too small to justify the use of Table 15 (Appendix); however, we illustrate the computations.

Example 11.3.3.1.1. Apply Friedman's all-pairwise-comparison procedure to the hyperactivity data of Example 10.4.2.1. From Table 15 of the Appendix, $QP_{0.95}(4) = 3.633$, while $\sqrt{g(g+1)/12n} = 0.645$; hence, a difference in mean ranks must be at least $(3.633)(0.645)$, or 2.34, in order to be significant at the 0.05 level. The various mean rank differences are:

Group	versus	Group	$\left\| \overline{R}_{c+} - \overline{R}_{d+} \right\|$
c		d	—
1		2	2.25
1		3	1.75
1		4	0
2		3	0.50
2		4	2.25
3		4	1.75

Hence, none of the pairs would be declared significantly different using this test procedure.

Table 11.12. Procedure for all Comparisons to a Control Following Friedman's Test

---

A. Data: y_{ij}, $i = 1, 2, \ldots, g$; $j = 1, 2, \ldots, n$, from Table 11.7.
B. Assumptions: Stated by assumptions 1–3 (Section 11.3.1) and $n \geq 15$.
C. Computations:
   1. Rank y_{ij} from smallest to largest in each individual block using midranks for tied observations.
   2. Denote these ranks as in Table 11.8.
   3. Let the control group be the first group; then compute

$$Z_{1d} = \frac{|\overline{R}_{1+} - \overline{R}_{d+}|}{\sqrt{g(g+1)/6n}} \qquad \text{for } d = 2, \ldots, g.$$

D. Two-tailed statistical test:
   1. Null hypothesis: $H_0: \tau_1 = \tau_d$
   2. Alternative hypothesis: $H_a: \tau_1 \neq \tau_d$
   3. Decision rule for an α-level test: Reject H_0 in favor of H_a if Z_{1d} exceeds $QC_{1-\alpha}(g-1)$ where $QC_{1-\alpha}(g-1)$ is from Table 16 of the Appendix.

11.3.3.2   All Treatments Compared to a Control

In order to compare all treatments to one particular treatment, the procedure outline in Table 11.12 is recommended. This procedure controls the error rate on an experimentwise basis.

An illustration may help describe the test procedure.

Example 11.3.3.2.1.   For the problem of Example 10.4.2.1, suppose the investigator wished to compare groups B, C, and D to group A, the comparison of B, C, and D among themselves being of no interest. From Table 16 of the Appendix, $QC_{0.95}(3) = 2.35$. In order for a difference to be significant, it must exceed $(2.35)\sqrt{g(g+1)/6n} = 2.145$. We notice that $|\overline{R}_{1+} - \overline{R}_{2+}| = 2.25$, $|\overline{R}_{1+} - \overline{R}_{3+}| = 1.75$, and $|\overline{R}_{1+} - \overline{R}_{4+}| = 0$. Hence, group B differs significantly from group A, while groups C and D do not.

11.4   SUMMARY

The analyses described in this chapter represent multiple-group-comparison procedures for interval- and ratio-scale data. These procedures may also be safely applied to ordinal-scale data provided the number of ties is not excessive. These rank test procedures may be viewed as multiple-group extensions of the rank tests described in Chapter 6.

While little attention has been given to the estimation of parameters in this chapter, it should be pointed out that the estimate of a treatment group difference may be obtained by applying the schemes of Chapter 6. In particular, for completely random designs, a given difference may be estimated by the Wilcoxon estimator in expressions (6.22) and (6.23). For the randomized complete block design, the estimator that logically fits with Friedman's procedure is the median of the pairwise differences between a pair of groups. Another estimator that could be employed in this situation is statistic (6.12). Hence, the full range of inferences, that is, both testing and estimation, are afforded by these techniques.

Exact tests for small sample sizes in CRD and RCBD designs can be found in the texts of Conover (1980) and Hollander and Wolfe (1973). These tests require extensive tables of critical values that are not included in this book.

The rank analyses of variance presented in this chapter are available in several statistical software packages. The procedure RANK in SAS changes the original values of the data into ranks. When a one-way analysis of variance procedure or a two-way ANOVA are applied to these ranks, by using the procedure General Linear Model (GLM), for example, the results are equivalent to the Kruskal–Wallis and Friedman tests, respectively.

The program P3S in BMDP can also perform these analysis.

PROBLEMS

11.1. To study the effect of sinoaortic deafferentation surgery (SAD) and decerebration on rats' heart rate and arterial pressure, six male healthy rats underwent SAD and then decerebration (operation I), eight rats had SAD surgery and then sham decerebration (operation II), and seven rats had sham SAD and then decerebration (operation III). After 2 hr of recovery, the heart rates (beats/min) are:

Operation	I	II	III
	370	432	413
	365	428	415
	381	438	409
	351	425	411
	377	427	408
	372	433	414
		434	412
		429	

(a) Compare the results of the operations using the Kruskal–Wallis test with $\alpha = 0.05$.

(b) Test all the pairwise comparisons among the operations.

11.2. Patients with subarachnoid hemmorrhage from a single intracranial aneurysm were randomized to four treatment groups: bed rest (BR), drug-induced hypotension (DIH), carotid ligation (CL), and intracranial surgery (ICS). Since bed rest therapy implies the disease follows its natural history, this group of patients is considered as a control group. The weeks to death observed in these patients are:

Treatment	BR	DIH	CL	ICS
	55	37	20	12
	32	49	16	19
	13	66	58	38
	34	21	34	25
	6	101	85	18
	48	38	67	54
	11	51	50	46

(a) Perform a test to evaluate the difference in time to death between these four groups.

(b) Test all treatment groups against the control.

11.3. In an experimental trial to identify the site of agents that activate cardiovascular response from the central nervous system, local injections of lidocaine were applied at different forebrain sites in rats treated with angiotensin, a peptid that increases arterial pressure. The diminution in arterial pressure (mm Hg) observed after 2 min of the injection was recorded as follows:

Site I	Site II	Site III	Site IV
26	7	39	27
24	9	33	29
21	4	29	19
27	6	32	18
25	8	36	26
22	5		20
23			24
20			

(a) At the 5% level of significance, is there any evidence to conclude that there is a difference between the four sites?

(b) Use a procedure to study all pairwise comparisons.

(c) If we consider the data for site II as a control group, compare the sites to site II.

(d) Do (a)–(c) when the values in site II are 18, 18, 18, 23, 23, and 23.

11.4. Seven patients in a psychiatric clinic received, in random order, four treatment drugs to control their depression. The depression scores observed are (low values correspond to low-depression symptoms):

	Drug			
Patient ID	I	II	III	IV
1	3	5	12	4
2	8	6	14	7
3	5	7	11	3
4	6	8	16	5
5	7	9	17	7
6	4	7	13	6
7	9	10	15	8

(a) Determine if the four drug treatments have significantly different effects by using Friedman's test procedure.

(b) Perform a test of all pairwise comparisons among the drug groups.

11.5. Regional vascular resistance response to graded doses of intravenous nitroglycerin were measured in seven rats with chronic sinoaortic deafferentation, as shown in the next table:

	Dose (μg/kg)			
Rat ID	10	30	100	300
1	8	19	37	45
2	6	25	30	50
3	10	23	28	39
4	7	24	29	42
5	12	23	29	40
6	15	25	33	55
7	5	20	32	53

(a) Perform Friedman's test to compare the four doses of nitroglycerin, with $\alpha = 0.05$.

(b) Obtain all pairwise comparisons.

(c) If a dose of 10 is used as the control, obtain conclusions.

REFERENCES

Conover, W. J. (1980). *Practical Nonparametric Statistics*, Wiley, New York.

Dunn, O. J. (1964). Multiple comparisons using rank sums, *Technometrics*, **6**, 241–252.

Friedman, M. (1937). The use of ranks to avoid the assumption of normality implicit in the analysis of variance, *J. Am. Statist. Assoc.*, **32**, 675–701.

Hollander, M., and D. A. Wolfe. (1973). *Nonparametric Statistical Methods*, Wiley, New York.

Kruskal, W. H., and W. A. Wallis. (1952). Use of ranks in one-criterion variance analysis, *J. Am. Statist. Assoc.*, **47**, 583–621.

Lehmann, E. L. (1975). *Nonparametrics: Statistical Methods Based on Ranks*, Holden-Day, San Francisco, CA.

Miller, R. J. Jr. (1981). *Simultaneous Statistical Inference*, Springer-Verlag, New York.

CHAPTER 12

Comparing More Than Two Groups of Observations: Chi-Square and Related Procedures

12.1 INTRODUCTION

The focus of the previous two chapters has been on the comparison of more than two groups of observations. However, the procedures discussed in Chapters 10 and 11 do not apply to categorical or nominal-scale data. The rank test procedures require data of at least an ordinal scale while the analysis-of-variance tests of Chapter 10 require a continuous distribution. This chapter is an extension of the procedures of Chapter 7. In particular, the g group comparison problem is addressed for the situation in which the data are of nominal (or ordinal) scale. Alternatively, the original responses may have been interval or ratio, but various categories of response may have been constructed for purposes of analysis.

The discussion of Chapter 10 regarding the problem of multiple comparisons and design considerations also applies to this chapter. Specifically, the experimental error rate would not be properly controlled if the data analyst performed all pairwise two-group tests as in Chapter 7. Procedures are required that permit the global comparison of the g groups.

As in Chapter 7, the case of two response categories is considered first.

12.2 CASE OF TWO RESPONSE CATEGORIES

For convenience, the two response categories are denoted by 0 and 1. Generally, 0 indicates the absence of the characteristic while 1 indicates its presence. There are two basic experimental designs for which a discussion of the statistical analysis is presented. The randomized complete block design, which is an extension of the matched-pairs design, and the completely random design, which is the g group extension of the two-independent-groups problem. The test for the randlmized complete block design is due to Cochran (1950).

12.2.1 Cochran's Test for Randomized Complete Block Design

Let us consider the following problem that arises frequently in psychiatric research.

Example 12.2.1.1. In a group of 12 psychiatric inpatients with different diagnoses, four resident physicians were asked to conduct a brief structured psychiatric interview of each patient. The order of interviewing was randomized, and each of the four residents interviewed each of the patients. One aspect of the interview was the residents' rating of a "thought disorder" in the patient. The following data resulted.

	Resident			
Patient	1	2	3	4
1	0	0	0	0
2	0	1	0	0
3	0	0	1	0
4	0	0	0	0
5	1	1	1	1
6	0	1	1	1
7	1	1	0	0
8	0	1	0	1
9	0	1	1	1
10	0	0	1	0
11	1	1	0	1
12	1	1	1	1

For this data 0 indicates no thought disorder and 1 indicates thought disorder. We would like to determine if there is evidence to conclude that any one of the residents is more likely to give a rating of thought disorder than any of the other residents.

It is evident from the example that the data are of the form of a randomized complete block design with a dichotomous response. The blocks in this case are the patients, while the treatment groups are the residents. The procedure for testing the hypothesis of equal treatment groups for such randomized complete block designs is called Cochran's test and is outlined in Table 12.1. Note that the procedure assumes that the

Table 12.1. Cochran's Test for Comparing g Groups of Dichotomous Response Data in a Randomized Complete Block Design

---

A. Data: $y_{ij} = 0$ or 1 for $i = 1, \ldots, g$; $j = 1, \ldots, n$; i.e., the general data structure is:

	Group			
Block	1	$\cdots$	g	Total
1	y_{11}	$\cdots$	y_{g1}	y_{+1}
$\vdots$	$\vdots$		$\vdots$	$\vdots$
n	y_{1n}	$\cdots$	y_{gn}	y_{+n}
Total	y_{1+}	$\cdots$	y_{g+}	y_{++}

B. Assumptions:
   1. The data in step A arose from a randomized complete block design.
   2. The y_{ij} are dichotomous variates.
   3. n is large.
C. Computations:
   1. Compute the number of "positives" for each block, $y_{+1}, \ldots, y_{+n}$ and compute the number of positives for each treatment group, $y_{1+}, \ldots, y_{g+}$.
   2. Compute the total number of positives y_{++}.
   3. Compute

$$Q = \frac{(g-1)\left[g\Sigma_{i=1}^{g} y_{i+}^2 - y_{++}^2 \right]}{gy_{++} - \Sigma_{j=1}^{n} y_{+j}^2}.$$

D. Statistical test:
   1. Null hypothesis: H_0: The probabilities of a positive response are the same for all g groups.
   2. Alternative hypothesis: H_a: The probabilities of a positive response are not all equal.
   3. Decision rule for an α-level test: Reject H_0 in favor of H_a if $Q > \chi_{1-\alpha}^2 (g-1)$, where $\chi_{1-\alpha}^2(g-1)$ is from Table 6 of the Appendix.

---

number of blocks is large as the test procedure is strictly a large-sample test procedure.

Let us apply the Cochran procedure to Example 12.2.1.1 (Table 12.2).

Cochran's Test is the multiple-group extension of the McNemar (1947) test of Chapter 7. For one or two planned treatment group comparisons, the McNemar test may be applied to the relevant pairs.

We now turn to the problem of comparing g groups in a completely random design.

Table 12.2. Worked Solution to Example 12.2.1.1 Using Cochran's Procedure

A. Data: The data are:

Patient	Resident 1	2	3	4	Total
1	0	0	0	0	0
2	0	1	0	0	1
3	0	0	1	0	1
4	0	0	0	0	0
5	1	1	1	1	4
6	0	1	1	1	3
7	1	1	0	0	2
8	0	1	0	1	2
9	0	1	1	1	3
10	0	0	1	0	1
11	1	1	0	1	3
12	1	1	1	1	4
Total	4	8	6	6	24

B. Assumptions:
   1. The data arose from a randomized block design.
   2. The variates are dichotomous.
   3. n is sufficiently large to justify the use of the chi-square distribution for the test.
C. Computations:
   1. The various totals are summarized as in step A.
   2. The test statistic Q is therefore given by

$$Q = \frac{3\left[4(4^2 + 8^2 + 6^2 + 6^2) - 24^2\right]}{4(24) - (0^2 + 1^2 + \cdots + 4^2)} = 3.69.$$

D. Statistical test:
   1. Null hypothesis: H_0: The probability of a positive response is the same for all g groups.
   2. Alternative hypothesis: H_a: The probabilities are not all equal.
   3. Decision rule for a 0.05 level test: Reject H_0 in favor of H_a if Q exceeds $\chi^2_{0.95}(3)$.
E. Action taken: Since $\chi^2_{0.95}(3) = 7.81$ and $Q = 3.69$, there is insufficient evidence to reject H_0 at the 0.05 level, meaning the number of positives does not differ significantly among these residents.

12.2.2 Chi-Square Tests for Completely Random Design

Let us commence with an example.

Example 12.2.2.1. In a recent follow-up study, schizophrenic, manic, and depressive patients were interviewed 30 years after their initial diagnosis. On the basis of the interviews, diagnoses were given to each patient. The resulting data are:

	Original Diagnosis		
Follow-up Diagnosis?	Schizophrenia	Mania	Depression
Same	56	5	16
Not same	37	20	18
Total	93	25	34

All follow-up diagnoses were made by the psychiatrist without knowledge of the person's initial diagnosis. Furthermore, the interview was conducted by an interviewer without knowledge of the patients' original diagnoses. On the basis of this data, is there sufficient evidence to conclude that the proportion of agreement between the follow-up diagnosis and the original diagnosis does not remain the same for the three original groups?

This example is typical of many problems involving the comparison of rates or proportions. The basic data for such problems is described as in Table 12.3.

The basic assumptions for the data are that:

1. The individual samples are independent random samples from their respective populations.
2. y_i has a binomial distribution with parameters n_i and p_i.

The principal hypotheses are the following:

$$H_0: p_1 = \cdots = p_g \quad \text{versus} \quad H_a: p_i \text{ are not all equal.} \quad (12.1)$$

Table 12.3. Basic Data Layout for a $2 \times g$ Table (y_i is the Number of Individuals Positive)

Response	Group 1	$\cdots$	Group g
Positive (1)	y_1	$\cdots$	y_g
Negative (0)	$n_1 - y_1$	$\cdots$	$n_g - y_g$
Total	n_1	$\cdots$	n_g

Table 12.4. Chi-square Test for Comparing g Groups of Dichotomous Response Data

A. Data: y_i, $i = 1, \ldots, g$, as in Table 12.3.
B. Assumptions: Stated by assumptions 1 and 2; also each E_{ij} below is at least 5.
C. Computations:
   1. Let

$$y_+ = \sum_{i=1}^{g} y_i, \qquad n_+ = \sum_{i=1}^{g} n_i;$$

   2. Let

$$E_{i1} = n_i \frac{y_+}{n_+}, \qquad E_{i2} = n_i \frac{n_+ - y_+}{n_+},$$

$$O_{i1} = y_i, \qquad O_{i2} = n_i - y_i.$$

   3. Let

$$\chi^2 = \sum_{i=1}^{g} \sum_{j=1}^{2} \frac{(O_{ij} - E_{ij})^2}{E_{ij}}.$$

Denote the sample proportions by $\hat{p}_i = y_i/n_i$ and $\hat{p} = y_+/n_+$; then a simpler form for χ^2 is

$$\sum_{i=1}^{g} \frac{n_i(\hat{p}_i - \hat{p})^2}{\hat{p}(1 - \hat{p})} = \frac{1}{\hat{p}(1 - \hat{p})} \left[\sum_{i=1}^{g} n_i \hat{p}_i^2 - n_+ \hat{p}^2 \right].$$

D. Statistical test:
   1. Null hypothesis: H_0: $p_1 = \cdots = p_g$.
   2. Alternative hypothesis: H_a: p_i not all equal.
   3. Decision Rule for an α-level test: Reject H_0 in favor of H_a if χ^2 in step C exceeds $\chi_{1-\alpha}^2(g - 1)$ from Table 6 of the Appendix.

The test procedure is described in Table 12.4.

The test procedure in Table 12.4 is sometimes called the chi-square test of homogeneity of proportions. We now apply this procedure to the data of Example 12.2.2.1. This is described in Table 12.5.

We note in passing that in Table 12.4 the E_{ij} are the expected cell entries if the hypothesis of homogeneity of proportions is true. If this hypothesis is true, then the best estimate of the common proportion of positives in each group is the grand total number of positives over the total sample size (see

Table 12.4). Also note that each E_{ij} is assumed to be at least 5, to ensure the validity of the chi-square approximation.

With regard to multiple comparisons among the p_i, Scheffé's procedure is recommended. The procedure is most easily implemented via confidence interval computation. In particular, in order to compare group c with group d, the $(1 - \alpha)$ 100% simultaneous confidence interval for $p_c - p_d$ is

$$(\hat{p}_c - \hat{p}_d) \pm \sqrt{\chi^2_{1-\alpha}(g - 1)} \sqrt{\frac{\hat{p}_c(1 - \hat{p}_c)}{n_c} + \frac{\hat{p}_d(1 - \hat{p}_d)}{n_d}}, \quad (12.2)$$

where $\hat{p}_c = y_c/n_c$, $\hat{p}_d = y_d/n_d$, and $\chi^2_{1-\alpha}(g - 1)$ is from Table 6 of the Appendix. The intervals (12.2) may be computed for any pair of groups, and the intervals are simultaneous confidence intervals in the sense discussed in Chapter 10. If zero is in an interval, then one concludes that $p_c = p_d$; otherwise, one concludes that $p_c \neq p_d$.

Example 12.2.2.2. For the study of Example 12.2.2.1, the patients were also assessed at follow-up regarding their psychiatric hospitalizations during the follow-up period. The following data arose:

Chronically Institutionalized?	Original Diagnosis		
	Schizophrenia	Mania	Depression
Yes	86	14	22
No	7	11	12
Total	93	25	34

Place 95% simultaneous confidence intervals on all pairwise comparisons of the groups.

The reader may verify that the proportions chronically institutionalized are 0.925, 0.560, and 0.647 for the three respective diagnostic groups. The corresponding pairwise confidence intervals (CI) are:

Group	versus	Group	Difference	95% CI
Schizophrenia		Manic	0.365	(0.113, 0.617)
Schizophrenia		Depressive	0.278	(0.066, 0.489)
Manic		Depressive	−0.087	(−0.402, 0.228)

Thus, the schizophrenics differ from both manics and depressives, while the manics and depressives do not differ from one another.

Table 12.5. Worked Solution of Example 12.2.2.1 Using Chi-Square Test

A. Data: The data are

Follow-up Diagnosis?	Group			Total
	Schizophrenia	Manic	Depressive	
Same	56	5	16	77
Not Same	37	20	18	75
Total	93	25	34	152

B. Assumptions:
  1. The data constitute three independent random samples.
  2. The number of persons with the same diagnosis follows a binomial distribution with parameters n_i, p_i for group i.
C. Computations:
  1. The observed and expected cell entries are given by:

$$O_{11} = 56, \quad E_{11} = 47.11; \qquad O_{21} = 5, \quad E_{21} = 12.66;$$

$$O_{31} = 16, \quad E_{31} = 17.22; \qquad O_{12} = 37, \quad E_{12} = 45.89;$$

$$O_{22} = 20, \quad E_{22} = 12.34; \qquad O_{32} = 18, \quad E_{32} = 16.78.$$

  2. Thus, the test statistic is $\chi^2 = (56 - 47.11)^2/47.11 + (5 - 12.66)^2/12.66 + \cdots + (18 - 16.78)^2/16.78 = 12.96$.
D. Statistical test:
  1. Null hypothesis: H_0: $p_1 = p_2 = p_3$.
  2. Alternative hypothesis: H_a: p_1, p_2, p_3 not all equal.
  3. Decision rule for a 0.05 level test: Reject H_0 in favor of H_a if χ^2 exceeds $\chi^2_{0.95}(2)$.
E. Action taken: Since $\chi^2_{0.95}(2) = 5.99$ while the computed test statistic is 12.96, the null hypothesis is rejected at the 0.05 level, i.e., we conclude that the proportion of agreement between the follow-up and the original diagnosis is not the same for the three groups.

12.3 CASE OF MORE THAN TWO RESPONSE CATEGORIES

12.3.1 Chi-Square Tests for Completely Random Design

The basic data layout is given in Table 12.6.

It is assumed that each of the g random samples arises from a multinomial distribution and that the ith random sample is multinomial with parameters n_i and cell probabilities $p_{i1}, \ldots, p_{ir}$ for the r respective re-

Table 12.6. Data Layout for r Responses for Comparing g Groups in Completely Random Design

Response	Group 1	$\cdots$	g	
1	y_{11}	$\cdots$	y_{g1}	y_{+1}
$\vdots$	$\vdots$		$\vdots$	$\vdots$
r	y_{1r}	$\cdots$	y_{gr}	y_{+r}
	n_1	$\cdots$	n_g	n_+

sponse categories. Furthermore, the g random samples are assumed to be independent random samples. To summarize, the key assumptions are as follows:

(a) The data are g independent random samples from multinomial populations;

(b) The probability of an individual falling into response category j is p_{ij} for a person in group i.

Clearly, for each i we have $\sum_{j=1}^{r} p_{ij} = 1$. The principal testing problem concerns the hypotheses

$$H_0 : \begin{pmatrix} p_{11} \\ \vdots \\ p_{1r} \end{pmatrix} = \cdots = \begin{pmatrix} p_{g1} \\ \vdots \\ p_{gr} \end{pmatrix} \quad \text{versus} \quad H_a : \text{Probability vectors not all equal.}$$

$$(12.3)$$

The test procedure is summarized in Table 12.7.

Example 12.3.1.1. In a study of the long-term social effects of schizophrenia and the affective disorders, the following long-term outcome data (40 years outcome) on the occupational outcome of the patient are reported:

OCCUPATIONAL

Outcome	Schizophrenia	Manic	Depressive
Good	65	58	142
Fair	14	7	33
Poor	107	21	37

Table 12.7. Chi-Square Test Procedure for Comparing g Groups with r Response Categories/Group

---

A. Data: y_{ij}, $i = 1, \ldots, g$; $j = 1, \ldots, r$, from Table 12.6.

B. Assumptions: Stated in assumptions (a) and (b); also, each E_{ij} below is at least 5.

C. Computations:

   1. Compute the expected cell entries by

$$E_{ij} = n_i \frac{y_{+j}}{n_+} \quad \text{for } i = 1, \ldots, g, \ j = 1, \ldots, r,$$

      where

$$y_{+j} = \sum_{i=1}^{g} y_{ij}; \qquad n_+ = \sum_{i=1}^{g} n_i.$$

   2. Denoting y_{ij} by O_{ij}, then compute

$$\chi^2 = \sum_{i=1}^{g} \sum_{j=1}^{r} \frac{(O_{ij} - E_{ij})^2}{E_{ij}}.$$

D. Statistical test:

   1. Null hypothesis: H_0 given by (12.3).

   2. Alternative hypothesis: H_a given by (12.3).

   3. Decision rule for an α-level test: Reject H_0 in favor of H_a if χ^2 exceeds $\chi^2_{1-\alpha} [(g - 1)(r - 1)]$ where $\chi^2_{1-\alpha}[(g - 1)(r - 1)]$ is from Table 6 of the Appendix.

The occupational outcome classifications are generally described as follows:

Good: the patient was gainfully employed full-time.

Fair: the patient was employed part-time.

Poor: the patient was unemployed due to incapacitating psychiatric illness.

Is there evidence to suggest that the occupational outcome distribution is different for the three diagnostic groups?

The worked solution to Example 12.3.1.1 is summarized in Table 12.8.

With regard to multiple comparisons among the p_{ij}, a Scheffé-type procedure is recommended (Grizzle, Starmer, and Koch, 1969). As in the previous section, the procedure is most easily implemented via a confidence

Table 12.8. Worked Solution to Example 12.3.1.1 Using Chi-Square Test Procedure

A. Data: The data are:

Occupational Outcome	Schizophrenia	Manic	Depressive	Total
Good	65	58	142	265
Fair	14	7	33	54
Poor	107	21	37	165
Total	186	86	212	484

B. Assumptions:
  1. The data are three independent random samples from multinomial populations.
  2. The multinomial probabilities are given by p_{ij}, where $\Sigma_{j=1}^{r} p_{ij} = 1$.
C. Computations:
  1. The observed and expected cell entries are:

Occupational Outcome	Schizophrenia		Manic		Depressive	
	O	E	O	E	O	E
Good	65	101.84	58	47.09	142	116.07
Fair	14	20.75	7	9.60	33	23.65
Poor	107	63.41	21	29.32	37	72.27

  2. The test statistic is therefore

$$\chi^2 = \frac{(65 - 101.84)^2}{101.84} + \cdots + \frac{(37 - 72.27)^2}{72.27} = 77.78.$$

D. Statistical test:

  1. Null hypothesis: H_0: $\begin{pmatrix} p_{11} \\ p_{12} \\ p_{13} \end{pmatrix} = \begin{pmatrix} p_{21} \\ p_{22} \\ p_{23} \end{pmatrix} = \begin{pmatrix} p_{31} \\ p_{32} \\ p_{33} \end{pmatrix}$.

  2. Alternative hypothesis: H_a: The proportions are not all equal.
  3. Decision rule for a 0.05 level test: Reject H_0 in favor of H_a if χ^2 exceeds $\chi^2_{0.95}(4)$, where $\chi^2_{0.95}(4)$ is taken from Table 6 of the Appendix.
E. Action taken: As $\chi^2_{0.95}(4) = 9.49$ and $\chi^2 = 77.78$, the null hypothesis is rejected, and it is concluded that the occupational distributions differ at the 5% level.

interval computation. Specifically, in order to compare the probability of response in category j between groups c and d, the $(1 - \alpha)$ 100% simultaneous confidence for $p_{cj} - p_{dj}$ is

$$
\left(\hat{p}_{cj} - \hat{p}_{dj}\right) \pm \sqrt{\chi^2_{1-\alpha}[(g-1)(r-1)]} \; \sqrt{\frac{\hat{p}_{cj}\left(1 - \hat{p}_{cj}\right)}{n_c} + \frac{\hat{p}_{dj}\left(1 - \hat{p}_{dj}\right)}{n_d}} \,,
$$

$$(12.4)$$

where $\hat{p}_{cj} = y_{cj}/n_c$, $\hat{p}_{dj} = y_{dj}/n_d$, and $\chi^2_{1-\alpha}[(g-1)(g-1)]$ is from Table 6 of the Appendix. The intervals (12.4) may be computed for any group comparison and for any particular response category. If zero is in an interval, then one concludes that $p_{cj} = p_{dj}$; if zero is not in the interval, then the conclusion is that $p_{cj} \neq p_{dj}$.

12.4 SUMMARY

The procedures of this chapter provide methods of analysis for the multiple-group comparison problem of categorical data. These techniques coupled with those of the previous two chapters provide a fairly extensive body of approaches for the data analyst.

For more reading on the topic of categorical data analysis, the reader may refer to Fleiss (1981), Bishop, Fienberg, and Holland (1975), or Forthofer and Lehnen (1981).

The computation of chi-square tests for the completely random design with two or more response categories can be performed using the procedure FREQ of the SAS statistical package or the program BMDP4F of BMDP. Cochran's test for the randomized complete block design can be done using the procedure MATRIX of SAS or by coding the algorithm presented in Table 12.1, part C, using BASIC or FORTRAN.

PROBLEMS

12.1. Ten patients with recent subarachnoid hemmorrhage were appraised by three physicians as to the degree of risk for a major surgical procedure. Coding 0 for low risk and 1 as high risk gave the following results:

Patient	Physician		
	I	II	III
1	0	1	1
2	1	1	1
3	0	0	0
4	0	1	0
5	0	0	0
6	1	1	0
7	0	1	0
8	0	1	1
9	1	1	0
10	0	1	0

Does the risk assessment differ among the physicians?

12.2. Sixteen students from a junior high school were classified by five of their teachers (mathematics, English, social science, music, and physical education) as either showing or not showing behavior problems in class. Coding a no-problem child as 0 and a behavior problem child as 1, we have the following results:

Student	Teacher				
	1	2	3	4	5
1	1	1	1	1	0
2	1	0	1	1	0
3	0	0	1	0	0
4	0	0	0	0	0
5	0	0	0	0	0
6	0	1	0	0	0
7	1	0	1	1	1
8	1	1	1	1	0
9	1	1	1	1	1
10	0	1	0	1	0
11	1	1	1	1	1
12	1	1	0	1	0
13	0	0	0	0	0
14	1	0	0	0	0
15	1	1	1	1	1
16	0	1	0	1	0

Does the behavior problem classification differ among the teachers?

12.3. Intra-arterial narrowing, interpreted as vasospasm by the attending physician, was reported in patients who had a recently ruptured intracranial internal carotid artery aneurysm (Nibbelink, Torner, and Henderson, 1981). The resulting neurologic condition was classified with the following codes: 1 = symptom free, 2 = minor symptoms (headache, meningeal irritation, diplopia), 3 = major neurologic deficit, 4 = impaired state of alertness, 5 = poorly responsive. The distribution of patients with and without vasospasm in each neurologic condition is presented in the next table. The number of deaths is indicated in parentheses in the bottom row of the table. Mortality was determined for all patients following administration of antihypertensive medication.

Vasospasm	Neurologic Condition					Total
	1	2	3	4	5	
Present	6	74	32	13	10	135
Absent	16	124	18	11	5	174
Total	22 (2)	198 (90)	50 (24)	24 (17)	15 (10)	309 (143)

Source: D. W. Nibbelink, J. C. Torner, and W. G. Henderson (1981). Randomized treatment study. Drug-induced hypotension. In A. L. Saks, D. W. Nibbelink, and J. C. Torner (eds.), *Aneurysmal Subarachnoid Hemorrhage*, Urban and Schwartzenberg, Baltimore–Munich. Reprinted with permission of the publishers.

(a) Is the presence of vasospasm different for the levels of neurologic condition?

(b) Obtain 95% simultaneous confidence intervals on all the pairwise comparisons among the neurologic conditions.

(c) Compare the mortality rates among the neurologic conditions.

12.4. Patients whose primary diagnosis was schizophrenia, senile dementia, or mental retardation with psychosis received pharmocologic doses of choline in an attempt to suppress their involuntary facial movements (tardive dyskinesia). The results of this experiment are:

Clinical Effect	Severity of Tardive Dyskinesia		
	Mild	Moderate	Severe
Improved	8	9	11
Not improved	12	6	7

(a) Is the clinical effect of the drug different for the severity groups defined in this table?

(b) Obtain 95% simultaneous confidence intervals on all the pairwise comparisons among the groups. Comment on your results.

12.5. Patients with schizophrenia and other mental disorders were evaluated with two tests to detect the presence of psychotic symptoms. The scales used are a reality testing scale (includes grandiosity, suspicion, persecution, and hallucination) and a behavioral disturbance scale (inappropriate affect, negativism, excitement, disorientation, etc.). The presence of significant symptoms in either of these subscales indicated psychosis. The results of the study are presented in the following table:

	Diagnosis	
Symptoms	Schizophrenia	Other
None	17	23
Some, not psychotic	9	12
Psychotic	12	0
No information	6	8

Source: N. E. Waxler. Is outcome of schizophrenia better in nonindustrial societies? *J. Nerv. Ment. Dis.*, 167, 144–158, copyright by Williams & Wilkins (1979).

Are the distributions for the symptoms different for the two diagnostic groups? Use $\alpha = 0.05$. Obtain the chi-square test with and without the last row of the table. Comment on your findings.

12.6. A sample of 373 adolescents (193 boys and 180 girls) from four different community school areas in a midwest city and 102 adolescents (53 boys and 49 girls) from a near rural sector was selected. From a personal interview with four psychiatrists, plus information gathered from their teachers, school advisers, and family doctors, a global evaluation of the mental health of each person in the sample was obtained with the following results:

	Urban			Rural		
Symptoms	Both Sexes	Boys	Girls	Both Sexes	Boys	Girls
None	112	59	53	29	14	15
Mild	122	60	62	43	23	20
Moderate	113	58	55	28	15	13
Marked	26	16	10	2	1	1

(a) Are the symptom distributions different for boys and girls within each geographic location?

(b) Are there urban–rural differences with respect to the symptom distributions?

12.7. For patients who were about to undergo a major surgical procedure related to their cerebrovascular accident, the risk for each patient was appraised using the rating scale of "good," "fair," and "poor" to define the patient's medical condition. The distribution of patients with respect to medical condition by age in decades is presented in the following table:

	Medical Condition		
Age	Good	Fair	Poor
30–39	12	11	5
40–49	16	13	7
50–59	11	4	14
60–69	9	8	10
70–79	1	2	3

Is there evidence that the condition distributions are different for the five ages?

REFERENCES

Bishop, Y. M. M., S. E. Fienberg, and P. W. Holland. (1975). *Discrete Multivariate Analysis: Theory and Practice*, MIT Press, Cambridge, MA.

Cochran, W. G. (1950). The comparisons of percentages in matched samples, *Biometrika*, **37**, 256–266.

Fleiss, J. L. (1981). *Statistical Methods for Rates and Proportions*, Wiley, New York.

Forthofer, R. N., and R. G. Lehnen. (1981). *Public Program Analysis: A New Categorical Data Approach*, Lifetime Learning, Belmont, CA.

Grizzle, J. E., C. F. Starmer, and G. G. Koch. (1969). Analysis of categorical data, *Biometrics*, **25**, 489–504.

McNemar, Q. (1947). Note on the sampling error of the difference between correlated proportions or percentages, *Psychometrika*, **12**, 153–157.

Nibbelink, D. W., J. C. Torner, and W. G. Henderson. (1981). Randomized treatment study. Drug-induced hypotension, in: *Aneurysmal Subarachnoid Hemorrhage*, A. L. Saks, D. W. Nibbelink, and T. C. Torner (eds.), Urban and Schwarzenberg, Baltimore-Munich.

CHAPTER 13

Special Topics in Analysis of Epidemiologic and Clinical Data: Studying Association between a Disease and a Characteristic

13.1 INTRODUCTION

There are certain statistical techniques that are frequently used in the analysis of epidemiologic data. Virtually all of these statistical methods may be applied to other types of data as well; however, it is expected that the student of epidemiology will find them of special interest. We use the word *clinical* in the chapter title since the techniques are also applicable to studies in clinical research that are not necessarily of an epidemiological nature.

Throughout this chapter and the next, we consider whether a dichotomous risk factor may be associated with a measurable outcome like the development of a particular disease, death due to the disease, length of time to death, or length of time in remission. This procedure has, in fact, two applications. In this chapter, we discuss the questions of measuring the association between a dichotomous risk factor and a dichotomous disease state. In Chapter 14, we discuss the question of studying the association between the dichotomous risk factor and the length of time to some endpoint, typically death or recurrence of the disease. The term *risk factor* is used to indicate the variable whose effect on the disease endpoint we wish to determine.

Before proceeding to the discussion of the actual methods, a word is in order regarding the general types of epidemiologic investigations. Interested readers should supplement these chapters by referring to a text on epidemiologic methods (e.g. Miettinen, 1985 or Kleinbaum, Kupper and Morgenstern, 1982).

13.2   TYPES OF STUDIES IN EPIDEMIOLOGY AND CLINICAL RESEARCH

For convenience, let us assume that the risk factor is denoted by the variable X and the outcome variable is denoted by Y. In the case of a dichotomous risk factor and a dichotomous response variable, we use the notation $[X = 0]$ to denote one level of the risk factor and $[X = 1]$ for the other level. Similarly, the two disease state responses are denoted by $[Y = 0]$ and $[Y = 1]$. The main question is whether there is an association between the variables X and Y. For example, in a family study of depression, the variable X may represent the presence or absence of a family history of depression, while the variable Y may represent the presence or absence of depression in the persons under study. How does one determine if there is an association between X and Y? In order to examine this question, it is first useful to determine what type of sampling scheme was used in the study. There are three basic sampling schemes: the prospective, the retrospective, and the cross-sectional sampling designs.

13.2.1   Prospective Study

The prospective study, either epidemiologic or purely clinical, can be a most difficult study to conduct. It typically involves a great cost in terms of both manpower and money. From the statistical standpoint, the prospective study involves the selection of a random sample of persons with risk factor at level $[X = 0]$ and the selection of another random, possibly matched, sample of persons with risk factor at level $[X = 1]$. If Y happens to be a dichotomous response variate indicating presence or absence of disease, then at the time of the selection of the samples, all those persons who already have the disease are discarded from the sample. This is done because one is interested, under this design, in following up a group of persons with and without a risk factor who do not have the disease at the start of the study. Thus, the sampling scheme of the prospective study is as depicted in Figure 13.1.

Hence, the prospective study is a forward-going study; it selects persons with and without the risk factor and then follows them in order to observe the distribution of the response variable Y. This is one type of study that

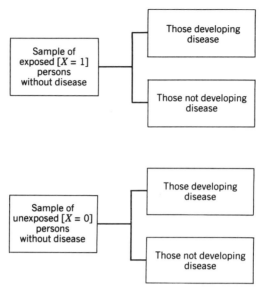

Figure 13.1. Schema of prospective study.

has been generally discussed in the text. In fact, we note that the $[X = 0]$ and $[X = 1]$ groups form the group-identifying labels, and the procedures of Chapters 6 and 7 may be applied to compare the response variable Y. Futhermore, it is easily seen that if the risk factor consisted of g rather than 2 levels, then the procedures of Chapters 10–12 may be applied to compare the distribution of the Y variable. Thus, the procedures that have been presented in detail in this text generally apply quite easily to prospective clinical or epidemiologic investigations.

The main problem in interpreting these analyses of epidemiologic data is in the original assignment of X labels: it is not done by random assignment but may be controlled by other, often unmeasured factors. In spite of this, the prospective study is generally regarded as a sound epidemiologic study design inasmuch as it is often relatively free of other biases when compared to the alternative cross-sectional or retrospective study design.

One of the easiest ways to perform a prospective study is to do it historically. That is, identify, if possible, two cohorts of persons, one with a characteristic and the other without the characteristic from an earlier time period; then perform the prospective study from this point. For example, in a study of the long-term (30–40 year) outcome of schizophrenia, mania, and depression, three diagnostic groups were identified from records of the

University of Iowa Psychiatric Hospital from 1935 to 1945. This study, conducted from 1973 to 1979, consisted of tracing these cohorts and assessing the outcome. The study was indeed prospective, but it was designed in such a way that the follow-up period had ended, thus negating the need to follow a new cohort for 30–40 years. Such a study is frequently termed an *historical prospective* study. It is still a prospective study since it is the characteristic variable X that is sampled, not the outcome variable Y.

13.2.2 Retrospective Study

The retrospective (or case control) study is the inverse of the prospective study. The samples are determined from the Y responses; then the researcher "looks back" to determine how many people in each Y category have the risk factor. These studies are generally less expensive but may be somewhat difficult to interpret. In a retrospective study, the data gathered are in the form of how X depends on Y. In many cases, the information gathered in a retrospective study can be turned around to study the results from the viewpoint of a prospective study; however, the interpretation of the results is somewhat more guarded.

A major reason for doing a retrospective rather than prospective study is that of cost. For example, if an investigator wished to study the question of whether schizophrenics have lower cancer rates than nonschizophrenic controls, the costs of doing a prospective study would be almost prohibitive. The rate of cancer is so low in the general population that an enormous sample of schizophrenics and controls is needed to have a sufficiently powerful test of the hypothesis. On the other hand, a retrospective study would select a random sample of known cancer cases and appropriate controls and then observe the presence or absence of schizophrenia in each person's medical history. The costs of conducting the latter study would surely be less than that of the prospective study.

The basic sampling scheme for the retrospective study is outlined in Figure 13.2 for the case of a dichotomous variable Y.

There is ample opportunity for biased data in a retrospective study. The selection of the samples with and without disease rather than on the basis of the characteristic raises the question of whether the samples are representative of the diseased population. If, for example, Y is a variable indicating cancer or not cancer, and X is a variable denoting presence or absence of schizophrenia, then an observed association between X and Y in a retrospective study must be interpreted in light of how representative these cancer cases are of all cancer cases. It may be that the desired

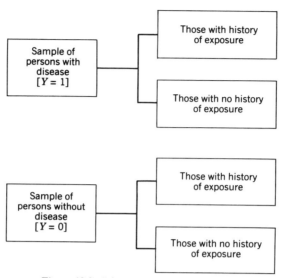

Figure 13.2. Schema of retrospective study.

association is completely distorted by the retrospective study design. See Schlesselman (1982) for a good discussion of such potential biases and methods for dealing with them.

13.2.3   Cross-Sectional Study

In some situations, the joint distribution of X and Y is observed by selecting a random sample from the general population. This type of study is illustrated in Figure 13.3.

In this situation, the variables X and Y are studied together as they appear in the population. To determine if social class, X, is associated with psychiatric illness, Y, one study that could be performed is to survey a well-defined population at a given point in time. Then the study could classify each person in the sample on the basis of social class (e.g., lower or not lower) and psychiatric diagnoses (e.g., schizophrenia or not schizophrenia). This type of study would be a cross-sectional study. This study is generally less expensive than the prospective study. The bias problem must again be carefully examined since it is possible that persons with, for example, both the disease and the characteristic are systematically excluded

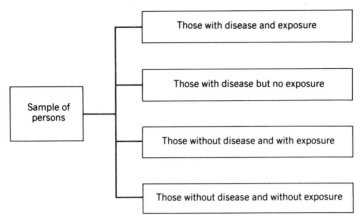

Figure 13.3. Schema of cross-sectional study.

from the sample. This could happen if this group had a lower study participation rate than the other groups.

If such biases can be discounted, the procedures of Chapter 8 are especially appropriate for the analysis of an association between X and Y.

It follows from this discussion of sample designs that data can be summarized in the form of a 2×2 table; for example,

$$
\begin{array}{c|cc}
 & Y = 1 & Y = 0 \\
\hline
X = 1 & A & C \\
X = 0 & B & D \\
\end{array}
\qquad (13.1)
$$

where A, B, C, and D are the numbers of persons in each category. Epidemiologic studies cannot be properly interpreted without first knowing the sampling scheme. Were the row margins fixed, as in a prospective study? Were the column margins fixed, as in a retrospective study? Or was only the total sample size fixed, as in a cross-sectional study? Only after the sampling design is understood can a data analyst begin the analysis.

After specifying the design, the possible biases must be carefully assessed before proceeding with the formal statistical analysis. The statistical analysis is really quite secondary to these more fundamental clinical and epidemiologic issues. Many of the questions of interest in a prospective and cross-sectional study are easily studied by the statistical methods of the previous chapters.

13.3 DICHOTOMOUS RESPONSE AND DICHOTOMOUS RISK FACTOR: 2 × 2 TABLES

The basic situation is described for the dichotomous response and risk factor problem by four probabilities in the sampled population:

$$p_{00} = \Pr[\,X = 0, Y = 0\,],$$

$$p_{01} = \Pr[\,X = 0, Y = 1\,],$$

$$\quad (13.2)$$

$$p_{10} = \Pr[\,X = 1, Y = 0\,],$$

$$p_{11} = \Pr[\,X = 1, Y = 1\,],$$

where p_{00} is the probability that a randomly selected person does not have the risk factor and does not have the disease, and so forth, until p_{11} is the probability that a randomly selected person has both the risk factor and the disease. Clearly, it follows that

$$p_{00} + p_{01} + p_{10} + p_{11} = 1, \quad (13.3)$$

as an individual must fall into one, and only one, of the four categories.

From the discussion of the previous section it is clear that only the cross-sectional study provides direct estimates of the quantities p_{00}, p_{01}, p_{10}, and p_{11}. The prospective and retrospective studies yield estimates of various conditional probabilities. Some additional notational would be useful. Let the marginal probabilities be denoted by

$$p_{0+} = \Pr[\,X = 0\,] = \Pr[\,X = 0, Y = 0\,] + \Pr[\,X = 0, Y = 1\,] = p_{00} + p_{01},$$

$$p_{1+} = \Pr[\,X = 1\,] = \Pr[\,X = 1, Y = 0\,] + \Pr[\,X = 1, Y = 1\,] = p_{10} + p_{11},$$

$$p_{+0} = \Pr[\,Y = 0\,] = \Pr[\,X = 0, Y = 0\,] + \Pr[\,X = 1, Y = 0\,] = p_{00} + p_{10},$$

$$p_{+1} = \Pr[\,Y = 1\,] = \Pr[\,X = 0, Y = 1\,] + \Pr[\,X = 1, Y = 1\,] = p_{01} + p_{11}.$$

$$\quad (13.4)$$

The various conditional probabilities may be computed directly from (13.2) and (13.4). For those probabilities of X given Y, we have

$$\Pr[X = 0 | Y = 0] = p_{00}/p_{+0},$$

$$\Pr[X = 1 | Y = 0] = p_{10}/p_{+0},$$

$$\Pr[X = 0 | Y = 1] = p_{01}/p_{+1},$$ (13.5)

$$\Pr[X = 1 | Y = 1] = p_{11}/p_{+1}.$$

The conditional probabilities of Y given X are given by

$$\Pr[Y = 0 | X = 0] = p_{00}/p_{0+},$$

$$\Pr[Y = 1 | X = 0] = p_{01}/p_{0+},$$

$$\Pr[Y = 0 | X = 1] = p_{10}/p_{1+},$$ (13.6)

$$\Pr[Y = 1 | X = 1] = p_{11}/p_{1+}.$$

For many epidemiologic and clinical studies, the prospective sampling design provides direct estimates of probabilities (13.6) while the retrospective design study provides direct estimates of probabilities (13.5). This assumption is made in the remainder of this chapter. The reader should be aware, however, that a more comprehensive treatment of this issue would require incorporation of the time period of the study into the discussion. Kleinbaum, Kupper, and Morgenstern (1982) or Breslow and Day (1980) provide these details and should be consulted for further elaboration.

Before discussing the question of what form an estimator of a measure of association will take (which will depend on the sampling design), it is of interest to discuss various possible measures of association between X and Y in the population.

13.3.1 Expressing Relationship between a Risk Factor and a Disease

There are many ways to exhibit the relationship between X and Y, even for this simple dichotomous situation. The choice of a particular measure for a study depends to some degree on the purposes of the investigation. One measure of association is the *risk difference*. It is defined by

$$\text{Risk difference} = \Pr[Y = 1 | X = 1] - \Pr[Y = 1 | X = 0]. \quad (13.7)$$

This quantity is the amount of the disease rate attributable to the risk factor. If one multiplies the risk difference (13.7) by a population figure like 100,000, the result is the expected number of individuals (of 100,000) who would not get the disease if the risk factor could be eliminated. This type of figure has been useful to public health workers who wish to express the number of lives that would be saved if, for example, pollution of the atmosphere was reduced or cigarette smoking eliminated. It has similar usage in psychiatry in terms of estimating the reduction in the number of psychiatric disorders if a particular risk factor were eliminated.

Another measure of association that is used frequently is the *relative risk* or *risk ratio*:

$$\text{Relative risk} = \frac{\Pr[Y = 1 | X = 1]}{\Pr[Y = 1 | X = 0]}. \tag{13.8}$$

It is the likelihood of the disease in those with the risk factor relative to the likelihood of the disease among those who do not have the risk factor. Clearly, a value of 1 indicates that the rates are equal in the two groups. This means that the probability of having the disease is the same if one has the risk factor or not. The relative risk is used frequently as a measure of association in epidemiologic studies. Relative risk is thought to be of greater value in etiological studies in which the goals are to identify risk factors related to disease.

The final measure of association that we include here is the *odds ratio*. Recall that the odds ratio is equal to 1 and the log odds ratio is equal to zero if there is no association between X and Y. The odds ratio, while defined in Chapter 8, is restated by the following equivalent expressions:

$$\text{OR} = \frac{\Pr[Y = 1 | X = 1] / \Pr[Y = 0 | X = 1]}{\Pr[Y = 1 | X = 0] / \Pr[Y = 0 | X = 0]}; \tag{13.9}$$

or

$$\text{OR} = \frac{\Pr[X = 1 | Y = 1] / \Pr[X = 0 | Y = 1]}{\Pr[X = 1 | Y = 0] / \Pr[X = 0 | Y = 0]}; \tag{13.10}$$

and from (13.5–13.6) it follows that (13.9) and (13.10) are equivalent to

$$\text{OR} = \frac{p_{00} p_{11}}{p_{10} p_{01}}. \tag{13.11}$$

Expressions (13.9) and (13.10) express the fact that the odds ratio is indeed a ratio of odds. For instance, ratio (13.9) is the odds of the disease

Table 13.1. Typical 2 × 2 Table of Sample Data[a]

	$Y = 1$	$Y = 0$	Total
$X = 1$	A	C	$A + C$
$X = 0$	B	D	$B + D$
Total	$A + B$	$C + D$	N

[a] Entries are number of persons.

among those with the risk factor, $[X = 1]$, divided by the odds of the disease among those without the risk factor, $[X = 0]$. Clearly (under the assumptions in this chapter) ratio (13.9) is directly estimated for the prospective or cross-sectional sampling designs, while ratio (13.10) is easily estimated for the retrospective study.

We will focus on the odds ratio and the relative risk as the measures of association. There are others that can be employed, but these two measures of association are among the most useful in epidemiologic or clinical research. Both of these measures are equal to 1 if there is no association between X and Y and are not equal to 1 if there is an association. The reader is referred to Miettinen (1985) and Kleinbaum et al. (1982) for a further account of the various measures of association.

13.3.2 Inference for Relative Risk and Odds Ratio for 2 × 2 Table: Unmatched Samples

Throughout this section, the sample data are assumed to be of the form given in Table 13.1.

13.3.2.1 Prospective Study: Two Independent Samples

13.3.2.1.1 Relative Risk
For this situation, we have two independent random samples: one of size $A + C$ and the other of size $B + D$. By formula (13.8), the relative risk is directly estimated by

$$\hat{R} = \frac{A/(A + C)}{B/(B + D)}. \tag{13.12}$$

The natural logarithm* of (13.12) is

$$\log \hat{R} = \log(A) + \log(B + D) - \log(B) - \log(A + C), \tag{13.13}$$

*Throughout this chapter, "log" will denote the natural logarithm.

which has an estimated variance of

$$\hat{\sigma}^2_{\log \hat{R}} = \frac{C}{A(A + C)} + \frac{D}{B(B + D)}. \tag{13.14}$$

As the relative risk (13.8) is equal to 1 if and only if the population disease rates are equal, it follows that a test of the hypothesis of no association is equivalent to testing that the logarithm of the relative risk is equal to zero (recall that $\log 1 = 0$). For large samples, the hypothesis may be tested with the statistic

$$\left(\log \hat{R}\right)^2 / \hat{\sigma}^2_{\log \hat{R}}, \tag{13.15}$$

as it is as approximately distributed as a chi-square variate with one degree of freedom when the null hypothesis of no association is true; thus, the null hypothesis of no association will be rejected for large values of expression (13.15).

A $(1 - \alpha)100\%$ confidence interval for the logarithm of the relative risk can be determined by

$$\log \hat{R} \pm Z_{1-\alpha/2}\hat{\sigma}_{\log \hat{R}}, \tag{13.16}$$

where $Z_{1-\alpha/2}$ is taken from Table 4 of the Appendix. A $(1 - \alpha)100\%$ confidence interval for the relative risk itself is obtained by taking antilogarithms of the endpoints of the interval determined by expression (13.16).

13.3.2.1.2   Odds Ratio
From ratio (13.9) and Table 13.1, the odds ratio for a prospective study is estimated by

$$\widehat{OR} = \frac{[A/(A + C)]/[C/(A + C)]}{[B/(B + D)]/[D/(B + D)]} = \frac{AD}{BC},$$

and thus the log odds ratio for a prospective study is estimated by

$$\log \widehat{OR} = \log(AD/BC); \tag{13.17}$$

the variance of the log odds ratio estimator is estimated by

$$\hat{\sigma}^2_{\log(\widehat{OR})} = \left(\frac{1}{A} + \frac{1}{B} + \frac{1}{C} + \frac{1}{D}\right). \tag{13.18}$$

In order to test the null hypothesis of no association between X and Y, the statistic

$$\left(\log \widehat{OR}\right)^2 \Big/ \hat{\sigma}^2_{\log(\widehat{OR})} \qquad (13.19)$$

can be compared to a chi-square distribution with one degree of freedom. Since the log of the population odds ratio is zero if there is no association between X and Y, the null hypothesis is rejected for large values of expression (13.19).

A $(1 - \alpha)100\%$ confidence interval for the log of odds ratio is given by

$$\log \widehat{OR} \pm Z_{1-\alpha/2}\hat{\sigma}_{\log(\widehat{OR})}, \qquad (13.20)$$

where $Z_{1-\alpha/2}$ is from Table 4 of the Appendix.

Taking antilogarithms of the endpoints obtained from (13.20) yields a $(1 - \alpha)100\%$ confidence interval for the odds ratio itself.

Consider the following example.

Example 13.3.2.1.2.1. In a long-term outcome study of psychiatric depression, 146 males and 148 females with a clinical diagnosis of depression were assessed with regard to their mental health and various social adjustment variates such as employment success. The following data resulted:

	Outcome (Y)		
	Poor	Not Poor	Total
Female Depressives	37	111	148
Male Depressives	24	122	146
Total	61	233	294

Using relative risk and/or odds ratio estimators, is there sufficient evidence to conclude that poor outcome is associated with the sex of a depressive patient?

From the data in the example, it is evident that $A = 37$, $B = 24$, $C = 111$, and $D = 122$. From the statistics in Sections 13.3.2.1.1 and 13.3.2.1.2, one readily obtains

$$\hat{R} = \frac{37/148}{24/146} = 1.52083,$$

$$\log \hat{R} = 0.41926,$$

$$\hat{\sigma}^2_{\log \hat{R}} = \frac{111}{148(37)} + \frac{122}{24(146)} = 0.055088,$$

and thus

$$\left(\log \hat{R}\right)^2 / \hat{\sigma}_{\log \hat{R}}^2 = (0.41926)^2/(0.055088) = 3.19$$

for the relative risk analysis; while one obtains

$$\widehat{OR} = \frac{37(122)}{24(111)} = 1.694444,$$

$$\log \widehat{OR} = 0.527355,$$

$$\hat{\sigma}_{\log(\widehat{OR})}^2 = \frac{1}{37} + \frac{1}{24} + \frac{1}{111} + \frac{1}{122} = 0.085899,$$

and thus

$$\frac{\left(\log \widehat{OR}\right)^2}{\hat{\sigma}_{\log(\widehat{OR})}^2} = \frac{(0.52735)^2}{0.08589} = 3.24$$

for the odds ratio analysis.

In neither case does the chi-square statistic reach the 3.84 value that would be required for a 0.05 level test. As $Z_{0.975} = 1.96$, a 95% confidence interval for the log-relative risk is $0.41926 \pm (1.96)(0.2347) = (-0.04075, 0.87927)$, while for the relative risk it is given by

$$\left(e^{-0.04075}, e^{0.87927}\right) = (0.9601, 2.4091). \tag{13.21}$$

Notice that the value of 1 is included in the interval (13.21), which agrees with the result of our chi-square test, but (13.21) also supports the hypothesis of an association as 1 is barely in the interval.

For the odds ratio, the 95% confidence interval for the log odds ratio is $0.52735 \pm (1.96)(0.29309) = (-0.04711, 1.10181)$, while for the odds ratio it is therefore given by

$$\left(e^{-0.04711}, e^{1.10181}\right) = (0.9540, 3.0096). \tag{13.22}$$

Notice that the value of 1 is in the interval (13.22), which agrees with the test result. Again, the value of 1 is barely in the interval.

It may happen that an entry in Table 13.1 is zero. In this situation, it is advisable to add 0.5 to each cell entry A, B, C, and D and then proceed to the analysis just described with these adjusted cell frequencies. The analyst must adjust each A, B, C, or D if any one is zero since the log of zero is $-\infty$.

Also notice that the analyses described do not yield identical results for the relative risk and the odds ratio.

13.3.2.2 Retrospective Study: Two Independent Samples

13.3.2.2.1 Odds Ratio as Approximate Relative Risk

Of the important developments in the analysis of retrospective data, few rival Cornfield's (1951), whose results we present in this section. Recall that a retrospective study provides direct estimates of expression (13.5) because the random samples are of cases and noncases rather than those with the risk factor and those without the risk factor. Let us suppose that an investigator would like to make an inference regarding the relative risk (13.8). Can this be done from the results of a retrospective study?

Below we address such a question. The reader is again reminded that this presentation is somewhat simplified here, as the time period of the study is not introduced. Again, epidemiologic methods texts such as Kleinbaum et al. (1982) may be consulted.

From basic probability, we know that

$$\Pr[Y = 1 | X = 1] = \frac{\Pr[X = 1, Y = 1]}{\Pr[X = 1]}. \tag{13.23}$$

Furthermore, we know that the numerator of expression (13.23) is

$$\Pr[X = 1, Y = 1] = \Pr[X = 1 | Y = 1]\Pr[Y = 1], \tag{13.24}$$

while the denominator is

$$\Pr[X = 1] = \Pr[X = 1 | Y = 1]\Pr[Y = 1] + \Pr[X = 1 | Y = 0]\Pr[Y = 0], \tag{13.25}$$

since $\Pr[X = 1] = \Pr[X = 1, Y = 1] + \Pr[X = 1, Y = 0]$. Since $\Pr[Y = 0] = 1 - \Pr[Y = 1]$, it follows that expression (13.25) can be written as

$$\Pr[X = 1] = \Pr[X = 1 | Y = 0] + \Pr[Y = 1]$$
$$\times \{\Pr[X = 1 | Y = 1] - \Pr[X = 1 | Y = 0]\}. \tag{13.26}$$

Thus, (13.23), using (13.24) for the numerator and (13.26) for the denominator, is

$$\Pr[Y = 1 | X = 1]$$
$$= \frac{\Pr[X = 1 | Y = 1]\Pr[Y = 1]}{\Pr[X = 1 | Y = 0] + \left(\Pr[Y = 1]\{\Pr[X = 1 | Y = 1] - \Pr[X = 1 | Y = 0]\}\right)}; \tag{13.27}$$

similarly, $\Pr[Y = 1 | X = 0]$ can be written as

$$\Pr[Y = 1 | X = 0]$$

$$= \frac{\Pr[X = 0 | Y = 1]\Pr[Y = 1]}{\Pr[X = 0 | Y = 0] - (\Pr[Y = 1]\{\Pr[X = 0 | Y = 0] - \Pr[X = 0 | Y = 1]\})} .$$

$$(13.28)$$

The ratio of probability (13.27) to probability (13.28) is the relative risk. At this point, Cornfield's approximation applies. If the overall disease rate, which is $\Pr[Y = 1]$, is very small, then the parenthesized expressions in the denominators of expressions (13.27) and (13.28) are very close to zero, since a very small term $(\Pr[Y = 1])$ is being multiplied by a term that is less than or equal to 1. Hence, let us treat those parenthetical terms as if they are negligible. Thus, from (13.27) and (13.28), we have

$$\Pr[Y = 1 | X = 1] \doteq \frac{\Pr[X = 1 | Y = 1]\Pr[Y = 1]}{\Pr[X = 1 | Y = 0]}, \qquad (13.29)$$

$$\Pr[Y = 1 | X = 0] \doteq \frac{\Pr[X = 0 | Y = 1]\Pr[Y = 1]}{\Pr[X = 0 | Y = 0]}. \qquad (13.30)$$

As the relative risk is defined by $\Pr[Y = 1 | X = 1] / \Pr[Y = 1 | X = 0]$, it follows from expressions (13.29) and (13.30) that the relative risk is approximately equal to the ratio of (13.29) to (13.30), that is,

$$RR \doteq \frac{\Pr[X = 1 | Y = 1]\Pr[X = 0 | Y = 0]}{\Pr[X = 1 | Y = 0]\Pr[X = 0 | Y = 1]}, \qquad (13.31)$$

and this approximation is good if the disease rate is small. Notice that the right side of (13.31) is made of terms that are directly estimable in a retrospective study. So this approximate relative risk may be estimated from a retrospective study.

Furthermore, comparing the right side of expression (13.31) to expression (13.10) shows that they are identical. That is, the odds ratio computed for a 2×2 table arising in a retrospective study is an estimate of the approximate relative risk. Hence, inference procedures for the odds ratio and the approximate relative risk are one and the same for a retrospective study if the disease rate is small. Frequently in presentations of retrospective study data, the adjective *approximate* is omitted from the discussion of relative risk. The reader should bear in mind that the odds ratio is, generally, only an approximation to the relative risk. For certain types of case control (i.e., retrospective) studies called "incidence-density" designs (Miettinen, 1976, and Greenland and Thomas, 1982), the rare-disease assumption is not required. The reader can refer to Kleinbaum et al. (1982) for a further account of this.

13.3.2.2.2 Estimation of and Tests of Hypotheses for Odds Ratio
For the retrospective study, the two random samples are of sizes $A + B$ and $C + D$ in the notation of Table 13.1. Thus, the following estimates of the conditional probabilities in (13.31) arise:

$$\Pr[X = 1|Y = 1] = A/(A + B),$$
$$\Pr[X = 1|Y = 0] = C/(C + D),$$
$$\Pr[X = 0|Y = 1] = B/(A + B),$$
$$\Pr[X = 0|Y = 0] = D/(C + D).$$
(13.32)

Substituting probability (13.32) directly into expression (13.31) results in

$$\widehat{OR} = AD/BC; \tag{13.33}$$

note that this expression is the same as that used for estimating the odds ratio in a prospective study.

The large-sample variance of $\log \widehat{OR}$ is estimated by

$$\hat{\sigma}^2_{\log(\widehat{OR})} = \frac{1}{A} + \frac{1}{B} + \frac{1}{C} + \frac{1}{D}. \tag{13.34}$$

As mentioned in the previous discussion regarding prospective studies, if any cell frequency is zero, each entry A, B, C, and D should have 0.5 added to it before proceeding to compute statistics (13.33) and (13.34).

A large-sample test of the hypothesis that the odds ratio is equal to 1 is given by comparing

$$\left(\log \widehat{OR}\right)^2 \Big/ \hat{\sigma}^2_{\log(\widehat{OR})} \tag{13.35}$$

to a chi-square distribution with one degree of freedom. A $(1 - \alpha)100\%$ confidence interval for the $\log OR$ is provided by

$$\log \widehat{OR} \pm Z_{1 - \alpha/2} \hat{\sigma}_{\log(\widehat{OR})}, \tag{13.36}$$

where $Z_{1-\alpha/2}$ is taken from Table 4 of the Appendix. A $(1 - \alpha)100\%$ confidence interval for the odds ratio itself is obtained via exponentiating the endpoints of expression (13.36).

It should be emphasized that for a retrospective study the sample odds ratio AD/BC is always an appropriate estimate of the population odds ratio, regardless of how well it estimates the population relative risk. In fact, the sample odds ratio AD/BC is an appropriate estimate of the population odds ratio for all three types of studies—prospective, retrospective, and cross-sectional—and thus a test of association can be based upon it for each type of study. As it turns out, the test of association using the sample odds ratio has the same form for all three types of studies.

Example 13.3.2.2.2.1. A retrospective study of clinical charts was conducted that involved 112 psychotic patients and 113 nonpsychotic "controls." The goal of the study was to determine if a positive family history of psychiatric illness was more likely to lead to a psychotic disorder. The data are:

	Positive Family History?	Y Psychosis	No Psychosis	Total
	Yes	39	25	64
X	No	73	88	161
	Total	112	113	225

At the 5% level of significance, is there sufficient evidence to conclude that there is an association? From these data it is clear that

$$\widehat{OR} = \frac{39(88)}{73(25)} = 1.88,$$

$$\log \widehat{OR} = 0.63156,$$

$$\hat{\sigma}^2_{\log(\widehat{OR})} = \frac{1}{39} + \frac{1}{73} + \frac{1}{25} + \frac{1}{88} = 0.09070,$$

and thus

$$\left(\log \widehat{OR}\right)^2 \big/ \hat{\sigma}^2_{\log(\widehat{OR})} = 4.398.$$

From Table 6 of the Appendix, $\chi^2_{0.95}(1) = 3.84$; hence, there is sufficient evidence to conclude that there is an association between familial history and psychotic disorder. As $Z_{0.975} = 1.96$, a 95% confidence interval for $\log OR$ is $0.63156 \pm 1.96(0.30116) = (0.04129, 1.22183)$, or for the actual odds ratio is

$$\left(e^{0.04129}, e^{1.22183} \right) = (1.0422, 3.3934). \tag{13.37}$$

Notice that 1 is not in the interval (13.37), which agrees with the results of the statistical test.

13.3.2.3   Cross-Sectional Study

The statistical analysis for the relative risk and the odds ratio for a cross-sectional study follows that found in Section 13.3.2.1 for the prospective study. There are no differences between these two studies with regard to the formal statistical analysis of relative risk or odds ratio. The principal difference arises in the interpretation of the results in light of the bias potential of a cross-sectional study relative to the prospective study.

13.3.3   Inference for Odds Ratio from S Independent 2 × 2 Tables: Unmatched Samples

Since the statistical inference procedures for the odds ratio are the same for the three basic sampling designs, we focus on this particular measure of association in this section. The problem we now wish to address is that of determining an overall estimate of the odds ratio from a series of S independent 2 × 2 tables. There is no need to distinguish between the three types of studies for this particular problem, since we focus on the odds ratio (see Section 13.3.2). The basic data layout is shown in Table 13.2.

Example 13.3.3.1.   Suppose a study was performed in which the presence or absence of disease was observed in addition to the presence or absence of

Table 13.2. Data Layout for S Independent 2 × 2 Tables

	$Y = 1$	$Y = 0$	Total
$X = 1$	A_i	C_i	M_{1i}
$X = 0$	B_i	D_i	M_{0i}
Total	R_{1i}	R_{0i}	N_i
	for $i = 1, 2, \ldots, S$		

a characteristic. These observations were made on both males and females. The resulting data are as follows:

	Males				Females		
	$Y = 1$	$Y = 0$			$Y = 1$	$Y = 0$	
$X = 1$	118	42	160	$X = 1$	111	25	136
$X = 0$	83	165	248	$X = 0$	78	69	147
	201	207	408		189	94	283

Determine an overall estimate of the association between X and Y.

In this example, it is clear that $S = 2$ and that the S tables are independent of one another. In this section, we discuss two procedures for estimating the assumed common odds ratio for examples like 13.3.3.1, for testing its departure from unity, and for placing confidence intervals on the common odds ratio. The reader should bear in mind that throughout this section it is assumed that the data are unmatched.

The two procedures we discuss are the Mantel–Haenszel procedure and a procedure based on the weighted regression ideas of Chapter 9.

13.3.3.1   Mantel–Haenszel (1959) Procedure

This procedure may easily be one of the most widely used tools in the analysis of epidemiologic data. For data in the form of Table 13.2, this procedure produces an overall test for association between X and Y, it produces an estimate of the common odds ratio, and it is applicable to tables in which a particular cell entry, that is, A_i, B_i, C_i, or D_i, is zero. It must be noted, however, that proper application of this procedure requires that the population odds ratios do not vary greatly among the S 2×2 tables. Hence, if there is appreciable variation in these quantities, then the combined estimator is really of little value and the procedures of this section should not be performed.

The rationale of the test procedure is as follows: under the null hypothesis that the common odds ratio is unity, the mean or expected value of A_i is given by

$$E(A_i) = \frac{M_{1i}R_{1i}}{N_i},$$

(13.38)

while its variance* is given by

$$V(A_i) = \frac{R_{1i}R_{0i}M_{1i}M_{0i}}{N_i^2(N_i - 1)}.$$
(13.39)

The Mantel–Haenszel continuity-corrected test statistic is then given by

$$\chi^2_{\text{M-H}} = \frac{\left(\left|\sum_{i=1}^S A_i - \sum_{i=1}^S E(A_i)\right| - 1/2\right)^2}{\sum_{i=1}^S V(A_i)},$$
(13.40)

which has an approximate chi-square distribution with one degree of freedom under the null hypothesis. Large values of expression (13.40) lead to rejection of the null hypothesis that the odds ratio is unity. Recall that the odds ratio is the approximate relative risk for a retrospective study, thus the statistic (13.40) may also be viewed as a test statistic for the relative risk in retrospective studies.

An estimate of the common odds ratio for the Mantel–Haenszel procedure is provided by the expression

$$\widehat{\text{OR}}_{\text{M-H}} = \frac{\left(\sum_{i=1}^S A_i D_i\right)/N_i}{\left(\sum_{i=1}^S B_i C_i\right)/N_i},$$
(13.41)

with approximate large-sample variance given by

$$\hat{\sigma}^2_{\text{OR}_{\text{M-H}}} = \left(\widehat{\text{OR}}_{\text{M-H}}\right)^2 \left[\left(\sum_{i=1}^S T_i^2/w_i\right)\Big/\left(\sum_{i=1}^S T_i\right)^2\right],$$
(13.42)

where

$$T_1 = \left(\frac{1}{R_{1i}} + \frac{1}{R_{0i}}\right)^{-1} \frac{B_i}{R_{1i}} \frac{C_i}{R_{0i}} \quad \text{and} \quad w_i^{-1} = \left(\frac{A_i B_i}{R_{1i}}\right)^{-1} + \left(\frac{C_i D_i}{R_{0i}}\right)^{-1}.$$

Expression (13.42) is due to Hauck (1979). This estimator of variance is valid in the case in which the N_i are large and the number of tables, S, is fixed. Other estimators of the variance have been proposed by Breslow and Liang (1982, 1984).

---

*The variance (13.39) is quite similar to a binomial variance but is computed under the assumption that A_i has a hypergeometric distribution. We may think of (13.39) as the binomial-variance times a finite population correction term that is close to 1.

Table 13.3. Worked Solution to Example 13.3.3.1 Using Mantel–Haenszel Procedure

A. Data: The data are:

Males

$A_1 = 118$	$C_1 = 42$	$M_{11} = 160$
$B_1 = 83$	$D_1 = 165$	$M_{01} = 248$
$R_{11} = 201$	$R_{01} = 207$	$N_1 = 408$

Females

$A_2 = 111$	$C_2 = 25$	$M_{12} = 136$
$B_2 = 78$	$D_2 = 69$	$M_{02} = 147$
$R_{12} = 189$	$R_{02} = 94$	$N_2 = 283$

B. Assumptions:
   1. It is assumed that the two 2×2 tables are independent of one another and that each table did not arise in a matched-sample study.
   2. It is further assumed that the odds ratio in the population of males is comparable to that in the population of females.
C. Computations:
   1. From the data the following summary is obtained:

	$A_i D_i / N_i$	$B_i C_i / N_i$	$E(A_i)$	$V(A_i)$
Males ($i = 1$)	47.72	8.54	78.82	24.37
Females ($i = 2$)	27.06	6.89	90.83	15.73
Total	74.78	15.43	169.65	40.10

   2. The estimate of the odds ratio is therefore given by $\widehat{OR}_{M\text{-}H} = 74.78/15.43 = 4.85$.
   3. The test statistic is

$$\chi^2_{M\text{-}H} = \frac{(|(229 - 169.65)| - 1/2)^2}{40.10} = 86.37$$

D. Statistical test:
   1. Null hypothesis: H_0: Odds ratio = 1
   2. Alternative hypothesis: H_a: Odds ratio $\neq 1$
   3. Decision rule for a 0.05 level test: Reject H_0 in favor of H_a if $\chi^2_{M\text{-}H}$ exceeds $\chi^2_{0.95}(1)$.
E. Action taken: Since $\chi^2_{M\text{-}H} = 86.37$ while $\chi^2_{0.95}(1) = 3.84$, the null hypothesis is rejected, and one concludes that there is an association between X and Y.

Table 13.4. Summary of Weighted Least-Squares Procedure for Computing and Testing Hypotheses for Common Odds Ratio from S 2 × 2 Tables

A. Data: The data are given in Table 13.2.
B. Assumptions: The S 2 × 2 tables are independent unmatched samples from populations with common odds ratio.
C. Computations:
1. Compute the estimated odds ratio and its natural logarithm for each table; i.e.,

$$\widehat{OR}_i = A_i D_i / B_i C_i \qquad (13.43)$$

$$\log \widehat{OR}_i = \log(A_i D_i / B_i C_i) \qquad (13.44)$$

If any value of A_i, B_i, C_i, or D_i is zero, then add 0.5 to each cell entry in that particular 2 × 2 table; then proceed with calculating (13.43) and (13.44) with the revised cell entries.

2. Compute the estimated large-sample variance of each log OR; these variances are

$$\hat{\sigma}^2_{\log(\widehat{OR}_i)} = \frac{1}{A_i} + \frac{1}{B_i} + \frac{1}{C_i} + \frac{1}{D_i}. \qquad (13.45)$$

3. Determine the chi-square statistic for each 2 × 2 table via

$$\chi_i^2 = \frac{\left(\log \widehat{OR}_i \right)^2}{\hat{\sigma}^2_{\log(\widehat{OR}_i)}} \qquad (13.46)$$

4. Determine the "pooled estimator" of the log odds ratio by weighting each $\log \widehat{OR}_i$ by the inverse of its variance, $\hat{\sigma}^2_{\log(\widehat{OR}_i)}$; the estimate is

$$\log \widehat{OR}_p = \frac{\sum_{i=1}^{S} \log \widehat{OR}_i / \hat{\sigma}^2_{\log(\widehat{OR}_i)}}{\sum_{i=1}^{S} 1 / \hat{\sigma}^2_{\log(\widehat{OR}_i)}} ; \qquad (13.47)$$

the large-sample variance of (13.47) is

$$\hat{\sigma}^2_{\log(\widehat{OR}_p)} = \left(\sum_{i=1}^{S} \frac{1}{\hat{\sigma}^2_{\log(\widehat{OR}_i)}} \right)^{-1} \qquad (13.48)$$

5. To test the null hypothesis that the common odds ratio is equal to 1, the test statistic is

$$\chi^2_{pooled} = \frac{\left(\log \widehat{OR}_p \right)^2}{\hat{\sigma}^2_{\log(\widehat{OR}_p)}} \qquad (13.49)$$

Table 13.4. (*continued*)

---

which has a chi-square distribution with one degree of freedom under the null hypothesis.

6. To test the null hypothesis that the odds ratios are equal in the S groups, the chi-square test statistic is

$$\chi^2_{\text{difference}} = \chi^2_{\text{sum}} - \chi^2_{\text{pooled}} \qquad (13.50)$$

where $\chi^2_{\text{sum}} = \sum_{i=1}^{S} \chi^2_i$; $\chi^2_{\text{difference}}$ has a chi-square distribution with $S - 1$ degree of freedom if the null hypothesis of homogeneity is true.

D. Test of homogeneity of odds ratios:
   1. Null hypothesis: H_0: The S odds ratios are equal.
   2. Alternative hypothesis: H_a: The S odds ratios are not all equal.
   3. Decision rule for an α-level test: Reject H_0 if $\chi^2_{\text{difference}}$ exceeds $\chi^2_{1-\alpha}(S - 1)$, where this latter value is from Table 6 of the Appendix.

E. Test that common odds ratio is unity:
   1. Null hypothesis: H_0: Common odds ratio = 1.
   2. Alternative hypothesis: H_a: Common odds ratio $\neq$ 1.
   3. Decision rule for an α-level test: Reject H_0 if χ^2_{pooled} exceeds $\chi^2_{1-\alpha}(1)$, where this value is from Table 6 of the Appendix.

Let us consider the application of these methods to the data of Example 13.3.3.1 (Table 13.3).

Note that the individual estimates of the odds ratio for the males and females are 5.59 and 3.93. The Mantel–Haenszel estimator is 4.85, which is between the two estimates.

13.3.3.2 *Weighted Least-Squares Procedure*

An alternative to the Mantel–Haenszel procedure is founded on a weighted least-squares approach. The procedure has the advantage of testing the homogeneity of the S odds ratios as part of the analysis. The procedure is based on the weighted squares methods described in Section 9.6 and is a special case of the general methodology of Grizzle, Starmer, and Koch (1969). The analysis is based on the natural logarithm of the odds ratio and its estimated variance for each 2×2 table. The procedure is not to be recommended if the cell frequencies are close to zero, although (as noted in Chapter 9) adding 0.5 to each cell frequency helps if an occasional A_i, B_i, C_i, or D_i is close to zero. The procedure is described in Table 13.4.

The test for homogeneity should be performed first; if homogeneity of the S odds ratio is rejected, there is little point in proceeding.

A $(1 - \alpha)$ 100% confidence interval for the log odds ratio is

$$\log \widehat{OR}_p \pm Z_{1-\alpha/2} \hat{\sigma}_{\log(\widehat{OR}_p)}, \tag{13.51}$$

where $Z_{1-\alpha/2}$ is from Table 4 of the Appendix. Taking the exponent of the endpoints of interval (13.51) results in a $(1 - \alpha)$ 100 % interval for the odds ratio.

A further comment in regard to the test of homogeneity of the S odds ratios has to do with the question of multiple comparisons. If the test for homogeneity yields a statistically significant result, this indicates that there are differences between the groups. From Chapter 10, a Scheffé-type contrast may be performed to generate $(1 - \alpha)$ 100% simultaneous confidence intervals. The procedure is to specify the set of coefficients, $c_1, \ldots, c_S$, for the contrast, and then a $(1 - \alpha)$ 100% confidence interval for $\sum_{i=1}^{S} c_i \log OR_i$ is given by

$$\sum_{i=1}^{S} c_i \log \widehat{OR}_i \pm \sqrt{\chi^2_{1-\alpha}(S - 1)} \sqrt{\sum_{i=1}^{S} c_i^2 \hat{\sigma}^2_{\log(\widehat{OR}_i)}}, \tag{13.52}$$

where $\sum_{i=1}^{S} c_i = 0$ and $\chi^2_{1-\alpha}(S - 1)$ is from Table 6 of the Appendix. The intervals (13.52) are simultaneous confidence intervals (Grizzle et al., 1969) in the sense of Chapter 10. The data analyst is free to perform as many of the confidence interval computations (13.52) as he or she wishes.

Let us now illustrate the applications of the methods of Table 13.4 to the data of Example 13.3.3.1 (Table 13.5).

In the situation in which the S groups are ordered categories, such as age or dosage of drug or increasing levels of a factor, the weighted regression procedures of Chapter 9 can be applied to develop a regression equation for the log odds ratio as a function of this factor. For groups in an ordered category, the response variable would be

$$y_i = \log \frac{A_i D_i}{B_i C_i}. \tag{13.53}$$

The weights W_i are

$$W_i = \left(\frac{1}{A_i} + \frac{1}{B_i} + \frac{1}{C_i} + \frac{1}{D_i} \right)^{-1}, \tag{13.54}$$

and finally X_i would be the value of the factor for the ith group. If this

Table 13.5. Worked Solution to Example 13.3.3.1 Using Weighted Least-Squares Procedure

A. Data: The data are:

	Males ($i = 1$)			Females ($i = 2$)	
	$Y = 1$	$Y = 0$		$Y = 1$	$Y = 0$
$X = 1$	118	42	$X = 1$	111	25
$X = 0$	83	165	$X = 0$	78	69

B. Assumptions:

1. It is assumed that the two 2×2 tables are independent of one another, and the data did not arise in a matched-sample study.
2. Assumption 1 is required for the tests of homogeneity of odds ratios and for the tests that the common odds ratio is 1. To test for equality to unity in the common odds ratio, it is assumed that the S odds ratios are homogeneous.

C. Computations:

1. From the data one computes the following:

Males	Females
$\widehat{OR_1} = 5.59$	$\widehat{OR_2} = 3.93$
$\log \widehat{OR_1} = 1.72098$	$\log \widehat{OR_2} = 1.36864$
$\sigma^2_{\log \widehat{OR_1}} = 0.0504$	$\sigma^2_{\log \widehat{OR_2}} = 0.0763$

$$\chi_1^2 = \frac{(1.72098)^2}{0.0504} = 58.7653 \qquad \chi_2^2 = \frac{(1.36864)^2}{0.0763} = 24.5501$$

2. It follows that $\chi_{\text{sum}}^2 = 58.7653 + 24.5501 = 83.3154$,

$$\log \widehat{OR_p} = \frac{1.72098/0.0504 + 1.36864/0.0763}{1/0.0504 + 1/0.0763}$$

i.e., $\log \widehat{OR_p} = 1.58082$
(notice that the pooled estimator of the common odds ratio is therefore $e^{1.58082}$, or 4.86);

$$\hat{\sigma}^2_{\log(OR_p)} = \frac{1}{1/0.0504 + 1/0.0763} = 0.03035;$$

thus,

$$\chi_{\text{pooled}}^2 = \frac{(1.58082)^2}{(0.03035)} = 82.3391.$$

3.

$$\chi_{\text{difference}}^2 = 83.3154 - 82.3391 = 0.9763.$$

424

Table 13.5. (*continued*)

D. Test for homogeneity:
  1. Null hypothesis: H_0: The $S = 2$ odds ratios are equal.
  2. Alternative hypothesis: H_a: The odds ratios are not equal.
  3. Decision rule for an α-level test: Reject H_0 in favor of H_a if $\chi^2_{\text{difference}}$ exceeds $\chi^2_{1-\alpha}(S-1)$.
E. Test for equality of common odds ratio equal to 1:
  1. Null hypothesis: H_0: Common odds ratio is 1.
  2. Alternative hypothesis: H_a: Common odds ratio is not 1.
  3. Decision rule for an α-level test: Reject H_0 in favor of H_a if χ^2_{pooled} exceeds $\chi^2_{1-\alpha}(1)$.
F. Action taken: As $\chi^2_{\text{difference}} = 0.9763$ and $S = 2$, the critical value is $\chi^2_{0.95}(1) = 3.84$; hence, we accept that the two odds ratios are equal. The test of the null hypothesis that the common odds ratio is equal to 1 yields $\chi^2_{\text{pooled}} = 82.34$, which is highly significant; thus, we reject this null hypothesis.

---

factor is a variable like age—for example, the age range for group 1 is 20–30 and for group 2 is 30–40—it is customary to use the midpoint of interval i as the value of X_i in the regression analysis. The analysis proceeds as it does in Chapter 9 with $\log(A_iD_i/B_iC_i)$ replacing (9.28) and $1/A_i + 1/B_i + 1/C_i + 1/D_i$ replacing (9.29). As we have mentioned at various points in this section, if any of A_i, B_i, C_i, or D_i is zero, the entries are adjusted by adding 0.5 to each of them.

Table 13.6. Possible 2×2 Tables for each Pair in a Pair-Matched Design for Retrospective Studies

	Possibility 1				Possibility 2		
	$Y_i = 1$	$Y_i = 0$			$Y_i = 1$	$Y_i = 0$	
$X_i = 1$	1	1	2	$X_i = 1$	1	0	1
$X_i = 0$	0	0	0	$X_i = 0$	0	1	1
	1	1	2		1	1	2

	Possibility 3				Possibility 4		
	$Y_i = 1$	$Y_i = 0$			$Y_i = 1$	$Y_i = 0$	
$X_i = 1$	0	1	1	$X_i = 1$	0	0	0
$X_i = 0$	1	0	1	$X_i = 0$	1	1	2
	1	1	2		1	1	2

13.3.4   Inference for Odds Ratio with Pair-Matched Data for Retrospective Studies

As in Section 13.3.3, we continue to focus our attention on the odds ratio as the measure of association. Pair-matched data are frequently gathered, particularly in retrospective study designs. The problems we wish to address are again the questions of estimating the odds ratio (or its logarithm) and testing the hypothesis that the odds ratio is equal to 1. The retrospective pair-matched study design in actuality gives rise to a set of 2×2 tables like Table 13.2, with $R_{1i} = R_{0i} = 1$. In fact, each pair is a 2×2 table in which $N_i = 2$. Thus, it seems quite natural to examine the Mantel–Haenszel procedure applied to S pairs of individuals. No examination of the weighted least-squares approach is considered since each and every 2×2 table has two zero entries. In fact, the possible 2×2 tables are summarized in Table 13.6. Note that for each table, the margins of Y are equal to 1; that is, a nondiseased ($Y = 0$) subject is matched with a diseased ($Y = 1$) subject in each pair.

In the Mantel–Haenszel framework, possibility 1 and possibility 4 of Table 13.6 yield $A_i D_i = B_i C_i = V(A_i) = 0$. Therefore, these two tables contribute nothing to the analysis. That is, the concordant pairs do not contribute to this analysis. We conclude that all of the odds ratio information is contained in the discordant pairs, possibilities 2 and 3.

Also, for possibilities 1, 2, 3, and 4 of Table 13.6, note that:

	Possibility			
	1	2	3	4
$E(A_i)$	1	$\frac{1}{2}$	$\frac{1}{2}$	0
A_i	1	1	0	0
$A_i - E(A_i)$	0	$\frac{1}{2}$	$-\frac{1}{2}$	0
$V(A_i)$	0	$\frac{1}{4}$	$\frac{1}{4}$	0
Denote number of pairs by:	F	H	Q	J

Recall the Mantel–Haenszel estimator of the odds ratio from (13.41) is

$$\widehat{\text{OR}}_{\text{M-H}} = \frac{\left(\sum_{i=1}^{S} A_i D_i \right) / N_i}{\left(\sum_{i=1}^{S} B_i C_i \right) / N_i}.$$

Furthermore, note that $N_i = 2$ for all tables in Table 13.6, and also note that for the discordant pairs $A_i D_i = 1$ if the case ($Y_i = 1$) has the risk factor while the control ($Y_i = 0$) does not. Similarly, $B_i C_i = 1$ if the case does not have the risk factor while the control does; thus, for the matched-pair study,

$$\widehat{OR}_{M\text{-}H}$$

$$= \frac{\text{Number of pairs in which case has risk factor, control does not}}{\text{Number of pairs in which case does not have risk factor, control does}}$$

and thus

$$\widehat{OR}_{M\text{-}H} = H/Q. \tag{13.55}$$

From the above tabulation it follows that

$$\sum_{i=1}^{S} A_i = H + F,$$

$$\sum_{i=1}^{S} E(A_i) = F + \tfrac{1}{2}(Q + H), \tag{13.56}$$

$$\sum_{i=1}^{S} V(A_i) = \tfrac{1}{4}(Q + H);$$

thus, the Mantel–Haenszel test statistic (13.40) is

$$\chi^2_{M\text{-}H} = \frac{(|Q - H| - 1)^2}{Q + H}. \tag{13.57}$$

This statistic is identical to McNemar's chi-square statistic of Table 7.4. Thus, for matched-pair data, the test of the hypothesis that the odds ratio is 1 is based on McNemar's test.

As mentioned, the estimate of the odds ratio is expression (13.55), while the estimate of the log odds ratio is

$$\log \widehat{OR}_{M\text{-}H} = \log(H/Q), \tag{13.58}$$

and the variance is

$$\hat{\sigma}^2_{\log(\widehat{OR}_{M\text{-}H})} = 1/H + 1/Q; \tag{13.59}$$

thus, a $(1 - \alpha)$ 100% confidence interval for the log odds ratio is

$$\log \widehat{OR}_{\text{M-H}} \pm Z_{1-\alpha/2} \hat{\sigma}_{\log(\widehat{OR}_{\text{M-H}})}, \tag{13.60}$$

where $Z_{1-\alpha/2}$ is from Table 4 of the Appendix. The $(1 - \alpha)$ 100% confidence interval for the odds ratio is therefore obtained by taking the exponent of the endpoints of (13.60).

Example 13.3.4.1. Take a retrospective study in which patients and controls were pair matched; 14 pairs were such that both patient and control had the risk factor in question, 16 were such that the control had the risk factor but the patient did not, 59 were such that the patient had the risk factor but the control did not, while in 28 pairs neither had the risk factor. Is there evidence to conclude that the risk factor is associated with the disease?

From these data, it is clear that $H = 59$, $F = 14$, $Q = 16$, and $J = 28$; thus, $\widehat{OR}_{\text{M-H}} = \frac{59}{16} = 3.69$ is the estimate of the approximate relative risk, while the McNemar chi-square is $\chi^2_{\text{M-H}} = (|16 - 59| - 1)^2/(16 + 59) = 23.52$, which is quite significant when compared to the tabled value of the chi-square distribution with one degree of freedom. In terms of a 95% confidence interval for the log odds ratio, we have $1.30562 \pm (1.96)\left(\sqrt{\frac{1}{59} + \frac{1}{16}}\right) = (0.75316, 1.85808)$; thus for the odds ratio itself, it is $(e^{0.75316}, e^{1.85808}) = (2.12, 6.41)$.

From Section 13.3.3, we noted that inference from the odds ratio is the same for all three sampling designs if the study samples are not matched. This is also the case with pair-matched data. This is quite evident by inspecting Table 13.6 and reviewing its associated discussion. Only possibilities 2 and 3 contribute to the odds ratio analysis; thus, the analysis performed in Section 13.3.4 also applies to prospective and cross-sectional studies.

13.3.5 Standardization and Adjustment of Rates

In prospective and cross-sectional studies, two groups of individuals are compared with regard to the disease outcome. For some situations, there are S subgroups, similar to Table 13.2, and it is of interest to compare the two study groups while adjusting for the subgroup classification. Consider the data in Example 13.3.5.1.

Example 13.3.5.1. Consider the results of a cohort study of the number of cigarettes smoked per day and the death rate due to cancer of the lung or bronchus. The data are as follows:

| Age | Number of Deaths per Person-Years of Follow-Up | |
	Nonsmokers	Smokers (1–2 packs/day)
35–44	0/35,200	4/ 40,600
45–54	0/15,100	10/ 12,800
55–64	25/214,000	245/ 103,000
65–74	49/171,000	194/ 50,000
75 +	4/8490	7/ 1270
Total rounded)	78/443,790	460/ 207,670

Source: Miettinen (1972).

One question that could be asked of data like the above is whether the mortality rate is higher in smokers as compared to nonsmokers. While it is intuitively clear that it is higher for the smokers, the example does indicate that the distribution of person-years of follow-up by age is different for smokers as compared to nonsmokers. In particular, the relative frequency distributions of the person-years of follow-up for nonsmokers and for smokers are shown in the following table:

RELATIVE FREQUENCY DISTRIBUTIONS OF PERSON - YEARS OF FOLLOW - UP

Age	Nonsmokers	Smokers
35–44	0.0793	0.1955
45–54	0.0340	0.0616
55–64	0.4822	0.4960
65–74	0.3853	0.2408
75 +	0.0191	0.0061

From its relative frequency distribution, it is observed that the smoker group has relatively more persons in the 35–44 age group and relatively fewer in the 65–74 and 75 + age groups. Thus, this group would be expected to have fewer cancer deaths than the nonsmokers if smoking were not a mortality risk factor. It is evident that if the crude mortality rates of 78 per 443,790 and 460 per 207,670 were merely compared, it would not produce an unbiased estimate of the real effect of smoking. The question becomes one of adjusting the two rates so that the confounding effect of age on the mortality difference can be reduced. There are numerous ways to accomplish such a task. Two ways that we shall discuss are the direct and the indirect methods of adjustment. Some general notation is required. The

Table 13.7. Data Layout for Standardization of Rates

Age Group or Stratum	Study Group 0			Study Group 1		
	Events	At Risk	Rate	Events	At Risk	Rate
1	d_{01}	n_{01}	r_{01}	d_{11}	n_{11}	r_{11}
2	d_{02}	n_{02}	r_{02}	d_{12}	n_{12}	r_{12}
$\vdots$	$\vdots$	$\vdots$	$\vdots$	$\vdots$	$\vdots$	$\vdots$
S	d_{0S}	n_{0S}	r_{0S}	d_{1S}	n_{1S}	r_{1S}
Total	d_{0+}	n_{0+}	$r_{0+} = d_{0+}/n_{0+}$	d_{1+}	n_{1+}	$r_{1+} = d_{1+}/n_{1+}$

basic data layout is generally assumed to be of the form of Table 13.7, while the data from a standard or reference population are assumed to be of the form of Table 13.8. In Table 13.7, d_{ij} is the number of events in group i ($i = 0, 1$) and in age group or stratum j ($j = 1, 2, \ldots, S$), n_{ij} is the number at risk, while $r_{ij} = d_{ij}/n_{ij}$. In the standard population, D_j, N_j, and R_j are the corresponding number of events, number at risk, and rate in stratum j. The standard population may be chosen in a number of ways; one way is to use the combined data from the two groups, that is, $D_j = d_{0j} + d_{1j}$, and $N_j = n_{0j} + n_{1j}$, $R_j = (d_{0j} + d_{1j})/(n_{0j} + n_{1j})$. Alternatively, vital statistics data from the state or geographical catchment area of the study may be used.

In actual fact, the direct method only needs the data of Table 13.7 and the number in the at-risk column of Table 13.8. The indirect method of rate adjustment needs Table 13.8 and only the numbers at risk in Table 13.7. So neither method requires the entirety of both tables.

A further comment is in order regarding the terminology. Suppose the event of interest is death. The term *at risk* refers to an appropriate denominator for the number of events, that is, the number of deaths. It may

Table 13.8. Standard Population Data

Age Group or Stratum	Events	At Risk	Rate
1	D_1	N_1	R_1
2	D_2	N_2	R_2
$\vdots$	$\vdots$	$\vdots$	$\vdots$
S	D_S	N_S	R_S
Total	D_+	N_+	$R_+ = D_+/N_+$

be the number of persons exposed to the risk of death in that age group, or more typically it is the *person-years* at risk contributed by the cohort in that particular age group. The rate computed for each age group is termed an *age-specific rate*; it is specific for that particular age group. The total number of deaths divided by the total number at risk obtained by adding over the age groups is called a *crude rate*. Thus, r_{0+}, r_{1+}, and R_+ are crude rates, while r_{ij} and R_j are age-specific rates. We use the term age-specific rate; a more generally appropriate term is *stratum-specific rate*.

The main reason for adjusting two rates, that is, constructing standardized rates, is to obtain an accurate index of the rate difference between the two study groups. If the two arrays of at risk populations, namely, $n_{01}, \ldots, n_{0S}$ and $n_{11}, \ldots, n_{1S}$, were such that $n_{01}/n_{11} = \cdots = n_{0S}/n_{1S}$, then there is no need to adjust, as the age distributions are equivalent. On the other hand, if the preceding ratios are not constant, then the age groups' crude rates reflect this difference as well as the mortality rate difference.

The principal caution in interpreting a standardized rate is that it may conceal an "interaction" between age and the rates. For example, if the differences $r_{0j} - r_{1j}$ are fairly constant for the S age groups, then a comparison of standardized rates will generally be a fair measure of the study groups' difference. If these age-specific rate differences are not constant, then the comparison of the standardized rates may be rather misleading. Consider the picture in Figure 13.4, in which the rates for the two younger age groups are higher in group 0 than in group 1. For the two older age groups the reverse holds. A comparison of two standardized rates would probably result in a statement of no difference between the study groups. This result would be incorrect. Standardization should not be

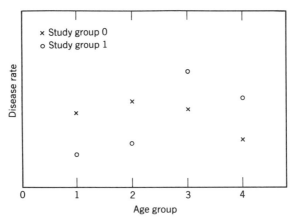

Figure 13.4. Situation where standardization of rates is inappropriate.

applied to data like Figure 13.4. The comparison should be restricted to a comparison of the groups for the two younger ages; then another analysis for the two older age groups should be undertaken.

In the next two sections we use the notation of Tables 13.7 and 13.8.

13.3.5.1 Indirect Method

The main reasons for using this method are that the n_{ij} may be small and/or the r_{ij} are unknown. The procedure is quite simple. The rationale is to determine the "expected number" of deaths in each study group if they had been subjected to the mortality rates of the standard population from Table 13.8. These expected numbers are

$$e_0 = \sum_{j=1}^{S} R_j n_{0j} \quad \text{and} \quad e_1 = \sum_{j=1}^{S} R_j n_{1j} \tag{13.61}$$

for groups 0 and 1. The *indirect standardized* rates are then defined by

$$S_0 = R_+ \frac{d_{0+}}{e_0} \quad \text{and} \quad S_1 = R_+ \frac{d_{1+}}{e_1} \tag{13.62}$$

for the zeroth and first groups. The quantities d_{0+}/e_0 and d_{1+}/e_1 are termed the *standardized mortality ratios* (SMRs); they are the observed divided by the expected numbers of deaths, that is, $\text{SMR}_0 = d_{0+}/e_0$ and $\text{SMR}_1 = d_{1+}/e_1$.

There are two inference questions that are generally of interest. Do the two indirect adjusted rates differ significantly from one another, and is either SMR significantly different from 1? The second question is easily answered by using the test statistic

$$\chi^2_{\text{SMR}_0} = \frac{(d_{0+} - e_0)^2}{e_0} \tag{13.63}$$

for group 0 and the statistic

$$\chi^2_{\text{SMR}_1} = \frac{(d_{1+} - e_1)^2}{e_1} \tag{13.64}$$

for group 1. Each of these statistics has a chi-square distribution with one degree of freedom. Hence, if the computed statistic exceeds $\chi^2_{1-\alpha}(1)$, then the hypothesis that the SMR equals 1 is rejected. Comparing two indirect adjusted rates is equivalent to comparing the two SMRs. An appropriate test statistic is

$$\chi^2_{compare} = \frac{(\log SMR_0 - \log SMR_1)^2}{1/e_0 + 1/e_1}.$$ (13.65)

This statistic has a large-sample chi-square distribution with one degree of freedom under the null hypothesis of equal SMRs. A comment is in order regarding the assumptions. Before using the test statistics (13.63), (13.64), and (13.65), the reader should note that a key assumption is that the ratio of the population age-specific rate for study group 0 to the standard population-specific rate is a constant. That is, if we denote the population age-specific rates for group 0 by π_{0J} (the r_{0j} estimate these), then it is assumed that

$$\frac{\pi_{01}}{R_1} = \frac{\pi_{02}}{R_2} = \cdots = \frac{\pi_{0S}}{R_S} = \Theta_0.$$ (13.66)

Analogously, for study group 1, it is assumed that the population age-specific rates π_{1j} satisfy

$$\frac{\pi_{11}}{R_1} = \frac{\pi_{12}}{R_2} = \cdots = \frac{\pi_{1S}}{R_S} = \Theta_1.$$ (13.67)

In this situation, the statistic (13.63) is testing the null hypothesis that $\Theta_0 = 1$, (13.64) tests $\Theta_1 = 1$, while (13.65) tests $\Theta_0 = \Theta_1$. If assumptions (13.66) and (13.67) do not hold, then the two SMRs may not be mutually comparable.

Example 13.3.5.1.1. In the study mentioned in Example 13.3.5.1, let us consider the nonsmoker group as the standard population. Further, let us include an additional group of "occasional" smokers and let us compute the indirect adjusted rates for the occasional smokers and the 1–2-pack/day group. The complete data are:

Age	Study Group 0 (Occasional)	Study Group 1 (1–2 Packs)	Standard Population
35–44	2/71,700	4/40,600	0/35,200
45–54	2/20,800	10/12,800	0/15,100
55–64	220/212,000	245/103,000	25/214,000
65–74	293/149,000	194/50,000	49/171,000
75 +	21/6300	7/1270	4/8490
Total	538/459,800	460/207,670	78/443,790

Source: Miettinen (1972).

Following the formulas presented above, it is clear that

$$e_0 = \left[71,700\left(\frac{0}{35,200} \right) + \cdots + 6300\left(\frac{4}{8490} \right) \right] = 70.43,$$

$$e_1 = \left[40,600\left(\frac{0}{35,200} \right) + \cdots + 1270\left(\frac{4}{8490} \right) \right] = 26.96,$$

$$SMR_0 = \frac{538}{70.43} = 7.64,$$

$$SMR_1 = \frac{460}{26.96} = 17.1,$$

$$S_0 = 7.64\left(\frac{78}{443,790} \right) = 0.001342,$$

$$S_1 = 17.1\left(\frac{78}{443,790} \right) = 0.003004.$$

Thus, the two indirect adjusted rates differ considerably. To test the hypothesis that each SMR is equal to unity, we have

$$\chi^2_{SMR_0} = \frac{(538 - 70.43)^2}{70.43} = 3104.10,$$

$$\chi^2_{SMR_1} = \frac{(460 - 26.96)^2}{26.96} = 6955.62.$$

In both cases, the results are highly significant since each of the two statistics has a chi-square distribution with one degree of freedom. In order to compare the two SMRs, we compute

$$\log SMR_0 = 2.0334 \quad \text{and} \quad \log SMR_1 = 2.8391;$$

hence,

$$\chi^2_{compare} = \frac{(2.0334 - 2.8391)^2}{(1/70.43 + 1/26.96)} = 12.66,$$

which when compared to the tabled value of the chi-square distribution with one degree of freedom is highly significant. We conclude that the two SMRs differ from one another, meaning the SMR for group 1 (1–2 packs) is significantly larger than the SMR for group 0 (occasional smoking).

13.3.5.2 Direct Method
The direct adjusted rate is defined by

$$T_0 = \sum_{j+1}^{S} \frac{N_j}{N_+} r_{0j} \quad \text{and} \quad T_1 = \sum_{j=1}^{S} \frac{N_j}{N_+} r_{1j} \tag{13.68}$$

for groups 0 and 1, respectively, where T_0 is the death rate in the standard population if they were subjected to the mortality experience of study group 0, and T_1 is defined analogously. The difference in two direct adjusted rates is

$$T_0 - T_1 = \sum_{j=1}^{S} \frac{N_j}{N_+} (r_{0j} - r_{1j}). \tag{13.69}$$

If one assumes that r_{0j} and r_{1j} have independent binomial distributions with $\pi_{0j} = \pi_{1j}$, and if N_j/N_+ is regarded as nonrandom (as in the case of a very large standard population), then the variance of $T_0 - T_1$ is

$$\hat{\sigma}^2_{(T_0 - T_1)} = \sum_{j=1}^{S} \left(\frac{N_j}{N_+} \right)^2 \left[\frac{\bar{r}_j (1 - \bar{r}_j)}{n_{0j} n_{1j}} (n_{0j} + n_{1j}) \right], \tag{13.70}$$

where $\bar{r}_j = (d_{0j} + d_{1j})/(n_{0j} + n_{1j})$. The equality of two direct adjusted rates may be tested via

$$\chi^2 = \frac{(T_0 - T_1)^2}{\hat{\sigma}^2_{(T_0 - T_1)}}, \tag{13.71}$$

which follows a chi-square distribution with one degree of freedom under the hypothesis of equality.

Example 13.3.5.2.1. In a clinical trial of a pharmacological agent for the treatment of depression, 79 patients were assigned to one of two treatment groups: drug + ECT and drug alone. After the course of treatment, Hamilton scale ratings for depression were obtained for each patient and compared to their original ratings. As the patients differed in the severity of illness, this variable was used for stratification. The data are as follows:

Severity of Depression at Admission	n_{0j}	Drug Alone		n_{1j}	Drug + ECT	
		Number Improved	No Change or Worse (d_{0j})		Number Improved	No Change or Worse (d_{1j})
Extremely severe	28	5	23	25	7	18
Moderately severe	12	4	8	16	13	3
Mild	1	0	1	2	1	1

Of the last 1000 patients with psychotic depression who were admitted to this clinic, 618 were extremely severely ill, 335 were moderately severely ill, while 47 were mildly ill. Using these data as the standard population, compare the two direct adjusted rates.

We choose to work with the rate of no change or worsening rather than the rate of improvement. The summary computations are:

j Group	N_j/N_+	Drug Alone			Drug + ECT		
		n_{0j}	d_{0j}	r_{0j}	n_{1j}	d_{1j}	r_{1j}
1	0.618	28	23	0.8214	25	18	0.7200
2	0.335	12	8	0.6667	16	3	0.1875
3	0.047	1	1	1.0000	2	1	0.5000

Therefore, $T_0 = 0.618(0.8214) + 0.335(0.6667) + (0.047)(1) = 0.77797$, $T_1 = 0.618(0.7200) + 0.335(0.1875) + 0.047(0.5000) = 0.53127$, and $T_0 - T_1 = 0.2467$. For the variance computations, we determine

j	$d_{0j} + d_{1j}$	$n_{0j} + n_{1j}$	$\bar{r}_j$	$\bar{r}_j(1 - \bar{r}_j)$	$\dfrac{N_j^2}{N_+^2} \dfrac{\bar{r}_j(1 - \bar{r}_j)(n_{0j} + n_{1j})}{n_{0j} n_{1j}}$
1	41	53	0.7736	0.1751	0.005063
2	11	28	0.3929	0.2385	0.003903
3	2	3	0.6667	0.2222	0.000736
					0.009702

and $\hat{\sigma}_{(T_0 - T_1)}^2 = 0.0097$. From (13.71), we obtain $\chi^2 = (0.2467)^2/0.0097 = 6.27$. This exceeds 3.84 ($= \chi_{0.95}^2(1)$); thus, we conclude that there is a difference at the 5% level. This result means that the direct adjusted rate of no change or worsening for the drug-alone group (0.77797) is significantly larger than the direct adjusted rate of no change or worsening for the drug + ECT group (0.53127).

13.4 SUMMARY

The procedures of this chapter are generally useful for the analysis of dichotomous disease outcome data. These procedures apply to prospective, retrospective, and cross-sectional study designs. The reader is encouraged to complement the reading and study of these methods with readings on epidemiologic methods and interpretation, like the texts of Kleinbaum, et al. (1982), Schlesselman (1982), Breslow and Day (1980), and Miettinen (1985).

PROBLEMS

13.1. In a prospective and randomized study, 5 mg of diazepam (prior to contrast media injection) was given to glioma patients undergoing cerebral tomography to assess its effect in reducing the incidence of contrast media-associated seizures. The observed results are (Pagani et al., 1984):

Group	Seizure Yes	No
Control	14	72
Diazepam	2	81

(a) Compute the odds ratio and the estimated variance of its logarithm.
(b) Perform the large-sample test of the hypothesis H_0: OR = 1.
(c) Obtain a 95% confidence interval for the odds ratio.
(d) Draw conclusions about the treatment.

13.2. In a study on infants born in a rural community, all live births and perinatal deaths were ascertained from the health registry records. Smoking habits of the mother were obtained from a personal interview. The resulting information is presented in the following table, where death means stillbirth or death in the first week of life, and survival means alive at the end of the first week of life.

| | | Mortality Status | |
		Death	Survival
Mother	Smoker	31	130
	Nonsmoker	27	213

To assess the possible association between smoking status and perinatal mortality,

(a) obtain an estimate of the relative risk;

(b) obtain a 95% confidence interval for the relative risk and interpret.

13.3. In a retrospective study of endometrial cancer and estrogen use, 265 cases were compared with two types of controls: 280 women admitted to the hospital for dilatation and curettage (D & C), and 345 community women. The number of cases and controls, according to socioeconomic status, are:

High Socioeconomic Status:

| Estrogen | Cases | Controls | |
		D & C	Community
Yes	59	60	61
No	132	129	185
	191	189	246

Low Socioeconomic Status:

| Estrogen | Cases | Controls | |
		D & C	Community
Yes	9	10	10
No	65	81	89
	74	91	99

(a) Use the Mantel–Haenszel procedure to estimate the common odds ratio and to test the null hypothesis of no association between endometrial cancer and estrogen use when the controls are the D & C women.

(b) Same as (a) but with the community controls.

(c) Comment on the conclusions of these tests.

(d) Repeat the analyses using the weighted least-squares procedure.

13.4. In a cross-sectional study to determine the prevalence of previously unknown diabetes mellitus in an adult community, 4654 participants with ages between 30 and 95 years had their fasting plasma glucose (FPG) determined. Previously unknown diabetes was defined as FPG equal to 140 mg/dL or more. Known diabetes, defined by history, was present in 223 adults. The distribution of unknown diabetes, per sex and age intervals, was found to be (Barrett-Connor, 1980):

Age, 30–39:	Unknown Diabetes	
	Yes	No
Male	3	260
Female	2	305

Age, 40–49:		
	Yes	No
Male	11	219
Female	6	267

Age, 50–59:		
	Yes	No
Male	27	285
Female	13	458

Age, 60–69:		
	Yes	No
Male	27	617
Female	27	840

Age, 70 + :		
	Yes	No
Male	18	542
Female	11	493

It is of interest for the researchers to determine the possible association of male sex with unknown diabetes in this community sample.

(a) Obtain estimates of the odds ratio in each stratum with the corresponding 95% confidence interval.

(b) Obtain an estimate of the common odds ratio with the Mantel–Haenszel procedure and a 95% confidence interval.

(c) Test H_0: odds ratio = 1 with the Mantel–Haenszel chi-square procedure.

(d) Test the homogeneity of the odds ratios obtained in (a).

13.5. Women whose pregnancy ended in perinatal death (cases) were pair matched with women whose child was alive for at least one week after delivery (control). Their smoking habits during pregnancy were obtained from hospital records and written questionnaires. The data collected on these pairs is summarized in the following table:

		Controls	
		+	−
Cases	+	26	38
	−	18	69

where + means that the risk factor (smoking) was present during pregnancy, and − means that the risk factor was absent.

(a) Obtain an estimate of the odds ratio.

(b) Perform a Mantel–Haenszel test of the null hypothesis of no association between the risk factor and the pregnancy outcome.

(c) Obtain a 95% confidence interval for the estimate in (a).

13.6. The prevalence of diabetes, by place of residence and sex, was ascertained from health records in a U.S. region, resulting in the following data (diabetes cases per population) stratified by age (years):

Age	Urban Counties			Rural Counties		
	Female	Male	Total	Female	Male	Total
0–19	$\dfrac{57}{55,000}$	$\dfrac{75}{54,000}$	$\dfrac{132}{109.000}$	$\dfrac{32}{30,000}$	$\dfrac{35}{31,000}$	$\dfrac{67}{61,000}$
20–39	$\dfrac{171}{57,000}$	$\dfrac{165}{55,000}$	$\dfrac{336}{112,000}$	$\dfrac{61}{20,000}$	$\dfrac{56}{19,000}$	$\dfrac{117}{39,000}$
40–59	$\dfrac{509}{41,000}$	$\dfrac{558}{40,000}$	$\dfrac{1067}{81,000}$	$\dfrac{179}{11,000}$	$\dfrac{202}{11,000}$	$\dfrac{381}{22,000}$
60 +	$\dfrac{574}{17,000}$	$\dfrac{260}{7,000}$	$\dfrac{834}{24,000}$	$\dfrac{201}{5,000}$	$\dfrac{334}{6,000}$	$\dfrac{535}{11,000}$

(a) Obtain the relative frequency distribution of the population by age, for each sex and residence combination.

(b) Define as the standard population the combined data of urban and rural counties and use the indirect method of standardization to compare the prevalance rates by sex and place of residence.

REFERENCES

Barrett-Connor, E. (1980). The prevalence of diabetes mellitus in an adult community as determined by history or fasting hyperglycemia, *Am. J. Epidemiol.* **111**, 705–712.

Breslow, N. E., and N. E. Day. (1980). *Statistical Methods in Cancer Research*, Vol. 1, *The Analysis of Case-Control Studies*, International Agency for Research on Cancer, Scientific Publications No. 32, Lyon.

Breslow, N. E., and K. Y. Liang. (1982). The variance of the Mantel–Haenszel estimator, *Biometrics*, **38**, 943–952.

Breslow, N. E., and K. Y. Liang. (1984). Correction Note, *Biometrics*, **40**, 1217.

Cornfield, J. (1951). A method of estimating comparative rates from clinical data. Applications to cancer of the lung, breast and cervix, *J. Natl. Canc. Inst.*, **11**, 1269–1275.

Greenland, S., and D. C. Thomas. (1982). On the need for the rare disease assumption in case-control studies, *Am. J. Epidemiol.*, **116**, 547–553.

Grizzle, J. E., C. E. Starmer, and G. G. Koch. (1969). Analysis of categorical data by linear models, *Biometrics*, **25**, 489–504.

Hauck, W. W. (1979). The large sample variance of the Mantel–Haenszel estimator of a common odds ratio, *Biometrics*, **35**, 817–819.

Kleinbaum, D. G., L. L. Kupper, and H. Morgenstern. (1982). *Epidemiologic Research: Principles and Quantitative Methods*, Lifetime Learning, Belmont, CA.

Miettinen, O. S. (1976). Estimability and estimation in case-reference studies, *Am. J. Epidemiol.*, **103**, 226–235.

Miettinen, O. S. (1972). Standardization of risk ratios, *Am. J. Epidemiol.*, **96**, 383–388.

Miettinen, O. S. (1985). *Theoretical Epidemiology: Principles of Occurrence, Research in Medicine*, Wiley, New York.

Pagani, J. J., L. A. Hayman, R. H. Bigelow, H. I. Libshitz, and R. A. Lepke. (1984). Prophylactic diazepam in prevention of contrast media-associated seizures in glioma patients undergoing cerebral computed tomography, *Cancer*, **54**, 2200–2204.

Schlesselman, J. J. (1982). *Case-Control Studies: Design, Conduct, Analysis*, Oxford University Press, New York.

CHAPTER 14

Estimation and Comparison of Survival Curves

14.1 INTRODUCTION

In Chapter 13, we discussed various statistical procedures for assessing the association between a dichotomous risk factor and a dichotomous disease state (e.g., presence or absence of the disease). In Chapter 14, we discuss selected statistical procedures for analyzing survival time data. We use the term *survival time*, but the reader should understand that the methods are more generally applicable to other time response data, such as length of time in disease remission or length of stay as a psychiatric inpatient. Several issues pertain to time response data. One issue is estimation of the survival curve and the determination of standard errors for the curve at various time points. Another issue is the comparison of the survival curves for two independent groups of individuals. In regard to the latter, this chapter may be viewed as a continuation of Chapter 13. The techniques we describe are generally applicable to prospective-type studies, medical follow-up studies, and clinical trials.

A discussion of time response data may not appear to warrant separate treatment. For example, why not use the two-group comparison methods of Chapters 6 and 7 for the group comparisons? An example and the subsequent discussion may help illustrate why special techniques should be applied.

Example 14.1.1. Consider some hypothetical survival data for male residents of Iowa with primary bladder cancer. All of the patients were diagnosed sometime between July 1, 1982 and June 30, 1987 and were followed through June 30, 1987.

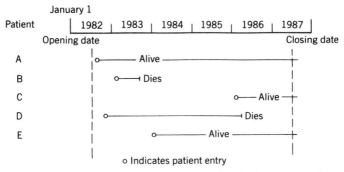

Figure 14.1. Five typical patient entries into the bladder cancer study.

This example is quite typical of the way in which a clinical follow-up study would be conducted. In particular, there is a beginning date for admitting patients to the sample and an ending date after which no new patients are entered into the study. There is also a closing date for the study, which may coincide with the ending date for allowing new patient entries. Generally, the closing date for the study is some administrative endpoint (e.g., the day study funding ceases). In Figure 14.1, we have depicted five patients who may have entered into this bladder cancer study.

The point 0 in Figure 14.1 represents the patient's date of diagnosis. Notice that patient *A* was diagnosed at the very start of the study and was alive at the closing date of the study; this patient survived at least five years after diagnosis. Death being a certainty, we know for sure that this patient's time from diagnosis to death is a number of years that is greater than 5. The closing date of our study has "censored" our view of the actual number of years; thus, we refer to this patient as a "censored observation" or a patient who "withdraws alive." In spite of the fact that we do not know the precise number of years until this person's death, we should use the available information that the patient survived five years. Patient *B* is a different story. For this patient, the actual time to death is known, but this patient was first diagnosed in 1983, not at the start of the study. Variable entry times do not cause problems, provided there have been no radical changes in therapy or diagnostic specificity or sensitivity that would indicate that patients admitted in one year are different than the previous or other years. Obviously, good clinical and medical judgment are required to resolve such a question. Certainly, if the time interval of the study was particularly long with regard to entry times, then the assumption of patient homogeneity and diagnostic stability over time would be suspect. Patients *C* and *E* are two additional censored observations with, however, variable entry times. Patient *D* is similar to patient *B* in as much as death occurs during the follow-up period, and the entry time into the study is after the opening date for admissions. We now summarize the features of Example 14.1.1.

Methodological Characteristics of Clinical Follow-Up Study

1. There is a clear well-defined starting point for each patient (date of diagnosis).
2. There is a clear well-defined endpoint (death or closing date of the study) for each patient.
3. The patients are a sample from a common population.

Reasons for Special Techniques Required

1. The censored observations do not provide the exact time to death.
2. The follow-up time varies for the patients.

We need to discuss statistical analysis procedures that will permit the conditions of methodological characteristics 1–3.

A further comment regarding characteristic 3 is in order. In particular, it is extraordinary in a clinical investigation to think of the sample of patients as a homogeneous group in all respects. We assume that patients have been or can be separated into subgroups, within which the patients may be regarded as similar. The analyses we are discussing then assume that we are dealing with each of these subgroups as a unit by itself.

If characteristics 1–3 are reasonable for a set of clinical data like Example 14.1.1, then Figure 14.1 may be revised as in Figure 14.2. Notice

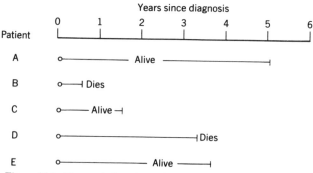

Figure 14.2. Five typical patients plotted from date of diagnosis.

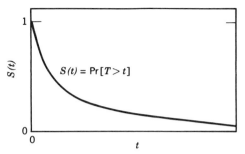

Figure 14.3. A typical population survival curve.

that this figure uses the well-defined starting and ending times for each patient and simplifies Figure 14.1 by eliminating the calendar year.

14.2   SURVIVAL CURVE FOR A POPULATION

14.2.1   Definition

If we regard the survival time variable as T, then the objective in most survival studies is to estimate the probability that an individual survives beyond a specified time, say t. That is, the main interest is in the function,

$$S(t) = \Pr[T > t]. \tag{14.1}$$

Graphically, if we observed a very large population until each one died, the function $S(t)$ is a decreasing function in t. It ranges from 1 to 0 as in Figure 14.3.

Given a set of sample data with possibly censored data points, then how should $S(t)$ be estimated? We discuss two procedures, one for ungrouped data and the other for grouped data.

14.2.2   Estimation from Ungrouped Data

To motivate the estimator of the survival function $S(t)$, let us consider a simple modification of Example 14.1.1. Suppose the study was only a two-year study (e.g., July 1, 1982–June 30, 1984) and one of the main goals of the study was to estimate the probability that a person would survive more than two years [i.e., $S(2)$]. Further, suppose that 500 people entered the study on July 1, 1982. Of these 500 persons, 300 die in the year while 200 are alive as of June 30, 1983. On July 1, 1983, an additional 1000 persons enter the study, and at the close of the study on June 30, 1984, 650 of these 1000 have died while 350 survive. Of the original 500 who were admitted on July 1, 1982, 125 die during the period July 1, 1983–June 30, 1984. How does one then estimate the probability of surviving more than two years? At least two procedures suggest themselves. The first is to simply estimate $S(2)$, the probability of surviving more than two years by using only the 500 patients admitted on July 1, 1982. This estimate of $S(2)$ would be $\tilde{S}(2) = \frac{75}{500} = 0.150$. This does not seem to make the best use of all of the data. We can utilize the data from the patients who entered on July 1, 1983, by noting that

$$\Pr[T > 2] = \Pr[T > 2 | T > 1]\Pr[T > 1], \qquad (14.2)$$

where the first term on the right side of (14.2) is the conditional probability of surviving greater than two years, given survival greater than one year. Clearly, the estimate of $\Pr[T > 2 | T > 1]$ is 75/200, while the estimate of $\Pr[T > 1]$ is $(200 + 350)/500 + 1000) = 0.367$; hence, the estimate of $\Pr[T > 2]$ is $(75/200)(0.367) = 0.138$. This type of estimator is called the *product limit estimator* of the survival curve and was originated by Kaplan and Meier (1958). The more general form of this product limit estimator is described in Table 14.1.

Table 14.1. Procedure for Estimating Survivorship Curve and Its Standard Error Estimate with Product Limit Estimator

---

1. Order the N follow-up times, either to death or censoring, and denote these by $t_1 \leq t_2 \leq \cdots \leq t_N$.
2. Denote by δ_i an indicator variable, taking value 1 if the observation at t_i is a death and 0 if censored.
3. The product limit estimator of the survival curve at time t is then given by

$$\hat{S}(t) = \prod_{i : t_i \leq t} \frac{N - i + 1 - \delta_i}{N - i + 1} \qquad (14.3)$$

for all $t \leq t_N$, where the product is over all i for which $t_i \leq t$. If t_N is a death, then $\hat{S}(t) = 0$ for $t > t_N$; if t_N is a censored observation, then $\hat{S}(t)$ is not defined beyond t_N, although it is between 0 and $\hat{S}(t_N)$.
4. The standard error of the estimate $\hat{S}(t)$ is estimated with

$$\hat{\sigma}_{S(t)} = \hat{S}(t) \left[\sum_{t_i \leq t} \frac{\delta_i}{(N - i)(N - i + 1)} \right]^{1/2} \qquad (14.4)$$

Strictly speaking, this is a large-sample estimate of the standard error of $\hat{S}(t)$.

Example 14.2.2.1. In a small clinical study, a psychiatrist wished to estimate the survival time distribution for a sample of severely depressed patients. For simplicity of presentation, we consider a sample of eight such patients. The data are as follows:

Patient (i)	Time (yr) from Diagnosis To Death or Censoring	Death (1) or Censored (0)
1	.5	1
2	1.0	0
3	2.0	0
4	3.0	1
5	5.0	1
6	7.0	0
7	9.0	1
8	12.0	0

Let us estimate the survival curve using the product limit estimator $\hat{S}(t)$. The estimate using (14.3) is:

$$\hat{S}(t) = \begin{cases} 1 & t < 0.5, \\ \frac{7}{8} & 0.5 \leq t < 3.0, \\ \left(\frac{7}{8}\right)\left(\frac{4}{5}\right) = \frac{7}{10} & 3.0 \leq t < 5.0, \\ \left(\frac{7}{8}\right)\left(\frac{4}{5}\right)\left(\frac{3}{4}\right) = \frac{21}{40} & 5.0 \leq t < 9.0, \\ \left(\frac{7}{8}\right)\left(\frac{4}{5}\right)\left(\frac{3}{4}\right)\left(\frac{1}{2}\right) = \frac{21}{80} & 9.0 \leq t < 12.0, \\ \text{Undefined} & 12.0 < t. \end{cases}$$

Graphically, the survival curve may then be plotted as in Figure 14.4.

To compute the standard error for the estimate, the following computations are required:

t	$\displaystyle\sum_{t_i \leq t} \frac{\delta_i}{(N - i)(N - i + 1)}$	$\hat{S}(t)$	$\hat{\sigma}_{\hat{S}(t)}$
$t < 0.5$	0	1	0
$0.5 \leq t < 3.0$	$\dfrac{1}{8(7)}$	$\dfrac{7}{8}$	0.1169
$3.0 \leq t < 5.0$	$\dfrac{1}{8(7)} + \dfrac{1}{4(5)}$	$\dfrac{7}{10}$	0.1823
$5.0 \leq t < 9.0$	$\dfrac{1}{8(7)} + \dfrac{1}{4(5)} + \dfrac{1}{3(4)}$	$\dfrac{21}{40}$	0.2041
$9.0 \leq t \leq 12.0$	$\dfrac{1}{8(7)} + \dfrac{1}{4(5)} + \dfrac{1}{3(4)} + \dfrac{1}{1(2)}$	$\dfrac{21}{80}$	0.2118

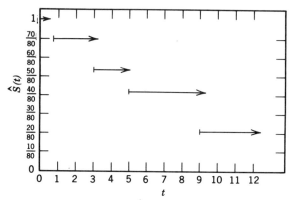

Figure 14.4. Plot of survival curve estimate of Example 14.2.2.1.

These standard errors could now be used to place standard error bars on the survival estimates in Figure 14.4. In addition, large-sample $(1 - \alpha)$ 100% confidence limits may be placed on the true survival curve at a point t by

$$\hat{S}(t) \pm Z_{1-\alpha/2}\hat{\sigma}_{\hat{S}(t)}, \tag{14.5}$$

where $Z_{1-\alpha/2}$ is from Table 4 of the Appendix. Obviously, if an endpoint of interval (14.5) is less than 0 or exceeds 1, the endpoint is set equal to 0 or 1 respectively.

14.2.3   Estimation from Grouped Data

In many situations, the data are reported in categories of time or the number of patients is so large that a grouping would simplify the computation and presentation of the data. In either situation, the question arises as to the procedure for estimating the survival curve. Cutler and Ederer (1958) describe a procedure for estimating the survival curve from such "life-table" data. Let us consider an example of hypothetical data for 231 larynx carcinoma patients as summarized in Table 14.2.

Combining these seven cohorts of patients gives Table 14.3.

The problem of estimating the survival curve is really straightforward, the only complication being the handling of the censored individuals. In particular, how much of the interval from 0 to 1 year are the 37 censored patients in active follow-up? The usual procedure, and it is somewhat arbitrary, is to assume that each of the 37 patients are followed for half of the interval. Similarly, the 36 censored patients in the 1–2-year interval are

Table 14.2. Survival Data for 231 Larynx Cancer Patients

Years After Diagnosis (Y)	Number of Patients Alive at Start of Interval (A)	Number of Patients Dying in Interval (B)	Number of Patients Censored or Withdrawn Alive in Interval (C)
Patients Diagnosed in 1978			
0–1	17	3	0
1–2	14	2	1
2–3	11	1	2
3–4	8	1	3
4–5	4	0	2
5–6	2	1	0
6–7	1	0	1
Patients Diagnosed in 1979			
0–1	32	9	2
1–2	21	2	6
2–3	13	1	4
3–4	8	0	3
4–5	5	0	3
5–6	2	0	2
Patients Diagnosed in 1980			
0–1	39	10	5
1–2	24	6	3
2–3	15	2	6
3–4	7	1	4
4–5	2	0	2
Patients Diagnosed in 1981			
0–1	50	21	6
1–2	23	7	10
2–3	6	0	4
3–4	2	·0	2
Patients Diagnosed in 1982			
0–1	41	12	3
1–2	26	8	10
2–3	8	1	7
Patients Diagnosed in 1983			
0–1	33	14	10
1–2	9	3	6
Patients Diagnosed in 1984			
0–1	19	8	11

Table 14.3. Combined Life Table from Table 14.2

Years After Diagnosis	Number of Patients Alive at Start of Interval	Number Dying in the Interval	Number Censored or Withdrawn Alive in Interval
0–1	231	77	37
1–2	117	28	36
2–3	53	5	23
3–4	25	2	12
4–5	11	0	7
5–6	4	1	2
6–7	1	0	1

assumed to be followed for half of the interval and so forth. Thus, the probability of survival is easily estimated as:

$\hat{S}_1$ = probability of surviving to end of interval 1: $\dfrac{\left(231 - \frac{37}{2}\right) - 77}{\left(231 - \frac{37}{2}\right)}$

and using (14.2)

$\hat{S}_2$ = probability of surviving to end of interval 2: $\hat{S}_1 \dfrac{\left(117 - \frac{36}{2}\right) - 28}{\left(117 - \frac{36}{2}\right)},$

$\hat{S}_3$ = probability of surviving to end of interval 3: $\hat{S}_2 \dfrac{\left(53 - \frac{23}{2}\right) - 5}{\left(53 - \frac{23}{2}\right)},$

$\hat{S}_4$ = probability of surviving to end of interval 4: $\hat{S}_3 \dfrac{\left(25 - \frac{12}{2}\right) - 2}{\left(25 - \frac{12}{2}\right)},$

$\hat{S}_5$ = probability of surviving to end of interval 5: $\hat{S}_4 \dfrac{\left(11 - \frac{7}{2}\right) - 0}{\left(11 - \frac{7}{2}\right)},$

$\hat{S}_6$ = probability of surviving to end of interval 6: $\hat{S}_5 \dfrac{\left(4 - \frac{2}{2}\right) - 1}{\left(4 - \frac{2}{2}\right)},$

$\hat{S}_7$ = probability of surviving to end of interval 7: $\hat{S}_6 \dfrac{\left(1 - \frac{1}{2}\right) - 0}{\left(1 - \frac{1}{2}\right)}.$

Table 14.4. General Notation for Life Table Data

Interval of Follow-Up (i)	Number of Patients Alive at Start of Interval i	Number of Patients Dying during Interval i	Number of Patients Censored during Interval i	Probability of Surviving to End of Interval i
1	a_1	d_1	c_1	$\hat{S}_1$
2	a_2	d_2	c_2	$\hat{S}_2$
$\vdots$	$\vdots$	$\vdots$	$\vdots$	$\vdots$
I	a_I	d_I	c_I	$\hat{S}_i$

These estimates are referred to as life-table estimates of the survival probability. For convenience, some general notation is in order. For data like Table 14.3, we shall establish the notational scheme in Table 14.4.

In Table 14.4, we define

$$\hat{S}_1 = \frac{(a_1 - c_1/2) - d_1}{a_1 - c_1/2},$$

$$\hat{S}_2 = \hat{S}_1 \frac{(a_2 - c_2/2) - d_2}{a_2 - c_2/2},$$

$$\vdots$$

$$\hat{S}_I = \hat{S}_{I-1} \frac{(a_I - c_I/2) - d_I}{(a_I - c_I/2)}. \tag{14.6}$$

The large-sample standard error estimate for S_i is given by

$$\hat{\sigma}_{\hat{S}_i} = \hat{S}_i \left[\sum_{j=1}^{i} \frac{d_j}{(a_j - c_j/2)(a_j - c_j/2 - d_j)} \right]^{1/2} \tag{14.7}$$

Notice that statistic (14.7) is really quite similar to the ungrouped data estimator given in (14.4). A $(1 - \alpha)$ 100% for the true value of the probability of surviving to the end of interval i is given by

$$\hat{S}_i \pm Z_{1-\alpha/2}\hat{\sigma}_{\hat{S}_i}, \tag{14.8}$$

where $Z_{1-\alpha/2}$ is from Table 4 of the Appendix. In Table 14.5, we apply these methods to the data of Table 14.3.

Table 14.5. Life Table Computed for Data of Table 14.3

(i)	Interval of Follow-up (yr)	Number of Patients Alive at Start of Interval (a_i)	Number of Deaths during Interval (d_i)	Number Censored during Interval (c_i)	$(\hat{S}_i)$	$\dfrac{d_i}{(a_i - c_i/2)(a_i - c_i/2 - d_i)}$	$\hat{\sigma}_{\hat{S}_i}$
1	(0–1)	231	77	37	0.6376	0.00267	0.03295
2	(1–2)	117	28	36	0.4573	0.00398	0.03729
3	(2–3)	53	5	23	0.4022	0.00330	0.04012
4	(3–4)	25	2	12	0.3599	0.00619	0.04572
5	(4–5)	11	0	7	0.3599	0	0.04572
6	(5–6)	4	1	2	0.2399	0.16666	0.10257
7	(6–7)	1	0	1	0.2399	0	0.10257

Hence, the five-year survival rate is estimated as 0.360, with a standard error of 0.0457.

Two final points are essential to this discussion. The first point is that the data analyst should be aware of the distinction between a censored observation and a person who is lost to follow-up. Qualitatively they are quite different. The latter are usually classified as censored observations with respect to the life table computations; however, they are very different types of incomplete data. If there are more than just a few lost-to-follow-up patients, the entire study is quite unlikely to provide meaningful survival information. Thus, every attempt should be made to minimize the number of such lost cases.

The second comment is to note that the type of life table we have presented in this section is sometimes referred to as a *cohort* (or clinical) *life table*. Epidemiologists and demographers frequently require a different life table procedure to use on age-specific mortality rates. For example, given the survival mortality statistics (age-specific rates) for the state of Iowa, it may be of interest to generate a life table in order to determine the probability that a person survives until age X. This type of life table would then be used to predict survival for a hypothetical cohort of persons who might be subject to these age-specific mortality rates. This type of life table is called a *current life table*. The computations for such tables are slightly different from those of this section; however, the basic concepts are identical. An account of such life table computations may be found in Chiang's (1968) text.

14.3 COMPARISON OF TWO SURVIVAL CURVES

14.3.1 Ungrouped Data

Numerous procedures have been proposed for the comparison of two independent survival curves. One procedure was developed by Mantel (1966) and later studied by others, particularly Peto and Peto (1972). The procedure is sometimes called the Peto and Peto log-rank test, Mantel's log-rank test, or simply the log-rank test. We shall refer to it as the log-rank test. The test is a direct by-product of the Mantel–Haenszel procedure of Chapter 13. The assumptions required for the test are:

1. The two samples (group 0 and group 1) are two independent random samples.
2. The censoring patterns for the observations are the same for the two groups.
3. The two population survival curves are $S_0(t)$ and $S_1(t)$, and $S_1(t) = [S_0(t)]^\theta$ for all values of t ($\theta > 0$).

Assumption 3 states that the relative risk of death for group 1 comparable to group 0 is given by the relative risk parameter θ. The test should not be applied if the relative risk of death is dependent on t. A quick way to check assumption 3 is to determine the product limit estimates of $S_1(t)$ and $S_0(t)$ using statistic (14.3). Denote these by $\hat{S}_1(t)$ and $\hat{S}_0(t)$. Plot $\log_e[-\log_e \hat{S}_1(t)]$ against t, and also plot $\log_e[-\log_e \hat{S}_0(t)]$ against t. The resulting figures should be approximately parallel with the differences resulting from $\log_e[-\log_e \hat{S}_0(t)] - \log_e[-\log_e \hat{S}_1(t)]$ being fairly constant as a function of t. If this is the case, then assumption 3 is valid.

The log-rank test is suitable for testing the hypothesis that

$$H_0: \theta = 1 \quad \text{versus} \quad H_a: \theta \neq 1; \tag{14.9}$$

that is, that the relative risk is unity versus the alternative that it is not 1. From the discussions in earlier chapters, it should come as no surprise that the Mantel–Haenszel procedure would be applicable to test (14.9). The procedure is described in Table 14.6.

Let us consider an example.

Example 14.3.1.1. Sixteen patients with stomach carcinoma are randomized to receive one of two chemotherapies (Group 0 or Group 1). From treatment, the survival times, in weeks, are the following, with "plus" indicating a censored time:

Group 0. 63, 59, 57 + , 40, 37, 33, 21 + , 11.
Group 1. 57, 51, 44 + , 32, 27, 20 + , 10, 6.

The log-rank test will be used to test the hypothesis (14.9). Following Table 14.6 we have:

t_i	d_i	d_{0i}	n_{0i}	n_{1i}	n_i	$E(d_{0i})$	$V(d_{0i})$
6	1	0	8	8	16	0.5000	0.2500
10	1	0	8	7	15	0.5333	0.2489
11	1	1	8	6	14	0.5714	0.2449
27	1	0	6	5	11	0.5454	0.2479
32	1	0	6	4	10	0.6000	0.2400
33	1	1	6	3	9	0.6666	0.2222
37	1	1	5	3	8	0.6250	0.2344
40	1	1	4	3	7	0.5714	0.2449
51	1	0	3	2	5	0.6000	0.2400
57	1	0	3	1	4	0.7500	0.1875
59	1	1	2	0	2	1.0000	0
63	1	1	1	0	1	1.0000	0.0
		6				7.9631	2.3647

Therefore,

$$\chi^2_{\text{M-H}} = \frac{\left(|6 - 7.9631| - \frac{1}{2}\right)^2}{2.3647} = 0.9053.$$

As $\chi^2_{0.95}(1) = 3.84$, the result is not significant. Of course, the sample sizes were small for this illustration. The test procedure in Table 14.6 is valid only for large sample sizes.

Gehan (1965) has proposed an alternative test procedure that we now describe. This test is a modification of the Wilcoxon rank sum for censored data.

Here every observation, censored or not, of group 0 is compared with every observation of group 1, censored or not. Let $t_{01} \leq t_{02} \leq \cdots \leq t_{0n_0}$ and $t_{11} \leq t_{12} \leq \cdots \leq t_{1n_1}$ be the follow-up times until death or censoring for group 0 and group 1, respectively. Furthermore, if the follow-up time is censored, it will be primed. For example, if the follow-up times for group 0 were 2, 4 + , and 5, then $t_{01} = 2$, $t'_{02} = 4$, and $t_{03} = 5$. Then a score U_{ij} is

Table 14.6. Summary of Log-Rank Test Procedure

1. Start with two independent random samples of sizes N_0 and N_1.
2. Suppose that there are D distinct times of death in the combined samples, which will be denoted by $t_1 < t_2 < \cdots < t_D$.
3. At t_i let there be d_i deaths of which d_{0i} (d_{1i}) are in group 0 (group 1).
4. Just an infinitesimal amount of time before t_i, let n_{0i} (n_{1i}) be the number of persons in group 0(1). These are the number "at risk." Let $n_i = n_{0i} + n_{1i}$.
5. At t_i, set up the following 2×2 table:

	Group 0	Group 1	Total
Deaths	d_{0i}	d_{1i}	d_i
Survivors	$n_{0i} - d_{0i}$	$n_{1i} - d_{1i}$	$n_i - d_i$
At Risk	n_{0i}	n_{1i}	n_i

6. Now follow the Mantel–Haenszel procedure of Chapter 13 and compute:

$$E(d_{0i}) = n_{0i}\frac{d_i}{n_i},$$

$$V(d_{0i}) = \frac{d_i(n_i - d_i)n_{0i}n_{1i}}{n_i^2(n_i - 1)} = \frac{n_{0i}d_i}{n_i}\frac{(n_i - d_i)n_{1i}}{n_i(n_i - 1)}.$$

7. The test statistic is then

$$\chi^2_{\text{M-H}} = \frac{\left[|\Sigma_{i=1}^D d_{0i} - \Sigma_{i=1}^D n_{0i}d_i/n_i| - 1/2\right]^2}{\Sigma_{i=1}^D V(d_{0i})}.$$

8. Reject H_0 if $\chi^2_{\text{M-H}}$ exceeds $\chi^2_{1-\alpha}(1)$.

assigned according to the scheme

$$U_{ij} = \begin{cases} -1 & \text{if } t_{0i} < t_{1j} \text{ or } t_{0i} \le t'_{1j}, \\ 0 & \text{if } t_{0i} = t_{1j} \text{ or } t'_{0i} < t_{1j} \text{ or } t_{0i} > t'_{1j}, \\ & \text{or both observations are censored,} \\ 1 & \text{if } t_{0i} > t_{1j} \text{ or } t'_{0i} \ge t_{1j}. \end{cases}$$

With these scores, the Gehan (1965) test statistic is defined as $U = \Sigma_{i=1}^{n_0}\Sigma_{j=1}^{n_1}U_{ij}$. Under H_0: $S_0(t) = S_1(t)$, U may be viewed as having a normal distribution with mean zero and variance

$$\text{Var}(U) = \tfrac{1}{3}n_0 n_1(n_0 + n_1 + 1)$$

if there are no ties or censored observations. The variance is more complex with ties and censoring. Fortunately, there is an alternative way to compute U and $\text{Var}(U)$ that is less difficult (Mantel, 1967). Here the two samples of sizes n_0 and n_1 are pooled into a single $n_0 + n_1$ sample and ordered from lowest to highest values. A score U_i, $i = 1, 2, \ldots, n_0 + n_1$, is calculated for each t_i observation as the difference between the number of survival times that are lower than t_i and the number that are greater than t_i. If t_i is censored, at least we can count the number of uncensored observations that are lower than t_i. If t_i and t_j are censored, we do not have information to order them. If t_i is not censored then it is clearly less than any censored t_j that is greater than t_i. Any censored t_j that is less than an uncensored t_i cannot be ordered.

Then the statistic U of Gehan's test can be computed by summing the scores assigned to group 0:

$U = \Sigma_i U_i$, where i ranges over group 0.

As before, U can be considered as a normal random variable with zero mean and variance

$$\text{Var}(U) = \frac{n_0 n_1}{(n_0 + n_1)(n_0 + n_1 - 1)} \sum_{i=1}^{n_0 + n_1} U_i^2.$$

The following table shows the calculation of U_i for Example 14.3.1.1:

t_i	Known to be Lower than t_i	Known to be Greater than t_i	U_i	Group Indicator
6	0	15	-15	1
10	1	14	-13	1
11	2	13	-11	0
20 +	3	0	3	1
21 +	3	0	3	0
27	3	10	-7	1
32	4	9	-5	1
33	5	8	-3	0
37	6	7	-1	0
40	7	6	1	0
44 +	8	0	8	1
51	8	4	4	1
57	9	3	6	1
57 +	10	0	10	0
59	10	1	·9	0
63	11	0	11	0

Therefore,

$$U = -11 + 3 - 3 - 1 + 1 + 10 + 9 + 11 = 19,$$

$$\text{Var}(U) = \frac{(8)(8)}{(8+8)(8+8-1)}\left((-15)^2 + (-13)^2 + \cdots + 9^2 + 11^2\right)$$

$$= (0.2666)(1036) = 276.27,$$

and by the normality of U we have $Z = U/\sqrt{\text{Var}(U)} = 1.14$, a nonsignificant value.

14.3.2 Grouped Data

For grouped data, the two independent survival curve estimates $\hat{S}_{0,1}, \ldots, \hat{S}_{0,I}$ for group 0 and $\hat{S}_{1,1}, \ldots, \hat{S}_{1,I}$ for group 1 are readily compared in the ith interval by computing

$$\frac{\hat{S}_{0,i} - \hat{S}_{1,i}}{\sqrt{\hat{\sigma}^2_{\hat{S}_{0,i}} + \hat{\sigma}^2_{\hat{S}_{1,i}}}} \tag{14.10}$$

from (14.6) and (14.7) and comparing it to $Z_{1-\alpha/2}$ from Table 4 of the Appendix. This would provide, for example, a test that the ith year survival rates are equal to one another. The test procedure assumes that sample sizes are large.

14.4 SAMPLE SIZE CONSIDERATIONS

We restrict attention to the case of comparing two groups of equal sample size with the log-rank test. Freedman (1982) has developed tables for this problem and has shown that the sample size requirements depend on the total number of events (deaths), d, to be observed in the combined groups and the risk ratio, $\theta(14.9)$, that one wishes to detect. For a given significance level α and power $1 - \beta$, the total number of events d needed to be observed (in the combined groups) to detect a risk ratio θ in the trial is

$$d = \left(Z_{1-\alpha^*} + Z_{1-\beta}\right)^2 \left(\frac{1+\theta}{1-\theta}\right)^2,$$

where α^* is α for a one-tailed test and $\alpha^* = \alpha/2$ for a two-tailed test. If the survival rate expected at the end of the study is P_i for group i ($i = 1, 2$), then the total sample size n is

$$n = \frac{2d}{2 - P_1 - P_2},$$

where it is assumed that $n/2$ will be assigned to each treatment group.

Tables 14.7 and 14.8 indicate the number of patients n and the number of events d required to detect specified differences between the two study groups. Table 14.7 is for a one-tailed test while Table 14.8 is for a two-tailed test.(Tables reproduced by permission of author and publishers.) An example will illustrate the use of the tables.

Table 14.7. Number of Patients (number of events) Required to Detect an Improvement $(P_2 - P_1)$ in Survival Rate over a Baseline Survival Rate (P_1), When (i) $\alpha = 5\%$, $1 - \beta = 80\%$, (ii) $\alpha = 5\%$, $1 - \beta = 90\%$, (iii) $\alpha = 1\%$, $1 - \beta = 95\%$, 1-tailed test $P_2 - P_1$

P_1	0.05	0.10	0.15	0.20	0.25	0.30	0.35	0.40	0.45	0.50
	391 (362)	137 (123)	79 (69)	55 (46)	42 (34)	34 (27)	29 (22)	25 (19)	23 (16)	21 (14)
0.05	542 (501)	189 (170)	109 (95)	75 (64)	58 (48)	47 (38)	40 (31)	35 (26)	31 (22)	28 (20)
	997 (922)	348 (313)	200 (175)	138 (117)	106 (87)	86 (69)	73 (56)	64 (48)	57 (41)	52 (36)
	759 (664)	232 (198)	122 (101)	80 (64)	58 (45)	45 (34)	37 (27)	32 (22)	28 (18)	24 (16)
0.10	1051 (920)	322 (273)	169 (139)	110 (88)	80 (62)	62 (47)	51 (37)	43 (30)	38 (25)	34 (22)
	1934 (1692)	592 (503)	311 (256)	202 (161)	146 (113)	114 (86)	93 (68)	79 (55)	69 (46)	61 (39)
	1115 (919)	320 (256)	161 (124)	101 (75)	71 (51)	54 (38)	43 (29)	36 (23)	31 (19)	27 (16)
0.15	1544 (1273)	443 (354)	222 (172)	139 (104)	98 (71)	75 (52)	60 (40)	50 (32)	42 (26)	37 (22)
	2840 (2343)	815 (652)	408 (316)	255 (191)	180 (130)	137 (95)	109 (73)	90 (59)	77 (48)	67 (40)
	1439 (1115)	398 (298)	194 (140)	118 (83)	82 (55)	61 (40)	48 (30)	40 (24)	33 (19)	29 (16)
0.20	1993 (1545)	551 (413)	268 (194)	163 (114)	113 (76)	84 (55)	66 (41)	54 (32)	46 (26)	40 (22)
	3668 (2843)	1013 (760)	492 (357)	300 (210)	207 (140)	154 (100)	121 (76)	99 (59)	83 (48)	72 (39)
	1723 (1249)	464 (325)	221 (149)	133 (86)	90 (56)	66 (40)	52 (30)	42 (23)	35 (18)	30 (15)
0.25	2386 (1730)	643 (450)	306 (206)	183 (119)	124 (78)	92 (55)	71 (41)	58 (31)	48 (25)	41 (20)
	4391 (3183)	1182 (827)	562 (379)	336 (218)	228 (142)	168 (100)	130 (75)	105 (58)	87 (46)	75 (37)
	1960 (1323)	518 (336)	242 (151)	143 (86)	96 (55)	70 (38)	54 (28)	43 (21)	36 (17)	31 (14)
0.30	2714 (1832)	717 (466)	335 (209)	198 (119)	133 (76)	97 (53)	74 (39)	60 (30)	49 (23)	42 (19)
	4995 (3371)	1319 (857)	616 (385)	364 (218)	244 (140)	177 (97)	136 (71)	108 (54)	90 (42)	76 (34)
	2147 (1371)	559 (335)	258 (148)	151 (83)	100 (52)	72 (36)	55 (26)	44 (20)	36 (15)	31 (12)
0.35	2973 (1858)	774 (464)	357 (205)	208 (114)	138 (72)	100 (50)	76 (36)	60 (27)	50 (21)	42 (16)
	5471 (3419)	1423 (853)	656 (377)	382 (210)	253 (133)	182 (91)	138 (65)	110 (49)	90 (38)	76 (30)
	2281 (1312)	586 (322)	268 (140)	155 (77)	102 (48)	73 (33)	55 (23)	44 (17)	36 (13)	30 (10)
0.40	3159 (1816)	812 (446)	370 (194)	214 (107)	140 (66)	100 (45)	76 (32)	60 (24)	49 (18)	41 (14)
	5814 (3343)	1493 (821)	680 (357)	392 (196)	257 (122)	183 (82)	138 (58)	109 (43)	88 (33)	74 (26)
	2363 (1240)	600 (300)	271 (129)	155 (70)	101 (43)	72 (28)	54 (20)	43 (15)	35 (11)	30 (9)
0.45	3272 (1718)	831 (415)	375 (178)	214 (96)	140 (59)	99 (39)	74 (28)	58 (20)	47 (15)	40 (12)
	6022 (3161)	1529 (764)	689 (327)	393 (177)	255 (108)	180 (72)	135 (50)	105 (37)	85 (27)	71 (21)

Table 14.7. (*continued*)

P_1	0.05	0.10	0.15	0.20	0.25	0.30	0.35	0.40	0.45	0.50
	2391 (1135)	601 (270)	269 (114)	153 (61)	99 (37)	70 (24)	52 (17)	41 (12)	33 (9)	
0.50	3311 (1572)	832 (374)	372 (158)	211 (84)	136 (51)	95 (33)	71 (23)	56 (16)	45 (12)	
	6092 (2894)	1530 (688)	683 (290)	386 (154)	248 (93)	174 (60)	129 (42)	100 (30)	80 (22)	
	2365 (1005)	588 (235)	261 (97)	146 (51)	94 (30)	66 (19)	49 (13)	38 (9)		
0.55	3275 (1391)	814 (325)	360 (135)	202 (70)	129 (42)	90 (27)	67 (18)	52 (13)		
	6025 (2561)	1497 (598)	661 (248)	370 (129)	236 (76)	163 (49)	120 (33)	92 (23)		
	2285 (856)	562 (196)	246 (80)	137 (41)	87 (24)	61 (15)	45 (10)			
0.60	3164 (1186)	778 (272)	340 (110)	189 (56)	120 (33)	83 (20)	61 (13)			
	5821 (2183)	1429 (500)	624 (202)	345 (103)	217 (59)	149 (37)	109 (24)			
	2151 (699)	523 (156)	226 (62)	125 (31)	79 (17)	54 (10)				
0.65	2979 (968)	723 (216)	312 (85)	171 (42)	107 (24)	74 (14)				
	5481 (1781)	1328 (398)	572 (157)	312 (78)	194 (43)	132 (26)				
	1965 (540)	470 (117)	201 (45)	109 (21)	68 (12)					
0.70	2721 (748)	650 (162)	276 (62)	149 (29)	93 (16)					
	5005 (1376)	1193 (298)	505 (113)	271 (54)	166 (29)					
	1726 (388)	405 (81)	169 (29)	91 (13)						
0.75	2389 (537)	559 (111)	233 (40)	124 (18)						
	4395 (988)	1025 (205)	424 (74)	222 (33)						
	1436 (251)	327 (49)	134 (16)							
0.80	1986 (347)	450 (67)	182 (22)							
	3652 (639)	824 (123)	329 (41)							
	1094 (136)	238 (23)								
0.85	1513 (189)	326 (32)								
	2778 (347)	592 (59)								
	705 (52)									
0.90	972 (72)									
	1778 (133)									

(i) Example: To detect an improvement from 0.5 to 0.7 using a 1-tailed test consult the cell in the table which is shaded.

(ii) Note: For numbers to detect smaller but realistic differences in the bottom left-hand corner use formulae:

$$d = (Z_1 + Z_2)^2 (1 + \theta)^2/(1 - \theta)^2; \quad n = 2d/(2 - P_1 - P_2)$$

Example 14.4.1. Freedman (1982) discusses the planning of a trial of superficial bladder cancer. The control treatment yields a two-year recurrence-free rate of 0.50. It is hoped that a new therapy will increase this recurrence-free rate to 0.70. Referring to Table 14.7, it seems that 153, 211, or 386 patients (one half to each group) are required for a one-tailed test at $\alpha = 0.05$ for powers of 80, 90, and $\alpha = 0.01$ for power of 95% respectively.

14.5 SUMMARY

These estimation and test procedures provide introductory techniques for the comparison and estimation of survival curves. There are numerous more advanced techniques available for the estimation of survival curves using the regression ideas of Chapter 9. The reader is referred to the texts of Kalbfleisch and Prentice (1980), Cox and Oakes (1984), and Lee (1980) for an account of these procedures and further exemplifications.

To solve numerically the survival methods presented in this chapter, the reader can use BMDP and SAS, among other statistical software.

In BMDP, there are two programs for survival analysis: P1L and P2L. The program P1L can produce a life table analysis using the time of survival as input, it can generate the product limit estimate of the survival curve, and it can plot this estimate. For testing the equality of survival distributions, two tests are used: the generalized Savage test (Mantel–Cox

Table 14.8. Number of Patients (number of events) Required to Detect an Improvement $(P_2 - P_1)$ in Survival Rate over a Baseline Survival Rate (P_1), When (i) $\alpha = 5\%$, $1 - \beta = 80\%$, (ii) $\alpha = 5\%$, $1 - \beta = 90\%$, (iii) $\alpha = 1\%$, $1 - \beta = 95\%$, 2-tailed test $P_2 - P_1$

P_1	$P_2 - P_1$									
	0.05	0.10	0.15	0.20	0.25	0.30	0.35	0.40	0.45	0.50
0.05	497 (459)	174 (156)	100 (87)	69 (59)	53 (44)	43 (34)	37 (28)	32 (24)	29 (21)	26 (18)
	664 (615)	232 (209)	133 (116)	92 (78)	71 (58)	58 (46)	49 (38)	43 (32)	38 (27)	35 (24)
	1126 (1042)	393 (354)	225 (197)	156 (133)	119 (98)	97 (78)	82 (64)	72 (54)	64 (46)	58 (41)
0.10	963 (843)	295 (251)	155 (128)	101 (30)	73 (57)	57 (43)	47 (34)	40 (28)	35 (23)	31 (20)
	1289 (1128)	395 (335)	207 (171)	135 (108)	98 (76)	76 (57)	63 (45)	53 (37)	46 (31)	41 (26)
	2185 (1912)	668 (568)	351 (289)	228 (182)	165 (123)	129 (97)	105 (76)	89 (62)	77 (52)	69 (44)
0.15	1415 (1167)	406 (325)	204 (158)	127 (95)	90 (65)	68 (48)	55 (37)	46 (29)	39 (24)	34 (20)
	1894 (1562)	544 (435)	272 (211)	170 (128)	120 (87)	91 (64)	73 (49)	61 (39)	52 (32)	45 (27)
	3209 (2648)	921 (737)	461 (357)	288 (216)	203 (147)	154 (108)	123 (83)	102 (66)	87 (54)	76 (45)
0.20	1827 (1416)	505 (379)	245 (178)	150 (105)	104 (70)	77 (50)	61 (38)	50 (30)	42 (24)	36 (20)
	2445 (1895)	676 (507)	328 (238)	200 (140)	138 (93)	103 (67)	81 (51)	66 (40)	56 (32)	48 (26)
	4144 (3212)	1145 (858)	556 (403)	339 (237)	234 (158)	174 (113)	137 (85)	112 (67)	94 (54)	81 (44)
0.25	2187 (1585)	589 (412)	280 (189)	168 (109)	114 (71)	84 (50)	65 (37)	53 (29)	44 (23)	38 (19)
	2927 (2122)	788 (551)	375 (253)	224 (146)	152 (95)	112 (67)	87 (50)	70 (39)	59 (31)	50 (25)
	4961 (3597)	1335 (934)	634 (428)	380 (247)	258 (161)	189 (113)	147 (84)	118 (65)	99 (52)	84 (42)
0.30	2487 (1679)	657 (427)	307 (192)	182 (109)	122 (70)	89 (49)	68 (36)	55 (27)	45 (21)	39 (17)
	3330 (2247)	879 (571)	411 (257)	243 (145)	163 (93)	118 (65)	91 (47)	73 (36)	60 (28)	51 (23)
	5643 (3809)	1490 (968)	696 (435)	411 (246)	275 (158)	200 (110)	153 (80)	122 (61)	101 (48)	86 (38)
0.35	2724 (1703)	709 (425)	327 (188)	191 (105)	127 (66)	91 (45)	70 (33)	55 (25)	46 (19)	39 (17)
	3647 (2279)	949 (569)	438 (251)	255 (140)	169 (89)	122 (61)	93 (44)	74 (33)	60 (25)	51 (20)
	6181 (3863)	1607 (964)	741 (426)	432 (237)	286 (150)	205 (102)	156 (74)	124 (55)	101 (43)	85 (34)
0.40	2895 (1665)	744 (409)	339 (178)	196 (98)	129 (61)	92 (41)	70 (29)	55 (22)	45 (17)	38 (13)
	3876 (2228)	995 (547)	454 (238)	262 (131)	172 (81)	123 (55)	93 (39)	73 (29)	60 (22)	50 (17)
	6569 (3777)	1687 (927)	769 (403)	443 (221)	290 (138)	207 (93)	156 (66)	122 (49)	99 (37)	83 (29)
0.45	2999 (1574)	762 (381)	344 (163)	197 (88)	128 (54)	91 (36)	68 (25)	54 (18)	44 (14)	37 (11)
	4014 (2107)	1019 (509)	460 (218)	263 (118)	171 (72)	121 (48)	91 (34)	71 (24)	58 (18)	48 (14)
	6804 (3572)	1727 (863)	779 (370)	444 (200)	288 (122)	203 (81)	152 (57)	119 (41)	96 (31)	80 (24)

Table 14.8. (*continued*)

P_1	P_2-P_1 0.05	0.10	0.15	0.20	0.25	0.30	0.35	0.40	0.45	0.50
	3034 (1441)	763 (343)	341 (145)	193 (77)	125 (46)	88 (30)	65 (21)	51 (15)	42 (11)	
0.50	4061 (1929)	1020 (459)	456 (193)	258 (103)	166 (62)	116 (40)	87 (28)	67 (20)	55 (15)	
	6883 (3269)	1728 (777)	771 (327)	436 (174)	280 (105)	196 (68)	145 (47)	112 (33)	90 (24)	
	3001 (1275)	746 (298)	330 (123)	185 (64)	119 (38)	83 (24)	61 (17)	48 (12)		
0.55	4017 (1707)	998 (399)	441 (165)	247 (86)	158 (51)	110 (33)	81 (22)	63 (15)		
	6808 (2893)	1691 (676)	746 (280)	417 (146)	266 (86)	184 (55)	135 (37)	104 (26)		
	2900 (1087)	713 (249)	312 (101)	173 (52)	110 (30)	76 (19)	56 (12)			
0.60	3881 (1455)	953 (333)	417 (135)	231 (69)	146 (40)	101 (25)	74 (16)			
	6577 (2466)	1615 (565)	705 (229)	389 (116)	245 (67)	168 (42)	122 (27)			
	2730 (887)	663 (198)	286 (78)	157 (39)	99 (22)	68 (13)				
0.65	3654 (1187)	886 (265)	382 (105)	209 (52)	131 (29)	39 (17)				
	6192 (2012)	1500 (450)	646 (177)	352 (88)	219 (49)	148 (29)				
	2493 (685)	596 (149)	253 (57)	137 (27)	85 (15)					
0.70	3337 (917)	796 (199)	338 (76)	182 (36)	112 (19)					
	5654 (1555)	1347 (336)	570 (128)	306 (61)	187 (32)					
	2190 (492)	512 (102)	214 (37)	114 (17)						
0.75	2930 (659)	684 (136)	284 (49)	150 (22)						
	4965 (1117)	1157 (231)	478 (83)	250 (37)						
	1821 (318)	413 (62)	168 (21)							
0.80	2436 (426)	551 (82)	222 (27)							
	4125 (722)	930 (139)	371 (46)							
	1387 (173)	300 (30)								
0.85	1854 (231)	398 (39)								
	3138 (392)	668 (66)								
	892 (66)									
0.90	1189 (89)									
	2007 (150)									

test) [Mantel (1966)], which is equivalent to the log-rank test of this chapter, and the Gehan test. The program P2L includes more advanced topics. The analysis of survival data now is dependent on explanatory variables, called prognostic factors or covariates. This analysis is based on the proportional hazards regression model of Cox (1972). A similar type of analysis can be obtained from the SAS statistical package, version 5. The procedure LIFETEST computes the product limit estimate or the life table estimate of the survival distribution. Several plots can be requested: the estimated survival function, its logarithm, the estimated hazard function and the estimated probability density function. The log-rank test and the Gehan test are used to compare survival curves. The procedure LIFEREG can be used to fit parametric models for time to failure data that may be right censored. The possible models in this procedure are the negative exponential, Weibull, lognormal, and log logistic. The SAS Supplemental Library (SUGI) also includes survival software. The procedures are SURVTEST, for testing differences between survival curves using the Gehan–Wilcoxon test, the log-rank test, or the likelihood ratio test; PHGLM, to estimate survival and hazard functions with the Kaplan–Meier estimators or the proportional hazard model estimators and to perform Cox's proportional hazards regression, and COXREGR, to perform regression analysis using Cox's model.

PROBLEMS

14.1. Eleven patients with chronic leukemia in remission are randomized into two groups of maintenance therapy. The tumor-free times, in weeks, are:

> Group 1, Drug A: 6, 11, 13, 20 + , 22.
> Group 2, Drug B: 5, 14, 23, 31, 39 + , 50.

(a) Plot the survival curve for each group.
(b) Compute the product limit estimator of these curves and the corresponding standard errors for each observed time.
(c) Compare the survival curves with the log-rank test.
(d) Compare the survival curves with the Gehan test.
(e) Comment on the results.

14.2. To compare two treatments for solid tumors, two groups of rats were inoculated with a highly malignant neoplasm, and after randomization into the treatments, the survival (days) was observed as follows:

> Group 1, Drug A: 12, 16, 16, 18 + , 19 + , 20, 28.
> Group 2, Drug B: 10, 14, 15, 18, 18, 20 + , 21.

(a) Plot the survival curve for each group.
(b) Compute the product limit estimator of these curves and the corresponding standard errors for each observed time.
(c) Compare the survival curves.
(d) Comment on the results.

14.3. Two groups of rats were exposed to a toxic chemical added to their food and water, in two doses, low and moderate. The survival times (weeks since exposure to death) for these two groups are:

Group 0 (low dose): 18, 23, 25, 26, +29, 30, 30, 31, +31, +32.
Group 1 (moderate): 13, 13, 15, 17, +17, 18, 18, 21, 23, +23, 24, 25, 25.

(a) Plot the survival curve for each group using the product limit estimator for these curves.
(b) Compare these survival curves with the log-rank test.
(c) Compare these survival curves with the Gehan test.

14.4. From a follow-up study, 88 cases of soft-tissue sarcomas were collected. Their survival times after treatment are as follows, according to sex:

Years Since Treatment	Number Patients Alive at Start of Interval	Number Dying in the Interval	Number Censored or Withdrawn Alive
Sex: Male			
0–1	18	3	0
1–2	15	1	1
2–3	13	0	0
3–4	13	0	2
4–5	11	0	0
5–6	11	0	1
6–7	10	0	0
7–8	10	0	2
8–9	8	0	0
9–10	8	0	0
10–11	8	0	0
11–12	8	0	0
12–13	8	0	0
Sex: Female			
0–1	70	4	1
1–2	65	5	1
2–3	59	6	2
3–4	51	5	0
4–5	46	6	1
5–6	39	3	0
6–7	36	2	1
7–8	33	4	0
8–9	29	1	1
9–10	27	2	0
10–11	25	1	1
11–12	23	2	0
12–13	21	1	0

(a) With these data, estimate the survival curve for each group of patients.

(b) Plot both curves.

(c) Complete these life tables with an estimate for the standard error of the survival curve estimators.

14.5. Using Freedman tables, recommend sample sizes for a clinical trial to detect an improvement of 0.10 in survival rate over a baseline survival rate of 0.35 when comparing two treatments. Use the two-tailed test table.

REFERENCES

Chiang, C. L. (1968). *Introduction to Stochastic Processes in Biostatistics*, Wiley, New York.

Cox, D. R. (1972). Regression models and life tables, *J. Roy. Statist. Soc. Ser. B*, **34**, 187–220.

Cox, D. R., and D. Oakes. (1984). *Analysis of Survival Data*, Chapman and Hall, London.

Cutler, S. J., and F. Ederer. (1958). Maximum utilization of the life table method in analyzing survival, *J. Chron. Dis.*, **8**, 669–712.

Freedman, L. S. (1982). Tables of the number of patients required in clinical trials using the log-rank test, *Statist. Med.*, **1**, 121–129.

Gehan, E. A. (1965). A generalized Wilcoxon test for comparing arbitrarily simply-censored samples, *Biometrika*, **52**, 203–223.

Kalbfleisch, J. D., and R. L. Prentice. (1980). *The Statistical Analysis of Failure Time Data*, Wiley, New York.

Kaplan, E. L., and P. Meier. (1958). Nonparametric estimation from incomplete observations, *J. Am. Statist. Assoc.*, **53**, 457–481.

Lee, E. T. (1980). *Statistical Methods for Survival Data Analysis*, Lifetime Learning, Belmont, CA.

Mantel, N. (1966). Evaluation of survival data and two new rank order statistics arising in its consideration, *Canc. Chemother. Rep.*, **50**, 163–170.

Mantel, N. (1967). Ranking procedures for arbitrarily restricted observations, *Biometrics*, **23**, 65–78.

Peto, R., and J. Peto. (1972). Asymptotically efficient rank invariant procedures, *J. Roy. Statist. Soc., Ser. A*, **135**, 185–207.

Appendix

Table 1. Table of Random Digits[a]

	00-04	05-09	10-14	15-19	20-24	25-29	30-34	35-39	40-44	45-49
0	41396	62881	79285	30352	34334	75023	14390	32858	26501	53597
1	52523	31982	76947	62848	48361	93224	38012	09099	05116	86719
2	61882	41643	24745	15098	85576	21390	17387	83590	16855	77983
3	65627	72463	26617	92616	58883	16425	94844	95676	51496	10151
4	57198	95035	22564	19930	03526	95154	03995	58140	87311	86976
5	66144	40040	13827	75883	47776	57787	65099	47400	96027	41238
6	37043	86368	33482	76860	52103	00745	71175	83456	53173	19972
7	27815	08752	21966	20606	42134	02339	57087	24899	53465	35583
8	23241	98094	76168	55183	52326	41297	77712	02228	17175	12241
9	51135	82554	81198	54108	50998	63915	94304	64093	81671	59414
10	72968	74602	47813	44613	11751	22547	61441	38827	53395	16292
11	23637	23789	85682	13276	04872	59329	39509	93603	29738	76379
12	32561	13052	69507	35645	27687	52388	84103	16737	85749	82735
13	37091	45153	32398	76970	50918	65931	26301	84332	37219	18020
14	76755	67678	55909	04955	12742	71926	17730	60013	12196	80796
15	94734	70616	33296	34011	23686	66398	59888	85855	70986	04328
16	16582	47595	97636	60139	19504	05057	50264	75229	29803	60770
17	66959	66674	28686	07224	78839	98782	92589	42162	04065	32047
18	86879	43414	00996	74066	64430	19254	94784	57352	67637	97781
19	90768	36462	99844	39892	44737	53751	35497	50236	20467	92069
20	01259	32405	46093	89563	17042	95742	68669	92403	68975	70745
21	48663	40208	82439	88891	47905	98569	43994	62925	36408	33895
22	01561	98920	04271	80809	54348	04395	51846	62748	33534	10143
23	25421	11355	65784	51899	18787	23945	70693	97646	18784	25964
24	12756	06041	15230	09597	81699	47479	76340	73002	47909	16698
25	90082	68744	14862	18531	71283	83575	42532	44523	47770	12626
26	48912	24180	14363	62406	53946	95319	32811	44363	70526	56059
27	23430	87962	07432	55562	51709	00966	10101	28222	49426	76875
28	32221	88549	14870	14841	24772	06072	26195	35372	99519	11569
29	58230	18440	89996	14758	03047	37446	45508	76384	79222	15498
30	74727	19023	28082	49716	74886	69125	51536	63822	40643	87481
31	83895	68705	18488	49762	23154	94451	82199	37792	09017	67966
32	55737	72642	32355	97281	62953	64513	39503	07341	37933	55081
33	30946	71806	99617	97378	45425	17846	88647	10579	22559	99666
34	86119	13525	42600	81211	91297	30913	78370	52089	25671	13639
35	03627	24857	17557	79646	19027	45576	85266	38238	53501	67334
36	88345	41313	77201	15212	67791	66726	14736	87265	26753	80851
37	95811	36519	76352	53140	47150	21013	36005	34055	54764	33753
38	35328	94856	52958	29254	27403	09841	48517	90161	86441	41913
39	57167	27052	68924	13587	39328	51696	91497	07159	30439	77838
40	67343	08603	43883	45589	67641	78449	50302	23382	16307	03404
41	18265	21197	59773	99379	90523	58190	84606	74761	12259	72516
42	21038	44202	61975	61642	04710	61794	79905	53097	43699	37401
43	83179	84606	99860	27630	12527	59910	05324	53399	83584	54240
44	71791	52210	53621	60123	04504	85307	49893	91694	77786	03596
45	10247	03987	42806	61453	51923	37971	02911	16059	26874	97521
46	71214	85592	47656	17139	42588	06337	24073	12576	51997	56774
47	20051	18015	05817	00188	57170	76847	60335	54426	79974	38858

465

Table 1. (*continued*)

	00-04	05-09	10-14	15-19	20-24	25-29	30-34	35-39	40-44	45-49
48	57060	91476	52880	67940	92685	04269	32781	46913	52366	34761
49	07736	07579	29237	79224	27786	92317	19479	83435	43209	79762
50	66375	86340	42001	09388	69452	03412	03611	44489	64316	37214
51	74780	27712	10670	95366	87634	16950	83932	81966	05533	07465
52	56350	63842	02259	77840	03159	55108	61464	44189	24690	34158
53	89205	18211	87522	92772	41746	17338	42291	57906	83583	98504
54	98351	84903	13997	82198	44630	47645	18984	86184	32546	91679
55	25474	13902	22037	67984	37984	14200	94906	71747	32503	24338
56	60138	59658	62014	24584	89455	43756	67032	04550	08446	57160
57	67769	52456	68386	73576	04976	61454	81722	68880	43696	95745
58	48698	80001	55366	52903	34863	57905	55656	19173	15567	25878
59	89529	24505	17065	68941	30957	87837	50727	74441	78633	59223
60	32077	99251	11855	89952	50810	83615	12186	75357	10007	42061
61	91632	94275	08517	15652	09435	73569	42195	67682	05973	86038
62	94823	19276	01729	33643	89842	20647	15758	70298	90411	19498
63	07467	28848	45663	34936	72311	38092	32552	49730	85584	86842
64	08049	86850	45582	25285	76214	67471	15657	48534	67359	95625
65	80212	50399	58765	30912	35483	92587	81823	01211	69417	86206
66	60877	56923	41243	16251	12247	73431	48189	17394	09020	04942
67	09662	53424	26365	90588	86618	80841	03396	58691	98965	93330
68	25291	23205	26364	61913	76544	13700	07412	77750	70311	43318
69	53722	67768	50159	65316	08479	08356	62497	03370	68077	35152
70	61445	81093	55738	76951	24498	04801	63189	12317	00703	66777
71	75146	68645	25784	69407	58658	80849	25665	17919	86409	24981
72	73681	39569	18476	36766	94951	69090	81827	56864	65446	25232
73	00454	70467	99623	75154	92891	53693	61131	49906	03879	24505
74	80221	44932	27078	36138	32324	45104	05844	64531	73207	58254
75	60527	39157	56945	09212	48495	07917	01918	51850	91459	79461
76	30336	17120	96966	42414	01642	49046	51803	67398	81577	30257
77	34701	69221	47186	80966	09122	42178	35495	75117	50567	30781
78	39376	41910	06023	41944	01424	98077	74291	70333	95402	74287
79	85348	51663	50761	24767	18357	25698	88796	14528	51794	37893
80	31157	65290	55782	00460	33857	89401	82239	07926	90671	46994
81	67320	26366	16801	47333	55494	57222	24140	23016	41957	09142
82	57096	67359	48517	83418	42069	81168	73326	27467	40711	99663
83	93390	87208	71525	30570	60223	65781	09962	73221	62712	42844
84	24584	96224	30346	34066	33397	52468	44552	55205	58813	60480
85	09734	36272	17964	51449	36935	66700	40904	38315	02965	73299
86	57539	41785	18776	52996	42333	16163	27515	10387	15958	04425
87	05752	57497	36670	01081	17278	02587	74922	17150	13268	77812
88	76939	69101	71733	12560	18959	93894	02635	02111	00817	74201
89	99225	45821	48534	50643	68954	25451	25689	58331	59040	10777
90	23585	75945	54264	14752	33370	80712	09370	59451	16757	81862
91	75333	74070	75859	70239	80934	84156	39639	28622	70003	55328
92	87839	84512	82848	99690	25598	38870	56624	81494	02449	78665
93	08879	91961	64607	03225	69624	87142	80668	55869	72382	54931
94	97223	20401	52019	25534	21457	98662	40890	87367	65064	77223
95	12062	74867	54653	50998	11456	16330	34831	05594	68317	11990
96	41517	29475	28630	79350	87876	87840	34012	07922	11944	60802
97	58586	01904	65950	15129	26773	47072	51344	12622	86627	26643
98	04237	75525	62474	15202	83589	08602	41885	30669	83778	27749
99	85195	73101	90302	85333	01050	93621	03852	55659	58423	12970

	50–54	55–59	60–64	65–69	70–74	75–79	80–84	85–89	90–94	95–99
0	57229	95135	44690	03663	26836	59549	08198	21855	66052	63743
1	98669	54483	40683	37376	36491	17620	17425	31469	18525	69938
2	55979	03209	86377	49473	81842	07020	44662	25623	05247	92743
3	06007	07878	02685	89615	22582	21984	44628	13243	83447	68709
4	90251	19503	66066	09600	88291	77914	30976	83254	25381	54823
5	43413	52843	26722	47405	88055	47901	57605	86547	65088	83993
6	03423	70487	69457	56688	24457	03989	90722	64585	03894	91255
7	18534	14484	71649	76546	55348	19718	72200	76393	78894	97760
8	44413	12428	62145	63730	52198	94835	25645	58164	11946	86299
9	63196	05795	41454	73699	50421	80135	83882	71322	21431	56879
10	30667	51713	41996	61552	64609	43974	60292	81673	48487	22049
11	16571	84067	70317	47060	14450	34865	74196	83199	92870	78197
12	35018	10377	03488	04639	64117	71430	04420	69745	37396	29459
13	67146	23606	18338	88332	08536	39186	07050	72513	91285	91717
14	62883	90343	71727	53572	82328	42117	39577	86458	35584	42328
15	93655	58295	10948	40295	44390	83043	26090	80201	02934	49260
16	84349	09768	84387	25428	75783	83120	45680	58637	17672	15428
17	70832	32988	26333	95955	34950	36578	34960	07761	37237	74741
18	34591	83999	27660	93602	29788	91327	52341	82910	89415	38854
19	63794	98741	18971	96726	14390	74087	29088	91265	93366	03929
20	58079	35082	28653	82209	83028	45447	71235	16419	66290	77792
21	77754	62356	33152	01918	37188	88908	51816	22871	85582	43161
22	05868	22279	35868	89021	17377	67198	38927	59367	20324	86040
23	34745	39395	10953	75893	63528	06804	51975	66093	09094	55903
24	03645	03891	50830	37842	99979	17186	85847	85137	98131	52326
25	65154	93027	20534	78787	57701	08502	77029	45414	71218	85871
26	02526	86560	20854	80100	90594	44886	81610	94080	92495	20076
27	75917	73889	01855	80062	11935	00005	31926	51920	14138	11506
28	65147	05397	70276	62784	59039	03558	28320	20117	66261	37389
29	05415	14792	85196	04358	59939	30959	36403	79935	41311	47970
30	32129	08686	70364	44078	01308	26245	23212	20170	69882	50919
31	98842	07406	25478	45327	59886	38544	79161	43798	18121	04326
32	72269	24374	67837	37665	48417	91953	02365	51657	33079	41831
33	55261	59118	64889	96677	16182	35240	77613	72370	83576	41042
34	39112	28474	79293	33666	20693	78250	57881	40202	14288	25968
35	24427	11288	36452	94480	11376	06399	50036	63522	12808	04770
36	91123	90883	54756	21330	38576	99114	98990	18426	60911	46366
37	56565	33676	85295	49783	88653	50588	21510	26506	28087	74163
38	48061	74897	32800	02939	79663	52391	97378	92791	61467	75815
39	32450	32249	31166	03447	32848	79783	91864	77669	18836	50885
40	03199	05993	76202	92811	95033	62883	31368	61126	76286	49042
41	90401	43217	33835	44138	51903	54461	96884	14474	22568	28402
42	87022	31825	67334	60718	46424	22332	43417	60504	14777	11665
43	01091	67728	27365	05315	09984	89045	57233	42220	82808	78205
44	26520	71996	11534	82630	94820	76076	10117	80210	44741	23863
45	29720	17663	87270	10300	05002	29439	26792	08450	96133	39416
46	36652	98901	77565	86344	80944	78734	62194	94728	53333	29702
47	28309	13254	05608	10391	81199	44071	21600	83541	89463	39007
48	91209	49937	78748	10949	29825	02707	12669	01609	44219	49739
49	72431	82045	61219	25317	33096	79063	76673	18685	98795	59838

467

Table 1. (*continued*)

	50–54	55–59	60–64	65–69	70–74	75–79	80–84	85–89	90–94	95–99
50	40691	94868	96244	16417	96262	97031	04218	79207	75384	66805
51	98753	96369	77355	15603	35759	96313	60843	89234	33021	42751
52	78802	02529	03153	46272	86938	78374	98559	61806	85285	30654
53	41029	12853	84448	92826	83254	71931	78903	98920	41685	60612
54	31017	57394	90113	52332	14348	56569	59850	56022	58064	69718
55	95144	62675	72817	42375	84162	17027	67598	88319	92408	76088
56	04941	49479	80830	43643	31502	54926	69468	27619	59338	03332
57	77233	98393	84710	27568	50633	45556	42442	21293	83330	71423
58	01413	20950	69280	58772	53539	49385	43633	47228	88635	17277
59	48278	56991	79165	12178	14294	50495	40442	18105	60812	66490
60	78462	01275	07878	54934	45980	46343	07205	97155	23031	78803
61	61518	87982	44812	51537	83758	77114	10100	61677	04976	06937
62	33358	96658	26210	56747	10172	48280	87504	04779	74424	93688
63	70929	17945	07023	75323	42214	80566	44323	37982	60161	71807
64	45790	11343	60905	02554	42218	57469	60829	55327	37890	46047
65	02788	95626	83686	32984	49147	17783	50232	52528	31393	12497
66	43395	23212	49589	63798	38778	75516	94928	99155	03382	44474
67	94145	93715	90966	24371	38963	93998	55343	36598	18893	66990
68	03398	20163	62643	44488	65369	44646	28562	58779	18649	69499
69	31210	88808	84950	79758	49761	14824	13309	77234	60473	73020
70	20744	86135	64114	72510	87839	83158	44800	47211	28030	53291
71	64883	90155	80739	51283	52155	82673	16598	91791	49190	12354
72	80509	92969	61376	31894	93237	84452	62843	02907	45082	89259
73	77446	70671	21296	36077	38709	14903	13861	13571	74495	28082
74	13873	73046	37428	42648	37037	12249	59588	16684	11988	29532
75	45084	25599	86495	83328	08605	89190	56588	46512	51315	27519
76	96647	08917	12767	19179	69319	23957	25665	60996	63029	59347
77	26516	73616	34351	44611	64170	19894	01138	37617	49381	19822
78	07529	91609	37578	50924	80930	30976	41068	31162	15919	93304
79	96928	95868	68939	65247	25824	10062	73659	70951	31744	30588
80	02461	29583	47904	06965	68666	43210	38899	46467	46283	30033
81	91127	38760	29489	95312	40396	48695	35024	03016	86841	60500
82	29150	54637	11292	15523	07167	03790	91270	02377	87366	32557
83	99456	43574	75350	40785	41044	95383	89410	95771	88380	28106
84	03250	47587	76936	76819	39519	63063	80579	19487	15236	51751
85	07289	24378	74673	82543	25023	56853	44030	35066	26970	49142
86	76087	58057	52101	02787	25026	82779	88641	82069	60550	39160
87	75901	33812	83563	04224	26899	79551	81886	96069	27372	15977
88	37676	33585	00968	90162	72087	44831	95168	24072	18552	15206
89	65376	82878	12600	69973	86158	45824	20384	06239	23461	01068
90	72489	19839	59934	68589	14469	71304	53716	75911	31387	19488
91	20490	91375	43185	44486	95753	42390	52076	62573	03505	51966
92	79622	38649	44972	20776	19024	17682	73471	42932	56626	52971
93	71509	39928	72542	02769	93104	78293	82461	91893	57785	19223
94	56879	02851	84532	35237	25059	62195	79807	19781	47234	95426
95	40619	88471	98466	05637	39280	81171	49696	82567	14103	80099
96	61718	33868	49789	57886	97237	41273	43580	82145	17536	97561
97	52465	48340	24058	74523	93877	51641	59666	55673	17174	92269
98	99874	43192	01997	79619	53874	78660	02481	15672	56869	64439
99	66417	57021	10618	06510	29310	71344	34132	73673	09714	57467

[a] Computer-generated by Patricio B. Rojas.

Table 2. Table of Cumulative Binomial Distribution $\Pr(X \le x)^a$ where
$\Pr(X = x) = \binom{n}{x} p^x (1 - p)^{n-x}$

n	x	$p = 0.10$	$p = 0.20$	$p = 0.25$	$p = 0.30$	$p = 0.40$	$p = 0.50$
5	0	.59049	.32768	.23730	.16807	.07776	.03125
	1	.91854	.73728	.63281	.52822	.33696	.18750
	2	.99144	.94208	.89648	.83692	.68256	.50000
	3	.99954	.99328	.98438	.96922	.91296	.81250
	4	.99999	.99968	.99902	.99757	.98976	.96875
	5	1.0	1.0	1.0	1.0	1.0	1.0
6	0	.53144	.26214	.17798	.11765	.04666	.01562
	1	.88574	.65536	.53394	.42018	.23328	.10938
	2	.98415	.90112	.83057	.74431	.54432	.34375
	3	.99873	.98304	.96240	.92953	.82080	.65625
	4	.99995	.99840	.99536	.98906	.95904	.89063
	5		.99994	.99976	.99927	.99590	.98438
	6		1.0	1.0	1.0	1.0	1.0
7	0	.47830	.20972	.13348	.08235	.02799	.00781
	1	.85031	.57672	.44495	.32942	.15863	.06250
	2	.97431	.85197	.75641	.64707	.41990	.22656
	3	.99727	.96666	.92944	.87396	.71021	.50000
	4	.99982	.99533	.98712	.97120	.90374	.77344
	5	.99999	.99963	.99866	.99621	.98116	.93750
	6		.99999	.99994	.99978	.99836	.99219
	7		1.0	1.0	1.0	1.0	1.0
8	0	.43047	.16777	.10011	.05765	.01680	.00391
	1	.81310	.50332	.36708	.25530	.10638	.03516
	2	.96191	.79692	.67854	.55177	.31539	.14453
	3	.99498	.94372	.88618	.80590	.59409	.36328
	4	.99957	.98959	.97270	.94203	.82633	.63672
	5	.99998	.99877	.99577	.98871	.95019	.85547
	6		.99992	.99962	.99871	.99148	.96484
	7			.99998	.99993	.99934	.99609
	8			1.0	1.0	1.0	1.0
9	0	.38742	.13422	.07508	.04035	.01008	.00195
	1	.77484	.43621	.30034	.19600	.07054	.01953
	2	.94703	.73820	.60068	.46283	.23179	.08984
	3	.99167	.91436	.83427	.72966	.48261	.25391
	4	.99911	.98042	.95107	.90119	.73343	.50000
	5	.99994	.99693	.99001	.97471	.90065	.74609
	6		.99969	.99866	.99571	.97497	.91016
	7		.99998	.99989	.99957	.99620	.98047

469

Table 2. (*continued*)

n	x	$p = 0.10$	$p = 0.20$	$p = 0.25$	$p = 0.30$	$p = 0.40$	$p = 0.50$
	8				.99998	.99974	.99805
	9				1.0	1.0	1.0
10	0	.34868	.10737	.05631	.02825	.00605	.00098
	1	.73610	.37581	.24403	.14931	.04636	.01074
	2	.92981	.67780	.52559	.38278	.16729	.05469
	3	.98720	.87913	.77588	.64961	.38228	.17187
	4	.99837	.96721	.92187	.84973	.63310	.37695
	5	.99985	.99363	.98027	.95265	.83376	.62305
	6	.99999	.99914	.99649	.98941	.94524	.82813
	7		.99992	.99958	.99841	.98771	.94531
	8			.99997	.99986	.99832	.98926
	9				.99999	.99990	.99902
	10				1.0	1.0	1.0
15	0	.20589	.03518	.01336	.00475	.00047	.00003
	1	.54904	.16713	.08018	.03527	.00517	.00049
	2	.81594	.39802	.23609	.12683	.02711	.00369
	3	.94444	.64816	.46129	.29687	.09050	.01758
	4	.98728	.83577	.68649	.51549	.21728	.05923
	5	.99775	.93895	.85163	.72162	.40322	.15088
	6	.99969	.98194	.94338	.86886	.60981	.30362
	7	.99997	.99576	.98270	.94999	.78690	.50000
	8		.99922	.99581	.98476	.90495	.69638
	9		.99989	.99921	.99635	.96617	.84912
	10		.99999	.99988	.99933	.99065	.94077
	11			.99999	.99991	.99807	.98242
	12				.99999	.99972	.99631
	13					.99997	.99951
	14						.99997
	15						
20	0	.12158	.01153	.00317	.00080	.00004	.00000
	1	.39175	.06918	.02431	.00764	.00052	.00002
	2	.67693	.20608	.09126	.03548	.00361	.00020
	3	.86705	.41145	.22516	.10709	.01596	.00129
	4	.95683	.62965	.41484	.23751	.05095	.00591
	5	.98875	.80421	.61717	.41637	.12560	.02069
	6	.99761	.91331	.78578	.60801	.25001	.05766
	7	.99958	.96786	.89819	.77227	.41589	.13159
	8	.99994	.99002	.95907	.88667	.59560	.25172
	9	.99999	.99741	.98614	.95204	.75534	.41190
	10		.99944	.99606	.98286	.87248	.58810
	11		.99990	.99906	.99486	.94347	.74828

n	x	$p = 0.10$	$p = 0.20$	$p = 0.25$	$p = 0.30$	$p = 0.40$	$p = 0.50$
	12		.99998	.99982	.99872	.97897	.86841
	13			.99997	.99974	.99353	.94234
	14				.99996	.99839	.97931
	15				.99999	.99968	.99409
	16					.99995	.99871
	17					.99999	.99980
	18						.99998
	19						
	20						
25	0	.07179	.00378	.00075	.00013	.00000	
	1	.27121	.02739	.00702	.00157	.00005	.00000
	2	.53709	.09823	.03211	.00896	.00043	.00001
	3	.76359	.23399	.09621	.03324	.00237	.00008
	4	.90201	.42067	.21374	.09047	.00947	.00046
	5	.96660	.61669	.37828	.19349	.02936	.00204
	6	.99052	.78004	.56110	.34065	.07357	.00732
	7	.99774	.89088	.72651	.51185	.15355	.02164
	8	.99954	.95323	.85056	.67693	.27353	.05388
	9	.99992	.98267	.92867	.81056	.42462	.11476
	10	.99999	.99445	.97033	.90220	.58577	.21218
	11		.99846	.98927	.95575	.73228	.34502
	12		.99963	.99663	.98253	.84623	.50000
	13		.99992	.99908	.99401	.92220	.65498
	14		.99999	.99979	.99822	.96561	.78782
	15			.99996	.99955	.98683	.88524
	16			.99999	.99990	.99567	.94612
	17				.99998	.99879	.97836
	18					.99972	.99268
	19					.99995	.99796
	20					.99999	.99954
	21						.99992
	22						.99999
	23						
	24						
	25						
30	0	.04239	.00124	.00018	.00002		
	1	.18370	.01052	.00196	.00031	.00000	
	2	.41135	.04418	.01060	.00211	.00005	
	3	.64744	.12271	.03745	.00932	.00031	.00000
	4	.82451	.25523	.09787	.03015	.00151	.00003

Table 2. (*continued*)

n	x	p = 0.10	p = 0.20	p = 0.25	p = 0.30	p = 0.40	p = 0.50
	5	.92681	.42751	.20260	.07659	.00566	.00016
	6	.97417	.60697	.34805	.15952	.01718	.00072
	7	.99222	.76079	.51429	.28138	.04352	.00261
	8	.99798	.87135	.67360	.43152	.09401	.00806
	9	.99955	.93891	.80341	.58881	.17629	.02139
	10	.99991	.97438	.89427	.73037	.29147	.04937
	11	.99998	.99051	.94934	.84068	.43109	.10024
	12		.99689	.97841	.91553	.57847	.18080
	13		.99910	.99182	.95995	.71450	.29233
	14		.99977	.99725	.98306	.82463	.42777
	15		.99995	.99918	.99363	.90294	.57223
	16		.99999	.99978	.99788	.95189	.70767
	17			.99995	.99937	.97876	.81920
	18			.99999	.99984	.99170	.89976
	19				.99996	.99715	.95063
	20				.99999	.99914	.97861
	21					.99978	.99194
	22					.99995	.99739
	23					.99999	.99928
	24						.99984
	25						.99997
	26						
	27						
	28						
	29						
	30						
50	0	.00515	.00001	.00000			
	1	.03379	.00019	.00001			
	2	.11173	.00129	.00009	.00000		
	3	.25029	.00566	.00050	.00003		
	4	.43120	.01850	.00211	.00017		
	5	.61612	.04803	.00705	.00072	.00000	
	6	.77023	.10340	.01939	.00249	.00001	
	7	.87785	.19041	.04526	.00726	.00006	
	8	.94213	.30733	.09160	.01825	.00023	
	9	.97546	.44374	.16368	.04023	.00076	.00000
	10	.99065	.58356	.26220	.07885	.00220	.00001
	11	.99678	.71067	.38162	.13904	.00569	.00005
	12	.99900	.81394	.51099	.22287	.01325	.00015
	13	.99971	.88941	.63704	.32788	.02799	.00047
	14	.99993	.93928	.74808	.44683	.05396	.00130
	15	.99998	.96920	.83692	.56918	.09550	.00330

n	x	p = 0.10	p = 0.20	p = 0.25	p = 0.30	p = 0.40	p = 0.50
	16		.98556	.90169	.68388	.15609	.00767
	17		.99374	.94488	.78219	.23688	.01642
	18		.99749	.97127	.85944	.33561	.03245
	19		.99907	.98608	.91520	.44648	.05946
	20		.99968	.99374	.95224	.56103	.10132
	21		.99990	.99738	.97491	.67014	.16112
	22		.99997	.99898	.98772	.76602	.23994
	23		.99999	.99963	.99441	.84383	.33591
	24			.99988	.99763	.90219	.44386
	25			.99996	.99907	.94266	.55614
	26			.99999	.99966	.96859	.66409
	27				.99988	.98397	.76006
	28				.99996	.99238	.83888
	29				.99999	.99664	.89868
	30					.99863	.94054
	31					.99948	.96755
	32					.99982	.98358
	33					.99994	.99233
	34					.99998	.99670
	35						.99870
	36						.99953
	37						.99985
	38						.99995
	39						.99999
	40						
	41						
	42						
	43						
	44						
	45						
	46						
	47						
	48						
	49						
	50						
100	0	.00003					
	1	.00032					
	2	.00194					
	3	.00784					
	4	.02371	.00000				
	5	.05758	.00002				

Table 2. (*continued*)

n	x	p = 0.10	p = 0.20	p = 0.25	p = 0.30	p = 0.40	p = 0.50
	6	.11716	.00008				
	7	.20605	.00028	.00000			
	8	.32087	.00086	.00001			
	9	.45129	.00233	.00004			
	10	.58316	.00570	.00014	.00000		
	11	.70303	.01257	.00039	.00001		
	12	.80182	.02533	.00103	.00002		
	13	.87612	.04691	.00246	.00006		
	14	.92743	.08044	.00542	.00016		
	15	.96011	.12851	.01108	.00040		
	16	.97940	.19234	.02111	.00097		
	17	.98999	.27119	.03763	.00216		
	18	.99542	.36209	.06301	.00452	.00000	
	19	.99802	.46016	.09953	.00889	.00001	
	20	.99919	.55946	.14883	.01646	.00002	
	21	.99969	.65403	.21144	.02883	.00004	
	22	.99989	.73893	.28637	.04787	.00011	
	23	.99996	.81091	.37108	.07553	.00025	
	24	.99999	.86865	.46167	.11357	.00056	
	25		.91252	.55347	.16313	.00119	
	26		.94417	.64174	.22440	.00240	
	27		.96585	.72238	.29637	.00460	.00000
	28		.97998	.79246	.37678	.00843	.00001
	29		.98875	.85046	.46234	.01478	.00002
	30		.99394	.89621	.54912	.02478	.00004
	31		.99687	.93065	.63311	.03985	.00009
	32		.99845	.95540	.71072	.06150	.00020
	33		.99926	.97241	.77926	.09125	.00044
	34		.99966	.98357	.83714	.13034	.00089
	35		.99985	.99059	.88392	.17947	.00176
	36		.99994	.99482	.92012	.23861	.00332
	37		.99998	.99725	.94695	.30681	.00602
	38		.99999	.99860	.96602	.38219	.01049
	39			.99931	.97901	.46208	.01760
	40			.99968	.98750	.54329	.02844
	41			.99985	.99283	.62253	.04431
	42			.99994	.99603	.69674	.06661
	43			.99997	.99789	.76347	.09667
	44			.99999	.99891	.82110	.13563
	45				.99946	.86891	.18410
	46				.99974	.90702	.24206
	47				.99988	.93621	.30865
	48				.99995	.95770	.38218

n	x	$p = 0.10$	$p = 0.20$	$p = 0.25$	$p = 0.30$	$p = 0.40$	$p = 0.50$
	49				.99998	.97290	.46021
	50				.99999	.98324	.53979
	51					.98999	.61782
	52					.99424	.69135
	53					.99680	.75794
	54					.99829	.81590
	55					.99912	.86437
	56					.99956	.90333
	57					.99979	.93339
	58					.99990	.95569
	59					.99996	.97156
	60					.99998	.98240
	61					.99999	.98951
	62						.99398
	63						.99668
	64						.99824
	65						.99911
	66						.99956
	67						.99980
	68						.99991
	69						.99996
	70						.99998
	71						.99999
	72						
	73						
	74						
	75						
	76						
	77						
	78						
	79						
	80						
	81						
	82						
	83						
	84						
	85						
	86						
	87						
	88						
	89						

Table 2. (*continued*)

n	x	p = 0.10	p = 0.20	p = 0.25	p = 0.30	p = 0.40	p = 0.50
	90						
	91						
	92						
	93						
	94						
	95						
	96						
	97						
	98						
	99						
	100						

[a] For tests in text, for $e \leq 0.5$, $B_e(n, p)$ is that value y such that $P[X \leq y] \leq e$ and $P[X \leq y + 1] \geq e$. For $e > 0.5$, $B_e(n, p)$ is that value y such that $P[X \geq y] \leq 1 - e$ and $P[X \geq y - 1] \geq 1 - e$. Computer-generated by Patricio B. Rojas.

Table 3. Cumulative Distribution of Poisson Random Variable $\Pr(X \le x)^a$

$$\Pr(X \le x) = \sum_{i=0}^{x} \frac{\lambda^i e^{-\lambda}}{i!}$$

$\lambda = E(X)$

x	0.5	1.0	1.5	2.0	2.5	3.0	4.0	5.0	6.0	7.0	8.0	9.0	10.0
0	.60653	.36788	.22313	.13534	.08208	.04979	.01832	.00674	.00248	.00091	.00034	.00012	.00005
1	.90980	.73576	.55783	.40601	.28730	.19915	.09158	.04043	.01735	.00730	.00302	.00123	.00050
2	.98561	.91970	.80885	.67668	.54381	.42319	.23810	.12465	.06197	.02964	.01375	.00623	.00277
3	.99825	.98101	.93436	.85712	.75758	.64723	.43347	.26503	.15120	.08177	.04238	.02123	.01034
4	.99983	.99634	.98142	.94735	.89118	.81526	.62884	.44049	.28506	.17299	.09963	.05496	.02925
5	.99999	.99941	.99554	.98344	.95798	.91608	.78513	.61596	.44568	.30071	.19124	.11569	.06709
6		.99992	.99907	.99547	.98581	.96649	.88933	.76218	.60630	.44971	.31337	.20678	.13014
7		.99999	.99983	.99890	.99575	.98810	.94887	.86663	.74398	.59871	.45296	.32390	.22022
8			.99997	.99976	.99886	.99620	.97864	.93191	.84724	.72909	.59255	.45565	.33282
9				.99995	.99972	.99890	.99187	.96817	.91608	.83050	.71662	.58741	.45793
10				.99999	.99994	.99971	.99716	.98630	.95738	.90148	.81589	.70599	.58304
11					.99999	.99993	.99908	.99455	.97991	.94665	.88808	.80301	.69678
12						.99998	.99973	.99798	.99117	.97300	.93620	.87577	.79156
13							.99992	.99930	.99637	.98719	.96582	.92615	.86446
14							.99998	.99977	.99860	.99428	.98274	.95853	.91654
15								.99993	.99949	.99759	.99177	.97796	.95126
16								.99998	.99983	.99904	.99628	.98889	.97296
17								.99999	.99994	.99964	.99841	.99468	.98572
18									.99998	.99987	.99935	.99757	.99281
19									.99999	.99996	.99975	.99894	.99655
20										.99999	.99991	.99956	.99841
21											.99997	.99983	.99930
22											.99999	.99993	.99970
23												.99998	.99988
24												.99999	.99995

^{a} Computer-generated by Patricio B. Rojas

Table 4. Distribution of Normal Distribution with Mean 0, Variance 1[a]

z	.00	.01	.02	.03	.04	.05	.06	.07	.08	.09
.0	.5000	.4960	.4920	.4880	.4840	.4801	.4761	.4721	.4681	.4641
.1	.4602	.4562	.4522	.4483	.4443	.4404	.4364	.4325	.4286	.4247
.2	.4207	.4168	.4129	.4090	.4052	.4013	.3974	.3936	.3897	.3859
.3	.3821	.3783	.3745	.3707	.3669	.3632	.3594	.3557	.3520	.3483
.4	.3446	.3409	.3372	.3336	.3300	.3264	.3228	.3192	.3156	.3121
.5	.3085	.3050	.3015	.2981	.2946	.2912	.2877	.2843	.2810	.2776
.6	.2743	.2709	.2676	.2643	.2611	.2578	.2546	.2514	.2483	.2451
.7	.2420	.2389	.2358	.2327	.2296	.2266	.2236	.2206	.2177	.2148
.8	.2119	.2090	.2061	.2033	.2005	.1977	.1949	.1922	.1894	.1867
.9	.1841	.1814	.1788	.1762	.1736	.1711	.1685	.1660	.1635	.1611
1.0	.1587	.1562	.1539	.1515	.1492	.1469	.1446	.1423	.1401	.1379
1.1	.1357	.1335	.1314	.1292	.1271	.1251	.1230	.1210	.1190	.1170
1.2	.1151	.1131	.1112	.1093	.1075	.1056	.1038	.1020	.1003	.0985
1.3	.0968	.0951	.0934	.0918	.0901	.0885	.0869	.0853	.0838	.0823
1.4	.0808	.0793	.0778	.0764	.0749	.0735	.0721	.0708	.0694	.0681
1.5	.0668	.0655	.0643	.0630	.0618	.0606	.0594	.0582	.0571	.0559
1.6	.0548	.0537	.0526	.0516	.0505	.0495	.0485	.0475	.0465	.0455
1.7	.0446	.0436	.0427	.0418	.0409	.0401	.0392	.0384	.0375	.0367
1.8	.0359	.0351	.0344	.0336	.0329	.0322	.0314	.0307	.0301	.0294
1.9	.0287	.0281	.0274	.0268	.0262	.0256	.0250	.0244	.0239	.0233
2.0	.0228	.0222	.0217	.0212	.0207	.0202	.0197	.0192	.0188	.0183
2.1	.0179	.0174	.0170	.0166	.0162	.0158	.0154	.0150	.0146	0143
2.2	.0139	.0136	.0132	.0129	.0125	.0122	.0119	.0116	.0113	.0110
2.3	.0107	.0104	.0102	.0099	.0096	.0094	.0091	.0089	.0087	.0084
2.4	.0082	.0080	.0078	.0075	.0073	.0071	.0069	.0068	.0066	.0064
2.5	.0062	.0060	.0059	.0057	.0055	.0054	.0052	.0051	.0049	.0048
2.6	.0047	.0045	.0044	.0043	.0041	.0040	.0039	.0038	.0037	.0036
2.7	.0035	.0034	.0033	.0032	.0031	.0030	.0029	.0028	.0027	.0026
2.8	.0026	.0025	.0024	.0023	.0023	.0022	.0021	.0021	.0020	.0019
2.9	.0019	.0018	.0018	.0017	.0016	.0016	.0015	.0015	.0014	.0014
3.0	.0013	.0013	.0013	.0012	.0012	.0011	.0011	.0011	.0010	.0010
3.1	.0010	.0009	.0009	.0009	.0008	.0008	.0008	.0008	.0007	.0007
3.2	.0007	.0007	.0006	.0006	.0006	.0006	.0006	.0005	.0005	.0005
3.3	.0005	.0005	.0005	.0004	.0004	.0004	.0004	.0004	.0004	.0003
3.4	.0003	.0003	.0003	.0003	.0003	.0003	.0003	.0003	.0003	.0002
3.6	.0002	.0002	.0001	.0001	.0001	.0001	.0001	.0001	.0001	.0001
3.9	.0000									

[a]Entries are probability that Z is greater than or equal to z: $P(Z \geq z)$.
Reprinted from R. Steel and J. Torrie, (1960). *Principles and Procedures of Statistics*, McGraw Hill, p. 434, with permission of the authors and the publisher.

Table 5. Percentage Points of t Distribution

df	Probability of a larger value of t, sign ignored								
	0.5	0.4	0.3	0.2	0.1	0.05	0.02	0.01	0.001
1	1.000	1.376	1.963	3.078	6.314	12.706	31.821	63.657	636.619
2	.816	1.061	1.386	1.886	2.920	4.303	6.965	9.925	31.598
3	.765	.978	1.250	1.638	2.353	3.182	4.541	5.841	12.941
4	.741	.941	1.190	1.533	2.132	2.776	3.747	4.604	8.610
5	.727	.920	1.156	1.476	2.015	2.571	3.365	4.032	6.859
6	.718	.906	1.134	1.440	1.943	2.447	3.143	3.707	5.959
7	.711	.896	1.119	1.415	1.895	2.365	2.998	3.499	5.405
8	.706	.889	1.108	1.397	1.860	2.306	2.896	3.355	5.041
9	.703	.883	1.100	1.383	1.833	2.262	2.821	3.250	4.781
10	.700	.879	1.093	1.372	1.812	2.228	2.764	3.169	4.587
11	.697	.876	1.088	1.363	1.796	2.201	2.718	3.106	4.437
12	.695	.873	1.083	1.356	1.782	2.179	2.681	3.055	4.318
13	.694	.870	1.079	1.350	1.771	2.160	2.650	3.012	4.221
14	.692	.868	1.076	1.345	1.761	2.145	2.624	2.977	4.140
15	.691	.866	1.074	1.341	1.753	2.131	2.602	2.947	4.073
16	.690	.865	1.071	1.337	1.746	2.120	2.583	2.921	4.015
17	.689	.863	1.069	1.333	1.740	2.110	2.567	2.898	3.965
18	.688	.862	1.067	1.330	1.734	2.101	2.552	2.878	3.922
19	.688	.861	1.066	1.328	1.729	2.093	2.539	2.861	3.883
20	.687	.860	1.064	1.325	1.725	2.086	2.528	2.845	3.850
21	.686	.859	1.063	1.323	1.721	2.080	2.518	2.831	3.819
22	.686	.858	1.061	1.321	1.717	2.074	2.508	2.819	3.792
23	.685	.858	1.060	1.319	1.714	2.069	2.500	2.807	3.767
24	.685	.857	1.059	1.318	1.711	2.064	2.492	2.797	3.745
25	.684	.856	1.058	1.316	1.708	2.060	2.485	2.787	3.725
26	.684	.856	1.058	1.315	1.706	2.056	2.479	2.779	3.707
27	.684	.855	1.057	1.314	1.703	2.052	2.473	2.771	3.690
28	.683	.855	1.056	1.313	1.701	2.048	2.467	2.763	3.674
29	.683	.854	1.055	1.311	1.699	2.045	2.462	2.756	3.659
30	.683	.854	1.055	1.310	1.697	2.042	2.457	2.750	3.646
40	.681	.851	1.050	1.303	1.684	2.021	2.423	2.704	3.551
60	.679	.848	1.046	1.296	1.671	2.000	2.390	2.660	3.460
120	.677	.845	1.041	1.289	1.658	1.980	2.358	2.617	3.373
∞	.674	.842	1.036	1.282	1.645	1.960	2.326	2.576	3.291
df	0.25	0.2	0.15	0.1	0.05	0.025	0.01	0.005	0.0005
	Probability of a larger value of t, sign considered								

Reprinted from R. Steel and J. Torrie, (1960). *Principles and Procedures of Statistics*, McGraw-Hill, p. 433, with permission of the authors and publisher. This Table is adapted from Table III of R. A. Fisher and F. Yates' (1974) Statistical Tables for Biological, Agricultural and Medical Research published by Longman Group UK Ltd., London (previously published by Oliver and Boyd Ltd., Edinburgh) by permission of the authors and publishers.

Table 6. Percentage Points of χ^2 Distribution

$p = \Pr[X \le x]$

d.f.	0.005	0.010	0.025	0.050	0.10	0.20	0.25	0.50	0.75	0.80	0.90	0.950	0.975	0.990	0.995	0.999
1	0.00	0.00	0.00	0.00	0.02	0.06	0.10	0.45	1.32	1.64	2.71	3.84	5.02	6.63	7.88	10.83
2	0.01	0.02	0.05	0.10	0.21	0.45	0.58	1.39	2.77	3.22	4.61	5.99	7.38	9.21	10.60	13.82
3	0.07	0.11	0.22	0.35	0.58	1.01	1.21	2.37	4.11	4.64	6.25	7.81	9.35	11.34	12.84	16.27
4	0.21	0.30	0.48	0.71	1.06	1.65	1.92	3.36	5.39	5.99	7.78	9.49	11.14	13.28	14.86	18.47
5	0.41	0.55	0.83	1.15	1.61	2.34	2.67	4.35	6.63	7.29	9.24	11.07	12.83	15.09	16.75	20.51
6	0.68	0.87	1.24	1.64	2.20	3.07	3.45	5.35	7.84	8.56	10.64	12.59	14.45	16.81	18.55	22.46
7	0.99	1.24	1.69	2.17	2.83	3.82	4.25	6.35	9.04	9.80	12.02	14.07	16.01	18.48	20.28	24.32
8	1.34	1.65	2.18	2.73	3.49	4.59	5.07	7.34	10.22	11.03	13.36	15.51	17.53	20.09	21.95	26.12
9	1.73	2.09	2.70	3.33	4.17	5.38	5.90	8.34	11.39	12.24	14.68	16.92	19.02	21.67	23.59	27.88
10	2.16	2.56	3.25	3.94	4.87	6.18	6.74	9.34	12.55	13.44	15.99	18.31	20.48	23.21	25.19	29.59
11	2.60	3.05	3.82	4.57	5.58	6.99	7.58	10.34	13.70	14.63	17.28	19.68	21.92	24.72	26.76	31.26
12	3.07	3.57	4.40	5.23	6.30	7.81	8.44	11.34	14.85	15.81	18.55	21.03	23.34	26.22	28.30	32.91
13	3.57	4.11	5.01	5.89	7.04	8.63	9.30	12.34	15.98	16.98	19.81	22.36	24.74	27.69	29.82	34.53
14	4.07	4.66	5.63	6.57	7.79	9.47	10.17	13.34	17.12	18.15	21.06	23.68	26.12	29.14	31.32	36.12
15	4.60	5.23	6.26	7.26	8.55	10.31	11.04	14.34	18.25	19.31	22.31	25.00	27.49	30.58	32.80	37.70
16	5.14	5.81	6.91	7.96	9.31	11.15	11.91	15.34	19.37	20.47	23.54	26.30	28.85	32.00	34.27	39.25
17	5.70	6.41	7.56	8.67	10.09	12.00	12.79	16.34	20.49	21.61	24.77	27.59	30.19	33.41	35.72	40.79
18	6.26	7.01	8.23	9.39	10.86	12.86	13.68	17.34	21.60	22.76	25.99	28.87	31.53	34.81	37.16	42.31
19	6.84	7.63	8.91	10.12	11.65	13.72	14.56	18.34	22.72	23.90	27.20	30.14	32.85	36.19	38.58	43.82
20	7.43	8.26	9.59	10.85	12.44	14.58	15.45	19.34	23.83	25.04	28.41	31.41	34.17	37.57	40.00	45.31
21	8.03	8.90	10.28	11.59	13.24	15.44	16.34	20.34	24.93	26.17	29.62	32.67	35.48	38.93	41.40	46.80
22	8.64	9.54	10.98	12.34	14.04	16.31	17.24	21.34	26.04	27.30	30.81	33.92	36.78	40.29	42.80	48.27
23	9.26	10.20	11.69	13.09	14.85	17.19	18.14	22.34	27.14	28.43	32.01	35.17	38.08	41.64	44.18	49.73
24	9.89	10.86	12.40	13.85	15.66	18.06	19.04	23.34	28.24	29.55	33.20	36.42	39.36	42.98	45.56	51.18

25	10.52	11.52	13.12	14.61	16.47	18.94	19.94	24.34	29.34	30.68	34.38	37.65	40.65	44.31	46.93	52.62
26	11.16	12.20	13.84	15.38	17.29	19.82	20.84	25.34	30.43	31.79	35.56	38.89	41.92	45.64	48.29	54.05
27	11.81	12.88	14.57	16.15	18.11	20.70	21.75	26.34	31.53	32.91	36.74	40.11	43.19	46.96	49.64	55.48
28	12.46	13.56	15.31	16.93	18.94	21.59	22.66	27.34	32.62	34.03	37.92	41.34	44.46	48.28	50.99	56.89
29	13.12	14.26	16.05	17.71	19.77	22.48	23.57	28.34	33.71	35.14	39.09	42.56	45.72	49.59	52.34	58.30
30	13.79	14.95	16.79	18.49	20.60	23.36	24.48	29.34	34.80	36.25	40.26	43.77	46.98	50.89	53.67	59.70
32	15.13	16.36	18.29	20.07	22.27	25.15	26.30	31.34	36.97	38.47	42.58	46.19	49.48	53.49	56.33	62.49
34	16.50	17.79	19.81	21.66	23.95	26.94	28.14	33.34	39.14	40.68	44.90	48.60	51.97	56.06	58.96	65.25
36	17.89	19.23	21.34	23.27	25.64	28.73	29.97	35.34	41.30	42.88	47.21	51.00	54.44	58.62	61.58	67.99
38	19.29	20.69	22.88	24.88	27.34	30.54	31.81	37.34	43.46	45.08	49.51	53.38	56.90	61.16	64.18	70.70
40	20.71	22.16	24.43	26.51	29.05	32.34	33.66	39.34	45.62	47.27	51.81	55.76	59.34	63.69	66.77	73.40
42	22.14	23.65	26.00	28.14	30.77	34.16	35.51	41.34	47.77	49.46	54.09	58.12	61.78	66.21	69.34	76.08
44	23.58	25.15	27.57	29.79	32.49	35.97	37.36	43.34	49.91	51.64	56.37	60.48	64.20	68.71	71.89	78.75
46	25.04	26.66	29.16	31.44	34.22	37.80	39.22	45.34	52.06	53.82	58.64	62.83	66.62	71.20	74.44	81.40
48	26.51	28.18	30.75	33.10	35.95	39.62	41.08	47.34	54.20	55.99	60.91	65.17	69.02	73.68	76.97	84.04
50	27.99	29.71	32.36	34.76	37.69	41.45	42.94	49.33	56.33	58.16	63.17	67.50	71.42	76.15	79.49	86.66
52	29.48	31.25	33.97	36.44	39.44	43.28	44.81	51.33	58.47	60.33	65.42	69.83	73.81	78.62	82.00	89.27
54	30.98	32.79	35.59	38.12	41.18	45.12	46.68	53.33	60.60	62.50	67.67	72.15	76.19	81.07	84.50	91.87
56	32.49	34.35	37.21	39.80	42.94	46.96	48.55	55.33	62.73	64.66	69.92	74.47	78.57	83.51	86.99	94.46
58	34.01	35.91	38.84	41.49	44.70	48.80	50.42	57.33	64.86	66.82	72.16	76.78	80.94	85.95	89.48	97.04
60	35.53	37.48	40.48	43.19	46.46	50.64	52.29	59.33	66.98	68.97	74.40	79.08	83.30	88.38	91.95	99.61
62	37.07	39.06	42.13	44.89	48.23	52.49	54.17	61.33	69.10	71.13	76.63	81.38	85.65	90.80	94.42	102.17
64	38.61	40.65	43.78	46.59	50.00	54.34	56.05	63.33	71.23	73.28	78.86	83.68	88.00	93.22	96.88	104.72
66	40.16	42.24	45.43	48.29	51.77	56.19	57.93	65.33	73.34	75.42	81.09	85.96	90.35	95.63	99.33	107.26
68	41.71	43.84	47.09	50.02	53.55	58.04	59.81	67.33	75.46	77.57	83.31	88.25	92.69	98.03	101.78	109.79
70	43.28	45.44	48.76	51.74	55.33	59.90	61.70	69.33	77.58	79.71	85.53	90.53	95.02	100.43	104.21	112.32
80	51.17	53.54	57.15	60.39	64.28	69.21	71.14	79.33	88.13	90.41	96.58	101.88	106.63	112.33	116.32	124.84
90	59.20	61.75	65.65	69.13	73.29	78.56	80.62	89.33	98.65	101.05	107.57	113.15	118.14	124.12	128.30	137.21
100	67.33	70.06	74.22	77.93	82.36	87.95	90.13	99.33	109.14	111.67	118.50	124.34	129.56	135.81	140.17	149.45

Parts of this table are reprinted from Table IV of R. A. Fisher and F. Yates' (1974) Statistical Tables for Biological, Agricultural and Medical Research published by Longman Group UK Ltd., London (previously published by Oliver and Boyd Ltd., Edinburgh) and by permission of the authors and publishers.

Table 7. Percentage Points of F Distribution

Denominator df	Probability of a larger F	Numerator df								
		1	2	3	4	5	6	7	8	9
1	.100	39.86	49.50	53.59	55.83	57.24	58.20	58.91	59.44	59.86
	.050	161.4	199.5	215.7	224.6	230.2	234.0	236.8	238.9	240.5
	.025	647.8	799.5	864.2	899.6	921.8	937.1	948.2	956.7	963.3
	.010	4052	4999.5	5403	5625	5764	5859	5928	5982	6022
	.005	16211	20000	21615	22500	23056	23437	23715	23925	24091
2	.100	8.53	9.00	9.16	9.24	9.29	9.33	9.35	9.37	9.38
	.050	18.51	19.00	19.16	19.25	19.30	19.33	19.35	19.37	19.38
	.025	38.51	39.00	39.17	39.25	39.30	39.33	39.36	39.37	39.39
	.010	98.50	99.00	99.17	99.25	99.30	99.33	99.36	99.37	99.39
	.005	198.5	199.0	199.2	199.2	199.3	199.3	199.4	199.4	199.4
3	.100	5.54	5.46	5.39	5.34	5.31	5.28	5.27	5.25	5.24
	.050	10.13	9.55	9.28	9.12	9.01	8.94	8.89	8.85	8.81
	.025	17.44	16.04	15.44	15.10	14.88	14.73	14.62	14.54	14.47
	.010	34.12	30.82	29.46	28.71	28.24	27.91	27.67	27.49	27.35
	.005	55.55	49.80	47.47	46.19	45.39	44.84	44.43	44.13	43.88
4	.100	4.54	4.32	4.19	4.11	4.05	4.01	3.98	3.95	3.94
	.050	7.71	6.94	6.59	6.39	6.26	6.16	6.09	6.04	6.00
	.025	12.22	10.65	9.98	9.60	9.36	9.20	9.07	8.98	8.90
	.010	21.20	18.00	16.69	15.98	15.52	15.21	14.98	14.80	14.66
	.005	31.33	26.28	24.26	23.15	22.46	21.97	21.62	21.35	21.14
5	.100	4.06	3.78	3.62	3.52	3.45	3.40	3.37	3.34	3.32
	.050	6.61	5.79	5.41	5.19	5.05	4.95	4.88	4.82	4.77
	.025	10.01	8.43	7.76	7.39	7.15	6.98	6.85	6.76	6.68
	.010	16.26	13.27	12.06	11.39	10.97	10.67	10.46	10.29	10.16
	.005	22.78	18.31	16.53	15.56	14.94	14.51	14.20	13.96	13.77
6	.100	3.78	3.46	3.29	3.18	3.11	3.05	3.01	2.98	2.96
	.050	5.99	5.14	4.76	4.53	4.39	4.28	4.21	4.15	4.10
	.025	8.81	7.26	6.60	6.23	5.99	5.82	5.70	5.60	5.52
	.010	13.75	10.92	9.78	9.15	8.75	8.47	8.26	8.10	7.98
	.005	18.63	14.54	12.92	12.03	11.46	11.07	10.79	10.57	10.39
7	.100	3.59	3.26	3.07	2.96	2.88	2.83	2.78	2.75	2.72
	.050	5.59	4.74	4.35	4.12	3.97	3.87	3.79	3.73	3.68
	.025	8.07	6.54	5.89	5.52	5.29	5.12	4.99	4.90	4.82
	.010	12.25	9.55	8.45	7.85	7.46	7.19	6.99	6.84	6.72
	.005	16.24	12.40	10.88	10.05	9.52	9.16	8.89	8.68	8.51
8	.100	3.46	3.11	2.92	2.81	2.73	2.67	2.62	2.59	2.56
	.050	5.32	4.46	4.07	3.84	3.69	3.58	3.50	3.44	3.39
	.025	7.57	6.06	5.42	5.05	4.82	4.65	4.53	4.43	4.36
	.010	11.26	8.65	7.59	7.01	6.63	6.37	6.18	6.03	5.91
	.005	14.69	11.04	9.60	8.81	8.30	7.95	7.69	7.50	7.34
9	.100	3.36	3.01	2.81	2.69	2.61	2.55	2.51	2.47	2.44
	.050	5.12	4.26	3.86	3.63	3.48	3.37	3.29	3.23	3.18
	.025	7.21	5.71	5.08	4.72	4.48	4.32	4.20	4.10	4.03
	.010	10.56	8.02	6.99	6.42	6.06	5.80	5.61	5.47	5.35
	.005	13.61	10.11	8.72	7.96	7.47	7.13	6.88	6.69	6.54
10	.100	3.29	2.92	2.73	2.61	2.52	2.46	2.41	2.38	2.35
	.050	4.96	4.10	3.71	3.48	3.33	3.22	3.14	3.07	3.02
	.025	6.94	5.46	4.83	4.47	4.24	4.07	3.95	3.85	3.78
	.010	10.04	7.56	6.55	5.99	5.64	5.39	5.20	5.06	4.94
	.005	12.83	9.43	8.08	7.34	6.87	6.54	6.30	6.12	5.97
11	.100	3.23	2.86	2.66	2.54	2.45	2.39	2.34	2.30	2.27
	.050	4.84	3.98	3.59	3.36	3.20	3.09	3.01	2.95	2.90
	.025	6.72	5.26	4.63	4.28	4.04	3.88	3.76	3.66	3.59
	.010	9.65	7.21	6.22	5.67	5.32	5.07	4.89	4.74	4.63
	.005	12.23	8.91	7.60	6.88	6.42	6.10	5.86	5.68	5.54
12	.100	3.18	2.81	2.61	2.48	2.39	2.33	2.28	2.24	2.21
	.050	4.75	3.89	3.49	3.26	3.11	3.00	2.91	2.85	2.80
	.025	6.55	5.10	4.47	4.12	3.89	3.73	3.61	3.51	3.44
	.010	9.33	6.93	5.95	5.41	5.06	4.82	4.64	4.50	4.39
	.005	11.75	8.51	7.23	6.52	6.07	5.76	5.52	5.35	5.20
13	.100	3.14	2.76	2.56	2.43	2.35	2.28	2.23	2.20	2.16
	.050	4.67	3.81	3.41	3.18	3.03	2.92	2.83	2.77	2.71
	.025	6.41	4.97	4.35	4.00	3.77	3.60	3.48	3.39	3.31
	.010	9.07	6.70	5.74	5.21	4.86	4.62	4.44	4.30	4.19
	.005	11.37	8.19	6.93	6.23	5.79	5.48	5.25	5.08	4.94
14	.100	3.10	2.73	2.52	2.39	2.31	2.24	2.19	2.15	2.12
	.050	4.60	3.74	3.34	3.11	2.96	2.85	2.76	2.70	2.65
	.025	6.30	4.86	4.24	3.89	3.66	3.50	3.38	3.29	3.21
	.010	8.86	6.51	5.56	5.04	4.69	4.46	4.28	4.14	4.03
	.005	11.06	7.92	6.68	6.00	5.56	5.26	5.03	4.86	4.72

			Numerator df									
10	12	15	20	24	30	40	60	120	∞	P	df
60.19	60.71	61.22	61.74	62.00	62.26	62.53	62.79	63.06	63.33	.100	1
241.9	243.9	245.9	248.0	249.1	250.1	251.1	252.2	253.3	254.3	.050	
968.6	976.7	984.9	993.1	997.2	1001	1006	1010	1014	1018	.025	
6056	6106	6157	6209	6235	6261	6287	6313	6339	6366	.010	
24224	24426	24630	24836	24940	25044	25148	25253	25359	25465	.005	
9.39	9.41	9.42	9.44	9.45	9.46	9.47	9.47	9.48	9.49	.100	2
19.40	19.41	19.43	19.45	19.45	19.46	19.47	19.48	19.49	19.50	.050	
39.40	39.41	39.43	39.45	39.46	39.46	39.47	39.48	39.49	39.50	.025	
99.40	99.42	99.43	99.45	99.46	99.47	99.47	99.48	99.49	99.50	.010	
199.4	199.4	199.4	199.4	199.5	199.5	199.5	199.5	199.5	199.5	.005	
5.23	5.22	5.20	5.18	5.18	5.17	5.16	5.15	5.14	5.13	.100	3
8.79	8.74	8.70	8.66	8.64	8.62	8.59	8.57	8.55	8.53	.050	
14.42	14.34	14.25	14.17	14.12	14.08	14.04	13.99	13.95	13.90	.025	
27.23	27.05	26.87	26.69	26.60	26.50	26.41	26.32	26.22	26.13	.010	
43.69	43.39	43.08	42.78	42.62	42.47	42.31	42.15	41.99	41.83	.005	
3.92	3.90	3.87	3.84	3.83	3.82	3.80	3.79	3.78	3.76	.100	4
5.96	5.91	5.86	5.80	5.77	5.75	5.72	5.69	5.66	5.63	.050	
8.84	8.75	8.66	8.56	8.51	8.46	8.41	8.36	8.31	8.26	.025	
14.55	14.37	14.20	14.02	13.93	13.84	13.75	13.65	13.56	13.46	.010	
20.97	20.70	20.44	20.17	20.03	19.89	19.75	19.61	19.47	19.32	.005	
3.30	3.27	3.24	3.21	3.19	3.17	3.16	3.14	3.12	3.10	.100	5
4.74	4.68	4.62	4.56	4.53	4.50	4.46	4.43	4.40	4.36	.050	
6.62	6.52	6.43	6.33	6.28	6.23	6.18	6.12	6.07	6.02	.025	
10.05	9.89	9.72	9.55	9.47	9.38	9.29	9.20	9.11	9.02	.010	
13.62	13.38	13.15	12.90	12.78	12.66	12.53	12.40	12.27	12.14	.005	
2.94	2.90	2.87	2.84	2.82	2.80	2.78	2.76	2.74	2.72	.100	6
4.06	4.00	3.94	3.87	3.84	3.81	3.77	3.74	3.70	3.67	.050	
5.46	5.37	5.27	5.17	5.12	5.07	5.01	4.96	4.90	4.85	.025	
7.87	7.72	7.56	7.40	7.31	7.23	7.14	7.06	6.97	6.88	.010	
10.25	10.03	9.81	9.59	9.47	9.36	9.24	9.12	9.00	8.88	.005	
2.70	2.67	2.63	2.59	2.58	2.56	2.54	2.51	2.49	2.47	.100	7
3.64	3.57	3.51	3.44	3.41	3.38	3.34	3.30	3.27	3.23	.050	
4.76	4.67	4.57	4.47	4.42	4.36	4.31	4.25	4.20	4.14	.025	
6.62	6.47	6.31	6.16	6.07	5.99	5.91	5.82	5.74	5.65	.010	
8.38	8.18	7.97	7.75	7.65	7.53	7.42	7.31	7.19	7.08	.005	
2.54	2.50	2.46	2.42	2.40	2.38	2.36	2.34	2.32	2.29	.100	8
3.35	3.28	3.22	3.15	3.12	3.08	3.04	3.01	2.97	2.93	.050	
4.30	4.20	4.10	4.00	3.95	3.89	3.84	3.78	3.73	3.67	.025	
5.81	5.67	5.52	5.36	5.28	5.20	5.12	5.03	4.95	4.86	.010	
7.21	7.01	6.81	6.61	6.50	6.40	6.29	6.18	6.06	5.95	.005	
2.42	2.38	2.34	2.30	2.28	2.25	2.23	2.21	2.18	2.16	.100	9
3.14	3.07	3.01	2.94	2.90	2.86	2.83	2.79	2.75	2.71	.050	
3.96	3.87	3.77	3.67	3.61	3.56	3.51	3.45	3.39	3.33	.025	
5.26	5.11	4.96	4.81	4.73	4.65	4.57	4.48	4.40	4.31	.010	
6.42	6.23	6.03	5.83	5.73	5.62	5.52	5.41	5.30	5.19	.005	
2.32	2.28	2.24	2.20	2.18	2.16	2.13	2.11	2.08	2.06	.100	10
2.98	2.91	2.85	2.77	2.74	2.70	2.66	2.62	2.58	2.54	.050	
3.72	3.62	3.52	3.42	3.37	3.31	3.26	3.20	3.14	3.08	.025	
4.85	4.71	4.56	4.41	4.33	4.25	4.17	4.08	4.00	3.91	.010	
5.85	5.66	5.47	5.27	5.17	5.07	4.97	4.86	4.75	4.64	.005	
2.25	2.21	2.17	2.12	2.10	2.08	2.05	2.03	2.00	1.97	.100	11
2.85	2.79	2.72	2.65	2.61	2.57	2.53	2.49	2.45	2.40	.050	
3.53	3.43	3.33	3.23	3.17	3.12	3.06	3.00	2.94	2.88	.025	
4.54	4.40	4.25	4.10	4.02	3.94	3.86	3.78	3.69	3.60	.010	
5.42	5.24	5.05	4.86	4.76	4.65	4.55	4.44	4.34	4.23	.005	
2.19	2.15	2.10	2.06	2.04	2.01	1.99	1.96	1.93	1.90	.100	12
2.75	2.69	2.62	2.54	2.51	2.47	2.43	2.38	2.34	2.30	.050	
3.37	3.28	3.18	3.07	3.02	2.96	2.91	2.85	2.79	2.72	.025	
4.30	4.16	4.01	3.86	3.78	3.70	3.62	3.54	3.45	3.36	.010	
5.09	4.91	4.72	4.53	4.43	4.33	4.23	4.12	4.01	3.90	.005	
2.14	2.10	2.05	2.01	1.98	1.96	1.93	1.90	1.88	1.85	.100	13
2.67	2.60	2.53	2.46	2.42	2.38	2.34	2.30	2.25	2.21	.050	
3.25	3.15	3.05	2.95	2.89	2.84	2.78	2.72	2.66	2.60	.025	
4.10	3.96	3.82	3.66	3.59	3.51	3.43	3.34	3.25	3.17	.010	
4.82	4.64	4.46	4.27	4.17	4.07	3.97	3.87	3.76	3.65	.005	
2.10	2.05	2.01	1.96	1.94	1.91	1.89	1.86	1.83	1.80	.100	14
2.60	2.53	2.46	2.39	2.35	2.31	2.27	2.22	2.18	2.13	.050	
3.15	3.05	2.95	2.84	2.79	2.73	2.67	2.61	2.55	2.49	.025	
3.94	3.80	3.66	3.51	3.43	3.35	3.27	3.18	3.09	3.00	.010	
4.60	4.43	4.25	4.06	3.96	3.86	3.76	3.66	3.55	3.44	.005	

Table 7. (*continued*)

Denominator df	Probability of a larger F	Numerator df								
		1	2	3	4	5	6	7	8	9
15	.100	3.07	2.70	2.49	2.36	2.27	2.21	2.16	2.12	2.09
	.050	4.54	3.68	3.29	3.06	2.90	2.79	2.71	2.64	2.59
	.025	6.20	4.77	4.15	3.80	3.58	3.41	3.29	3.20	3.12
	.010	8.68	6.36	5.42	4.89	4.56	4.32	4.14	4.00	3.89
	.005	10.80	7.70	6.48	5.80	5.37	5.07	4.85	4.67	4.54
16	.100	3.05	2.67	2.46	2.33	2.24	2.18	2.13	2.09	2.06
	.050	4.49	3.63	3.24	3.01	2.85	2.74	2.66	2.59	2.54
	.025	6.12	4.69	4.08	3.73	3.50	3.34	3.22	3.12	3.05
	.010	8.53	6.23	5.29	4.77	4.44	4.20	4.03	3.89	3.78
	.005	10.58	7.51	6.30	5.64	5.21	4.91	4.69	4.52	4.38
17	.100	3.03	2.64	2.44	2.31	2.22	2.15	2.10	2.06	2.03
	.050	4.45	3.59	3.20	2.96	2.81	2.70	2.61	2.55	2.49
	.025	6.04	4.62	4.01	3.66	3.44	3.28	3.16	3.06	2.98
	.010	8.40	6.11	5.18	4.67	4.34	4.10	3.93	3.79	3.68
	.005	10.38	7.35	6.16	5.50	5.07	4.78	4.56	4.39	4.25
18	.100	3.01	2.62	2.42	2.29	2.20	2.13	2.08	2.04	2.00
	.050	4.41	3.55	3.16	2.93	2.77	2.66	2.58	2.51	2.46
	.025	5.98	4.56	3.95	3.61	3.38	3.22	3.10	3.01	2.93
	.010	8.29	6.01	5.09	4.58	4.25	4.01	3.84	3.71	3.60
	.005	10.22	7.21	6.03	5.37	4.96	4.66	4.44	4.28	4.14
19	.100	2.99	2.61	2.40	2.27	2.18	2.11	2.06	2.02	1.98
	.050	4.38	3.52	3.13	2.90	2.74	2.63	2.54	2.48	2.42
	.025	5.92	4.51	3.90	3.56	3.33	3.17	3.05	2.96	2.88
	.010	8.18	5.93	5.01	4.50	4.17	3.94	3.77	3.63	3.52
	.005	10.07	7.09	5.92	5.27	4.85	4.56	4.34	4.18	4.04
20	.100	2.97	2.59	2.38	2.25	2.16	2.09	2.04	2.00	1.96
	.050	4.35	3.49	3.10	2.87	2.71	2.60	2.51	2.45	2.39
	.025	5.87	4.46	3.86	3.51	3.29	3.13	3.01	2.91	2.84
	.010	8.10	5.85	4.94	4.43	4.10	3.87	3.70	3.56	3.46
	.005	9.94	6.99	5.82	5.17	4.76	4.47	4.26	4.09	3.96
21	.100	2.96	2.57	2.36	2.23	2.14	2.08	2.02	1.98	1.95
	.050	4.32	3.47	3.07	2.84	2.68	2.57	2.49	2.42	2.37
	.025	5.83	4.42	3.82	3.48	3.25	3.09	2.97	2.87	2.80
	.010	8.02	5.78	4.87	4.37	4.04	3.81	3.64	3.51	3.40
	.005	9.83	6.89	5.73	5.09	4.68	4.39	4.18	4.01	3.88
22	.100	2.95	2.56	2.35	2.22	2.13	2.06	2.01	1.97	1.93
	.050	4.30	3.44	3.05	2.82	2.66	2.55	2.46	2.40	2.34
	.025	5.79	4.38	3.78	3.44	3.22	3.05	2.93	2.84	2.76
	.010	7.95	5.72	4.82	4.31	3.99	3.76	3.59	3.45	3.35
	.005	9.73	6.81	5.65	5.02	4.61	4.32	4.11	3.94	3.81
23	.100	2.94	2.55	2.34	2.21	2.11	2.05	1.99	1.95	1.92
	.050	4.28	3.42	3.03	2.80	2.64	2.53	2.44	2.37	2.32
	.025	5.75	4.35	3.75	3.41	3.18	3.02	2.90	2.81	2.73
	.010	7.88	5.66	4.76	4.26	3.94	3.71	3.54	3.41	3.30
	.005	9.63	6.73	5.58	4.95	4.54	4.26	4.05	3.88	3.75
24	.100	2.93	2.54	2.33	2.19	2.10	2.04	1.98	1.94	1.91
	.050	4.26	3.40	3.01	2.78	2.62	2.51	2.42	2.36	2.30
	.025	5.72	4.32	3.72	3.38	3.15	2.99	2.87	2.78	2.70
	.010	7.82	5.61	4.72	4.22	3.90	3.67	3.50	3.36	3.26
	.005	9.55	6.66	5.52	4.89	4.49	4.20	3.99	3.83	3.69
25	.100	2.92	2.53	2.32	2.18	2.09	2.02	1.97	1.93	1.89
	.050	4.24	3.39	2.99	2.76	2.60	2.49	2.40	2.34	2.28
	.025	5.69	4.29	3.69	3.35	3.13	2.97	2.85	2.75	2.68
	.010	7.77	5.57	4.68	4.18	3.85	3.63	3.46	3.32	3.22
	.005	9.48	6.60	5.46	4.84	4.43	4.15	3.94	3.78	3.64
26	.100	2.91	2.52	2.31	2.17	2.08	2.01	1.96	1.92	1.88
	.050	4.23	3.37	2.98	2.74	2.59	2.47	2.39	2.32	2.27
	.025	5.66	4.27	3.67	3.33	3.10	2.94	2.82	2.73	2.65
	.010	7.72	5.53	4.64	4.14	3.82	3.59	3.42	3.29	3.18
	.005	9.41	6.54	5.41	4.79	4.38	4.10	3.89	3.73	3.60
27	.100	2.90	2.51	2.30	2.17	2.07	2.00	1.95	1.91	1.87
	.050	4.21	3.35	2.96	2.73	2.57	2.46	2.37	2.31	2.25
	.025	5.63	4.24	3.65	3.31	3.08	2.92	2.80	2.71	2.63
	.010	7.68	5.49	4.60	4.11	3.78	3.56	3.39	3.26	3.15
	.005	9.34	6.49	5.36	4.74	4.34	4.06	3.85	3.69	3.56
28	.100	2.89	2.50	2.29	2.16	2.06	2.00	1.94	1.90	1.87
	.050	4.20	3.34	2.95	2.71	2.56	2.45	2.36	2.29	2.24
	.025	5.61	4.22	3.63	3.29	3.06	2.90	2.78	2.69	2.61
	.010	7.64	5.45	4.57	4.07	3.75	3.53	3.36	3.23	3.12
	.005	9.28	6.44	5.32	4.70	4.30	4.02	3.81	3.65	3.52

				Numerator df								
10	12	15	20	24	30	40	60	120	∞	P	df
2.06	2.02	1.97	1.92	1.90	1.87	1.85	1.82	1.79	1.76	.100	15
2.54	2.48	2.40	2.33	2.29	2.25	2.20	2.16	2.11	2.07	.050	
3.06	2.96	2.86	2.76	2.70	2.64	2.59	2.52	2.46	2.40	.025	
3.80	3.67	3.52	3.37	3.29	3.21	3.13	3.05	2.96	2.87	.010	
4.42	4.25	4.07	3.88	3.79	3.69	3.58	3.48	3.37	3.26	.005	
2.03	1.99	1.94	1.89	1.87	1.84	1.81	1.78	1.75	1.72	.100	16
2.49	2.42	2.35	2.28	2.24	2.19	2.15	2.11	2.06	2.01	.050	
2.99	2.89	2.79	2.68	2.63	2.57	2.51	2.45	2.38	2.32	.025	
3.69	3.55	3.41	3.26	3.18	3.10	3.02	2.93	2.84	2.75	.010	
4.27	4.10	3.92	3.73	3.64	3.54	3.44	3.33	3.22	3.11	.005	
2.00	1.96	1.91	1.86	1.84	1.81	1.78	1.75	1.72	1.69	.100	17
2.45	2.38	2.31	2.23	2.19	2.15	2.10	2.06	2.01	1.96	.050	
2.92	2.82	2.72	2.62	2.56	2.50	2.44	2.38	2.32	2.25	.025	
3.59	3.46	3.31	3.16	3.08	3.00	2.92	2.83	2.75	2.65	.010	
4.14	3.97	3.79	3.61	3.51	3.41	3.31	3.21	3.10	2.98	.005	
1.98	1.93	1.89	1.84	1.81	1.78	1.75	1.72	1.69	1.66	.100	18
2.41	2.34	2.27	2.19	2.15	2.11	2.06	2.02	1.97	1.92	.050	
2.87	2.77	2.67	2.56	2.50	2.44	2.38	2.32	2.26	2.19	.025	
3.51	3.37	3.23	3.08	3.00	2.92	2.84	2.75	2.66	2.57	.010	
4.03	3.86	3.68	3.50	3.40	3.30	3.20	3.10	2.99	2.87	.005	
1.96	1.91	1.86	1.81	1.79	1.76	1.73	1.70	1.67	1.63	.100	19
2.38	2.31	2.23	2.16	2.11	2.07	2.03	1.98	1.93	1.88	.050	
2.82	2.72	2.62	2.51	2.45	2.39	2.33	2.27	2.20	2.13	.025	
3.43	3.30	3.15	3.00	2.92	2.84	2.76	2.67	2.58	2.49	.010	
3.93	3.76	3.59	3.40	3.31	3.21	3.11	3.00	2.89	2.78	.005	
1.94	1.89	1.84	1.79	1.77	1.74	1.71	1.68	1.64	1.61	.100	20
2.35	2.28	2.20	2.12	2.08	2.04	1.99	1.95	1.90	1.84	.050	
2.77	2.68	2.57	2.46	2.41	2.35	2.29	2.22	2.16	2.09	.025	
3.37	3.23	3.09	2.94	2.86	2.78	2.69	2.61	2.52	2.42	010	
3.85	3.68	3.50	3.32	3.22	3.12	3.02	2.92	2.81	2.69	.005	
1.92	1.87	1.83	1.78	1.75	1.72	1.69	1.66	1.62	1.59	.100	21
2.32	2.25	2.18	2.10	2.05	2.01	1.96	1.92	1.87	1.81	.050	
2.73	2.64	2.53	2.42	2.37	2.31	2.25	2.18	2.11	2.04	.025	
3.31	3.17	3.03	2.88	2.80	2.72	2.64	2.55	2.46	2.36	.010	
3.77	3.60	3.43	3.24	3.15	3.05	2.95	2.84	2.73	2.61	.005	
1.90	1.86	1.81	1.76	1.73	1.70	1.67	1.64	1.60	1.57	.100	22
2.30	2.23	2.15	2.07	2.03	1.98	1.94	1.89	1.84	1.78	.050	
2.70	2.60	2.50	2.39	2.33	2.27	2.21	2.14	2.08	2.00	.025	
3.26	3.12	2.98	2.83	2.75	2.67	2.58	2.50	2.40	2.31	.010	
3.70	3.54	3.36	3.18	3.08	2.98	2.88	2.77	2.66	2.55	.005	
1.89	1.84	1.80	1.74	1.72	1.69	1.66	1.62	1.59	1.55	.100	23
2.27	2.20	2.13	2.05	2.01	1.96	1.91	1.86	1.81	1.76	.050	
2.67	2.57	2.47	2.36	2.30	2.24	2.18	2.11	2.04	1.97	.025	
3.21	3.07	2.93	2.78	2.70	2.62	2.54	2.45	2.35	2.26	.010	
3.64	3.47	3.30	3.12	3.02	2.92	2.82	2.71	2.60	2.48	.005	
1.88	1.83	1.78	1.73	1.70	1.67	1.64	1.61	1.57	1.53	.100	24
2.25	2.18	2.11	2.03	1.98	1.94	1.89	1.84	1.79	1.73	.050	
2.64	2.54	2.44	2.33	2.27	2.21	2.15	2.08	2.01	1.94	.025	
3.17	3.03	2.89	2.74	2.66	2.58	2.49	2.40	2.31	2.21	.010	
3.59	3.42	3.25	3.06	2.97	2.87	2.77	2.66	2.55	2.43	.005	
1.87	1.82	1.77	1.72	1.69	1.66	1.63	1.59	1.56	1.52	.100	25
2.24	2.16	2.09	2.01	1.96	1.92	1.87	1.82	1.77	1.71	.050	
2.61	2.51	2.41	2.30	2.24	2.18	2.12	2.05	1.98	1.91	.025	
3.13	2.99	2.85	2.70	2.62	2.54	2.45	2.36	2.27	2.17	.010	
3.54	3.37	3.20	3.01	2.92	2.82	2.72	2.61	2.50	2.38	.005	
1.86	1.81	1.76	1.71	1.68	1.65	1.61	1.58	1.54	1.50	.100	26
2.22	2.15	2.07	1.99	1.95	1.90	1.85	1.80	1.75	1.69	.050	
2.59	2.49	2.39	2.28	2.22	2.16	2.09	2.03	1.95	1.88	.025	
3.09	2.96	2.81	2.66	2.58	2.50	2.42	2.33	2.23	2.13	.010	
3.49	3.33	3.15	2.97	2.87	2.77	2.67	2.56	2.45	2.33	.005	
1.85	1.80	1.75	1.70	1.67	1.64	1.60	1.57	1.53	1.49	.100	27
2.20	2.13	2.06	1.97	1.93	1.88	1.84	1.79	1.73	1.67	.050	
2.57	2.47	2.36	2.25	2.19	2.13	2.07	2.00	1.93	1.85	.025	
3.06	2.93	2.78	2.63	2.55	2.47	2.38	2.29	2.20	2.10	.010	
3.45	3.28	3.11	2.93	2.83	2.73	2.63	2.52	2.41	2.29	.005	
1.84	1.79	1.74	1.69	1.66	1.63	1.59	1.56	1.52	1.48	.100	28
2.19	2.12	2.04	1.96	1.91	1.87	1.82	1.77	1.71	1.65	.050	
2.55	2.45	2.34	2.23	2.17	2.11	2.05	1.98	1.91	1.83	.025	
3.03	2.90	2.75	2.60	2.52	2.44	2.35	2.26	2.17	2.06	.010	
3.41	3.25	3.07	2.89	2.79	2.69	2.59	2.48	2.37	2.25	.005	

Denomi-nator *df*	Probability of a larger *F*	Numerator *df*								
		1	2	3	4	5	6	7	8	9
29	.100	2.89	2.50	2.28	2.15	2.06	1.99	1.93	1.89	1.86
	.050	4.18	3.33	2.93	2.70	2.55	2.43	2.35	2.28	2.22
	.025	5.59	4.20	3.61	3.27	3.04	2.88	2.76	2.67	2.59
	.010	7.60	5.42	4.54	4.04	3.73	3.50	3.33	3.20	3.09
	.005	9.23	6.40	5.28	4.66	4.26	3.98	3.77	3.61	3.48
30	.100	2.88	2.49	2.28	2.14	2.05	1.98	1.93	1.88	1.85
	.050	4.17	3.32	2.92	2.69	2.53	2.42	2.33	2.27	2.21
	.025	5.57	4.18	3.59	3.25	3.03	2.87	2.75	2.65	2.57
	.010	7.56	5.39	4.51	4.02	3.70	3.47	3.30	3.17	3.07
	.005	9.18	6.35	5.24	4.62	4.23	3.95	3.74	3.58	3.45
40	.100	2.84	2.44	2.23	2.09	2.00	1.93	1.87	1.83	1.79
	.050	4.08	3.23	2.84	2.61	2.45	2.34	2.25	2.18	2.12
	.025	5.42	4.05	3.46	3.13	2.90	2.74	2.62	2.53	2.45
	.010	7.31	5.18	4.31	3.83	3.51	3.29	3.12	2.99	2.89
	.005	8.83	6.07	4.98	4.37	3.99	3.71	3.51	3.35	3.22
60	.100	2.79	2.39	2.18	2.04	1.95	1.87	1.82	1.77	1.74
	.050	4.00	3.15	2.76	2.53	2.37	2.25	2.17	2.10	2.04
	.025	5.29	3.93	3.34	3.01	2.79	2.63	2.51	2.41	2.33
	.010	7.08	4.98	4.13	3.65	3.34	3.12	2.95	2.82	2.72
	.005	8.49	5.79	4.73	4.14	3.76	3.49	3.29	3.13	3.01
120	.100	2.75	2.35	2.13	1.99	1.90	·1.82	1.77	1.72	1.68
	.050	3.92	3.07	2.68	2.45	2.29	2.17	2.09	2.02	1.96
	.025	5.15	3.80	3.23	2.89	2.67	2.52	2.39	2.30	2.22
	.010	6.85	4.79	3.95	3.48	3.17	2.96	2.79	2.66	2.56
	.005	8.18	5.54	4.50	3.92	3.55	3.28	3.09	2.93	2.81
∞	.100	2.71	2.30	2.08	1.94	1.85	1.77	1.72	1.67	1.63
	.050	3.84	3.00	2.60	2.37	2.21	2.10	2.01	1.94	1.88
	.025	5.02	3.69	3.12	2.79	2.57	2.41	2.29	2.19	2.11
	.010	6.63	4.61	3.78	3.32	3.02	2.80	2.64	2.51	2.41
	.005	7.88	5.30	4.28	3.72	3.35	3.09	2.90	2.74	2.62

				Numerator df								
10	12	15	20	24	30	40	60	120	∞	P	df
1.83	1.78	1.73	1.68	1.65	1.62	1.58	1.55	1.51	1.47	.100	29
2.18	2.10	2.03	1.94	1.90	1.85	1.81	1.75	1.70	1.64	.050	
2.53	2.43	2.32	2.21	2.15	2.09	2.03	1.96	1.89	1.81	.025	
3.00	2.87	2.73	2.57	2.49	2.41	2.33	2.23	2.14	2.03	.010	
3.38	3.21	3.04	2.86	2.76	2.66	2.56	2.45	2.33	2.21	.005	
1.82	1.77	1.72	1.67	1.64	1.61	1.57	1.54	1.50	1.46	.100	30
2.16	2.09	2.01	1.93	1.89	1.84	1.79	1.74	1.68	1.62	.050	
2.51	2.41	2.31	2.20	2.14	2.07	2.01	1.94	1.87	1.79	.025	
2.98	2.84	2.70	2.55	2.47	2.39	2.30	2.21	2.11	2.01	.010	
3.34	3.18	3.01	2.82	2.73	2.63	2.52	2.42	2.30	2.18	.005	
1.76	1.71	1.66	1.61	1.57	1.54	1.51	1.47	1.42	1.38	.100	40
2.08	2.00	1.92	1.84	1.79	1.74	1.69	1.64	1.58	1.51	.050	
2.39	2.29	2.18	2.07	1.94	2.20	1.88	1.80	1.72	1.64	.025	
2.80	2.66	2.52	2.37	2.29	2.20	2.11	2.02	1.92	1.80	.010	
3.12	2.95	2.78	2.60	2.50	2.40	2.30	2.18	2.06	1.93	.005	
1.71	1.66	1.60	1.54	1.51	1.48	1.44	1.40	1.35	1.29	.100	60
1.99	1.92	1.84	1.75	1.70	1.65	1.59	1.53	1.47	1.39	.050	
2.27	2.17	2.06	1.94	1.88	1.82	1.74	1.67	1.58	1.48	.025	
2.63	2.50	2.35	2.20	2.12	2.03	1.94	1.84	1.73	1.60	.010	
2.90	2.74	2.57	2.39	2.29	2.19	2.08	1.96	1.83	1.69	.005	
1.65	1.60	1.55	1.48	1.45	1.41	1.37	1.32	1.26	1.19	.100	120
1.91	1.83	1.75	1.66	1.61	1.55	1.50	1.43	1.35	1.25	.050	
2.16	2.05	1.94	1.82	1.76	1.69	1.61	1.53	1.43	1.31	.025	
2.47	2.34	2.19	2.03	1.95	1.86	1.76	1.66	1.53	1.38	.010	
2.71	2.54	2.37	2.19	2.09	1.98	1.87	1.75	1.61	1.43	.005	
1.60	1.55	1.49	1.42	1.38	1.34	1.30	1.24	1.17	1.00	.100	∞
1.83	1.75	1.67	1.57	1.52	1.46	1.39	1.32	1.22	1.00	.050	
2.05	1.94	1.83	1.71	1.64	1.57	1.48	1.39	1.27	1.00	.025	
2.32	2.18	2.04	1.88	1.79	1.70	1.59	1.47	1.32	1.00	.010	
2.52	2.36	2.19	2.00	1.90	1.79	1.67	1.53	1.36	1.00	.005	

Table 8A. Exact Two-sided $100\% \times (1 - \alpha)$ Confidence Limits for Binomial Proportions. $\alpha = .05$

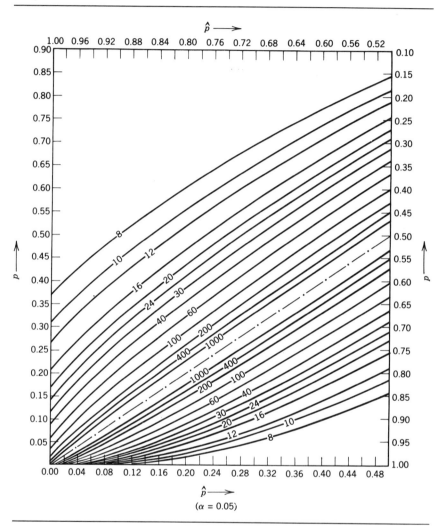

$\hat{p} \longrightarrow$

$(\alpha = 0.05)$

488

Table 8B. Exact Two-Sided $(1 - \alpha)100\%$ Confidence Limits for Binomial Proportions. $\alpha = .01$

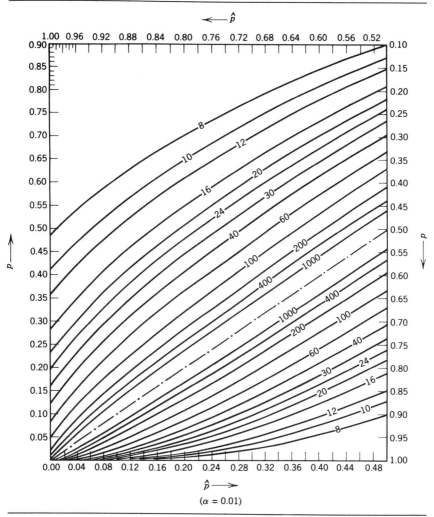

$(\alpha = 0.01)$

Table 9. Cumulative Distribution of Wilcoxon Signed-Rank Statistic [$\Pr(T \leq t)$]

t \ n	1	2	3	4	5	6	7
0	.5000	.2500	.1250	.0625	.0313	.0156	.0078
1	1.0000	.5000	.2500	.1250	.0625	.0313	.0156
2		.7500	.3750	.1875	.0938	.0469	.0234
3		1.0000	.6250	.3125	.1563	.0781	.0391
4			.7500	.4375	.2188	.1094	.0547
5			.8750	.5625	.3125	.1563	.0781
6			1.0000	.6875	.4063	.2188	.1094
7				.8125	.5000	.2813	.1484
8				.8750	.5937	.3438	.1875
9				.9375	.6875	.4219	.2344
10				1.0000	.7812	.5000	.2891
11					.8437	.5781	.3438
12					.9062	.6562	.4063
13					.9375	.7187	.4688
14					.9687	.7812	.5312

t \ n	8	9	10	11	12	13	14
0	.0039	.0020	.0010	.0005	.0002	.0001	.0001
1	.0078	.0039	.0020	.0010	.0005	.0002	.0001
2	.0117	.0059	.0029	.0015	.0007	.0004	.0002
3	.0195	.0098	.0049	'0024	.0012	.0006	.0003
4	.0273	.0137	.0068	.0034	.0017	.0009	.0004
5	.0391	.0195	.0098	.0049	.0024	.0012	.0006
6	.0547	.0273	.0137	.0068	.0034	.0017	.0009
7	.0742	.0371	.0186	.0093	.0046	.0023	.0012
8	.0977	.0488	.0244	.0122	.0061	.0031	.0015
9	.1250	.0645	.0322	.0161	.0081	.0040	.0020
10	.1563	.0820	.0420	.0210	.0105	.0052	.0026
11	.1914	.1016	.0527	.0269	.0134	.0067	.0034
12	.2305	.1250	.0654	.0337	.0171	.0085	.0043
13	.2734	.1504	.0801	.0415	.0212	.0107	.0054
14	.3203	.1797	.0967	.0508	.0261	.0133	.0067
15	.3711	.2129	.1162	.0615	.0320	.0164	.0083
16	.4219	.2480	.1377	.0737	.0386	.0199	.0101
17	.4727	.2852	.1611	.0874	.0461	.0239	.0123
18	.5273	.3262	.1875	.1030	.0549	.0287	.0148
19	.5781	.3672	.2158	.1201	.0647	.0341	.0176
20	.6289	.4102	.2461	.1392	.0757	.0402	.0209
21	.6797	.4551	.2783	.1602	.0881	.0471	.0247
22	.7266	.5000	.3125	.1826	.1018	.0549	.0290
23	.7695	.5449	.3477	.2065	.1167	.0636	.0338
24	.8086	.5898	.3848	.2324	.1331	.0732	.0392
25	.8437	.6328	.4229	.2598	.1506	.0839	.0453
26	.8750	.6738	.4609	.2886	.1697	.0955	.0520
27	.9023	.7148	.5000	.3188	.1902	.1082	.0594
28	.9258	.7520	.5391	.3501	.2119	.1219	.0676
29	.9453	.7871	.5771	.3823	.2349	.1367	.0765
30	.9609	.8203	.6152	.4155	.2593	.1527	.0863
31	.9727	.8496	.6523	.4492	.2847	.1698	.0969
32	.9805	.8750	.6875	.4829	.3110	.1879	.1083

t \ n	8	9	10	11	12	13	14
33	.9883	.8984	.7217	.5171	.3386	.2072	.1206
34	.9922	.9180	.7539	.5508	.3667	.2274	.1338
35	.9961	.9355	.7842	.5845	.3955	.2487	.1479
36	1.0000	.9512	.8125	.6177	.4250	.2709	.1629
37		.9629	.8389	.6499	.4548	.2939	.1788
38		.9727	.8623	.6812	.4849	.3177	.1955
39		.9805	.8838	.7114	.5151	.3424	.2131
40		.9863	.9033	.7402	.5452	.3677	.2316
41		.9902	.9199	.7676	.5750	.3934	.2508
42		.9941	.9346	.7935	.6045	.4197	.2708
43		.9961	.9473	.8174	.6333	.4463	.2915
44		.9980	.9580	.8398	.6614	.4730	.3129
45		1.0000	.9678	.8608	.6890	.5000	.3349
46			.9756	.8799	.7153	.5270	.3574
47			.9814	.8970	.7407	.5537	.3804
48			.9863	.9126	.7651	.5803	.4039
49			.9902	.9263	.7881	.6066	.4276
50			.9932	.9385	.8098	.6323	.4516
51			.9951	.9492	.8303	.6576	.4758
52			.9971	.9585	.8494	.6823	.5000

t \ n	15	16	17	18	19	20
0	.0000	.0000	.0000	.0000	.0000	.0000
1	.0001	.0000	.0000	.0000	.0000	.0000
2	.0001	.0000	.0000	.0000	.0000	.0000
3	.0002	.0001	.0000	.0000	.0000	.0000
4	.0002	.0001	.0001	.0000	.0000	.0000
5	.0003	.0002	.0001	.0000	.0000	.0000
6	.0004	.0002	.0001	.0001	.0000	.0000
7	.0006	.0003	.0001	.0001	.0000	.0000
8	.0008	.0004	.0002	.0001	.0000	.0000
9	.0010	.0005	.0003	.0001	.0001	.0000
10	.0013	.0007	.0003	.0002	.0001	.0000
11	.0017	.0008	.0004	.0002	.0001	.0001
12	.0021	.0011	.0005	.0003	.0001	.0001
13	.0027	.0013	.0007	.0003	.0002	.0001
14	.0034	.0017	.0008	.0004	.0002	.0001
15	.0042	.0021	.0010	.0005	.0003	.0001
16	.0051	.0026	.0013	.0006	.0003	.0002
17	.0062	.0031	.0016	.0008	.0004	.0002
18	.0075	.0038	.0019	.0010	.0005	.0002
19	.0090	.0046	.0023	.0012	.0006	.0003
20	.0108	.0055	.0028	.0014	.0007	.0004
21	.0128	.0065	.0033	.0017	.0008	.0004
22	.0151	.0078	.0040	.0020	.0010	.0005
23	.0177	.0091	.0047	.0024	.0012	.0006
24	.0206	.0107	.0055	.0028	.0014	.0007
25	.0240	.0125	.0064	.0033	.0017	.0008
26	.0277	.0145	.0075	.0038	.0020	.0010
27	.0319	.0168	.0087	.0045	.0023	.0012

Table 9. (*continued*)

n t	15	16	17	18	19	20
28	.0365	.0193	.0101	.0052	.0027	.0014
29	.0416	.0222	.0116	.0060	.0031	.0016
30	.0473	.0253	.0133	.0069	.0036	.0018
31	.0535	.0288	.0153	.0080	.0041	.0021
32	.0603	.0327	.0174	.0091	.0047	.0024
33	.0677	.0370	.0198	.0104	.0054	.0028
34	.0757	.0416	.0224	.0118	.0062	.0032
35	.0844	.0467	.0253	.0134	.0070	.0036
36	.0938	.0523	.0284	.0152	.0080	.0042
37	.1039	.0583	.0319	.0171	.0090	.0047
38	.1147	.0649	.0357	.0192	.0102	.0053
39	.1262	.0719	.0398	.0216	.0115	.0060
40	.1384	.0795	.0443	.0241	.0129	.0068
41	.1514	.0877	.0492	.0269	.0145	.0077
42	.1651	.0964	.0544	.0300	.0162	.0086
43	.1796	.1057	.0601	.0333	.0180	.0096
44	.1947	.1156	.0662	.0368	.0201	.0107
45	.2106	.1261	.0727	.0407	.0223	.0120
46	.2271	.1372	.0797	.0449	.0247	.0133
47	.2444	.1489	.0871	.0494	.0273	.0148
48	.2622	.1613	.0950	.0542	.0301	.0164
49	.2807	.1742	.1034	.0594	.0331	.0181
50	.2997	.1877	.1123	.0649	.0364	.0200
51	.3193	.2019	.1218	.0708	.0399	.0220
52	.3394	.2166	.1317	.0770	.0437	.0242
53	.3599	.2319	.1421	.0837	.0478	.0266
54	.3808	.2477	.1530	.0907	.0521	.0291
55	.4020	.2641	.1645	.0982	.0567	.0319
56	.4235	.2809	.1764	.1061	.0616	.0348
57	.4452	.2983	.1889	.1144	.0668	.0379
58	.4670	.3161	.2019	.1231	.0723	.0413
59	.4890	.3343	.2153	.1323	.0782	.0448
60	.5110	.3529	.2293	.1419	.0844	.0487
61	.5330	.3718	.2437	.1519	.0909	.0527
62	.5548	.3910	.2585	.1624	.0978	.0570
63	.5765	.4104	.2738	.1733	.1051	.0615
64	.5980	.4301	.2895	.1846	.1127	.0664
65	.6192	.4500	.3056	.1964	.1206	.0715
66	.6401	.4699	.3221	.2086	.1290	.0768
67	.6606	.4900	.3389	.2211	.1377	.0825
68	.6807	.5100	.3559	.2341	.1467	.0884
69	.7003	.5301	.3733	.2475	.1562	.0947
70	.7193	.5500	.3910	.2613	.1660	.1012
71	.7378	.5699	.4088	.2754	.1762	.1081
72	.7556	.5896	.4268	.2899	.1868	.1153
73	.7729	.6090	.4450	.3047	.1977	.1227
74	.7894	.6282	.4633	.3198	.2090	.1305
75	.8053	.6471	.4816	.3353	.2207	.1387
76	.8204	.6657	.5000	.3509	.2327	.1471
77	.8349	.6839	.5184	.3669	.2450	.1559
78	.8486	.7017	.5367	.3830	.2576	.1650
79	.8616	.7191	.5550	.3994	.2706	.1744

t \ n	15	16	17	18	19	20
80	.8738	.7359	.5732	.4159	.2839	.1841
81	.8853	.7523	.5912	.4325	.2974	.1942
82	.8961	.7681	.6090	.4493	.3113	.2045
83	.9062	.7834	.6267	.4661	.3254	.2152
84	.9156	.7981	.6441	.4831	.3397	.2262
85	.9243	.8123	.6611	.5000	.3543	.2375
86	.9323	.8258	.6779	.5169	.3690	.2490
87	.9397	.8387	.6944	.5339	.3840	.2608
88	.9465	.8511	.7105	.5507	.3991	.2729
89	.9527	.8628	.7262	.5675	.4144	.2853
90	.9584	.8739	.7415	.5841	.4298	.2979
91	.9635	.8844	.7563	.6006	.4453	.3108
92	.9681	.8943	.7707	.6170	.4609	.3238
93	.9723	.9036	.7847	.6331	.4765	.3371
94	.9760	.9123	.7981	.6491	.4922	.3506
95	.9794	.9205	.8111	.6647	.5078	.3643
96	.9823	.9281	.8236	.6802	.5235	.3781
97	.9849	.9351	.8355	.6953	.5391	.3921
98	.9872	.9417	.8470	.7101	.5547	.4062
99	.9892	.9477	.8579	.7246	.5702	.4204
100	.9910	.9533	.8683	.7387	.5856	.4347
101	.9925	.9584	.8782	.7525	.6009	.4492
102	.9938	.9630	.8877	.7659	.6160	.4636
103	.9949	.9673	.8966	.7789	.6310	.4782
104	.9958	.9712	.9050	.7914	.6457	.4927
105	.9966	.9747	.9129	.8036	.6603	.5073

Reprinted from E. L. Lehmann, (1975). *Nonparametrics: Statistical Methods Based on Ranks*, Holden-Day, pp. 418–421, by permission of the author and the publisher.

Table 10. Cumulative Distribution of Wilcoxon Rank Sum Statistic, $\Pr[T_1 - n_1(n_1 + 1)/2 \le t]$

n_1	t	$n_2 = 3$	$n_2 = 4$	$n_2 = 5$	$n_2 = 6$	$n_2 = 7$	$n_2 = 8$	$n_2 = 9$	$n_2 = 10$	$n_2 = 11$	$n_2 = 12$
3	0	.0500	.0286	.0179	.0119	.0083	.0061	.0045	.0035	.0027	.0022
	1	.1000	.0571	.0357	.0238	.0167	.0121	.0091	.0070	.0055	.0044
	2	.2000	.1143	.0714	.0476	.0333	.0242	.0182	.0140	.0110	.0088
	3	.3500	.2000	.1250	.0833	.0583	.0424	.0318	.0245	.0192	.0154
	4	.5000	.3143	.1964	.1310	.0917	.0667	.0500	.0385	.0302	.0242
	5	.6500	.4286	.2857	.1905	.1333	.0970	.0727	.0559	.0440	.0352
	6	.8000	.5714	.3929	.2738	.1917	.1394	.1045	.0804	.0632	.0505
	7	.9000	.6857	.5000	.3571	.2583	.1879	.1409	.1084	.0852	.0681
	8	.9500	.8000	.6071	.4524	.3333	.2485	.1864	.1434	.1126	.0901
	9	1.0000	.8857	.7143	.5476	.4167	.3152	.2409	.1853	.1456	.1165
	10		.9429	.8036	.6429	.5000	.3879	.3000	.2343	.1841	.1473
	11		.9714	.8750	.7262	.5833	.4606	.3636	.2867	.2280	.1824
	12		1.0000	.9286	.8095	.6667	.5394	.4318	.3462	.2775	.2242
	13			.9643	.8690	.7417	.6121	.5000	.4056	.3297	.2681
	14			.9821	.9167	.8083	.6848	.5682	.4685	.3846	.3165
	15			1.0000	.9524	.8667	.7515	.6364	.5315	.4423	.3670
	16				.9762	.9083	.8121	.7000	.5944	.5000	.4198
	17				.9881	.9417	.8606	.7591	.6538	.5577	.4725
	18				1.0000	.9667	.9030	.8136	.7133	.6154	.5275
4	0		.0143	.0079	.0048	.0030	.0020	.0014	.0010	.0007	.0005
	1		.0286	.0159	.0095	.0061	.0040	.0028	.0020	.0015	.0011
	2		.0571	.0317	.0190	.0121	.0081	.0056	.0040	.0029	.0022
	3		.1000	.0556	.0333	.0212	.0141	.0098	.0070	.0051	.0038
	4		.1714	.0952	.0571	.0364	.0242	.0168	.0120	.0088	.0066
	5		.2429	.1429	.0857	.0545	.0364	.0252	.0180	.0132	.0099
	6		.3429	.2063	.1286	.0818	.0545	.0378	.0270	.0198	.0148
	7		.4429	.2778	.1762	.1152	.0768	.0531	.0380	.0278	.0209
	8		.5571	.3651	.2381	.1576	.1071	.0741	.0529	.0388	.0291
	9		.6571	.4524	.3048	.2061	.1414	.0993	.0709	.0520	.0390
	10		.7571	.5476	.3810	.2636	.1838	.1301	.0939	.0689	.0516
	11		.8286	.6349	.4571	.3242	.2303	.1650	.1199	.0886	.0665
	12		.9000	.7222	.5429	.3939	.2848	.2070	.1518	.1128	.0852
	13		.9429	.7937	.6190	.4636	.3414	.2517	.1868	.1399	.1060
	14		.9714	.8571	.6952	.5364	.4040	.3021	.2268	.1714	.1308
	15		.9857	.9048	.7619	.6061	.4667	.3552	.2697	.2059	.1582
	16		1.0000	.9444	.8238	.6758	.5333	.4126	.3177	.2447	.1896
	17			.9683	.8714	.7364	.5960	.4699	.3666	.2857	.2231
	18			.9841	.9143	.7939	.6586	.5301	.4196	.3304	.2604
	19			.9921	.9429	.8424	.7152	.5874	.4725	.3766	.2995
	20			1.0000	.9667	.8848	.7697	.6448	.5275	.4256	.3418
	21				.9810	.9182	.8162	.6979	.5804	.4747	.3852
	22				.9905	.9455	.8586	.7483	.6334	.5253	.4308
	23				.9952	.9636	.8929	.7930	.6823	.5744	.4764
	24				1.0000	.9788	.9232	.8350	.7303	.6234	.5236

n_1	t	$n_2=5$	$n_2=6$	$n_2=7$	$n_2=8$	$n_2=9$	$n_2=10$
5	0	.0040	.0022	.0013	.0008	.0005	.0003
	1	.0079	.0043	.0025	.0016	.0010	.0007
	2	.0159	.0087	.0051	.0031	.0020	.0013
	3	.0278	.0152	.0088	.0054	.0035	.0023
	4	.0476	.0260	.0152	.0093	.0060	.0040
	5	.0754	.0411	.0240	.0148	.0095	.0063
	6	.1111	.0628	.0366	.0225	.0145	.0097
	7	.1548	.0887	.0530	.0326	.0210	.0140
	8	.2103	.1234	.0745	.0466	.0300	.0200
	9	.2738	.1645	.1010	.0637	.0415	.0276
	10	.3452	.2143	.1338	.0855	.0559	.0376
	11	.4206	.2684	.1717	.1111	.0734	.0496
	12	.5000	.3312	.2159	.1422	.0949	.0646
	13	.5794	.3961	.2652	.1772	.1199	.0823
	14	.6548	.4654	.3194	.2176	.1489	.1032
	15	.7262	.5346	.3775	.2618	.1818	.1272
	16	.7897	.6039	.4381	.3108	.2188	.1548
	17	.8452	.6688	.5000	.3621	.2592	.1855
	18	.8889	.7316	.5619	.4165	.3032	.2198
	19	.9246	.7857	.6225	.4716	.3497	.2567
	20	.9524	.8355	.6806	.5284	.3986	.2970
	21	.9722	.8766	.7348	.5835	.4491	.3393
	22	.9841	.9113	.7841	.6379	.5000	.3839
	23	.9921	.9372	.8283	.6892	.5509	.4296
	24	.9960	.9589	.8662	.7382	.6014	.4765
	25	1.0000	.9740	.8990	.7824	.6503	.5235
6	0		.0011	.0006	.0003	.0002	.0001
	1		.0022	.0012	.0007	.0004	.0002
	2		.0043	.0023	.0013	.0008	.0005
	3		.0076	.0041	.0023	.0014	.0009
	4		.0130	.0070	.0040	.0024	.0015
	5		.0206	.0111	.0063	.0038	.0024
	6		.0325	.0175	.0100	.0060	.0037
	7		.0465	.0256	.0147	.0088	.0055
	8		.0660	.0367	.0213	.0128	.0080
	9		.0898	.0507	.0296	.0180	.0112
	10		.1201	.0688	.0406	.0248	.0156
	11		.1548	.0903	.0539	.0332	.0210
	12		.1970	.1171	.0709	.0440	.0280
	13		.2424	.1474	.0906	.0567	.0363
	14		.2944	.1830	.1142	.0723	.0467
	15		.3496	.2226	.1412	.0905	.0589
	16		.4091	.2669	.1725	.1119	.0736
	17		.4686	.3141	.2068	.1361	.0903
	18		.5314	.3654	.2454	.1638	.1099
	19		.5909	.4178	.2864	.1942	.1317
	20		.6504	.4726	.3310	.2280	.1566
	21		.7056	.5274	.3773	.2643	.1838
	22		.7576	.5822	.4259	.3035	.2139
	23		.8030	.6346	.4749	.3445	.2461
	24		.8452	.6859	.5251	.3878	.2811
	25		.8799	.7331	.5741	.4320	.3177
	26		.9102	.7774	.6227	.4773	.3564
	27		.9340	.8170	.6690	.5227	.3962
	28		.9535	.8526	.7136	.5680	.4374
	29		.9675	.8829	.7546	.6122	.4789
	30		.9794	.9097	.7932	.6555	.5211

n_1	t	$n_2=7$	$n_2=8$	$n_2=9$	$n_2=10$
7	0	.0003	.0002	.0001	.0001
	1	.0006	.0003	.0002	.0001
	2	.0012	.0006	.0003	.0002
	3	.0020	.0011	.0006	.0004
	4	.0035	.0019	.0010	.0006
	5	.0055	.0030	.0017	.0010
	6	.0087	.0047	.0026	.0015
	7	.0131	.0070	.0039	.0023
	8	.0189	.0103	.0058	.0034
	9	.0265	.0145	.0082	.0048
	10	.0364	.0200	.0115	.0068
	11	.0487	.0270	.0156	.0093
	12	.0641	.0361	.0209	.0125
	13	.0825	.0469	.0274	.0165
	14	.1043	.0603	.0356	.0215
	15	.1297	.0760	.0454	.0277
	16	.1588	.0946	.0571	.0351
	17	.1914	.1159	.0708	.0439
	18	.2279	.1405	.0869	.0544
	19	.2675	.1678	.1052	.0665
	20	.3100	.1984	.1261	.0806
	21	.3552	.2317	.1496	.0966
	22	.4024	.2679	.1755	.1148
	23	.4508	.3063	.2039	.1349
	24	.5000	.3472	.2349	.1574
	25	.5492	.3894	.2680	.1819
	26	.5976	.4333	.3032	.2087
	27	.6448	.4775	.3403	.2374
	28	.6900	.5225	.3788	.2681
	29	.7325	.5667	.4185	.3004
	30	.7721	.6106	.4591	.3345
	31	.8086	.6528	.5000	.3698
	32	.8412	.6937	.5409	.4063
	33	.8703	.7321	.5815	.4434
	34	.8957	.7683	.6212	.4811
	35	.9175	.8016	.6597	.5189

Table 10. (*continued*)

n_1	t	$n_2 = 8$	$n_2 = 9$	$n_2 = 10$	n_1	t	$n_2 = 9$	$n_2 = 10$	n	t	$n_2 = 10$
8	0	.0001	.0000	.0000	9	0	.0000	.0000	10	0	.0000
	1	.0002	.0001	.0000		1	.0000	.0000		1	.0000
	2	.0003	.0002	.0001		2	.0001	.0000		2	.0000
	3	.0005	.0003	.0002		3	.0001	.0001		3	.0000
	4	.0009	.0005	.0003		4	.0002	.0001		4	.0001
	5	.0015	.0008	.0004		5	.0004	.0002		5	.0001
	6	.0023	.0012	.0007		6	.0006	.0003		6	.0002
	7	.0035	.0019	.0010		7	.0009	.0005		7	.0002
	8	.0052	.0028	.0015		8	.0014	.0007		8	.0004
	9	.0074	.0039	.0022		9	.0020	.0011		9	.0005
	10	.0103	.0056	.0031		10	.0028	.0015		10	.0008
	11	.0141	.0076	.0043		11	.0039	.0021		11	.0010
	12	.0190	.0103	.0058		12	.0053	.0028		12	.0014
	13	.0249	.0137	.0078		13	.0071	.0038		13	.0019
	14	.0325	.0180	.0103		14	.0094	.0051		14	.0026
	15	.0415	.0232	.0133		15	.0122	.0066		15	.0034
	16	.0524	.0296	.0171		16	.0157	.0086		16	.0045
	17	.0652	.0372	.0217		17	.0200	.0110		17	.0057
	18	.0803	.0464	.0273		18	.0252	.0140		18	.0073
	19	.0974	.0570	.0338		19	.0313	.0175		19	.0093
	20	.1172	.0694	.0416		20	.0385	.0217		20	.0116
	21	.1393	.0836	.0506		21	.0470	.0267		21	.0144
	22	.1641	.0998	.0610		22	.0567	.0326		22	.0177
	23	.1911	.1179	.0729		23	.0680	.0394		23	.0216
	24	.2209	.1383	.0864		24	.0807	.0474		24	.0262
	25	.2527	.1606	.1015		25	.0951	.0564		25	.0315
	26	.2869	.1852	.1185		26	.1112	.0667		26	.0376
	27	.3227	.2117	.1371		27	.1290	.0782		27	.0446
	28	.3605	.2404	.1577		28	.1487	.0912		28	.0526
	29	.3992	.2707	.1800		29	.1701	.1055		29	.0615
	30	.4392	.3029	.2041		30	.1933	.1214		30	.0716
	31	.4796	.3365	.2299		31	.2181	.1388		31	.0827
	32	.5204	.3715	.2574		32	.2447	.1577		32	.0952
	33	.5608	.4074	.2863		33	.2729	.1781		33	.1088
	34	.6008	.4442	.3167		34	.3024	.2001		34	.1237
	35	.6395	.4813	.3482		35	.3332	.2235		35	.1399
	36	.6773	.5187	.3809		36	.3652	.2483		36	.1575
	37	.7131	.5558	.4143		37	.3981	.2745		37	.1763
	38	.7473	.5926	.4484		38	.4317	.3019		38	.1965
	39	.7791	.6285	.4827		39	.4657	.3304		39	.2179
	40	.8089	.6635	.5173		40	.5000	.3598		40	.2406
						41	.5343	.3901		41	.2644
						42	.5683	.4211		42	.2894
						43	.6019	.4524		43	.3153
						44	.6348	.4841		44	.3421
						45	.6668	.5159		45	.3697
										46	.3980
										47	.4267
										48	.4559
										49	.4853
										50	.5147

Reprinted from E. L. Lehmann, (1975). *Nonparametrics: Statistical Methods Based on Ranks*, Holden-Day, pp. 408–410, by permission of the author and the publisher.

Table 11. Fisher's Exact Test: Probabilities for 2 × 2 Tables

N	S₁	S₂	X	Obs.	Other	Total	N	S₁	S₂	X	Obs.	Other	Total	N	S₁	S₂	X	Obs.	Other	Total
2	1	1	0	.500	.500	1.000	7	3	3	0	.114	.029	.143	9	2	3	1	.583	.417	1.000
2	1	1	1	.500	.500	1.000	7	3	3	1	.628	.372	1.000	9	2	3	2	.083	.000	.083
3	1	1	0	.667	.333	1.000	7	3	3	2	.372	.114	.486	9	2	4	0	.278	.167	.444
3	1	1	1	.333	.000	.333	7	3	3	3	.029	.000	.029	9	2	4	1	.722	.278	1.000
4	1	1	0	.750	.250	1.000	8	1	1	0	.875	.125	1.000	9	2	4	2	.167	.000	.167
4	1	1	1	.250	.000	.250	8	1	1	1	.125	.000	.125	9	3	3	0	.238	.226	.464
4	1	2	0	.500	.500	1.000	8	1	2	0	.750	.250	1.000	9	3	3	1	1.000	.000	1.000
4	1	2	1	.500	.500	1.000	8	1	2	1	.250	.000	.250	9	3	3	2	.226	.238	.464
4	2	2	0	.167	.167	.333	8	1	3	0	.625	.375	1.000	9	3	3	3	.012	.000	.012
4	2	2	1	1.000	.000	1.000	8	1	3	1	.375	.000	.375	9	3	4	0	.012	.048	.060
4	2	2	2	.167	.167	.333	8	1	4	0	.500	.500	1.000	9	3	4	1	.488	.512	1.000
5	1	1	0	.800	.200	1.000	8	1	4	1	.500	.500	1.000	9	3	4	2	.405	.012	.417
5	1	1	1	.200	.000	.200	8	2	2	0	.536	.464	1.000	9	3	4	3	.048	.000	.048
5	1	2	0	.600	.400	1.000	8	2	2	1	.464	.536	1.000	9	4	4	0	.040	.008	.048
5	1	2	1	.400	.000	.400	8	2	2	2	.035	.000	.035	9	4	4	1	.357	.167	.524
5	2	2	0	.300	.100	.400	8	2	3	0	.357	.107	.464	9	4	4	2	.643	.357	1.000
5	2	2	1	.700	.300	1.000	8	2	3	1	.643	.357	1.000	9	4	4	3	.167	.040	.206
5	2	2	2	.100	.000	.100	8	2	3	2	.107	.000	.107	9	4	4	4	.008	.000	.008
6	1	1	0	.833	.167	1.000	8	2	4	0	.214	.214	.428	10	1	1	0	.900	.100	1.000
6	1	1	1	.167	.000	.167	8	2	4	1	1.000	.000	1.000	10	1	1	1	.100	.000	.100
6	1	2	0	.667	.333	1.000	8	2	4	2	.214	.214	.428	10	1	2	0	.800	.200	1.000
6	1	2	1	.333	.000	.333	8	3	3	0	.179	.018	.197	10	1	2	1	.200	.000	.200
6	1	3	0	.500	.500	1.000	8	3	3	1	.715	.286	1.000	10	1	3	0	.700	.300	1.000
6	1	3	1	.500	.500	1.000	8	3	3	2	.286	.179	.465	10	1	3	1	.300	.000	.300
6	2	2	0	.400	.067	.467	8	3	3	3	.018	.000	.018	10	1	4	0	.600	.400	1.000
6	2	2	1	.533	.467	1.000	8	3	4	0	.071	.071	.143	10	1	4	1	.400	.000	.400
6	2	2	2	.067	.000	.067	8	3	4	1	.500	.500	1.000	10	1	5	0	.500	.500	1.000
6	2	3	0	.200	.200	.400	8	3	4	2	.500	.500	1.000	10	1	5	1	.500	.500	1.000
6	2	3	1	1.000	.000	1.000	8	3	4	3	.071	.071	.143	10	2	2	0	.622	.378	1.000
6	2	3	2	.200	.200	.400	8	4	4	0	.014	.014	.029	10	2	2	1	.378	.000	.378
6	3	3	0	.050	.050	.100	8	4	4	1	.243	.243	.486	10	2	2	2	.022	.000	.022
6	3	3	1	.500	.500	1.000	8	4	4	2	1.000	.000	1.000	10	2	3	0	.467	.067	.533
6	3	3	2	.500	.500	1.000	8	4	4	3	.243	.243	.486	10	2	3	1	.533	.467	1.000
6	3	3	3	.050	.050	.100	8	4	4	4	.014	.014	.029	10	2	3	2	.067	.000	.067
7	1	1	0	.857	.143	1.000	9	1	1	0	.889	.111	1.000	10	2	4	0	.333	.133	.467
7	1	1	1	.143	.000	.143	9	1	1	1	.111	.000	.111	10	2	4	1	.667	.333	1.000
7	1	2	0	.714	.286	1.000	9	1	2	0	.778	.222	1.000	10	2	4	2	.133	.000	.133
7	1	2	1	.286	.000	.286	9	1	2	1	.222	.000	.222	10	2	5	0	.222	.222	.444
7	1	3	0	.571	.429	1.000	9	1	3	0	.667	.333	1.000	10	2	5	1	.778	.778	1.000
7	1	3	1	.429	.000	.429	9	1	3	1	.333	.000	.333	10	2	5	2	.222	.222	.444
7	2	2	0	.476	.524	1.000	9	1	4	0	.556	.444	1.000	10	3	3	0	.292	.183	.475
7	2	2	1	.524	.000	.524	9	1	4	1	.444	.000	.444	10	3	3	1	.708	.292	1.000
7	2	2	2	.048	.000	.048	9	2	2	0	.583	.417	1.000	10	3	3	2	.183	.000	.183
7	2	3	0	.286	.143	.429	9	2	2	1	.417	.000	.417	10	3	3	3	.008	.000	.008
7	2	3	1	.714	.286	1.000	9	2	2	2	.028	.000	.028	10	3	4	0	.167	.033	.200
7	2	3	2	.143	.000	.143	9	2	3	0	.417	.083	.500	10	3	4	1	.667	.333	1.000

Cumulative probabilities are given for deviations in the observed direction from equality and for deviation of the same size or greater in the opposite direction. The total probabilities can be used for two-tail tests. Tables are extracted from more extensive tables prepared by Donald Goyette and M. Ray Mickey, Health Sciences Computing Facility, UCLA. In the probability columns "Obs." refers to the probability of a deviation as large or larger in the observed direction and "Other" refers to the probability of a deviation as large or larger in the opposite direction.

S_1 is the smallest marginal total and S_2 is the next smallest; X is the frequency in the cell corresponding to the two smallest totals.

Table 11. (continued)

N	S₁	S₂	X	Obs.	Other	Total	N	S₁	S₂	X	Obs.	Other	Total	N	S₁	S₂	X	Obs.	Other	Total
				PROBABILITY							**PROBABILITY**							**PROBABILITY**		
10	3	4	2	.333	.167	.500	11	3	4	2	.279	.212	.491	12	3	3	1	.618	.382	1.000
10	3	4	3	.033	0	.033	11	3	4	3	.024	0	.024	12	3	3	2	.127	0	.127
10	3	5	0	.083	.083	.167	11	3	5	0	.121	.061	.182	12	3	3	3	.005	0	.005
10	3	5	1	.500	.500	1.000	11	3	5	1	.576	.424	1.000	12	3	4	0	.255	.236	.491
10	3	5	2	.500	.500	1.000	11	3	5	2	.424	.121	.545	12	3	4	1	.764	.745	1.000
10	3	5	3	.083	.083	.167	11	3	5	3	.061	0	.061	12	3	4	2	.236	.255	.491
10	4	4	0	.071	.005	.076	11	4	4	0	.106	.088	.194	12	3	4	3	.018	0	.018
10	4	4	1	.452	.119	.571	11	4	4	1	.530	.470	1.000	12	3	5	0	.159	.045	.205
10	4	4	2	.548	.452	1.000	11	4	4	2	.470	.106	.576	12	3	5	1	.636	.364	1.000
10	4	4	3	.119	.071	.190	11	4	4	3	.088	0	.088	12	3	5	2	.364	.159	.523
10	4	4	4	.005	0	.005	11	4	4	4	.003	0	.003	12	3	5	3	.045	0	.045
10	4	5	0	.024	.024	.048	11	4	5	0	.045	.015	.061	12	3	6	0	.091	.091	.182
10	4	5	1	.262	.262	.524	11	4	5	1	.348	.197	.545	12	3	6	1	.500	.500	1.000
10	4	5	2	.738	.738	1.000	11	4	5	2	.652	.348	1.000	12	3	6	2	.500	.500	1.000
10	4	5	3	.262	.262	.524	11	4	5	3	.197	.045	.242	12	3	6	3	.091	.091	.182
10	4	5	4	.024	.024	.048	11	4	5	4	.015	0	.015	12	4	4	0	.141	.067	.208
10	5	5	0	.004	.004	.008	11	5	5	0	.013	.002	.015	12	4	4	1	.594	.406	1.000
10	5	5	1	.103	.103	.206	11	5	5	1	.175	.067	.242	12	4	4	2	.406	.141	.547
10	5	5	2	.500	.500	1.000	11	5	5	2	.608	.392	1.000	12	4	4	3	.067	0	.067
10	5	5	3	.500	.500	1.000	11	5	5	3	.392	.175	.567	12	4	4	4	.002	0	.002
10	5	5	4	.103	.103	.206	11	5	5	4	.067	.013	.080	12	4	5	0	.071	.010	.081
10	5	5	5	.004	.004	.008	11	5	5	5	.002	0	.002	12	4	5	1	.424	.152	.576
11	1	1	0	.909	.091	1.000	12	1	1	0	.917	.083	1.000	12	4	5	2	.576	.424	1.000
11	1	1	1	.091	0	.091	12	1	1	1	.083	0	.083	12	4	5	3	.152	.071	.222
11	1	2	0	.818	.182	1.000	12	1	2	0	.833	.167	1.000	12	4	5	4	.010	0	.010
11	1	2	1	.182	0	.182	12	1	2	1	.167	0	.167	12	4	6	0	.030	.030	.061
11	1	3	0	.727	.273	1.000	12	1	3	0	.750	.250	1.000	12	4	6	1	.273	.273	.545
11	1	3	1	.273	0	.273	12	1	3	1	.250	0	.250	12	4	6	2	.727	.727	1.000
11	1	4	0	.636	.364	1.000	12	1	4	0	.667	.333	1.000	12	4	6	3	.273	.273	.545
11	1	4	1	.364	0	.364	12	1	4	1	.333	0	.333	12	4	6	4	.030	.030	.061
11	1	5	0	.545	.455	1.000	12	1	5	0	.583	.417	1.000	12	5	5	1	.247	.045	.293
11	1	5	1	.455	0	.455	12	1	5	1	.417	0	.417	12	5	5	2	.689	.311	1.000
11	2	2	0	.655	.345	1.000	12	1	6	0	.500	.500	1.000	12	5	5	3	.311	.247	.558
11	2	2	1	.345	0	.345	12	1	6	1	.500	.500	1.000	12	5	5	4	.045	.027	.072
11	2	2	2	.018	0	.018	12	2	2	0	.682	.318	1.000	12	5	5	5	.001	0	.001
11	2	3	0	.509	.055	.564	12	2	2	1	.318	0	.318	12	5	6	0	.008	.008	.015
11	2	3	1	.491	.509	1.000	12	2	2	2	.015	0	.015	12	5	6	1	.121	.121	.242
11	2	3	2	.055	0	.055	12	2	3	0	.545	.455	1.000	12	5	6	2	.500	.500	1.000
11	2	4	0	.382	.109	.491	12	2	3	1	.455	.545	1.000	12	5	6	3	.500	.500	1.000
11	2	4	1	.618	.382	1.000	12	2	3	2	.045	0	.045	12	5	6	4	.121	.121	.242
11	2	4	2	.109	0	.109	12	2	4	0	.424	.091	.515	12	5	6	5	.008	.008	.015
11	2	5	0	.273	.182	.455	12	2	4	1	.576	.424	1.000	12	6	6	0	.001	.001	.002
11	2	5	1	.727	.273	1.000	12	2	4	2	.091	0	.091	12	6	6	1	.040	.040	.080
11	2	5	2	.182	0	.182	12	2	5	0	.318	.152	.470	12	6	6	2	.284	.284	.567
11	3	3	0	.339	.152	.491	12	2	5	1	.682	.318	1.000	12	6	6	3	1.000	.000	1.000
11	3	3	1	.661	.339	1.000	12	2	5	2	.152	0	.152	12	6	6	4	.284	.284	.567
11	3	3	2	.152	0	.152	12	2	6	0	.227	.227	.455	12	6	6	5	.040	.040	.080
11	3	3	3	.006	0	.006	12	2	6	1	.773	.773	1.000	12	6	6	6	.001	.001	.002
11	3	4	0	.212	.024	.236	12	2	6	2	.227	.227	.455	13	1	1	0	.923	.077	1.000
11	3	4	1	.721	.279	1.000	12	3	3	0	.382	.127	.509							

498

N	S_1	S_2	X	Obs.	Other	Total	N	S_1	S_2	X	Obs.	Other	Total	N	S_1	S_2	X	Obs.	Other	Total
13	1	1	1	.077	0	.077	13	4	5	3	.119	.098	.217	14	2	5	1	.604	.396	1.000
13	1	2	0	.846	.154	1.000	13	4	5	4	.007	0	.007	14	2	5	2	.110	0	.110
13	1	2	1	.154	0	.154	13	4	6	0	.049	.021	.070	14	2	6	0	.308	.165	.473
13	1	3	0	.769	.231	1.000	13	4	6	1	.343	.217	.559	14	2	6	1	.692	.308	1.000
13	1	3	1	.231	0	.231	13	4	6	2	.657	.343	1.000	14	2	6	2	.165	0	.165
13	1	4	0	.692	.308	1.000	13	4	6	3	.217	.049	.266	14	2	7	0	.231	.231	.462
13	1	4	1	.308	0	.308	13	4	6	4	.021	0	.021	14	2	7	1	.769	.769	1.000
13	1	5	0	.615	.385	1.000	13	5	5	0	.044	.032	.075	14	2	7	2	.231	.231	.462
13	1	5	1	.385	0	.385	13	5	5	1	.315	.249	.565	14	3	3	0	.453	.093	.547
13	1	6	0	.538	.462	1.000	13	5	5	2	.685	.315	1.000	14	3	3	1	.547	.453	1.000
13	1	6	1	.462	0	.462	13	5	5	3	.249	.044	.293	14	3	3	2	.093	0	.093
13	2	2	0	.705	.295	1.000	13	5	5	4	.032	0	.032	14	3	3	3	.003	0	.003
13	2	2	1	.295	0	.295	13	5	5	5	.001	0	.001	14	3	4	0	.330	.176	.505
13	2	2	2	.013	0	.013	13	5	6	0	.016	.005	.021	14	3	4	1	.670	.330	1.000
13	2	3	0	.577	.423	1.000	13	5	6	1	.179	.086	.266	14	3	4	2	.176	0	.176
13	2	3	1	.423	0	.423	13	5	6	2	.587	.413	1.000	14	3	4	3	.011	0	.011
13	2	3	2	.038	0	.038	13	5	6	3	.413	.179	.592	14	3	5	0	.231	.027	.258
13	2	4	0	.462	.077	.538	13	5	6	4	.086	.016	.103	14	3	5	1	.725	.275	1.000
13	2	4	1	.538	.462	1.000	13	5	6	5	.005	0	.005	14	3	5	2	.275	.231	.505
13	2	4	2	.077	0	.077	13	6	6	0	.004	.001	.005	14	3	5	3	.027	0	.027
13	2	5	0	.359	.128	.487	13	6	6	1	.078	.025	.103	14	3	6	0	.154	.055	.209
13	2	5	1	.641	.359	1.000	13	6	6	2	.383	.209	.592	14	3	6	1	.615	.385	1.000
13	2	5	2	.128	0	.128	13	6	6	3	.617	.383	1.000	14	3	6	2	.385	.154	.538
13	2	6	0	.269	.192	.462	13	6	6	4	.209	.078	.286	14	3	6	3	.055	0	.055
13	2	6	1	.731	.269	1.000	13	6	6	5	.025	.004	.029	14	3	7	0	.096	.096	.192
13	2	6	2	.192	0	.192	13	6	6	6	.001	0	.001	14	3	7	1	.500	.500	1.000
13	3	3	0	.420	.108	.528	14	1	1	0	.929	.071	1.000	14	3	7	2	.500	.500	1.000
13	3	3	1	.580	.420	1.000	14	1	1	1	.071	0	.071	14	3	7	3	.096	.096	.192
13	3	3	2	.108	0	.108	14	1	2	0	.857	.143	1.000	14	4	4	0	.210	.041	.251
13	3	3	3	.003	0	.003	14	1	2	1	.143	0	.143	14	4	4	1	.689	.311	1.000
13	3	4	0	.294	.203	.497	14	1	3	0	.786	.214	1.000	14	4	4	2	.311	.210	.520
13	3	4	1	.706	.294	1.000	14	1	3	1	.214	0	.214	14	4	4	3	.041	0	.041
13	3	4	2	.203	0	.203	14	1	4	0	.714	.286	1.000	14	4	4	4	.001	0	.001
13	3	4	3	.014	0	.014	14	1	4	1	.286	0	.286	14	4	5	0	.126	.095	.221
13	3	5	0	.196	.035	.231	14	1	5	0	.643	.357	1.000	14	4	5	1	.545	.455	1.000
13	3	5	1	.685	.315	1.000	14	1	5	1	.357	0	.357	14	4	5	2	.455	.126	.538
13	3	5	2	.315	.196	.510	14	1	6	0	.571	.429	1.000	14	4	5	3	.095	0	.095
13	3	5	3	.035	0	.035	14	1	6	1	.429	0	.429	14	4	5	4	.005	0	.005
13	3	6	0	.122	.070	.192	14	1	7	0	.500	.500	1.000	14	4	6	0	.070	.015	.085
13	3	6	1	.563	.437	1.000	14	1	7	1	.500	.500	1.000	14	4	6	1	.406	.175	.580
13	3	6	2	.437	.122	.559	14	2	2	0	.725	.275	1.000	14	4	6	2	.594	.406	1.000
13	3	6	3	.070	0	.070	14	2	2	1	.275	0	.275	14	4	6	3	.175	.070	.245
13	4	4	0	.176	.052	.228	14	2	2	2	.011	0	.011	14	4	6	4	.015	0	.015
13	4	4	1	.646	.354	1.000	14	2	3	0	.604	.396	1.000	14	4	7	0	.035	.035	.070
13	4	4	2	.354	.176	.530	14	2	3	1	.396	0	.396	14	4	7	1	.280	.280	.559
13	4	4	3	.052	0	.052	14	2	3	2	.033	0	.033	14	4	7	2	.720	.720	1.000
13	4	4	4	.001	0	.001	14	2	4	0	.495	.066	.560	14	4	7	3	.280	.280	.559
13	4	5	0	.098	.007	.105	14	2	4	1	.505	.495	1.000	14	4	7	4	.035	.035	.070
13	4	5	1	.490	.119	.608	14	2	4	2	.066	0	.066	14	5	5	0	.063	.023	.086
13	4	5	2	.510	.490	1.000	14	2	5	0	.396	.110	.505	14	5	5	1	.378	.203	.580

Table 11. (*continued*)

N	S_1	S_2	X	Obs.	Other	Total	N	S_1	S_2	X	Obs.	Other	Total	N	S_1	S_2	X	Obs.	Other	Total
14	5	5	2	.622	.378	1.000	15	1	7	0	.533	.467	1.000	15	4	6	0	.092	.011	.103
14	5	5	3	.203	.063	.266	15	1	7	1	.467	0	.467	15	4	6	1	.462	.143	.604
14	5	5	4	.023	0	.023	15	2	2	0	.743	.257	1.000	15	4	6	2	.538	.462	1.000
14	5	5	5	.000	0	.000	15	2	2	1	.257	0	.257	15	4	6	3	.143	.092	.235
14	5	6	0	.028	.003	.031	15	2	2	2	.010	0	.010	15	4	6	4	.011	0	.011
14	5	6	1	.238	.063	.301	15	2	3	0	.629	.371	1.000	15	4	7	0	.051	.026	.077
14	5	6	2	.657	.343	1.000	15	2	3	1	.371	0	.371	15	4	7	1	.338	.231	.569
14	5	6	3	.343	.238	.580	15	2	3	2	.029	0	.029	15	4	7	2	.662	.338	1.000
14	5	6	4	.063	.028	.091	15	2	4	0	.524	.057	.581	15	4	7	3	.231	.051	.282
14	5	6	5	.003	0	.003	15	2	4	1	.476	.524	1.000	15	4	7	4	.026	0	.026
14	5	7	0	.010	.010	.021	15	2	4	2	.057	0	.057	15	5	5	0	.084	.017	.101
14	5	7	1	.133	.133	.266	15	2	5	0	.429	.095	.524	15	5	5	1	.434	.167	.600
14	5	7	2	.500	.500	1.000	15	2	5	1	.571	.429	1.000	15	5	5	2	.566	.434	1.000
14	5	7	3	.500	.500	1.000	15	2	5	2	.095	0	.095	15	5	5	3	.167	.084	.251
14	5	7	4	.133	.133	.266	15	2	6	0	.343	.143	.486	15	5	5	4	.017	0	.017
14	5	7	5	.010	.010	.021	15	2	6	1	.657	.343	1.000	15	5	5	5	.000	0	.000
14	6	6	0	.009	.000	.010	15	2	6	2	.143	0	.143	15	5	6	0	.042	.047	.089
14	6	6	1	.121	.016	.138	15	2	7	0	.267	.200	.467	15	5	6	1	.294	.287	.580
14	6	6	2	.471	.156	.627	15	2	7	1	.733	.267	1.000	15	5	6	2	.713	.706	1.000
14	6	6	3	.529	.471	1.000	15	2	7	2	.200	0	.200	15	5	6	3	.287	.294	.580
14	6	6	4	.156	.121	.277	15	3	3	0	.484	.081	.565	15	5	6	4	.047	.042	.089
14	6	6	5	.016	.009	.026	15	3	3	1	.516	.484	1.000	15	5	6	5	.002	0	.002
14	6	6	6	.000	0	.000	15	3	3	2	.081	0	.081	15	5	7	0	.019	.007	.026
14	6	7	0	.002	.002	.005	15	3	3	3	.002	0	.002	15	5	7	1	.182	.100	.282
14	6	7	1	.051	.051	.103	15	3	4	0	.363	.154	.516	15	5	7	2	.573	.427	1.000
14	6	7	2	.296	.296	.592	15	3	4	1	.637	.363	1.000	15	5	7	3	.427	.182	.608
14	6	7	3	.704	.704	1.000	15	3	4	2	.154	0	.154	15	5	7	4	.100	.019	.119
14	6	7	4	.296	.296	.592	15	3	4	3	.009	0	.009	15	5	7	5	.007	0	.007
14	6	7	5	.051	.051	.103	15	3	5	0	.264	.242	.505	15	6	6	0	.017	.011	.028
14	6	7	6	.002	.002	.005	15	3	5	1	.758	.736	1.000	15	6	6	1	.168	.119	.287
14	7	7	0	.000	.000	.001	15	3	5	2	.242	.264	.505	15	6	6	2	.545	.455	1.000
14	7	7	1	.015	.015	.029	15	3	5	3	.022	0	.022	15	6	6	3	.455	.168	.622
14	7	7	2	.143	.143	.286	15	3	6	0	.185	.044	.229	15	6	6	4	.119	.017	.136
14	7	7	3	.500	.500	1.000	15	3	6	1	.659	.341	1.000	15	6	6	5	.011	0	.011
14	7	7	4	.500	.500	1.000	15	3	6	2	.341	.185	.525	15	6	6	6	.000	0	.000
14	7	7	5	.143	.143	.286	15	3	6	3	.044	0	.044	15	6	7	0	.006	.001	.007
14	7	7	6	.015	.015	.029	15	3	7	0	.123	.077	.200	15	6	7	1	.084	.035	.119
14	7	7	7	.000	.000	.001	15	3	7	1	.554	.446	1.000	15	6	7	2	.378	.231	.608
15	1	1	0	.933	.067	1.000	15	3	7	2	.446	.123	.569	15	6	7	3	.622	.378	1.000
15	1	1	1	.067	0	.067	15	3	7	3	.077	0	.077	15	6	7	4	.231	.084	.315
15	1	2	0	.867	.133	1.000	15	4	4	0	.242	.033	.275	15	6	7	5	.035	.006	.041
15	1	2	1	.133	0	.133	15	4	4	1	.725	.275	1.000	15	6	7	6	.001	0	.001
15	1	3	0	.800	.200	1.000	15	4	4	2	.275	.242	.516	15	7	7	0	.001	.000	.001
15	1	3	1	.200	0	.200	15	4	4	3	.033	0	.033	15	7	7	1	.032	.009	.041
15	1	4	0	.733	.267	1.000	15	4	4	4	.001	0	.001	15	7	7	2	.214	.100	.315
15	1	4	1	.267	0	.267	15	4	5	0	.154	.077	.231	15	7	7	3	.595	.405	1.000
15	1	5	0	.667	.333	1.000	15	4	5	1	.593	.407	1.000	15	7	7	4	.405	.214	.619
15	1	5	1	.333	0	.333	15	4	5	2	.407	.154	.560	15	7	7	5	.100	.032	.132
15	1	6	0	.600	.400	1.000	15	4	5	3	.077	0	.077	15	7	7	6	.009	.001	.010
15	1	6	1	.400	0	.400	15	4	5	4	.004	0	.004	15	7	7	7	.000	0	.000

Table 12A. Sample Size per Group for Fisher's Exact Test (One Tailed), $\alpha = 0.05$

Upper Figure: Power = 0.90
Middle Figure: Power = 0.80
Lower Figure: Power = 0.50

P_2	P_1 0.95	0.9	0.8	0.7	0.6	0.5	0.4	0.3	0.2	0.1
0.9	503									
	371									
	184									
0.8	89	232								
	67	173								
	38	87								
0.7	42	74	338							
	34	56	249							
	19	31	121							
0.6	25	39	97	408						
	20	30	73	302						
	12	17	37	143						
0.5	18	25	47	111	445					
	14	19	36	84	321					
	9	11	19	43	155					
0.4	13	17	30	53	116	445				
	11	13	23	41	85	321				
	7	9	12	22	43	155				
0.3	10	12	18	31	53	111	408			
	9	10	15	23	41	84	302			
	6	6	9	12	22	43	143			
0.2	8	10	12	18	30	47	97	338		
	6	8	10	15	23	36	73	249		
	5	5	6	9	12	19	37	121		
0.1	6	8	10	12	17	25	39	74	232	
	5	6	8	10	13	19	30	56	173	
	3	3	5	6	9	11	17	31	87	
0.05	5	6	8	10	13	18	25	42	89	503
	5	5	6	9	11	14	20	34	67	371
	3	3	5	6	7	9	12	19	38	184

Reproduced from J. K. Haseman. Exact sample sizes for use with the Fisher–Irwin test for 2×2 tables, *Biometrics*, **34**, 106–109, 1978. With permission from the Biometric Society.

Table 12B. Sample Size per Group for Fisher's Exact Test (One Tailed), $\alpha = 0.01$

Upper Figure: Power = 0.90
Middle Figure: Power = 0.80
Lower Figure: Power = 0.50

P_2	P_1 0.95	0.9	0.8	0.7	0.6	0.5	0.4	0.3	0.2	0.1
0.9	745									
	583									
	333									
0.8	130	344								
	101	269								
	61	155								
0.7	60	108	503							
	49	86	393							
	32	52	221							
0.6	37	56	143	609						
	31	46	113	475						
	18	27	66	265						
0.5	25	35	69	163	667					
	20	29	55	129	519					
	14	18	34	73	235					
0.4	18	24	42	77	171	667				
	16	20	34	60	137	519				
	10	13	21	35	78	285				
0.3	14	18	28	43	77	163	609			
	12	15	22	35	60	129	475			
	9	10	13	22	35	73	265			
0.2	12	13	18	28	42	69	143	503		
	9	12	16	22	34	55	113	393		
	6	8	9	13	21	34	66	221		
0.1	9	9	13	18	24	35	56	108	344	
	8	9	12	15	20	29	46	86	269	
	6	6	8	10	13	18	27	52	155	
0.05	8	9	12	14	18	25	37	60	130	745
	6	8	9	12	16	20	31	49	101	583
	5	6	6	9	10	14	18	32	61	333

Reproduced from J. K. Haseman. Exact sample sizes for use with the Fisher–Irwin test for 2×2 tables, *Biometrics*, **34**, 106–109, 1978. With permission from the Biometric Society.

Table 13A. Dunnett's Statistic (One Sided)

| Error df | $1-\alpha$ | \multicolumn{9}{c}{p = number of treatment means, excluding control} |
		1	2	3	4	5	6	7	8	9
5	.95	2.02	2.44	2.68	2.85	2.98	3.08	3.16	3.24	3.30
	.99	3.37	3.90	4.21	4.43	4.60	4.73	4.85	4.94	5.03
6	.95	1.94	2.34	2.56	2.71	2.83	2.92	3.00	3.07	3.12
	.99	3.14	3.61	3.88	4.07	4.21	4.33	4.43	4.51	4.59
7	.95	1.89	2.27	2.48	2.62	2.73	2.82	2.89	2.95	3.01
	.99	3.00	3.42	3.66	3.83	3.96	4.07	4.15	4.23	4.30
8	.95	1.86	2.22	2.42	2.55	2.66	2.74	2.81	2.87	2.92
	.99	2.90	3.29	3.51	3.67	3.79	3.88	3.96	4.03	4.09
9	.95	1.83	2.18	2.37	2.50	2.60	2.68	2.75	2.81	2.86
	.99	2.82	3.19	3.40	3.55	3.66	3.75	3.82	3.89	3.94
10	.95	1.81	2.15	2.34	2.47	2.56	2.64	2.70	2.76	2.81
	.99	2.76	3.11	3.31	3.45	3.56	3.64	3.71	3.78	3.83
11	.95	1.80	2.13	2.31	2.44	2.53	2.60	2.67	2.72	2.77
	.99	2.72	3.06	3.25	3.38	3.48	3.56	3.63	3.69	3.74
12	.95	1.78	2.11	2.29	2.41	2.50	2.58	2.64	2.69	2.74
	.99	2.68	3.01	3.19	3.32	3.42	3.50	3.56	3.62	3.67
13	.95	1.77	2.09	2.27	2.39	2.48	2.55	2.61	2.66	2.71
	.99	2.65	2.97	3.15	3.27	3.37	3.44	3.51	3.56	3.61
14	.95	1.76	2.08	2.25	2.37	2.46	2.53	2.59	2.64	2.69
	.99	2.62	2.94	3.11	3.23	3.32	3.40	3.46	3.51	3.56
15	.95	1.75	2.07	2.24	2.36	2.44	2.51	2.57	2.62	2.67
	.99	2.60	2.91	3.08	3.20	3.29	3.36	3.42	3.47	3.52
16	.95	1.75	2.06	2.23	2.34	2.43	2.50	2.56	2.61	2.65
	.99	2.58	2.88	3.05	3.17	3.26	3.33	3.39	3.44	3.48
17	.95	1.74	2.05	2.22	2.33	2.42	2.49	2.54	2.59	2.64
	.99	2.57	2.86	3.03	3.14	3.23	3.30	3.36	3.41	3.45
18	.95	1.73	2.04	2.21	2.32	2.41	2.48	2.53	2.58	2.62
	.99	2.55	2.84	3.01	3.12	3.21	3.27	3.33	3.38	3.42
19	.95	1.73	2.03	2.20	2.31	2.40	2.47	2.52	2.57	2.61
	.99	2.54	2.83	2.99	3.10	3.18	3.25	3.31	3.36	3.40
20	.95	1.72	2.03	2.19	2.30	2.39	2.46	2.51	2.56	2.60
	.99	2.53	2.81	2.97	3.08	3.17	3.23	3.29	3.34	3.38
24	.95	1.71	2.01	2.17	2.28	2.36	2.43	2.48	2.53	2.57
	.99	2.49	2.77	2.92	3.03	3.11	3.17	3.22	3.27	3.31
30	.95	1.70	1.99	2.15	2.25	2.33	2.40	2.45	2.50	2.54
	.99	2.46	2.72	2.87	2.97	3.05	3.11	3.16	3.21	3.24
40	.95	1.68	1.97	2.13	2.23	2.31	2.37	2.42	2.47	2.51
	.99	2.42	2.68	2.82	2.92	2.99	3.05	3.10	3.14	3.18
60	.95	1.67	1.95	2.10	2.21	2.28	2.35	2.39	2.44	2.48
	.99	2.39	2.64	2.78	2.87	2.94	3.00	3.04	3.08	3.12
120	.95	1.66	1.93	2.08	2.18	2.26	2.32	2.37	2.41	2.45
	.99	2.36	2.60	2.73	2.82	2.89	2.94	2.99	3.03	3.06
∞	.95	1.64	1.92	2.06	2.16	2.23	2.29	2.34	2.38	2.42
	.99	2.33	2.56	2.68	2.77	2.84	2.89	2.93	2.97	3.00

Reproduced from C. W. Dunnett (1955), A multiple comparison procedure for comparing several treatments with a control, *Journal of American Statistical Association*, **50**, 1096–1121, by permission of the author and the editor.

Table 13B. Dunnett's Statistic (Two Sided)

Error df	$1 - \alpha$	p = number of treatment means, excluding control								
		1	2	3	4	5	6	7	8	9
5	.95	2.57	3.03	3.39	3.66	3.88	4.06	4.22	4.36	4.49
	.99	4.03	4.63	5.09	5.44	5.73	5.97	6.18	6.36	6.53
6	.95	2.45	2.86	3.18	3.41	3.60	3.75	3.88	4.00	4.11
	.99	3.71	4.22	4.60	4.88	5.11	5.30	5.47	5.61	5.74
7	.95	2.36	2.75	3.04	3.24	3.41	3.54	3.66	3.76	3.86
	.99	3.50	3.95	4.28	4.52	4.71	4.87	5.01	5.13	5.24
8	.95	2.31	2.67	2.94	3.13	3.28	3.40	3.51	3.60	3.68
	.99	3.36	3.77	4.06	4.27	4.44	4.58	4.70	4.81	4.90
9	.95	2.26	2.61	2.86	3.04	3.18	3.29	3.39	3.48	3.55
	.99	3.25	3.63	3.90	4.09	4.24	4.37	4.48	4.57	4.65
10	.95	2.23	2.57	2.81	2.97	3.11	3.21	3.31	3.39	3.46
	.99	3.17	3.53	3.78	3.95	4.10	4.21	4.31	4.40	4.47
11	.95	2.20	2.53	2.76	2.92	3.05	3.15	3.24	3.31	3.38
	.99	3.11	3.45	3.68	3.85	3.98	4.09	4.18	4.26	4.33
12	.95	2.18	2.50	2.72	2.88	3.00	3.10	3.18	3.25	3.32
	.99	3.05	3.39	3.61	3.76	3.89	3.99	4.08	4.15	4.22
13	.95	2.16	2.48	2.69	2.84	2.96	3.06	3.14	3.21	3.27
	.99	3.01	3.33	3.54	3.69	3.81	3.91	3.99	4.06	4.13
14	.95	2.14	2.46	2.67	2.81	2.93	3.02	3.10	3.17	3.23
	.99	2.98	3.29	3.49	3.64	3.75	3.84	3.92	3.99	4.05
15	.95	2.13	2.44	2.64	2.79	2.90	2.99	3.07	3.13	3.19
	.99	2.95	3.25	3.45	3.59	3.70	3.79.	3.86	3.93	3.99
16	.95	2.12	2.42	2.63	2.77	2.88	2.96	3.04	3.10	3.16
	.99	2.92	3.22	3.41	3.55	3.65	3.74	3.82	3.88	3.93
17	.95	2.11	2.41	2.61	2.75	2.85	2.94	3.01	3.08	3.13
	.99	2.90	3.19	3.38	3.51	3.62	3.70	3.77	3.83	3.89
18	.95	2.10	2.40	2.59	2.73	2.84	2.92	2.99	3.05	3.11
	.99	2.88	3.17	3.35	3.48	3.58	3.67	3.74	3.80	3.85
19	.95	2.09	2.39	2.58	2.72	2.82	2.90	2.97	3.04	3.09
	.99	2.86	3.15	3.33	3.46	3.55	3.64	3.70	3.76	3.81
20	.95	2.09	2.38	2.57	2.70	2.81	2.89	2.96	3.02	3.07
	.99	2.85	3.13	3.31	3.43	3.53	3.61	3.67	3.73	3.78
24	.95	2.06	2.35	2.53	2.66	2.76	2.84	2.91	2.96	3.01
	.99	2.80	3.07	3.24	3.36	3.45	3.52	3.58	3.64	3.69
30	.95	2.04	2.32	2.50	2.62	2.72	2.79	2.86	2.91	2.96
	.99	2.75	3.01	3.17	3.28	3.37	3.44	3.50	3.55	3.59
40	.95	2.02	2.29	2.47	2.58	2.67	2.75	2.81	2.86	2.90
	.99	2.70	2.95	3.10	3.21	3.29	3.36	3.41	3.46	3.50
60	.95	2.00	2.27	2.43	2.55	2.63	2.70	2.76	2.81	2.85
	.99	2.66	2.90	3.04	3.14	3.22	3.28	3.33	3.38	3.42
120	.95	1.98	2.24	2.40	2.51	2.59	2.66	2.71	2.76	2.80
	.99	2.62	2.84	2.98	3.08	3.15	3.21	3.25	3.30	3.33
∞	.95	1.96	2.21	2.37	2.47	2.55	2.62	2.67	2.71	2.75
	.99	2.58	2.79	2.92	3.01	3.08	3.14	3.18	3.22	3.25

Reproduced from C. W. Dunnett (1955). A multiple comparison procedure for comparing several treatments with a control, *Journal of the American Statistical Association*, **50**, 1096–1121, by permission of the author and the editor.

Table 14. Tukey's Statistic

Error df	α	2	3	4	5	6	7	8	9	10	g = number of 11
5	.05	3.64	4.60	5.22	5.67	6.03	6.33	6.58	6.80	6.99	7.17
	.01	5.70	6.97	7.80	8.42	8.91	9.32	9.67	9.97	10.24	10.48
6	.05	3.46	4.34	4.90	5.31	5.63	5.89	6.12	6.32	6.49	6.65
	.01	5.24	6.33	7.03	7.56	7.97	8.32	8.61	8.87	9.10	9.30
7	.05	3.34	4.16	4.68	5.06	5.36	5.61	5.82	6.00	6.16	6.30
	.01	4.95	5.92	6.54	7.01	7.37	7.68	7.94	8.17	8.37	8.55
8	.05	3.26	4.04	4.53	4.89	5.17	5.40	5.60	5.77	5.92	6.05
	.01	4.74	5.63	6.20	6.63	6.96	7.24	7.47	7.68	7.87	8.03
9	.05	3.20	3.95	4.42	4.76	5.02	5.24	5.43	5.60	5.74	5.87
	.01	4.60	5.43	5.96	6.35	6.66	6.91	7.13	7.32	7.49	7.65
10	.05	3.15	3.88	4.33	4.65	4.91	5.12	5.30	5.46	5.60	5.72
	.01	4.48	5.27	5.77	6.14	6.43	6.67	6.87	7.05	7.21	7.36
11	.05	3.11	3.82	4.26	4.57	4.82	5.03	5.20	5.35	5.49	5.61
	.01	4.39	5.14	5.62	5.97	6.25	6.48	6.67	6.84	6.99	7.13
12	.05	3.08	3.77	4.20	4.51	4.75	4.95	5.12	5.27	5.40	5.51
	.01	4.32	5.04	5.50	5.84	6.10	6.32	6.51	6.67	6.81	6.94
13	.05	3.06	3.73	4.15	4.45	4.69	4.88	5.05	5.19	5.32	5.43
	.01	4.26	4.96	5.40	5.73	5.98	6.19	6.37	6.53	6.67	6.79
14	.05	3.03	3.70	4.11	4.41	4.64	4.83	4.99	5.13	5.25	5.36
	.01	4.21	4.89	5.32	5.63	5.88	6.08	6.26	6.41	6.54	6.66
15	.05	3.01	3.67	4.08	4.37	4.60	4.78	4.94	5.08	5.20	5.31
	.01	4.17	4.83	5.25	5.56	5.80	5.99	6.16	6.31	6.44	6.55
16	.05	3.00	3.65	4.05	4.33	4.56	4.74	4.90	5.03	5.15	5.26
	.01	4.13	4.78	5.19	5.49	5.72	5.92	6.08	6.22	6.35	6.46
17	.05	2.98	3.63	4.02	4.30	4.52	4.71	4.86	4.99	5.11	5.21
	.01	4.10	4.74	5.14	5.43	5.66	5.85	6.01	6.15	6.27	6.38
18	.05	2.97	3.61	4.00	4.28	4.49	4.67	4.82	4.96	5.07	5.17
	.01	4.07	4.70	5.09	5.38	5.60	5.79	5.94	6.08	6.20	6.31
19	.05	2.96	3.59	3.98	4.25	4.47	4.65	4.79	4.92	5.04	5.14
	.01	4.05	4.67	5.05	5.33	5.55	5.73	5.89	6.02	6.14	6.25
20	.05	2.95	3.58	3.96	4.23	4.45	4.62	4.77	4.90	5.01	5.11
	.01	4.02	4.64	5.02	5.29	5.51	5.69	5.84	5.97	6.09	6.19
24	.05	2.92	3.53	3.90	4.17	4.37	4.54	4.68	4.81	4.92	5.01
	.01	3.96	4.54	4.91	5.17	5.37	5.54	5.69	5.81	5.92	6.02
30	.05	2.89	3.49	3.84	4.10	4.30	4.46	4.60	4.72	4.83	4.92
	.01	3.89	4.45	4.80	5.05	5.24	5.40	5.54	5.65	5.76	5.85
40	.05	2.86	3.44	3.79	4.04	4.23	4.39	4.52	4.63	4.74	4.82
	.01	3.82	4.37	4.70	4.93	5.11	5.27	5.39	5.50	5.60	5.69
60	.05	2.83	3.40	3.74	3.98	4.16	4.31	4.44	4.55	4.65	4.73
	.01	3.76	4.28	4.60	4.82	4.99	5.13	5.25	5.36	5.45	5.53
120	.05	2.80	3.36	3.69	3.92	4.10	4.24	4.36	4.48	4.56	4.64
	.01	3.70	4.20	4.50	4.71	4.87	5.01	5.12	5.21	5.30	5.38
∞	.05	2.77	3.31	3.63	3.86	4.03	4.17	4.29	4.39	4.47	4.55
	.01	3.64	4.12	4.40	4.60	4.76	4.88	4.99	5.08	5.16	5.23

treatment means									α	Error df
12	13	14	15	16	17	18	19	20		
7.32	7.47	7.60	7.72	7.83	7.93	8.03	8.12	8.21	.05	5
10.70	10.89	11.08	11.24	11.40	11.55	11.68	11.81	11.93	.01	
6.79	6.92	7.03	7.14	7.24	7.34	7.43	7.51	7.59	.05	6
9.49	9.65	9.81	9.95	10.08	10.21	10.32	10.43	10.54	.01	
6.43	6.55	6.66	6.76	6.85	6.94	7.02	7.09	7.17	.05	7
8.71	8.86	9.00	9.12	9.24	9.35	9.46	9.55	9.65	.01	
6.18	6.29	6.39	6.48	6.57	6.65	6.73	6.80	6.87	.05	8
8.18	8.31	8.44	8.55	8.66	8.76	8.85	8.94	9.03	.01	
5.98	6.09	6.19	6.28	6.36	6.44	6.51	6.58	6.64	.05	9
7.78	7.91	8.03	8.13	8.23	8.32	8.41	8.49	8.57	.01	
5.83	5.93	6.03	6.11	6.20	6.27	6.34	6.40	6.47	.05	10
7.48	7.60	7.71	7.81	7.91	7.99	8.07	8.15	8.22	.01	
5.71	5.81	5.90	5.99	6.06	6.14	6.20	6.26	6.33	.05	11
7.25	7.36	7.46	7.56	7.65	7.73	7.81	7.88	7.95	.01	
5.62	5.71	5.80	5.88	5.95	6.03	6.09	6.15	6.21	.05	12
7.06	7.17	7.26	7.36	7.44	7.52	7.59	7.66	7.73	.01	
5.53	5.63	5.71	5.79	5.86	5.93	6.00	6.05	6.11	.05	13
6.90	7.01	7.10	7.19	7.27	7.34	7.42	7.48	7.55	.01	
5.46	5.55	5.64	5.72	5.79	5.85	5.92	5.97	6.03	.05	14
6.77	6.87	6.96	7.05	7.12	7.20	7.27	7.33	7.39	.01	
5.40	5.49	5.58	5.65	5.72	5.79	5.85	5.90	5.96	.05	15
6.66	6.76	6.84	6.93	7.00	7.07	7.14	7.20	7.26	.01	
5.35	5.44	5.52	5.59	5.66	5.72	5.79	5.84	5.90	05	16
6.56	6.66	6.74	6.82	6.90	6.97	7.03	7.09	7.15	.01	
5.31	5.39	5.47	5.55	5.61	5.68	5.74	5.79	5.84	.05	17
6.48	6.57	6.66	6.73	6.80	6.87	6.94	7.00	7.05	.01	
5.27	5.35	5.43	5.50	5.57	5.63	5.69	5.74	5.79	.05	18
6.41	6.50	6.58	6.65	6.72	6.79	6.85	6.91	6.96	.01	
5.23	5.32	5.39	5.46	5.53	5.59	5.65	5.70	5.75	.05	19
6.34	6.43	6.51	6.58	6.65	6.72	6.78	6.84	6.89	.01	
5.20	5.28	5.36	5.43	5.49	5.55	5.61	5.66	5.71	.05	20
6.29	6.37	6.45	6.52	6.59	6.65	6.71	6.76	6.82	.01	
5.10	5.18	5.25	5.32	5.38	5.44	5.50	5.54	5.59	.05	24
6.11	6.19	6.26	6.33	6.39	6.45	6.51	6.56	6.61	.01	
5.00	5.08	5.15	5.21	5.27	5.33	5.38	5.43	5.48	.05	30
5.93	6.01	6.08	6.14	6.20	6.26	6.31	6.36	6.41	.01	
4.91	4.98	5.05	5.11	5.16	5.22	5.27	5.31	5.36	.05	40
5.77	5.84	5.90	5.96	6.02	6.07	6.12	6.17	6.21	.01	
4.81	4.88	4.94	5.00	5.06	5.11	5.16	5.20	5.24	.05	60
5.60	5.67	5.73	5.79	5.84	5.89	5.93	5.98	6.02	.01	
4.72	4.78	4.84	4.90	4.95	5.00	5.05	5.09	5.13	.05	120
5.44	5.51	5.56	5.61	5.66	5.71	5.75	5.79	5.83	.01	
4.62	4.68	4.74	4.80	4.85	4.89	4.93	4.97	5.01	.05	∞
5.29	5.35	5.40	5.45	5.49	5.54	5.57	5.61	5.65	.01	

Table 15. Friedman's Statistic for All Pairwise Comparisons[a]

g	.0001	.0005	.001	.005	.01	.025	.05	.10	.20
2	5.502	4.923	4.654	3.970	3.643	3.170	2.772	2.326	1.812
3	5.864	5.316	5.063	4.424	4.120	3.682	3.314	2.902	2.424
4	6.083	5.553	5.309	4.694	4.403	3.984	3.633	3.240	2.784
5	6.240	5.722	5.484	4.886	4.603	4.197	3.858	3.478	3.037
6	6.362	5.853	5.619	5.033	4.757	4.361	4.030	3.661	3.232
7	6.461	5.960	5.730	5.154	4.882	4.494	4.170	3.808	3.389
8	6.546	6.050	5.823	5.255	4.987	4.605	4.286	3.931	3.520
9	6.618	6.127	5.903	5.341	5.078	4.700	4.387	4.037	3.632
10	6.682	6.196	5.973	5.418	5.157	4.784	4.474	4.129	3.730
11	6.739	6.257	6.036	5.485	5.227	4.858	4.552	4.211	3.817
12	6.791	6.311	6.092	5.546	5.290	4.925	4.622	4.285	3.895
13	6.837	6.361	6.144	5.602	5.348	4.985	4.685	4.351	3.966
14	6.880	6.407	6.191	5.652	5.400	5.041	4.743	4.412	4.030
15	6.920	6.449	6.234	5.699	5.448	5.092	4.796	4.468	4.089
16	6.957	6.488	6.274	5.742	5.493	5.139	4.845	4.519	4.144
17	6.991	6.525	6.312	5.783	5.535	5.183	4.891	4.568	4.195
18	7.023	6.559	6.347	5.820	5.574	5.224	4.934	4.612	4.242
19	7.054	6.591	6.380	5.856	5.611	5.262	4.974	4.654	4.287
20	7.082	6.621	6.411	5.889	5.645	5.299	5.012	4.694	4.329
22	7.135	6.677	6.469	5.951	5.709	5.365	5.081	4.767	4.405
24	7.183	6.727	6.520	6.006	5.766	5.425	5.144	4.832	4.475
26	7.226	6.773	6.568	6.057	5.818	5.480	5.201	4.892	4.537
28	7.266	6.816	6.611	6.103	5.866	5.530	5.253	4.947	4.595
30	7.303	6.855	6.651	6.146	5.911	5.577	5.301	4.997	4.648
32	7.337	6.891	6.689	6.186	5.952	5.620	5.346	5.044	4.697
34	7.370	6.925	6.723	6.223	5.990	5.660	5.388	5.087	4.743
36	7.400	6.957	6.756	6.258	6.026	5.698	5.427	5.128	4.786
38	7.428	6.987	6.787	6.291	6.060	5.733	5.463	5.166	4.826
40	7.455	7.015	6.816	6.322	6.092	5.766	5.498	5.202	4.864
50	7.571	7.137	6.941	6.454	6.228	5.909	5.646	5.357	5.026
60	7.664	7.235	7.041	6.561	6.338	6.023	5.764	5.480	5.155
70	7.741	7.317	7.124	6.649	6.429	6.118	5.863	5.582	5.262
80	7.808	7.387	7.196	6.725	6.507	6.199	5.947	5.669	5.353
90	7.866	7.448	7.259	6.792	6.575	6.270	6.020	5.745	5.433
100	7.918	7.502	7.314	6.850	6.636	6.333	6.085	5.812	5.503

[a] For a given g and α, the tabled entry is $q(\alpha, g, \infty)$.

Reprinted from M. Hollander and D. Wolfe (1973), *Nonparametric Statistical Methods*, copyright © 1973, John Wiley & Sons, by permission of John Wiley & Sons, Inc., and from H. L. Harter, (1960), Tables of range and studentized range, *Ann. Math. Statist.*, **31**, 1122–1147, by permission of the author and the editor.

Table 16. Friedman's Statistic for Comparisons to a Control

$l = g - 1$	α	
	.01	.05
1	2.58	1.96
2	2.79	2.21
3	2.92	2.35
4	3.00	2.44
5	3.06	2.51
6	3.11	2.57
7	3.15	2.61
8	3.19	2.65
9	3.22	2.69
10	3.25	2.72
11	3.27	2.74
12	3.29	2.77
15	3.35	2.83
20	3.42	2.91

[a] For a given l and α, the tabular value is $|m|(\alpha, l, \frac{1}{2})$.

Reproduced from M. Hollander and D. Wolfe (1973), *Nonparametric Statistical Methods*, copyright © 1973, John Wiley & Sons, by permission of John Wiley & Sons, Inc. and from C. W. Dunnett, New tables for multiple comparisons with a control, *Biometrics*, **20**, 482–491, 1964. With permission from the Biometric Society.

Index